Essentials of Histology
Text/Atlas/Review

Essentials of Histology
Text/Atlas/Review

William J. Krause, Ph.D.
Professor of Anatomy, Department of Pathology and Anatomical Sciences,
University of Missouri School of Medicine, Columbia, Missouri

J. Harry Cutts, Ph.D.
Professor of Anatomy (Retired), Department of Pathology and Anatomical Sciences,
University of Missouri School of Medicine, Columbia, Missouri

Little, Brown and Company
Boston/New York/Toronto/London

Library of Congress Cataloging-in-Publication Data

Krause, William J.
    Essentials of histology : text/atlas/review / William J. Krause,
  J. Harry Cutts.
      p.   cm.
    Includes bibliographical references and index.
    ISBN 0-316-50351-7
    1. Histology.   2. Histology — Atlases.   3. Histology — Examinations,
  questions, etc.   I. Cutts, J. Harry, 1926–   . II. Title.
    [DNLM: 1. Histology.   QS 504 K913e   1994]
    QM551.K893   1994
    612′.018 — dc20
    DNLM/DLC
    for Library of Congress   93-42961
                                                                              CIP

Printed in the United States of America

MV-NY

Editorial: Evan R. Schnittman, Amy Mastrodomenico
Production Editor: Karen Feeney
Copyeditor: Elizabeth Willingham
Indexer: Betty Hallinger
Production Supervisor/Designer: Louis C. Bruno, Jr.
Cover Designer: Hannus Design Associates
Cover Artist: Peg Gerrity

Contents

Preface

The format of *Essentials of Histology* departs considerably from that of the usual textbooks of histology. In general, this text follows the traditional and logical sequence of cells to tissues to organs, but within this sequence the chapters on the eye and ear have been placed immediately following the coverage of nerve tissue. This seems a more logical arrangement because these two structures essentially are specialized nerve receptors. Similarly, it is more appropriate to consider mitosis with the cell and meiosis with the reproductive organs.

However, the most obvious differences are in the organization of the material within each chapter. Here the subject matter is broken down into smaller learning units, each of which is introduced by a list of **key words** appropriate to that unit. The key words are designed to introduce terminology (and are emphasized in the text by bold type); they also serve as a summary of the topic and provide a means for rapid review. In addition, each chapter contains a **functional summary,** where function is discussed and related to structure within each unit; a **review table,** in which the major structural features of that chapter are reduced to a single table; a **developmental segment** to summarize how tissues appear the way they do; and finally a **clinical correlations segment** to briefly present histology in a clinical setting.

A second obvious departure from the usual format occurs in the treatment of the illustrative material. Rather than scattering photographs throughout the text to illustrate one or two points of description, the photographs are collected and presented at the end of each chapter. This arrangement allows us to make best use of the illustrations to provide a systematic and **complete pictorial review** of the material already covered in narrative form and to integrate light, scanning, and transmission electron microscopy into a comprehensive study of histologic structure. Although we have tried to present material of high quality, we have not searched for the ideal but rather have attempted to depict what the student will ordinarily encounter in the usual sections. We also have used black and white illustrations rather than color. The latter, while pretty, actually present no advantage in depicting histologic detail and tend to encourage the student to use color rather than form in making a histologic assessment of structural details.

During preparation of the text, we were guided by three major considerations — that most curricula place considerable time constraints on the student, that function and structure are inextricably related, and that the learning process essentially is a matter of repetition and reinforcement. We believe that the format of this text meets these criteria and presents the vast material of histology in a concise and logical manner, without sacrificing the detail that is necessary for an understanding of the microscopic structure of the body. *Essentials of Histology* is written to meet students' needs both within a classical classroom and a problem based learning **(PBL)** setting. In addition, this text is especially designed for reviewing for national board and **USMLE** examinations. A series of discussion and objective questions is provided for each chapter to aid the student in this regard.

W.J.K.
J.H.C.

Acknowledgments

We would like to thank Tom Manning for his diligence and for bringing our textbook to the attention of Little, Brown and Company. We would also like to thank Evan R. Schnittman, Amy Mastrodomenico, and Karen Feeney for working closely with us during the production of *Essentials of Histology.*

Credits

We gratefully acknowledge the permission of S.T.E.M. Laboratories, Inc. for the use of several figures in the text, developed previously by W.J. Krause as 2 x 2 color projection slides in conjunction with S.T.E.M. Laboratories, Inc. Kansas City, Missouri.

The following publishers provided permission to use previously published illustrative materials (listed by author):

Andrews, P., Georgetown University, Washington, DC
Figure 16-5, from *American Journal of Anatomy* 140:81, 1974, Wistar Press;
Figures 16-7, 16-9, 16-10, & 16-21, from *Laboratory Investigation* 32:610, 1975, © U.S.-Canadian Division of the International Academy of Pathology.

Berdan, R.C., University of Calgary, Calgary, Canada
Figure 15-43, from *Journal of Ultrastructural Research* 90:55, 1985, Academic Press.

Breipohl, W., Univ des Gesamthochschule, Essen, West Germany
Figure 14-5, from *Cell and Tissue Research* 183:105, 1977, Springer-Verlag.

Brink, P.R., State University of New York, Stony Brook, New York
Figures 2-25 & 2-26, from *American Journal of Anatomy* 154:1, 1979, Wistar Press.

Browning, J., Flinders University, Bedford Park, South Australia

Figure 15-42, from *Biomedical Research* 5(3):245, 1984, Biomedical Research Foundation, Tokyo, Japan.

Chan, B.S.T., University of Hong Kong, Shatin, Hong Kong
Figure 5-14, from *Acta Haematologica* 42:258, 1969, S. Karger AG, Basel.

Fujita, T., Niigata University, Asahi-Machi, Niigata, Japan
Figures 12-20, 12-21, & 16-16, from *Archivum Histologicum Japonicum* vol 37, 1974, Japan Society of Histological Documentation.

Haggis, G.H., Canada Deparment of Agriculture, Ottawa, Canada
Figure 15-56, from *Laboratory Investigation* 29:60, 1973, © U.S.-Canadian Division of the International Academy of Pathology.

Hall, C.E.
Figure 5-15, from *Journal of Biological Chemistry* 179:857, 1949, © The American Society of Biological Chemists, Inc.

Hirakow, R., Saitama Medical School, Iruma-Gun, Saitama, Japan
Figures 7-20 through 7-23, from *Electron Microscopy Technique*, Ishiyaku Publishers, Inc., Tokyo, Japan.
Figures 11-15, 11-16, & 11-17, from *Anatomy and Embryology* 172:325, 1985, Springer-Verlag.

Huxley, H.E., University Medical School, Cambridge, England

Figures 7-12 & 7-13, from *Scientific American* vol 199, 1958, Scientific American.

Köling, A., Uppsala University, Uppsala, Sweden
Figure 1-28, from "Freeze fracture electron microscopy of the nuclear envelope of the human odontoblast." *Archives of Oral Biology* 30:691, Copyright 1985, Pergamon Journals Ltd.

Kuwabara, T., National Eye Institute, NIH, Bethesda, Maryland
Figures 9-21 & 9-22, from *Histology* by Weiss and Greep. Copyright © 1977 McGraw-Hill. Used with permission of McGraw-Hill Book Company.

Lenoir, M., University of Montpellier, Montpellier Cedex, France
Figures 10-12 & 10-13, from *Anatomy and Embryology* 175:477, 1987, Springer-Verlag.

Magney, J.E., University of Minnesota, Minneapolis, Minnesota
Figures 15-40 & 15-51, from *American Journal of Anatomy* 177:47, 1986, Alan R. Liss, Inc.

Murakami, T., Okayama University, Medical School, Okayama, Japan
Figure 16-6, from *Archivum Histologicum Japonicum* vol 34, 1972, Japan Society of Histological Japonicum.

Ojeda, J.L., Faculty of Medicine, University of Santander, Spain
Figure 11-18, from *Acta Anatomica* 119:1, 1984, S. Karger AG, Basel.

Palumbo, C., University of Modena, Modena, Italy
Figure 4-25, from *Cell and Tissue Research* 246:129, 1986, Springer-Verlag.

Satoh, Y., Asahikawa Medical College, Asahikawa, Japan
Figure 15-41, from *Anatomischer Anzeiger* 159:305, 1985, VEB Gustav Fischer Verlag, Jena, German Democratic Republic.

Stranock, S.D., Merchiston Castle School, Edinburgh, Scotland
Figure 1-23, from *Journal of Anatomy*, 129:885, 1979, Cambridge University Press.

Trotter, J.A., University of New Mexico, Albuquerque, New Mexico

Figures 7-14 & 7-15, from *Anatomical Record* 213:16 & 213:26, 1985, Alan R. Liss, Inc.

Tyson, G.E., Mississippi State University, Mississippi State, Mississippi
Figure 16-8, from *Vichows Archiv. B. Cell Pathology*, 25:105, 1977, Springer-Verlag.

The following publishers provided permission to use illustrative materials that we have previously published in their journals:

British Medical Asosciation
Figure 15-27, from *British Medical Journal* 2:1052, 1977.

Cambridge University Press — all from *Journal of Anatomy*
Figure 1-26, 123:21, 1977;
Figure 2-23, 104:467, 1969;
Figure 2-24, 125:85, 1978;
Figure 2-36, 122:293, 1976;
Figure 2-37, 122:449, 1976;
Figure 15-59, 120:191, 1975;
Figures 15-77 & 15-78, 122:293, 1976;
Figures 15-79, 15-80, & 15-82, 122:449, 1976;
Figure 15-86, 123:21, 1977;
Figures 16-15, 16-18, & 16-22, 129:459, 1979;
Figures 16-29 & 16-30, 129:377, 1979;
Figures 16-31 through 16-39, 129:459, 1979.

Japan Society of Histological Documentation
Figure 15-75, from *Archivum Histologicum Japonicum* vol 43, 1980.

S. Karger AG, Basel — all from *Acta Anatomica*
Figure 2-14, 92:28, 1975;
Figure 8-31, 120:93, 1984;
Figures 15-90, 15-96, & 15-97, 101:259, 1978.

The Wistar Press
Figure 1-12, from *American Journal of Anatomy* 132:147, 1971;
Figures 2-38 & 6-23 from *Journal of Morphology* 140:321, 1973;
Figure 14-16 from *American Journal of Anatomy* 146:181, 1976;
Figure 15-87 from *Anatomical Record* 172:603, 1972.

We thank the following individual contributors for the illustrative materials they have provided:

Allison, O.L., S.T.E.M. Laboratories, Inc. Kansas City, Missouri
Figures 4-12, 4-15, 5-2, 5-3, 5-5, 5-7, 5-11, 12-9, 15-5, 18-22, 18-23, 18-24

Campbell, G.T., University of Nebraska, Omaha, Nebraska
Figures 19-6, 19-7, 19-8, 19-9, 19-10

Decker, J.D., University of Missouri, Columbia, Missouri
Figures 8-33, 17-30, 17-31, 17-32, 19-27, 19-28, 19-29

Dow, P., University of British Coumbia, Vancouver, Canada
Figure 7-17

Dunkerly, G.B., University of Missouri, Columbia, Missouri
Figure 10-7

Engstrom, H.H., Uppsala University, Uppsala, Sweden
Figures 10-17, 10-18

Feeney-Burns, L., University of Missouri, Columbia, Missouri
Figures 9-11, 9-13, 9-14, 9-20, 9-23

King, J.S., Ohio State University, Columbus, Ohio
Figures 8-9, 8-18

Lenoir, M., University of Montpellier, Montpellier Cedex, France
Figure 10-8

Sherman, D.M., University of Missouri, Columbia, Missouri
Figures 2-19, 19-11, 19-26

Stachura, J., Institute of Pathology, Copernicus Medical Academy, Krakow, Poland
Figures 5-16, 11-9

Use of the Text

To understand histology, it is essential to learn a specialized vocabulary and to assimilate a large body of facts. Learning, as distinct from memorization, depends to a great degree on repetition and reinforcement and is made easier if the material to be learned can be presented in discrete, manageable segments. The format of **Essentials of Histology** is designed specifically to meet these requirements and, if used properly, will enable the student to master the discipline quickly and efficiently. From our experience, the text can be used most effectively by adopting a study plan similar to that suggested below.

1. Read the **key words** carefully; they introduce the main features of the subject to be discussed and provide the basic vocabulary for that unit. As each segment is read, again note the key words (identified by bold print) and how they contribute to the discussion.
2. After completing the text segment, return to the key words, using them as **prompts** to recall the details of the material just read.
3. As each chapter is completed, use the key word segments for rapid review of all the material covered. If a key word fails to prompt a response, it and its associated text can be found quickly from the **bold** type in the appropriate segment.
4. The **developmental summaries** describe how the adult tissues "got to be the way they are" and provide another means of reinforcement for an understanding of organ and tissue structure.
5. The **functional summaries** briefly outline the structural/functional relationships and serve to draw the information together and to provide an additional review of the topic.
6. Further understanding of normal histology can be acquired from the changes that occur in disease. The **clinical correlations** segment of each chapter introduces the student to some aspect or aspects of histopathology that emphasize the basic structure of tissues and organs in a clinical setting. The summaries of selected histopathologies provide reinforcement of normal histology as the cells and organs are described and examined in the light of their changes from normal.
7. When study of the descriptive material has been completed, the **atlases** at the end of each chapter provide a final pictorial review of structure. Each is introduced by a **table** in which the key points for identification of an organ/tissue are presented, offering the briefest possible summary. The atlases also are useful as laboratory guides and can be used when examining histologic preparations with the microscope. A series of **questions** is provided at the end of each chapter to assist student understanding of selected topics.
8. As a final short review, the **appendix** provides a few short tables that outline the basic differences of several structures that are frequently difficult to recognize. They, too, can be used, in conjunction with the atlas portions, as laboratory guides for the identification of tissues.

1 The Cell

Multicellular organisms are made up of two distinct structural elements: cells and those products of cells that form the intercellular substances. Cells are the fundamental units of living material and show a variety of functional specializations that are essential for the survival of the organism. Each cell is a distinct entity; each contains all the machinery necessary for independent existence and is separated from its surroundings by an individual plasma membrane.

Protoplasm

KEY WORDS: protein, carbohydrate, lipid, nucleic acid, inorganic material, water

Protoplasm, the living substance of a cell, consists of protein, carbohydrate, lipid, nucleic acids, and inorganic materials dispersed in water to form a complex, semifluid gel. The consistency of protoplasm differs in different cells and may change from a viscous to a more fluid state.

Protein, alone or combined with lipid or carbohydrate, forms the major structural component of the cell and the intercellular substances. Enzymes and many hormones are proteins. The major **carbohydrates** are glucose, which is the chief source of energy in mammalian cells, and glycogen, the storage form of glucose. Complexes of carbohydrates and proteins form the main constituents of intercellular substances that bind cells together. Other carbohydrate-protein complexes form some enzymes and antibodies. **Lipids** serve as an energy source; they also have important structural functions and are major components of the membrane systems of cells.

Nucleic acids are divided into two classes. Deoxyribonucleic acid (DNA) represents the genetic material and is found mainly in the nucleus. Ribonucleic acid (RNA) is present in the cytoplasm and nucleus and carries information from the nucleus to the cytoplasm. It also serves as a template for synthesis of proteins by the cell.

Inorganic materials are as much an integral component of protoplasm as proteins, carbohydrates, and lipids; without them physiologic processes are impossible. Among the inorganic constituents of protoplasm are calcium, potassium, sodium, and magnesium present as carbonates, chlorides, phosphates, and sulfates; small quantities of iron, copper, and iodine; and trace elements such as cobalt, manganese, zinc, and other metals. The inorganic materials have many functions, including maintenance of intracellular and extracellular osmotic pressures, transmission of nerve impulses, contraction of muscle, adhesiveness of cells, activation of enzymes, transport of oxygen, and maintenance of the rigidity of tissues such as bone.

Water makes up about 75 percent of protoplasm. Part of the water is free and available as a solvent for various metabolic processes and part is bound to protein.

1

Properties of Protoplasm

KEY WORDS: irritability, conductivity, contractility, absorption, metabolism, secretion, excretion, growth, reproduction

Protoplasm is characterized by several physiologic properties that distinguish it from inanimate material. All living cells show these properties, but in some cells a particular property may be emphasized.

Irritability is a fundamental property of all living cells and refers to the ability to respond to a stimulus.

Conductivity refers to the ability of a cell to transmit a stimulus from the point of origin to another point on the cell surface or to other cells. Conductivity also is a property of all cells but, like irritability, is most highly developed in nerve tissue.

Contractility is the ability of a cell to change shape in response to a stimulus and generally is indicated by a shortening of the cell in some direction. This property is most prominent in muscle.

Absorption involves transfer of materials across the cell membrane into the interior of the cell where it might be used in some manner. All cells show the ability to absorb material, some very selectively.

Metabolism refers to the ability of a cell to break down absorbed material to produce energy.

Secretion is the process by which cells elaborate and release materials for use elsewhere. **Excretion,** on the other hand, is the elimination from cells of metabolic waste products.

Growth of an organism can occur by increasing the amount of cytoplasm in existing cells or by increasing the number of cells. There are limits to the size a cell can attain without sacrificing the efficiency with which nutrients and oxygen reach the interior of the cell. Beyond a maximum size, increase in the amount of protoplasm occurs through **reproduction** (division) of cells.

Organization of Protoplasm

KEY WORDS: nucleus, nuclear envelope, cytoplasm, plasmalemma (cell membrane), organelle, inclusion, cytoskeleton, cytoplasmic matrix (hyaloplasm), karyolymph

Although cells differ in size, shape, and function, the protoplasm of each cell consists of two major components: nucleus and cytoplasm. The **nucleus** contains the hereditary or genetic material and is completely surrounded by cytoplasm, from which it is separated by a **nuclear envelope.** The **cytoplasm** is limited by a **plasmalemma (cell membrane),** which separates the cell from the external environment. Within the cytoplasm are several structures representing organelles and inclusions. **Organelles** are highly organized, living structural units of the cytoplasm that perform specific functions in the cell. **Inclusions** generally represent inert cell products or metabolites that often are only temporary components. Most, but not all, of the organelles are membranous structures whose size and concentration vary with the type and activity of the cell. The different organelles tend to be localized in discrete areas of the cytoplasm so that they and their associated metabolic processes remain separate from other components of the cell. Cell shape is maintained by a three-dimensional **cytoskeleton** that provides structural support for the cell and serves in cell motility and intracellular transport. The cytoskeleton consists of various microfilaments and microtubules.

The organelles and inclusions are suspended in an amorphous medium called the **cytoplasmic matrix (hyaloplasm).** Nuclear material also is suspended in a structureless ground substance called the **karyolymph.** Other than their differences in location, karyolymph and hyaloplasm appear to be equivalent.

Cytoplasmic Organelles

Organelles are specialized units of the cell that perform specific functions and constitute part of the living substance of the cell. Organelles include structures such as the plasmalemma, granular and smooth forms of endoplasmic reticulum, ribosomes, Golgi complexes, mitochondria, lysosomes, peroxisomes, filaments, microtubules, and centrioles. Many organelles are limited by membranes that are similar in structure to the boundary of the cell itself. These membranes, including the cell membrane, are metabolically active sheets that are essential to the life of the cell. In electron micrographs, the membranes exhibit a trilaminar structure consisting of inner and outer dense lines separated by a light zone. Because the trilaminar structure is representative of all biological membranes of a cell, it has been called a unit membrane. The thickness of the unit membrane varies from organelle to organelle and generally is greatest where it forms the plasmalemma. While the membranes of different organelles appear to have only minor cytologic variations, they vary considerably in the chemical composition, enzymatic properties, and functions.

Plasmalemma (Cell Membrane)

KEY WORDS: unit membrane, phospholipid bilayer, transmembrane protein, integral protein, glycocalyx, P-face, E-face, endocytosis, phagocytosis, pinocytosis, micropinocytosis, fluid phase micropinocytosis, adsorptive micropinocytosis, coated pit, coated vesicle, clathrin, exocytosis

Each cell is enclosed by a plasmalemma that is 8- to 10-nm thick and has the typical trilaminar structure of the **unit membrane.** It appears as two dense lines, each 3 nm wide, separated by a 2- to 4-nm clear zone (see atlas figures 1-11 and 1-27). The plasmalemma is composed of proteins, lipids, glycolipids, and carbohydrates; the lipids are mainly phospholipid with some neutral fat and cholesterol-like substances. Lipids form about 50 percent of the total mass of the plasmalemma. Structurally, the plasmalemma is thought to consist of a **phospholipid bilayer** in which the hydrocarbon chains are directed inward and the polar groups are directed outward. The plasmalemma acts as a fluid due to the movement of adjacent phospholipids. Therefore breaks and tears seal spontaneously due to the polar nature of the lipids. Cholesterol molecules within the plasmalemma tend to limit this movement, thereby contributing to its mechanical stability. **Transmembrane proteins** extend through the full thickness of the membrane and serve as sites of transmembrane transport, enzymatic activity, cell communication, and cell attachment. **Integral proteins** lie only partly within the lipid bilayer. Glycoproteins appear to be present on the external surface and form the **glycocalyx.** This coat varies in thickness depending on the type of cell with which it is associated.

Freeze-fracture, a procedure that splits the plasmalemma between the hydrocarbon chains of the phospholipid bilayers, allows observation of the interior of the plasmalemma (Fig. 1-1). The outwardly directed, inner half-membrane closest to the cytoplasm is the **P-face,** which generally shows numerous globular particles 6 to 9 nm in diameter. The **E-face,** closest to the external environment, is relatively smooth, and only occasional particles are present. These are thought to be proteins that reside within the plasmalemma.

The plasmalemma is selectively permeable and plays an active role in bringing material into the cell (**endocytosis**) and discharging it from the cell. It also has receptors for hormones, generates messenger molecules, contains ion pumps, and has a role in cell recognition.

Phagocytosis is a form of endocytosis in which particulate matter is taken into a cell. During its attachment phase, particles bind to receptors on the plasmalemma, while in its ingestion phase, the cytoplasm forms pseudopods that flow around the particles, engulf them, and take them into the cell in membrane-bound vacuoles. In a similar way, fluid may be incorporated into the cell in small cytoplasmic vesicles in a process called **pinocytosis.** Phagocytosis and pinocytosis can be seen by light microscopy.

Some materials may enter the cell in even smaller vesicles formed by minute invaginations of the cell surface. This process, called **micropinocytosis,** is visible only with the electron microscope. Nonselective, fluid phase, and selective adsorptive types of micropinocytosis have been recognized (see atlas figure 1-11). In most cells, **fluid phase micropinocytosis** occurs with formation of small vesicles from the plasmalemma. The vesicles, which contain fluid and anything dispersed in the fluid, traverse the cytoplasm to

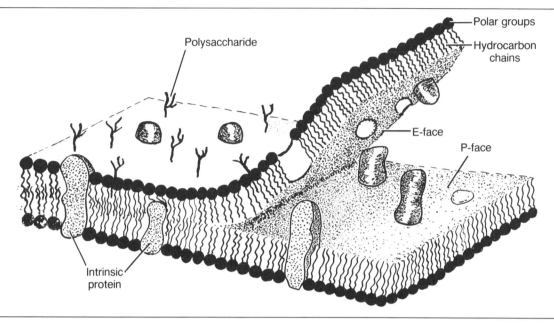

Fig. 1-1. Diagrammatic representation of the structure of the plasmalemma.

the opposite side of the cell, where they discharge their contents (Fig. 1-2A).

Adsorptive micropinocytosis is the selective uptake of specific macromolecules at certain receptor-binding sites in the cell membrane. This receptor-mediated micropinocytosis is important in the ingestion of regulatory and nutritional proteins. Short, bristlelike projections may be present on the cytoplasmic surface at these sites and form **coated pits** from which **coated vesicles** arise (Fig. 1-2B). The cytoplasmic surfaces of the vesicles are coated with **clathrin,** a protein that appears as radiating spikes that give a fuzzy appearance to the vesicles. Clathrin may prevent fusion of coated vesicles with membranous organelles; when the protein coat is lost, the vesicles fuse with lysosomes, Golgi complexes, other vesicles, or cell membranes.

Materials such as secretory granules are released from the cell by **exocytosis,** a process in which the limiting membranes of the granules fuse with the plasmalemma before discharging their contents.

Fig. 1-2. A. Diagrammatic representation of fluid phase micropinocytosis. B. Adsorptive micropinocytosis via coated vesicles.

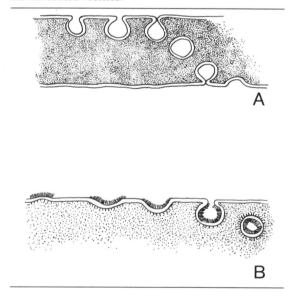

Endoplasmic Reticulum

KEY WORDS: tubule, cisternae, granular endoplasmic reticulum, ribosome, smooth endoplasmic reticulum

The cytoplasm of almost all cells contains a continuous, irregular network of membrane-bound channels called the endoplasmic reticulum. Typically, this organelle appears as anastomosing **tubules,** but the membranes also form parallel, flattened saccules called **cisternae.** Small vesicles not attached to tubules or cisternae may be present also and are considered to be part of the endoplasmic reticulum.

Smooth and granular forms of endoplasmic reticulum can be distinguished. **Granular endoplasmic reticulum** (GER) usually consists of an array of flattened cisternae bounded by a membrane (Fig. 1-3). The outer surface is studded with numerous particles of ribonucleoprotein called **ribosomes,** which synthesize proteins that generally are to be secreted by the cell. The proteins are synthesized on the external surface of the GER, then enter the lumen of the reticulum where they are isolated from the surrounding cytoplasm (see atlas figures 1-13 and 1-27). **Smooth endoplasmic reticulum** (SER) lacks ribosomes and consists primarily of a system of interconnecting tubules without cisternae (Fig. 1-4; see atlas figure 1-14).

In most cells, one form of endoplasmic reticulum usually predominates. Protein-secreting cells

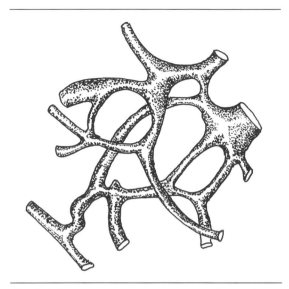

Fig. 1-4. Diagrammatic representation of smooth endoplasmic reticulum.

such as pancreatic acinar cells or plasma cells are characterized by an abundance of GER, whereas in cells that secrete steroid hormones, the smooth type predominates. In still other cells, such as liver cells, both types of endoplasmic reticulum are present in nearly equal amounts and may be continuous. Granular endoplasmic recticulum is known to be involved in the synthesis of protein, but the exact role of SER remains obscure. Smooth endoplasmic reticulum has been implicated in different functions in different cells: synthesis of steroid hormones in certain endocrine cells, synthesis of lipoproteins and detoxification of lipid-soluble drugs by liver cells, synthesis of triglycerides, and metabolism of lipid and cholesterol. It also has a role in the release and recapture of calcium ions during contraction and relaxation of striated muscle.

Ribosomes

KEY WORDS: ribonucleoprotein, free ribosome, polyribosome (polysome), messenger RNA, protein synthesis, codon, transfer RNA

Fig. 1-3. Diagrammatic representation of rough endoplasmic reticulum.

Ribosomes

Cisternae

Ribosomes are small, uniformly sized particles of **ribonucleoprotein** 12 to 15 nm in diameter and composed of large and small subunits. They may be attached to the membranes of the endoplasmic reticulum or be present as **free ribosomes** suspended in the cytoplasm, unassociated with membranes. Free ribosomes often occur in clusters called **polyribosomes (polysomes),** in which individual ribosomes are united by a thread of ribonucleic acid (RNA) called **messenger RNA** (mRNA). Free ribosomes are also sites of **protein synthesis,** the protein formed being used by the cell itself rather than secreted (see atlas figures 1-12 and 1-27). Individual free ribosomes are not active; only when they are attached to RNA to form polyribosomes do they become active in protein synthesis. Similarly, ribosomes on the endoplasmic reticulum must be associated with RNA before they engage in the synthesis of protein.

Messenger RNA is formed in the nucleus on a template of uncoiled deoxyribonucleic acid (DNA). It contains a message that is encoded as successive sets of three nucleotides called **codons** that specify the sequence in which amino acids are to be incorporated into newly forming protein. During synthesis, mRNA enters the cytoplasm and attaches to ribosomes that move along the mRNA, translating the code and assembling amino acids in the proper order. On reaching the end of the mRNA, ribosomes detach and simultaneously release the newly synthesized protein molecule. Amino acids are brought to the ribosomes for incorporation into the protein by **transfer RNA** (tRNA), another form of ribonucleoprotein. There is a specific tRNA for each of the amino acids. Ribosomal and tRNA are formed by transcription of specific segments of the DNA molecule. Formation of ribosomal RNA is directed by a specific region of a chromosome.

Golgi Complex

KEY WORDS: **negative image, saccule, forming face, maturing face, transport vesicle, condensing vacuole, secretory granule**

The Golgi complex (apparatus) does not stain in ordinary histological preparations, nor is it vis-

ible in living cells; it does sometime appear as a **negative image** — a nonstaining area of the cytoplasm usually close to the nucleus. The size and appearance of the Golgi complex varies with the type and activity of the cell and may be small and compact or large and netlike. Some cells contain multiple Golgi complexes.

In electron micrographs, the Golgi complex is seen to consist of several flattened **saccules** (cisternae), each limited by a smooth membrane (Fig. 1-5). The saccules are disc-shaped, slightly curved, and often appear to be compressed near the center and dilated at the edges. The saccules are arranged in stacks and are separated by spaces 20 to 30 nm wide. Because of the curvature of the saccules, the Golgi complex has convex and concave faces. The convex face usually is directed toward the nucleus and is called the **forming face;** the concave or **maturing face** is oriented toward the cell membrane. The forming face is associated with numerous small vesicles, and at this face the outer saccule is perforated by many small openings. The saccules at the maturing face tend to be more dilated than those at the concave face (see Fig. 1-5).

Secretory products are concentrated in the Golgi complex, whose size varies with the activity of the cell. In protein-secreting cells, peptides first accumulate within the lumen of the GER, then are transported to the Golgi complex in small **transport vesicles,** which are formed from ribosome-free areas of the GER adjacent to the Golgi complex. The vesicles carry small quantities

Fig. 1-5. Diagrammatic representation of the Golgi complex.

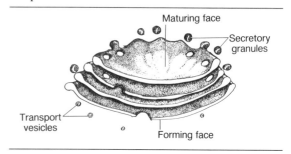

Maturing face

Secretory granules

Transport vesicles

Forming face

of protein to the Golgi body, where they coalesce with and contribute membrane to the developing outer saccule at the forming face (see atlas figure 1-15). Proteins accumulate within the cisternae of the Golgi membranes and are concentrated as they pass through the Golgi complex. At the maturing face, the saccules expand and bud off to form limiting membranes that enclose the protein in structures called **condensing vacuoles.** Addition of new membrane to the forming face balances loss of membrane from the maturing face. Secretory materials within the vacuoles become more concentrated and the condensing vacuoles eventually mature into **secretory granules.** Golgi membranes are able to synthesize carbohydrate and, depending on the cell type, may complex protein to newly synthesized carbohydrate to form a glycoprotein (see atlas figure 1-15). Proteins synthesized by the GER may be complexed to lipids that enter the Golgi cisternae from the SER; the resulting lipoproteins are released by the Golgi complex as membrane-bound granules.

During release of secretory products, the membranes of the secretory granules fuse with the plasmalemma and become incorporated into the cell membrane. The membranes of secretory granules must have some special properties since they fuse specifically with the plasmalemma and not with the membranes of other organelles.

There appears to be a continuous movement of membrane through the cell, from endoplasmic reticulum to transport vesicles, to Golgi complex, to secretory granules, and then to the plasmalemma. Internalization of plasmalemma occurs during phagocytosis, pinocytosis, and micropinocytosis.

Lysosomes

KEY WORDS: acid hydrolase, autolysis, primary lysosome, secondary lysosome, phagocytosis, heterophagy, phagosome, heterophagic vacuole, residual body, autophagy, cytolysosome, multivesicular body

Lysosomes are small, membrane-bound, dense bodies measuring 0.2 to 0.55 μm in diameter. More than 50 enzymes have been identified in lysosomes. Since they are active at an acid pH, lysosomal enzymes often are referred to as **acid hydrolases.** The limiting membrane of lysosomes protects the remainder of the cell from the effects of the contained enzymes which, if released into the cytoplasm, would digest or lyse the cell. Such an occurrence is called **autolysis** and is presumed to occur normally during such diverse events as resorption of tadpole tails at metamorphosis, regression of the mesonephros in kidney development, and regression of mammary tissue after cessation of lactation. Increased lysosomal activity occurs during the regression of some tumors.

The appearance of lysosomes varies according to the phase and activity state in which they are observed and their association with cell structures or material brought into the cell. **Primary lysosomes** are those that have been newly released at the Golgi complex and have not engaged in digestive activities. The enzymes of the primary lysosomes are synthesized in the GER, transported to the Golgi complex, and released from the maturing face as membrane-bound, electron-dense granules (see atlas figure 1-17). Primary lysosomes are formed similarly to secretory granules, but lysosomes usually remain within the cell and are not secreted. Some evidence suggests that primary lysosomes may form directly from smooth areas of the GER in the region of the Golgi complex. These regions have been called the Golgi-associated endoplasmic reticulum (GERL).

Secondary lysosomes are vacuolar structures that represent sites of past or current lysosomal activity and include heterophagic vacuoles, residual bodies, and cytolysosomes. The relationships of these structures are best understood from a description of the processes involved in **phagocytosis** (Fig. 1-6; see atlas figure 1-17).

Some cells, such as macrophages and some granular leukocytes of the blood, have a special capacity to engulf extracellular materials and destroy them. The process by which substances are taken into the cell from the exterior environment and broken down by lysosomal activity is called **heterophagy.** The process involves invagination of the cell membrane and containment of the material in a membrane-bound vacuole. Thus, the extracellular material taken into the cell is se-

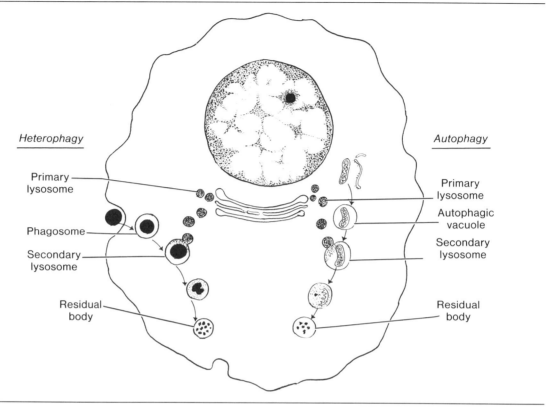

Fig. 1-6. Schematic representation of autophagy and heterophagy.

questered in a vacuole called a **phagosome** and remains isolated from the cytoplasm. As the phagosome moves through the cytoplasm of the cell, it encounters a primary lysosome. The membranes of the two structures fuse and the enzymes of the lysosome are discharged into the phagosome. The combined primary lysosome and phagosome is now called a **heterophagic vacuole,** a type of secondary lysosome. The material within the heterophagic vacuole is digested by the lysosomal enzymes, and any useful materials are transferred into the cytoplasm for use by the cell (see atlas figure 1-16). Nondegradable materials such as some dye particles, asbestos fibers, silica, or carbon may remain within the vacuole, now called a **residual body.** A residual body is another form of secondary lysosome which is thought by

some to be eliminated from the cell by exocytosis. However, in many cells the residual bodies accumulate and persist for long periods of time.

Autophagy refers to the lysosomal breakdown of cytoplasmic organelles in normal, viable cells (see Fig. 1-6). The lysosomal system is involved in the destruction of worn or damaged organelles and the remodeling of the cytoplasm. During the process a portion of the cytoplasm containing aged or damaged organelles becomes surrounded by a membrane to form an autophagic vacuole. The membrane is thought to be derived from SER. The vacuole fuses with a primary lysosome to form another type of secondary lysosome called a **cytolysosome.** The fate of the materials within the autophagic vacuoles (which may be the cell's own mitochondria, ribosomes, endoplasmic reticulum, and so forth) is the same as that of heterophagic vacuoles and again results in formation of residual bodies. In many cells, indigestible substances within autophagic vacuoles form a brownish material called lipofuscin pigment, the amount of which increases with age.

Another form of lysosome is the **multivesicular body,** a membrane bound vacuolar structure, 0.5 to 0.8 μm in diameter, that contains several small, clear vesicles. Its origin, function, and exact relationship to other lysosomes remain obscure (see atlas figure 1-18).

Peroxisomes

KEY WORDS: nucleoid, hydrogen peroxide

Peroxisomes or microbodies comprise another class of membrane-bound organelles. Usually larger than lysosomes, their internal structure varies and can be crystalline or dense. The crystalline structures are called **nucleoids** (see atlas figure 1-19). Peroxisomes lack acid hydrolases but do contain enzymes such as urate oxidase and D-amino acid oxidase that produce **hydrogen peroxide,** which, although essential for many cellular functions and capable of destroying microorganisms, in excess is lethal to cells. Peroxisomes contain the enzyme catalase, which degrades hydrogen peroxide to water. Peroxisomes have been implicated in the oxidation of substrates, particularly very long chain fatty acids, and also are abundant in cells involved in steroid synthesis and cholesterol metabolism.

Formation of peroxisomes does not appear to involve the Golgi complex. Inactive precursors of the peroxisomal enzymes are thought to be formed on free ribosomes, and their limiting membrane is believed to be derived from the budding of vesicles from smooth regions of the GER.

Mitochondria

KEY WORDS: outer mitochondrial membrane, inner mitochondrial membrane, cristae, membrane space, intracristal space, intercristal space, mitochondrial matrix, Krebs cycle, elementary particle, electron transfer, DNA, ribonucleoprotein, matrix granule

Mitochondria are membranous structures that play a vital role in the production of the energy required by cells. They are visible in living cells examined by phase contrast microscopy and can be stained in appropriately fixed tissues, where they appear as rods or thin filaments. They usually are not visible in routine tissue sections because of the lipid solvents used during tissue preparation.

Ultrastructurally, mitochondria show a variety of shapes and sizes, but all are enclosed by two membranes, each of which has the typical trilaminar substructure (Fig. 1-7). The **outer mitochondrial membrane** is a continuous, smooth structure that completely envelops the organelle. It contains specialized transport proteins that allow permeability to certain molecules from the cytosol. An **inner mitochondrial membrane** runs parallel to the outer membrane but is thrown into numerous folds, the **cristae,** that extend into the interior of the mitochondrion (see atlas figures 1-20 and 1-21).

The narrow space between inner and outer membranes, the **membrane space,** is continuous with the small **intracristal space** within each crista. The inner mitochondrial membrane sur-

Fig. 1-7. Structure of a mitochondrion.

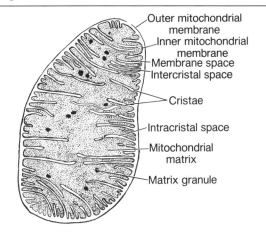

Outer mitochondrial membrane
Inner mitochondrial membrane
Membrane space
Intercristal space
Cristae
Intracristal space
Mitochondrial matrix
Matrix granule

rounds the larger **intercristal space** that contains a slightly more electron-dense material called the **mitochondrial matrix.** Enzymes of **Krebs cycle,** responsible for the final breakdown of fatty acids, monosugars, and some amino acids, reside within the mitochondrial matrix.

Cristae greatly increase the surface area of the inner mitochondrial membrane and may be either shelflike or tubular in shape; the tubular form is seen most often in cells involved in steroid synthesis. The inner mitochondrial membrane is the site of many enzymatic reactions and is studded with club-shaped structures called **elementary particles.** Each particle consists of a spherical head, 9 to 10 nm in diameter, attached to the inner mitochondrial membrane by a narrow stalk 5 nm long. Phosphorylating enzymes and enzymes of the **electron transfer** system are located either on the elementary particles or within the inner mitochondrial membranes that form the cristae. The inner mitochondrial membrane is impermeable to small ions, a feature essential for development of electrochemical gradients and the formation of high-energy metabolites. Energy released by the enzymes operating in the Krebs cycle is accepted by the electron transfer system of cytochromes and then incorporated into high-energy phosphate compounds such as adenosine triphosphate (ATP), the primary source of energy for cell activities. Thus, a primary function of mitochondria is synthesis of ATP, which reputedly then diffuses into the adjacent cytoplasm.

Mitochondria are unique among organelles since they contain their own complement of **DNA** and are capable of self-replication. Mitochondrial DNA differs from nuclear DNA in its lower molecular weight and is unusual in that it consists of branched filaments of variable thickness arranged in a circular manner. The mitochondrial matrix also contains small particles of **ribonucleoprotein** that are 12 nm in diameter and are similar in structure and function to cytoplasmic ribosomes. Messenger RNA and transfer RNA also have been identified in mitochondria. Scattered throughout the mitochondrial matrix are the more conspicuous **matrix granules,** which mea-

sure 30 to 50 nm in diameter. These granules are thought to regulate the internal ionic composition of the mitochondrion. In addition to the enzymes of Krebs cycle, enzymes involved in protein and lipid synthesis are present in the mitochondrial matrix of some cell types. Mitochondria also contain several enzymes associated with the synthesis of steroid hormones and at several steps in the synthetic pathway, substrate enters the mitochondrion for processing and then returns to other cytoplasmic compartments for the completion of additional steps. More than 50 enzymes have been localized to mitochondria.

Annulate Lamellae

The annulate lamellae are membranous organelles consisting of parallel cisternae arranged in stacks. At regular intervals along their lengths, the cisternae show numerous small pores that appear to be closed by thin, electron-dense diaphragms (see atlas figure 1-23). The cisternae are spaced uniformly throughout the stack, and the pores in successive cisternae may be aligned. Annulate lamellae often have a perinuclear location and might be continuous with elements of GER. They have been seen in germ cells, various somatic cells, and tumor cells.

Centrioles

KEY WORDS: centrosome, diplosome, microtubule, triplet, procentriole, centriolar satellite, basal body, ciliogenesis, procentriole organizer

Under the light microscope, centrioles appear as minute rods or granules usually located near the nucleus in a specialized region of the cytoplasm called the **centrosome.** In some cells centrioles are located between the nucleus and the free surface of the cell at some distance from the nucleus. Two centrioles usually are present in the nondividing cell and together form the **diplosome.** As seen in electron micrographs, the two centrioles that make up the diplosome are perpendicular to each other. The wall of each centriole consists of nine subunits, each of which is made up of three fused **microtubules;** the subunits are referred to as **triplets.** The nine sets of triplets are so arranged in the centriolar wall that they resemble a pinwheel when seen in cross section. The microtubules within each triplet are called the A, B, and C microtubules, the innermost being the A microtubule, the central tubule being the B, and the most peripheral tubule being the C (Fig. 1-8; see atlas figure 1-22). The clear center of the centriole contains a thin filament that passes in a helix immediately adjacent to the inner surface of the centriolar wall. Multinucleated cells contain several centrioles.

Centrioles are self-replicating organelles that duplicate just before cell division. A new centriole, called a **procentriole,** forms at right angles to each of the parent centrioles. Initially, the wall of the procentriole consists of a ring of amorphous material with no microtubules. As the procentriole elongates by addition of material at its distal end, microtubules appear in the wall and the new structure assumes the configuration of the parent centriole. Immediately after duplication, each parent centriole together with a newly formed daughter centriole migrates to the opposite poles of the cell, where they function in the development of the mitotic spindle. Small, dense bodies, the **centriolar satellites,** are associated with the centrioles and initiate the development and polymerization of microtubules during formation of the mitotic spindle.

Fig. 1-8. Diagrammatic representation of a centriole seen in cross section.

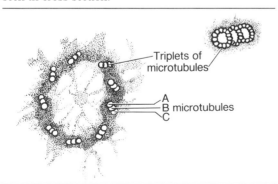

Triplets of microtubules

A
B microtubules
C

In some cells centrioles migrate close to the surface, where they form **basal bodies** from which arise cilia or flagella; these also are microtubule-containing structures. During the process of **ciliogenesis,** dense spherical bodies (**procentriole organizers**) appear in the cytoplasm and numerous procentrioles form around each. Multiple newly formed centrioles migrate to sites immediately beneath the plasmalemma and become oriented perpendicular to it. The two innermost microtubules (A and B) of each centriolar triplet begin a rapid polymerization of tubulin and serve as templates for formation of the microtubules of the axoneme. Elongation of the cilium is complete within one hour.

Cytoskeleton

The cytoskeleton gives structural support to the cytoplasm and consists of microfilaments, intermediate filaments, microtubules, and a microtrabecular lattice. Interaction between the cytoskeleton and the plasmalemma is essential for cell movement, endocytosis, focal mobility of the plasmalemma, maintenance of cell shape, stabilization of cell junctions, and spatial orientation of enzymes and other molecules in the hyaloplasm.

Microfilaments

KEY WORDS: actin, myosin

Cytoplasmic filaments are responsible for contractility, a property shown in some degree by almost all cells. Filaments are best developed in muscle cells, where the proteins **actin** and **myosin** form two different types of filaments whose interactions are responsible for the contractile properties of muscle cells.

Microfilaments have a diameter of 7 nm and usually are located immediately beneath the plasmalemma. **Actin** shows the same dimensions as the microfilaments and has been identified chemically in microfilaments. Actin is an important component of the cytoskeleton and occurs in several molecular forms depending on the cell type. Actin filaments may be organized into parallel bundles or randomly distributed to form an extensive, interwoven network. Linking proteins such as filamin link actin filaments together under certain conditions to form a stiff, supportive framework for the plasmalemma. Actin also may be linked to transmembrane proteins in specialized regions of the plasmalemma at junctional complexes contributing further to the cytoskeleton of individual cells. Under different conditions actin filaments participate in cell locomotion, ruffling of the cell membrane, invagination of the plasmalemma during endocytosis, and formation of the contraction ring of dividing cells. In this case, a thin layer of actin filaments located along the cytoplasmic surface of the cell membrane interacts with myosin. **Myosin** also is present in all cells and interacts with actin filaments to generate movement of the plasmalemma. Myosin is an actin-activated ATPase protein and may exist in monomeric forms. Actin/myosin interactions are involved in the movement of transport vesicles and certain organelles within the cell.

Intermediate Filaments

KEY WORDS: keratin, vimentin, desmin, neurofilament, glial filament

The thicker intermediate filaments measure 9 to 12 nm in diameter and form a more diverse population of filaments; they may be present as individual strands or loose bundles. Intermediate filaments often are attached to the internal surface of the plasmalemma at cell junctions and may contribute to the cytoskeleton of the cell, providing support. Microfilaments and intermediate filaments may occur in the same cell (see atlas figure 1-21).

Although indistinguishable structurally, five types of intermediate filaments have been identified by immunocytochemical means. Most cells contain only a single type, but occasionally a cell type may contain two. **Keratin** filaments are present in epithelial cells and form bundles that end in cell attachments. They are most abundant in the stratified squamous epithelia, especially in the skin. **Vimentin** filaments occur in fibroblasts and other cells derived from mesenchyme; **desmin** filaments are found in skeletal, cardiac, and smooth muscle cells and provide for the mechan-

ical integration of the contractile proteins actin and myosin; **neurofilaments** are found only in nerve cell bodies and their processes and often occur in bundles. **Glial filaments** are confined to the supporting (glial) cells of the central nervous system. A knowledge of this restricted distribution is often useful for the assessment of malignant tumors to determine their site of origin.

Microtubules

KEY WORDS: tubulin, centriole, cilia, flagella

Microtubules are straight or slightly curved, nonbranching tubules measuring 21 to 25 nm in diameter and several micrometers in length. Their walls, about 6 nm thick, consist of 13 parallel protein filaments, each 4 to 5 nm in diameter, arranged in a helix. The central zone is electron-lucent, so the structure appears to be hollow (see atlas figure 1-18). Microtubules are composed primarily of the protein **tubulin,** which occurs in alpha and beta forms. Small quantities of high molecular weight proteins called microtubule-associated proteins (MAPs) also have been isolated and are thought to correspond to the slender, lateral, filamentous projections of the microtubules.

Microtubules usually are scarce in resting cells but are present in large numbers in dividing cells, where they make up the mitotic spindle. After the cell has divided, most of the microtubules disappear. In interphase cells, microtubules form prominent components of **centrioles, cilia,** and **flagella,** and, in some cells, contribute to the cytoskeleton. Within platelets and nucleated red cells of nonmammalian species, microtubules form stiffening elements that help maintain cell shape. In nerve cells, microtubules are believed to be important for transport of material from one region of the cytoplasm to another. A transient increase in the number of microtubules is seen in nondividing cells during changes in shape associated with cell movement and during differentiation. It has been suggested that a three-dimensional framework (a microtrabecular lattice) in the hyaloplasm links the cell organelles and cytoskeleton into a coordinated functional unit during cell movement and other activities.

Cytoplasmic Inclusions

Inclusions are nonliving elements found in the cytoplasm and include such diverse materials as pigment granules, glycogen, lipid droplets, crystals, and secretory granules. They are not essential to the life or functioning of the cell and represent metabolic products, storage materials, or foreign substances taken into the cell from the environment.

Pigment Granules

KEY WORDS: melanin, melanosome, hemosiderin, lipofuscin

Naturally occurring pigments in human cells include melanin, hemosiderin, and lipofuscin, each of which has its own inherent color. **Melanin** is contained within **melanosomes,** which are membrane-bound granules formed and found in melanocytes and sometimes secondarily deposited in certain other cells, especially prominently at the skin's dermo-epidermal junction, contributing to the color of the skin. The pigment epithelium of the retina and iris and certain cells of the brain also contain melanin.

Hemosiderin is a golden brown pigment derived from breakdown of hemoglobin present in red blood cells. Phagocytic cells of the liver, bone marrow, and spleen normally contain this type of pigment.

Lipofuscin is found in many cells throughout the body, particularly in older persons. Sometimes called the "wear and tear" pigment, lipofuscin is light brown in color, increases with age, and represents an end product of lysosomal activity.

Glycogen

KEY WORDS: glucose polymer, beta particle, alpha particle

Glycogen is a large **glucose polymer** and is the storage form of carbohydrate. It cannot be seen in usual tissue preparations unless selectively stained. Ultrastructurally, glycogen appears either as **beta particles,** which are irregular, small, dense particles 15 to 45 nm in diameter, or as **alpha particles,** which measure 90 to 95 nm in diameter and represent several smaller particles of glycogen clumped to form rosettes (see atlas figures 1-19 and 1-25).

Fat

KEY WORDS: fat cell, lipid droplet

Fat cells are the chief storage sites for lipid, but many other cell types store fat as **lipid droplets** of various sizes. Lipid synthesized by a cell accumulates in cytoplasmic droplets that lack a limiting membrane. Intracellular lipid serves as a source of energy and as a supply of short-chain carbon compounds for the synthesis of membranes by the cell. During preparation of routine tissue sections, lipid usually is extracted and sites of lipid storage appear as clear vacuoles. In electron micrographs, preserved lipid droplets appear as homogeneous spheres of different densities (see atlas figure 1-25).

Crystals

Crystalline inclusions are normal constituents in several cell types and may be free in the cytoplasm or contained in secretory granules, mitochondria, endoplasmic reticulum, the Golgi complex, and even the nucleus. Many of the observed intracellular crystals are believed to represent a storage form of protein (see atlas figure 1-26).

Secretory Granules

Secretory granules are limited by a membrane and represent cell products that are to be secreted by the cell (see atlas figures 1-15 and 1-24). They are somewhat transitory, and some are formed as others are released. Depending on the type of cell producing them, secretory granules contain different products that serve different functions.

Nucleus

The nucleus is an essential organelle present in all complete cells. The only cytoplasmic structures in which nuclei are absent are mature mammalian erythrocytes and blood platelets; these should not be regarded as cells. Generally, each cell has a single nucleus but some, such as the parietal cells of the stomach, cardiac muscle cells, and liver cells, may possess two nuclei. Giant cells, such as the osteoclasts of bone, megakaryocytes of marrow, and skeletal muscle cells, may have several nuclei.

The shape of the nucleus varies and may be spherical, ovoid, or elongated corresponding to the cell shape, or it might be lobulated as in the granular leukocytes of the blood.

The nucleus contains all the information necessary to initiate and control the differentiation, maturation, and metabolic activities of each cell. The nondividing nucleus is enclosed in a nuclear envelope and contains the chromatin material and one or two nucleoli (see atlas figures 1-13 and 1-16). These are suspended in a nuclear ground substance called the karyolymph or nuclear matrix.

Chromatin and Chromosomes

KEY WORDS: karyosome, heterochromatin, histone, euchromatin, diploid, haploid, homologous chromosome, sex chromosome, autosome, karyotype, metacentric, acrocentric, submetacentric

Genetic information is stored in the molecules of DNA that make up the chromosomes. In nondividing nuclei, chromosomes are largely uncoiled and dispersed, but some regions of the chromosomes remain condensed, stain deeply, and are visible by the light microscope as chromatin. Ultrastructurally, chromatin appears as fibers of nucleoprotein, 20 to 30 nm in diameter. Each fiber consists of a double helix of DNA wrapped about a core of histone. Individual masses of chromatin are called **karyosomes** and, although not entirely constant, the chromatin masses do tend to be characteristic in size, pattern, and quantity for any given cell type. Collectively, the karyosomes form the **heterochromatin** of the nucleus and represent coiled portions of the chromosomes. Heterochromatin is believed to be complexed to **histones** and to be nonactive. His-

tones are simple proteins that contain a high proportion of basic amino acids. The dispersed regions of the chromosomes stain lightly and form **euchromatin,** which is active in controlling the metabolic processes of the cell (Fig. 1-9; see atlas figures 1-11 and 1-24). The distinction between heterochromatin and euchromatin disappears during cell division when all the chromatin condenses and becomes metabolically inert.

Chromosomes are permanent entities of the cell and are present at every stage of the cell cycle, but their appearance depends on the physiologic state of the cell. At interphase the chromosomes form delicate, tortuous threads, and it is only during cell division that they assume the appearance of discrete, solid, rodlike structures (see atlas figure 1-30). Analysis and study of chromosomes can be carried out most conveniently in dividing cells that have been arrested in metaphase. Alkaloids such as the vinca drugs and colchicine interfere with spindle formation and permit intracellular accumulation of metaphase chromosomes for study.

The number of chromosomes typically is con-

Fig. 1-9. Diagrammatic representation of nuclear structures.

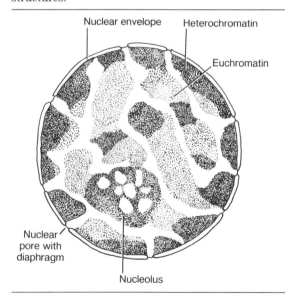

Nuclear envelope   Heterochromatin

Euchromatin

Nuclear pore with diaphragm

Nucleolus

stant for each species but varies considerably between species. In humans the chromosome number is 46 compared with 22 for the North American opossum, 32 in the alligator, and 78 in the dog. The figures given are for the **diploid** number in somatic cells. Germ cells (ova and sperm) contain half this number and are said to be **haploid.** The chromosomes present in somatic cells represent the inheritance of two sets of chromosomes, one from each male and female parent. In the male and female sets, chromosomes that are similar are called **homologous chromosomes.** In many diploid higher animals, a pair of **sex chromosomes** is specialized for and participates in the determination of sex; all other chromosomes are called **autosomes.** In humans there are 44 autosomes and a pair of sex chromosomes that are homologous (XX) in the female and heterologous (XY) in the male.

Homologous chromosomes can be recognized at metaphase and are arranged in groups representing the **karyotype** of a species. Individual chromosomes often can be identified by the length of their arms and the location of the centromere. If the centromere is in the middle of the chromosome and the arms (telomeres) are of equal length, the chromosome is said to be **metacentric.** If the centromere is close to one end, the chromosome is **acrocentric,** and if the centromere is between the midpoint and the end, the chromosome is **submetracentric.**

Nuclear Envelope

KEY WORDS: unit membrane, perinuclear space, nuclear pore, nuclear pore complex, lamins, fibrous lamina

The nuclear envelope consists of two concentric **unit membranes,** each 7.5 nm thick, separated by a **perinuclear space** 40 to 70 nm wide. The inner membrane is smooth, whereas the outer membrane often contains numerous ribosomes on its cytoplasmic surface and is continuous with the surrounding endoplasmic reticulum. At irregular intervals around the nucleus, the inner and outer membranes of the envelope become continuous with one another to form small oc-

tagonal openings called **nuclear pores** (see atlas figures 1-28 and 1-29). The pores measure about 50 nm in diameter and are closed by a **nuclear pore complex** that consists of two rings, one of which faces the cytoplasm. Eight radial spokes extend inward from the rings toward a central granule. The number and distribution of nuclear pores depends on the type of cell and its activity. The pores may be sites where materials are exchanged between the nucleus and cytoplasm, or they may be attachment sites for structural components of the nucleoplasm. A thin meshwork of filaments called **lamins** is made up of three polypeptides and lies along the inner surface of the nuclear membrane to form the **fibrous lamina.** The lamins are linked to specific membrane proteins in the inner nuclear membrane and act as a supporting framework for the nuclear envelope to aid in maintaining the shape of the nucleus.

Nucleolus

KEY WORDS: ribosomal RNA, nucleolus-organizing region, pars granulosa, pars fibrosa, nucleolus-associated chromatin

A nucleolus appears as a dense, well-defined body 1 to 3 nm in diameter, contained within a nucleus (see atlas figure 1-13). Nucleoli are sites where **ribosomal RNA** (rRNA) is synthesized. Since these sites (**nucleolus-organizing regions**) are located on five different chromosomes, any one cell may contain several nucleoli. Uusally only one or two large nucleoli are found, since the nucleolus-organizing regions tend to associate and the RNA produced at these regions aggregates into larger masses.

As seen in electron micrographs, nucleoli lie free in the nucleus, not limited by a membrane. They show two regions, each associated with a particular form of ribonucleoprotein. The dominant region, the **pars granulosa,** consists of dense granules of RNA 13 to 15 nm in diameter. The second region, the **pars fibrosa,** tends to be centrally placed and consists of dense masses of filaments 5 nm in diameter.

Deoxyribonucleoprotein also is associated with

the nucleolus and is present in filaments of chromatin that surround or extend into the nucleolus. This chromatin forms the **nucleolus-associated chromatin;** its DNA constitutes the template for synthesis of rRNA.

Nucleoli are found only in interphase nuclei and are especially prominent in cells that are actively synthesizing proteins. They are dispersed during cell division but reform at the nucleolus-organizing regions during reconstruction of the daughter nuclei after cell division.

Functional Summary

Cells are the fundamental units of structure of all tissues and organs and perform all of the activities necessary for the survival, growth, and reproduction of an organism. They carry out energy transformations and biosynthetic activities and are able to replicate themselves. The functional activities of a cell are carried out by specialized structures, the organelles, many of which consist of or are bounded by biological membranes essential to the organization of the cell. In addition to forming the interface between the cell and its external environment, they also are important in transportation of materials, organization of different energy transfer systems, transmission of stimuli, provision of selectively permeable barriers, and separating various intracellular spaces.

All materials that pass in or out of a cell must cross the plasmalemma; this structure is instrumental in selecting what enters and leaves the cell. Large molecules are taken in by pinocytosis, particulate matter can be incorporated into the cell by phagocytosis, and small molecules enter the cell by diffusion. The rate at which material diffuses into the cell depends on whether the material is soluble in lipid or water. Lipid-soluble materials readily dissolve in the lipid matrix of the plasmalemma and pass through the cell membrane relatively unhindered. The transmembrane proteins of the plasmalemma act as sites for passage of water-soluble substances and may serve as carrier proteins for materials such as glucose.

Although simple in microscopic appearance, the plasmalemma is very complex and variable in its molecular organization and function. Significant physiologic and biochemical differences may occur at specific regions of the plasmalemma according to the function of the cell. The plasmalemma contains special receptor sites that can react with agents such as hormones or neurotransmitters to transfer information to the cell and elicit specific responses. The structure and composition of the plasmalemma are important in determining the immunologic properties of the cell and its relationships and interactions with other cells. The plasmalemma may contain enzyme systems that act as ion pumps or initiate and control cellular activities by generating secondary messenger molecules. Membrane specializations also are involved in cell-to-cell attachments and communication.

The endoplasmic reticulum is associated with many synthetic activities of the cell. Smooth endoplasmic reticulum in liver cells is believed to serve in lipid and cholesterol metabolism, glycogen synthesis and storage, and detoxification of drugs. In endocrine cells, the SER has been implicated in the synthesis of steroid hormones. It plays an important role in muscle contraction, being responsible for the release and recapture of calcium ions. The GER is involved in the synthesis of proteins and provides a membrane for the transport vesicles that carry newly formed protein to the Golgi complex, where it is concentrated and packed into secretory granules. Golgi membranes are able to synthesize carbohydrate, complex it to protein, and form glycoproteins. The Golgi body also acts in the synthesis of lipoproteins, being responsible for complexing lipid to proteins produced by the GER. Synthesis of protein occurs in ribosomes, and protein formed by ribosomes attached to the GER usually is secreted by the cell, whereas that formed on free polysomes is used by the cell itself.

Mitochondria perform a number of functions, chiefly the production of energy for the cell. Pyruvate, produced by the degradation of glucose in the cytoplasm, enters the mitochondrion where, along with amino acids and fatty acids, it is processed by the enzymes of Krebs cycle located in the mitochondrial matrix. Transfer of electrons and hydrogen atoms to oxygen is mediated by enzymes of the electron transport system, which are located on the elementary particles or within the mitochondrial membrane that forms the cristae. Energy released by the oxidations is incorporated into the high-energy bonds of ATP, which then diffuses into the cytoplasm where it is available for use by the cell. Mitochondria also play a role in the synthesis of proteins, lipids, and steroids.

Lysosomes mainly function in intracellular digestion, which occurs in membrane-enclosed digestion vacuoles that isolate the lysosomal enzymes from the remainder of the cytoplasm. Materials may be taken into the cell during phagocytosis, or portions of cytoplasm containing aged or damaged organelles may be sequestered and digested by lysosomal activity. Usable end products diffuse into the cytoplasm, and the undigested residue remains within the vacuoles to form the residual bodies. Lysosomes might have other functions in normal cells. They have been implicated in the degradation of glycogen, in the removal from cells of excess substances such as unsecreted products, and in the release of thyroid hormone by splitting off the globulin to which the hormone is conjugated during its synthesis. Rupture of lysosomes in some cells may initiate mitosis.

Peroxisomes are similar in morphology to lysosomes but contain a number of enzymes capable of producing and degrading hydrogen peroxide. They play a role in the conversion of noncarbohydrate precursors to glucose and are instrumental in preventing the accumulation of lethal levels of hydrogen peroxide.

Microtubules, intermediate filaments, and microfilaments form the cytoskeleton of cells and perform a number of functions. Generally, intermediate filaments act as supporting elements. Microtubules contribute to the structure of cilia, flagella, and centrioles, provide supporting structures (stiffening rods) in some cells, have been implicated in intracellular transport of materials, and are essential for cell division and motility. Microfilaments (primarily actins) together with myosin function in cell movement, focal movements of cell membranes, and endocytosis and are responsible for the contraction ring during mitosis.

All the information needed to initiate and regulate the activities of a cell is encoded in the nucleus. This structure controls the growth, differentiation, maturation, and metabolic activities of the cell. The nucleus also is equipped to duplicate and pass on DNA to its daughter cells. The nucleolus, which is the site of production of rRNA and tRNA, plays a central role in the control of protein synthesis by the cell. All the nuclei in an individual contain identical genomes, but some portions are actively expressed in some cells and repressed in others. The differential activity of genes is due to differential activation, not to selective removal of genes.

Clinical Correlations

Cells respond to injury by undergoing degenerative changes. These vary in severity and may be reversible when the cause is removed. Otherwise, cell death results. Cloudy swelling is a common cellular reaction to most acute infections, anoxia, and toxic agents. It is the mildest of the degenerative changes and is reversible. The changes result from increased permeability of the plasmalemma with influx of water and sodium. The resulting reversible osmotic swelling of mitochondria gives a cloudy, granular appearance to the cytoplasm. Loss of matrix granules from mitochondria is an early indication of cellular damage. Hydropic degeneration also results from failure of the cell membrane, but there is a greater influx of water than in cloudy swelling and mitochondria are converted to water-filled vacuoles. Water also collects in and distends the cisternae of the endoplasmic reticulum and the cells appear pale, clear, and markedly swollen. Hyaline droplet degeneration represents accumulation of protein in cells, usually from abnormal storage of secretory products. Hyaline appears as homogeneous, refractile droplets in the cytoplasm.

Fatty degeneration results from accumulation of lipid in cells other than fat cells. Small droplets of fat collect in the cytoplasm and, even in advanced stages, tend to remain small and discrete and do not greatly enlarge the cell. The fat lies free in the cytoplasm with no limiting membrane. The cells most likely to undergo fatty change are those of the liver, skeletal muscle, and heart mucle. These are cells with high metabolic activity and specialized functions that obtain part of their energy from oxidation of lipids.

More than 24 "storage" diseases occur in humans. These are seen chiefly in infants and represent inheritable defects of lysosomes expressed by the absence of specific lysosomal enzymes. The substrate of the missing enzyme accumulates in autophagic vacuoles within the cytoplasm of various cells. Gaucher's disease is a storage disease marked by accumulation of glucocerebrosides in macrophages of the spleen, liver, bone marrow, and lymph nodes due to lack of the enzyme β-glucosidase. The macrophages increase in number and size and can displace or compress vital tissues. Neimann-Pick disease, a rare condition of early childhood that leads to mental deficiency and usually is fatal, represents a storage disease in which sphingomyelin and cholesterol accumulate in cells widespread throughout the body. The cells show a deficiency of the lysosomal enzyme sphyngomyelinase.

Although lysosomal storage diseases are perhaps the best documented diseases associated with a specific organelle (Table 1-1), peroxisomal disorders involving defects in the peroxisomal enzymes also have been documented. Impaired oxidation of long-chain fatty acids results in a variety of conditions that may involve the accumulation of abnormal lipids in specific cell populations. Likewise, diseases involving other organelles, such as mitochondria (mitochondrial cytopathy syndromes), are not uncommon.

Necrosis is the focal death of cells. It may occur suddenly, as in burns or exposure to corrosive chemicals, or may proceed gradually through degenerative changes. The nuclei of necrotic cells may be discernible only as a nuclear outline, reflecting karyolysis (hydrolysis of chromatin), or the chromatin may become fragmented and scattered (karyorrhexis) or shrink to form a dense, structureless mass (pyknosis). The swollen cells may be poorly outlined and show homogeneous or granular, acidophilic cytoplasm (coagulation necrosis) or absorb water and disintegrate, leaving little or no indication of their previous structure (liquefactive necrosis). Shrinkage necrosis results from gradual loss of water from the cell; the nucleus becomes condensed and the cytoplasm stains deeply because of the closer packing of organelles. Ultimately the cell becomes fragmented and phagocytes engulf the resulting debris.

An adult organ may increase in size because of an increase in the size of individual cells (hypertrophy) or an increase in the number of component cells (hyperplasia). Similarly, adult organs and tissues may decrease in size (atrophy) as a result of a reduction in the size or number of its cells. Aplasia refers to a deficiency of cell replacement so that little of the organ is left. It is ex-

Table 1-1 Lysosomal Storage Diseases

Disease	Missing enzyme	Accumulating substance
Sphingolipidoses		
Gaucher's disease	β-Glucosidase	Glucocerebroside
Fabry's disease	α-Galactosidase	Ceramide trihexoside
Krabbe's disease	β-Galactosidase	Galactocerebroside
Farber's disease	Acid ceramidase	Ceramide, gangliosides
Niemann-Pick disease	Sphingomyxelinase	Sphingomyelin
Tay-Sachs disease	N-Acetyl-β-glucosaminidase A	Ganglioside GM_2
Glycoproteinoses		
Fucosidosis	α-Fucosidase	Fucoglycoproteins
Sialidosis	Sialidase	Sialyl oligosaccharides
Mannosidosis	α-Mannosidase	Mannose-containing oligosaccharides
Mucolipidoses		
I cell disease	Severe deficiency of several hydrolases	Variety of undegraded substances
Mucolipidosis IV	Ganglioside sialidase	Gangliosides
Mucopolysaccharidoses		
Sanfilippo disease	Heparan-N-sulfatase	Heparan sulfate
Morquio's syndrome	N-acetyl-galactosamine-6-sulfatase, galactose-6-sulfatase	Keratan sulfate
Maroteaux-Lamy syndrome	Arylsulfatase	Dermatan sulfate
Sly syndrome	β-Glucuronidase	Heparan sulfate Dermatan sulfate
Other lysosomal storage diseases		
Pompe's disease	α-1,4-Glucosidase	Glycogen
Cystinosis	Defective transport system in lysosomal membrane	Cysteine disulfide
Wolman's disease	Acid lipase	Cholesterol esters, triglycerides

emplified by aplastic anemia, in which failure of the bone marrow to restore itself results in progressive anemia. Agenesis implies the complete absence of an organ because of faulty development.

Metaplasia refers to an abnormal transformation of fully differentiated adult cells to a different cell type. Epithelial metaplasia occurs where surface cells are exposed to unusual conditions as, for example, in the gallbladder, where the normal columnar epithelium becomes stratified squamous because of irritation from gallstones. Anaplasia is an important feature of tumor growth and means a loss of cell differentiation and specialization with increased capacity for growth. Neoplastic tumors can be defined as autonomous, abnormal masses that show progressive cellular growth without regard for normal replacement

needs. Benign tumors grow expansively but locally, and unless they grow in or compress vital
tissues, are well tolerated. Malignant tumors are
invasive and infiltrate surrounding tissues and
produce secondary (metastatic) tumors in sites
remote from the original tumor.

Mitosis

Nearly all multicellular organisms grow by increasing the number of cells. The zygote, which
is formed at conception, divides repeatedly and
gives rise to all the cells of the body. Every cell in
the resulting individual thus contains a nucleus,
and each nucleus possesses identical genetic information. In the adult, most cells have a finite
life span and must be replaced continuously. Proliferation of somatic cells is the result of mitosis,
which can be defined as the production of two
daughter cells with exactly the same number of
chromosomes and the same DNA content as the
original parent cell.

Mitosis usually lasts from 30 to 60 minutes and
involves division of the nucleus (karyokinesis)
and the cytoplasm (cytokinesis). Both events usually take place during mitosis, but karyokinesis
may occur without division of the cytoplasm, resulting in formation of multinucleated cells, such
as the megakaryocytes of bone marrow. Although
mitosis is a continuous process, for descriptive
purposes it is convenient to divide it into prophase, metaphase, anaphase, and telophase. The
time between successive mitotic divisions constitutes interphase and is the period when the
cell performs its usual functions, contributes to
the total economy of the body, and makes preparations for the next division.

Interphase

KEY WORDS: replication of DNA, centromere

Replication of DNA occurs during interphase,
before the cell visibly enters into mitosis. The
double helix of the chromosome unwinds, and
each strand acts as a template for the development of a complementary strand of DNA that contains an exact copy of the sequence of molecules

in the original DNA. A new double helix is formed
that contains a new strand and a parent strand
of DNA. Replication begins at the ends of the
chromosomes and progresses toward the center,
where a small area of the chromosome, the **centromere,** remains unduplicated. Shortly thereafter, the chromosomes begin to coil, shorten,
and become visible within the nucleus, and the
cell enters the prophase of mitosis.

Prophase

KEY WORDS: chromatid, centriole replication

In prophase, the cell assumes a more spherical
shape and appears more refractile, while in the
nucleus, chromosomes become visible and appear as threadlike structures (see atlas figure 1-
31A). At prophase each chromosome consists of
two coiled subunits called **chromatids** that are
closely associated along their lengths. Chromatids are the functional units of chromosomes,
and each contains a double strand of DNA. As
prophase progresses, the chromatids continue to
coil, thicken, and shorten, reaching about one-
twenty-fifth of their length by the end of prophase. The chromosomes then appear to approach the nuclear envelope.

As these events occur, nucleoli become smaller
and finally disappear, and the nuclear envelope
breaks down. When this occurs, the center of the
cell becomes more fluid and the chromosomes
move more freely, making their way to the equator of the cell. Simultaneous with the nuclear
events, the **centrioles replicate** and the resulting
pairs migrate to the opposite poles of the cell.

Metaphase

**KEY WORDS: mitotic spindle, equatorial plate,
continuous fiber, centromere (kinetochore),
chromosomal fiber, splitting of centromere**

The disappearance of the nuclear envelope marks
the end of prophase and the beginning of metaphase, which is characterized by formation of the
mitotic spindle and the alignment of chromosomes along the equator to form the **equatorial
plate** (see atlas figure 1-31B). The mitotic spindle

is a somewhat diffuse body formed mainly of microtubules; those that pass from pole to pole of the spindle are called **continuous fibers.** Other microtubules extend from the poles of the spindle to attach to the **centromere (kinetochore)** of each chromosome and form the **chromosomal fibers.** The centromere is a specialized region of unduplicated DNA and protein that holds together the chromatids of each chromosome and forms an attachment site for the chromosomal fibers.

The final act of metaphase is duplication of the DNA at the centromere, after which the **centromeres split.** The two chromatids of each chromosome separate and begin to migrate toward the centrioles at the opposite poles of the cell. Duplication of the centromeres and migration of chromatids occur simultaneously in all chromosomes of a given cell.

Anaphase

KEY WORDS: **telomere, daughter chromosome**

The initial separation of chromatids marks the beginning of anaphase (see atlas figure 1-32). As the chromatids move toward the opposite poles, the centromeres travel in advance of the **telomeres** (arms) of the chromosomes that trail behind. Movement of chromatids, which now are **daughter chromosomes,** is an active, dynamic process, but the mechanisms by which the movement is effected are not certain.

Telophase

KEY WORDS: **reforming nuclear envelope, nucleolus-organizing region, karyokinesis**

As the daughter chromosomes reach their respective poles, discontinuous portions of endoplasmic reticulum form around each group of chromosomes and begin to **reform the nuclear envelope** (see atlas figure 1-33). This event initiates telophase. When the nuclear envelope has been reformed completely, the chromosomes uncoil and become indistinct, and the two nuclei reassume the interphase configuration. The normal complement of nucleoli also reappears at this time. Their development is associated with specific **nucleolus-organizing regions** present on certain chromosomes. With this event **karyokinesis** is complete.

Cytokinesis

KEY WORDS: **interzonal fiber, midbody**

During telophase the mitotic spindle begins to disappear. The fibers between the two forming nuclei appear stretched and often are called **interzonal fibers** (see atlas figure 1-32B). Midway between the two nuclei, in the region formerly occupied by the equatorial plate, a constriction of the plasmalemma forms a furrow that extends around the equator of the cell. The constriction extends deeper into the cytoplasm, separating the daughter chromosomes until they are joined only by a thin protoplasmic bridge, called the **midbody,** that contains interzonal fibers. Eventually the daughter cells pull away from each other by ameboid movement, thus completing the separation of the cells and ending cytokinesis.

Cell organelles are evenly distributed between the two daughter cells. Immediately after division, the daughter cells enter a phase of active RNA and protein synthesis, resulting in an increase in the volume of the nucleus and cytoplasm. The endoplasmic reticulum and the Golgi complex are restored to their original concentrations, mitochondria reproduce by fission, and the centrioles replicate in the daughter cells just before the next division (Fig. 1-10).

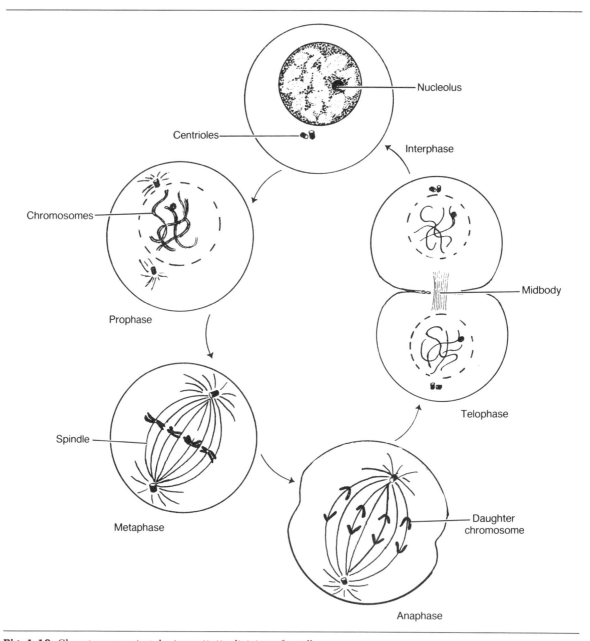

Fig. 1-10. Changes occurring during mitotic division of a cell.

Functional Summary

Mitosis produces daughter cells that have a genetic content identical to that of the parent cell. What determines if and when a cell divides is not known, but there are certain requirements that must be met before a cell can enter mitosis. There is some relationship between cell mass and cell division. For example, in *Amoeba proteus* mitosis can be prevented by periodic amputation of the cytoplasm. The cell then merely regenerates the lost cytoplasm without entering mitosis. In general, each daughter cell achieves the mass of the parent cell before it can divide. However, the relationship between cell growth and mitosis is not a causal one, and the two events can be separated in time. An example of this is seen in cleavage of ova, where growth of the cell occurs long before division takes place.

Duplication of the entire DNA complement is essential for cell division. Depriving cells of thymidine blocks DNA synthesis and prevents cells from entering mitosis. Provision of thymidine to such cells results in a wave of DNA synthesis followed by a wave of mitosis. Again, however, DNA duplication may be completed long before division occurs, and the existence and maintenance of polyploid cells argue against DNA synthesis being the trigger for mitosis.

The intense coiling and contracting of chromosomes at metaphase results in small, compact units that can be transported more easily to the poles of the cells. The destination of the chromosomes, their orderly arrangement at metaphase, and the plane of cell cleavage is determined by the mitotic spindle. It would seem reasonable that one of the preparations for mitosis must be synthesis of protein specifically for the formation of the spindle. Certain amino acid analogs result in synthesis of faulty spindle proteins, and cells cultured in the presence of these analogs fail to divide. When removed to normal media, the cells enter mitosis but only after a delay, during which the faulty spindle protein is replaced by newly synthesized normal protein.

Centrioles are responsible for polarization of the mitotic spindle and may play a role in assembling the spindle, but how this is achieved is unknown. Centrioles complete their duplication before mitosis begins, and cell division can be prevented by suppressing the replication of centrioles.

Mitosis must be an energy-consuming process, but cell division is not a period of intense respiratory activity. Restriction of energy sources and inhibition of respiration and oxidative phosphorylation do not stop mitosis once it has begun. Thus, it can be assumed that the energy needs are met during preparation for cell division.

Cell division often occurs in waves, with patches of cells or whole tissues undergoing synchronous division, implying some kind of cellular or tissue control. Substances that promote or initiate mitosis have been isolated from epidermis and salivary glands in several species, and other substances that appear to suppress mitosis (chalones) have been identified in a number of different tissues. Thus, the cell population and the rate of cell division may be governed by the reciprocal action of agents that control the rate of entry into mitosis either by stimulation or suppression of mitotic activity.

Clinical Correlations

Chromosomes can show abnormalities in number or configuration. An excess of chromosomes, usually some multiple of the haploid number, is called polyploidy. If the increase is by an uneven number, the cell is said to be aneuploid. Abnormal numbers of chromosomes frequently are found in tumors. In rare instances the centromere may split transversely rather than longitudinally, yielding chromosomes in which both arms are identical. Breaks may occur to give a fragment without a centromere; such fragments will not move to the poles at anaphase. Loss of the fragment and the genetic information it carries then occurs. Total absence of a chromosome from all body cells is lethal except in the case of the Y sex chromosome, which is absent in females. Persons with one X and no Y are phenotypically female but show a group of abnormalities (Turner's syndrome) that includes dwarfism and failure of ovarian development. An extra chromosome may occur, as in Down's syndrome, where there are three rather than two chromosomes designated No. 21. Individuals with Down's syndrome show a variety of physical and mental defects.

Atlas and Table of Key Features

Key Features of the Structural Components of the Cell

	Morphologic features	Function
Cytoplasmic constituents		
Membranous organelles		
Cell membrane (plasmalemma)	Electron-lucent layer (3.5–4.0 nm) separating two electron-dense layers (2.5–3.0 nm)	Selectively permeable membrane; cell-to-cell communication, receptors for hormones, cell recognition, ion pumps; generates messenger molecules
Granular endoplasmic reticulum	Network of membrane-bound tubules and cisternae; outer surface is covered with ribosomes	Site of synthesis of protein to be discharged from cell
Smooth endoplasmic reticulum	Network of branching, anastomosing, smooth, membrane-bound tubules	Varies with cell type; implicated in synthesis of steroid hormones, cholesterol, triglycerides, lipoproteins; detoxification of lipid-soluble drugs; acquisition or release of Ca^{++} ions
Golgi complex	Stacked, parallel array of several flattened, membrane-bound saccules (cisternae); convex surface is the forming face; concave surface is the maturing face	Site of concentration, modification, and packaging of secretory products; limited synthetic activity for complex carbohydrates and glycoproteins
Annulate lamellae	Parallel stacks of membranes enclosing cisternal lumina 30–50 nm in diameter; become continuous at regular intervals forming fenestrations (pores) in cisternae; pores often lie in register with one another	Unknown

Key Features of the Structural Components of the Cell (continued)

	Morphologic features	Function
Mitochondria	Size variable; usually round, oval, or rod-shaped; consist of two membranes: an outer smooth membrane enveloping a thinner, highly folded inner membrane; lamellar or tubular cristae projects into the interior (matrix); matrix granules prominent	Provide energy in form of phosphate bonds (ATP) for cell activities; involved in synthesis of steroid hormones in specific cell types
Lysosomes	Demonstration of acid phosphatases needed for confirmation	
Primary	Round, membrane-bound dense bodies 0.25–0.55 μm in diameter; interior variable in density	Yet to begin digestive activity
Secondary	Membrane-bound bodies, ovoid or irregular in outline, size variable. Usually contain material of some type (crystalloids, debris, organelle remnants, lipofusion pigment)	Currently or have been involved in digestive activity
Multivesicular body	Numerous small vesicles limited by a single, smooth membrane	Unknown
Peroxisomes	Spherical, membrane-bound bodies 0.2–0.4 μm in diameter; matrix may contain dense crystalline structures (nucleoids)	Oxidation of long-chain fatty acids
Nonmembranous organelles		
Ribosomes	Dense granules (15–25 nm) comprised of a large and small subunit. Polyribosomes are several ribosomes united by a strand of mRNA	Protein synthesis
Centrioles	Cylindrical structures (0.2 μm × 0.5 μm) with an electron-dense wall containing nine triplet microtubules surrounding an electron-lucent center; occur in pairs oriented at right angles	Essential for formation of microtubules of mitotic spindle, cilia, and flagella
Components of cytoskeleton		
Microtubules	Long, slender tubules 25 nm in diameter; wall 5–7 nm in width surrounding an electron-lucent lumen	Maintain cell shape and participate in shape changes; forms axonemes of cilia and flagella; intracellular transport
Microfilaments	Actin — 6-nm microfilament Myosin — 15 nm microfilament	Cell movment; control focal movement of plasmalemma or in endocytosis

Key Features of the Structural Components of the Cell (continued)

	Morphologic features	Function
Intermediate filaments	8–11 nm in diameter, subdivided immunocytochemically into five classes: 1. Keratin filaments — occur in epithelia 2. Desmin filaments — occur in three types of muscle 3. Vimentin filaments — occur in fibroblasts and mesenchymal cell derivatives 4. Neurofilaments — occur in nerve cells 5. Glial filaments — occur in glial cells	Stabilize cell shape and attachments
Cytoplasmic inclusions		
Glycogen	Beta particles (20–30 nm), occur singly and are irregular in outline; α particles are various-sized aggregates of the beta form	Storage form of glucose
Lipid	Spheroidal droplets of varying size and density; lack a limiting membrane	Primarily a storage form of short carbon chains (triglycerides)
Pigments		
Melanin	Dark brown; complexed in ellipsoidal melanosomes	Inert
Hemosiderin	Gold-brown; ultrastructurally appears as collections of 9-nm particles	Degradation product of hemoglobin; inert
Lipofuscin	Coarse, irregularly shaped, brown-gold granules	End product of lysosomal activity; inert
Crystalline structures	Vary considerably in size and structure; may occur in cytoplasmic matrix, organelles, or nucleus	Most thought to be a storage form of protein
Secretory granules	Membrane-bound; vary in size, density, and internal consistency	Material synthesized to be released by cell
Nuclear constituents		
Nuclear envelope	Consists of inner and outer membranes that become continuous around nuclear pores; outer membrane studded with ribosomes, inner membrane smooth; are separated by a perinuclear cistern; nuclear pore complex is associated with each pore	Specialized segment of endoplasmic reticulum that bounds nucleus; nuclear pores permit communication between cytoplasm and nucleoplasm

Key Features of the Structural Components of the Cell (continued)

	Morphologic features	Function
Fibrous lamina	Thin network of interwoven filaments	Stabilizes inner nuclear membrane; attachment site for components of nucleoplasm
Heterochromatin	Dense staining; condensed chromatin	Inactive; part of genome not being expressed
Euchromatin	Light staining; dispersed chromatin	Active; part of genome being expressed
Nucleolus	Conspicuous round body in nucleus; nucleolonema consists of dense granules in a matrix of filaments; amorphous component may be present	Synthesis of ribosomes

Organelles and Inclusions

Euchromatin

Heterochromatin

Plasmalemma

Micropinocytotic vesicles

Nucleus

Basal lamina

Fig. 1-11. A portion of a vascular capillary illustrating the nucleus and cytoplasm of an endothelial cell (human connective tissue). Note the limiting basal lamina. (TEM, ×6,000.)

Polyribosomes

Polyribosomes

Fig. 1-12. The cytoplasm of an immature human intestinal epithelial cell. Note the abundance of polyribosomes. (TEM, ×57,000.)

Secretory granule

Granular endoplasmic reticulum

Nucleolus

Nuclear envelope

Fig. 1-13. A portion of a chief cell taken from a human stomach illustrates regions of both the nucleus and cytoplasm. Note the abundance of granular endoplasmic reticulum and the nucleolus in this protein-secreting cell. (TEM, ×11,000.)

Mitochondrion

Tubular cristae

Polyribosomes

Smooth endoplasmic reticulum

Fig. 1-14. A region of cytoplasm from a cell of the adrenal cortex that contains numerous profiles of smooth endoplasmic reticulum. Mitochondria contain tubular cristae. Both features indicate a cell type engaged in the synthesis of steroid. (TEM, ×3,500.)

Cisternal lumen
of rough
endoplasmic
reticulum

Golgi
complex

Transport
vesicles

Limiting membrane
of secretory
granule

Secretory
granule

Golgi
complex

Transport
vesicles

Fig. 1-15. A portion of cytoplasm taken from a cell of the duodenal glands. This cell is actively involved in the synthesis and secretion of glycoprotein. Note the amorphous material (protein) within the cisternal lumen of the granular endoplasmic reticulum. The protein is transported to the Golgi complex, where it is complexed to carbohydrate. The formed glycoprotein is then "packaged" by surrounding Golgi membranes to form a secretory granule. (TEM, ×37,500.)

Nucleolus

Nucleus

Heterophagic vacuole

Mitochondria

Fig. 1-16. A macrophage from a human spleen that has phagocytosed foreign material. (TEM, ×2,500.)

Nucleus

Secondary lysosome

Golgi complex

Plasmalemma

Primary lysosomes

Fig. 1-17. A portion of a human gastric lining epithelial cell that contains five large secondary lysosomes. (TEM, ×12,000.)

Multivesicular body

Rough endoplasmic reticulum

Polyribosomes

Nucleus

Plasmalemma

Microtubules

Nuclear envelope

Fig. 1-18. A portion of a cell from the collecting tubule of a kidney illustrates several organelles. (TEM, ×12,000.)

Granular endoplasmic reticulum

Peroxisomes

Mitochondrion

Nucleus

Glycogen

Fig. 1-19. A region of hepatocyte cytoplasm that illustrates several organelles. (TEM, ×10,000.)

Fig. 1-20. The cytoplasm of two adjacent human intestinal epithelial cells. Note the abundance of mitochondria and the profiles of smooth endoplasmic reticulum. (TEM, ×10,000.)

Fig. 1-21. A region of cytoplasm taken from an immature ductal cell of a human submandibular gland. (TEM, ×50,000.)

Disrupted multivesicular body

Centriole

Polyribosomes

Centriole

Fig. 1-22. Centrioles form a submandibular gland ductal cell (A) and a human fibroblast (B) are shown in both longitudinal and cross-sectional profiles, respectively. (A. TEM, ×48,000. B. TEM, ×51,000.)

Annulate
lamellae

Fig. 1-23. An annulate lamella taken from a differentiating germ cell. (TEM, × 15,000.)

Heterochromatin

Granular endoplasmic reticulum

Nucleolus

Euchromatin

Plasmalemma

Secretory granules

Fig. 1-24. The apical region of a human pancreatic acinar cell illustrates numerous secretory granules, in addition to other organelles. (TEM, ×8,000.)

Granular endoplasmic reticulum

Mitochondria

Nucleus

Peroxisome

Lipid

Peroxisome

Glycogen

Fig. 1-25. The cytoplasm of two adjacent hepatocytes contains two inclusions: lipid droplets and glycogen. (TEM, ×15,000.)

Fig. 1-26. Crystalline inclusions of a proteinaceous nature shown in the cytoplasm of an intestinal epithelial cell. (TEM, × 15,000.)

Fig. 1-27. A region of cytoplasm (intestinal epithelial cell) illustrating parallel cisternae of granular endoplasmic reticulum, polyribosomes, a mitochondrion, and the plasmalemma at the lower right. (TEM, ×20,000.)

Fig. 1-28. A freeze-fracture replica of a human odontoblast that illustrates the nuclear envelope. Note the even distribution of nuclear pores. (×18,500.)

Fig. 1-29. A tangential section through the nucleus of a cell from the duodenal glands illustrates several nuclear pores. (TEM, ×11,000.)

Mitosis

Chromosomes

Plasmalemma

Fig. 1-30. A dividing cell taken from liver shows several distinct chromosomes. (TEM, ×5,000.)

Mitosis (Whitefish)

Fig. 1-31 to 1-33. Cells in division from a whitefish embryo. In addition to the different stages of mitosis shown, the chromosomes and spindle fibers can also be visualized with the light microscope.

Fig. 1-31. A. Prophase. (LM, ×400.) B. Metaphase. (LM, ×400.)

Fig. 1-32. A. Anaphase. (LM, ×400.) B. Anaphase. (LM, ×400.)

Fig. 1-33. A. Telophase. (LM, ×400.) B. Telophase. (LM, ×400.)

Review Questions & Answers

Questions

1. How do organelles differ from inclusions?
2. In what ways do mitochondria differ from other membrane-bound organelles?
3. Briefly discuss the role of the cytoplasmic microtubules.
4. What is a unit membrane? List structures bounded by a unit membrane.
5. What functions do mitochondria serve?
6. Trace the synthetic pathway of a glycoprotein.
7. Describe the cytoplasmic events that occur during mitosis. What is achieved by mitotic division?
7A. Identify the organelles shown in atlas figure 1-27.

Answers

1. Organelles are specialized, dynamic cellular units that perform specific roles in the functional activities, survival, and reproduction of cells; they constitute a part of the living substance of a cell. Inclusions, on the other hand, can be regarded as nonliving components. They make no contribution to the economy of the cell in which they are found and generally are either the end product of activities carried out by the organelles or foreign materials taken into the cell.

2. Mitochondria differ in several respects from other cell organelles. They are limited by two distinct membranes (each of which represents a unit membrane). They are capable of self-replication by fusion and contain their own complement of DNA. The mitochondrial DNA is unusual in that it has a circular rather than a linear (helical) arrangement. Although centrioles also are self-replicating organelles, they are not membrane-bound.

3. Microtubules are involved in the formation of the mitotic spindle, contribute to the cytoskeleton of the cell, and may be involved in the transport of materials from one part of a cell to another. They constitute the structural elements of centrioles, flagella, cilia, and ciliary basal bodies and have been implicated in the physical movement of cells.

4. The unit membrane is a trilaminar structure representative of all biological membranes. Morphologically it appears as two dense lines separated by a clear line, reflecting the molecular configuration of a phospholipid-lipid bilayer in which the hydrocarbon chains are directed inward and the polar groups outward. Although all the membranous structures of the cell have the configuration of the unit membrane, they vary in their enzymatic properties and functional activities in different locations. Structures bounded by unit membranes include the cell itself (the plasmalemma), the nucleus, mitochondria, lysosomes, peroxisomes, transport vesicles, and secretion granules. Unit membranes enclose the tubules and cisternae of the smooth and granular endoplasmic reticulum and form the Golgi saccules. Pinocytotic vesicles and phagocytic vacuoles also are bounded by unit membranes. The only organelles not enclosed by unit membranes are ribosomes, centrioles, filaments, and microtubules.

5. Mitochondria have been called the "power house" of the cell since ultimately, they provide the energy required for the metabolic activity of the cell. The enzymes of Krebs citric acid cycle, responsible for the oxidation of pyruvate to carbon dioxide and water, are present in the mitochondrial matrix. The energy released by this oxidation is accepted by the electron transfer system of cytochromes, which are capable of fixing the energy in the

high-energy bonds of ATP. The enzymes of this system are located in mitochondria either in the elementary particles or in the membranes that form the cristae. Mitochondria also contain several enzymes that implicate them in the synthesis of steroid hormones. Enzymes involved in protein and lipid synthesis also occur in the mitochondria.

6. Synthesis of the protein moiety of glycoprotein occurs on the ribosomes that are attached to granular endoplasmic reticulum. However, the ribosomes are inactive until they become associated with messenger RNA produced in the nucleus. The messenger RNA transmits the instructions for protein synthesis (encoded in the DNA of the nucleus) to the ribosomes, where it dictates the order in which amino acids are to be incorporated. The amino acids are transported to the ribosomes on yet another form of RNA, the transfer RNA, there being a specific transfer RNA for each amino acid. The ribosomes assemble the amino acids into the polypeptide chain and release it into the cisternae of the granular endoplasmic reticulum. The peptides are transported to the Golgi complex in small transport vesicles, the membranes of which are contributed by the endoplasmic reticulum. The protein material passes through the stacks of Golgi saccules, entering at the forming face and leaving at the maturing face. During passage through the Golgi, the protein is conjugated to carbohydrate synthesized by the Golgi. The newly formed glycoprotein is condensed and packaged into condensing vacuoles, which develop as the Golgi saccules at the maturing face bud off to form small vesicles that contain the glycoprotein product. The material is further condensed and the vacuoles eventually mature into secretory granules.

7. The nuclear changes taking place during mitosis are so dramatic and visible that the importance of the cytoplasmic events tends to be overlooked. As a cell enters mitosis it appears to round up and the cytoplasm becomes clear and less viscous. During prophase the centrioles replicate and the resulting pairs migrate to the opposite poles. The nuclear envelope breaks down and by the end of prophase has disappeared. The cytoplasm at metaphase is characterized by the appearance of numerous microtubules that form the mitotic spindle. Some of the spindle fibers extend from pole to pole as the continuous fibers; others extend from one pole to the centromere (kinetochore) of a chromosome as the chromosomal fibers. The microtubules of the spindle may contribute to the movement of chromosomes from the equatorial plate to the opposite poles of the dividing cells.

After the daughter chromosomes have completed their migration, discontinuous segments of the nuclear envelope begin to form from surrounding segments of the granular endoplasmic reticulum. The nuclear envelope becomes complete following the reappearance of nucleoli in the daughter nuclei. Simultaneous with these events, a cleavage furrow develops midway between the daughter nuclei as a result of an invagination (contraction) of the plasmalemma. The contraction continues until the daughter nuclei are united only by a slender cytoplasmic bridge that contains numerous spindle microtubules; ameboid movement also aids in separating the daughter cells. Before the appearance of the cleavage furrow, mitochondria migrate in nearly equal numbers to the opposite poles of the dividing cells, and they and the remainder of the cytoplasmic organelles are partitioned nearly equally between the two daughter cells.

Immediately following cytokinesis, the mitochondria replicate by fission to restore their numbers to that of the parent cell. The centrioles, also self-replicating organelles, duplicate in the period following cytoplasmic division. The daughter cells enter a period of metabolic activity following their separation, during which time the endoplasmic reticulum, Golgi membranes, and other organelles are restored to the concentrations found in the parent cell.

The end result of mitosis is the provision of two daughter cells, each with the identical genetic makeup of the parent cell and each with a complement of organelles necessary to carry out the normal cell activities and functions.

7A. Plasmalemma, mytochondrium, polyribosomes, and granular endoplasmic reticulum.

2 Epithelium

Epithelium is one of the four basic tissues, the others being connective, muscle, and nerve tissue. A basic tissue is a collection of cells of similar type that, together with their associated extracellular substances, are specialized to perform a common function or functions. Each basic tissue is present, in variable amounts, in the organs that collectively make up the entire organism.

The various epithelia consist of closely aggregated cells with only minimal amounts of intervening intercellular substances.

Structural Organization

KEY WORDS: sheet, basal lamina, lamina lucida, lamina densa, basement membrane, avascular, gland

The cells of an epithelium form **sheets** that cover the external surfaces of an organism and line the digestive, respiratory, cardiovascular, and urogenital tracts. Thus, substances that enter or leave the body must pass through an epithelial layer. Cells within an epithelial sheet are bound firmly together and resist forces that tend to separate them. The space between the membranes of adjacent epithelial cells is narrow (about 20 nm) and contains fibronectin and a small amount of proteoglycan that is rich in cations, chiefly calcium. Glycoproteins associated with the cell surface are integral membrane proteins that act as specialized adhesion molecules that aid in holding adjacent epithelial cell membranes in close opposition (see atlas figure 2-4).

Epithelial cells rest on a **basal lamina** that separates the epithelium from underlying connective tissue (see atlas figures 2-21 and 2-24). It consists of an electron-lucid **lamina lucida** immediately adjacent to the epithelium and a denser layer, the **lamina densa,** next to the connective tissue. The basal lamina, a product of the epithelial cells, consists of the glycoprotein laminin, a proteoglycan rich in heparan sulfate and type IV collagen. It is reinforced on the connective tissue side by a layer of reticular fibers embedded in proteoglycan. The basal lamina provides support and a surface for the attachment of the overlying epithelium. The basal lamina and the interface of the underlying connective tissue (reticular lamina) together make up the epithelial **basement membrane** that is visible with the light microscope (see atlas figure 2-7).

With rare exceptions, epithelium is **avascular** and depends on diffusion of substances across the basement membrane for its nutrition. Epithelial cells also occur in groups to form **glands** specialized for the secretion of various substances.

Classification of Epithelia

KEY WORDS: simple epithelium, stratified epithelium, squamous, cuboidal, columnar

The lining and covering forms of epithelium may consist of a single layer of cells, forming a **simple epithelium,** or multiple layers of cells may be present to form a **stratified epithelium.** The epithelial cells themselves can be divided into three types according to their shapes: **squamous** (thin, platelike cells), **cuboidal** (cells in which the height and width are approximately equal), and **columnar** (cells in which the height is greater than the width). Cells intermediate in height between cuboidal and columnar do occur and frequently are referred to as low columnar.

Simple Epithelia

KEY WORDS: simple squamous, simple cuboidal, simple columnar, pseudostratified columnar, apical surface, basal surface, lateral surface, polarity, mesothelium, endothelium

Epithelium consisting of a single layer of cells can be classified as **simple squamous, simple cuboidal,** or **simple columnar,** depending on the shape of the constituent cells (see atlas figures 2-4 through 2-8). A fourth type of simple epithelium, **pseudostratified columnar,** is composed of more than one type of cell whose nuclei are at different levels, falsely suggesting that the epithelium is made up of two or more layers (see atlas figure 2-9). While all the cells in this type of epithelium are in contact with the basement membrane, not all extend to the surface.

The surfaces of cells within an epithelial sheet show different orientations. The **apical surface** is free, the opposite or **basal surface** is directed toward the underlying connective tissue, and the **lateral surfaces** face adjacent epithelial cells. Differences in the orientation of the plasmalemma (i.e., apical, basal, or lateral) may be associated with differences in cell function and morphology. Organelles, including the nucleus, frequently take up preferred locations in the cell, in which case the cell is said to show **polarity.** An epithelial cell may be polarized apically, basally, or laterally with respect to the distribution of its organelles, depending on the functional status of the cell.

The term **mesothelium** is the special name given to the simple squamous epithelia that form the serous membranes of the pleura, pericardium, and peritoneum (see atlas figure 2-4). A specific name, **endothelium,** is given to the simple squamous epithelium that lines the cardiovascular and lymph vascular systems.

Stratified Epithelia

KEY WORDS: stratified squamous, stratified cuboidal, stratified columnar, keratinized stratified squamous, nonkeratinized stratified squamous, transitional epithelium, germinal epithelium

Stratified epithelia are classified according to the shape of the superficial (surface) cells, regardless of the shapes of the cells in the deeper layers. Except for those in the basal layer, cells of stratified epithelia are not in contact with the basement membrane, and only the most superficial cells have a free surface. In the thicker stratified types, the deeper cells often are irregular in shape. The types of stratified epithelia are **stratified squamous, stratified cuboidal,** and **stratified columnar.**

In regions where the surface is dry or subject to mechanical abrasion, the outer layers of cells may be transformed into a nonliving substance called keratin. Keratin is an especially tough protein that is resistant to mechanical injury and is relatively impervious to bacterial invasion or water loss. This type of stratified epithelium is referred to as **keratinized stratified squamous** epithelium (see atlas figure 2-11). The keratinized layer of cells at the surface is constantly being shed and replaced. In other regions the stratified squamous type of epithelium is moist, and recognizable, intact cells rather than flat, keratin-filled cells are sloughed from the surface. This type of epithelium is called a wet or **non-keratinized stratified squamous** epithelium (see atlas figure 2-10).

Transitional and germinal epithelia are not classified according to the cells of the surface layer. **Transitional epithelium** (uroepithelium) is restricted to the lining of the urinary passages and extends from the minor calyces of the kidneys to the urethra. Its appearance varies considerably, depending on the degree of distention to which it is subjected. The superficial cells of a nondistended organ appear rounded or dome-shaped and often show a free convex border that bulges into the lumen (see atlas figure 2-12). In the distended organ, the superficial cells may vary in shape from squamous to cuboidal. **Germinal epithelium** in the seminiferous tubules of the testes is a complex, stratified epithelium that consists of supporting cells and spermatogenic cells.

A classification of epithelia and the locations where each type can be found is presented in Table 2-1.

Cell Attachments

In addition to the intercellular matrix, several attachment points or junctions occur between neighboring epithelial cells and are thought to aid in holding adjacent cell membranes close to-

gether. They also serve as anchoring sites for the intermediate filaments of the cytoskeleton, which assists in stabilizing the cell shape.

Junctional Complexes

KEY WORDS: **terminal bar, zonula occludens (tight junction), zonula adherens, macula adherens (demosome), plaque, tonofilament, punctum adherens, hemidesmosome**

Terminal bars occur along the apical, lateral interfaces of most simple cuboidal and columnar epithelial cells that border on luminal surfaces. They are visible under the light microscope as short, dense lines. In electron micrographs a terminal bar is seen to form an area of specialization

Table 2-1. Classification of Epithelia

Type of epithelium	Location	Specialization
Simple squamous	Endothelium, mesothelium, parietal layer of Bowman's capsule, thin segment of loop of Henle, rete testis, pulmonary alveoli	
Simple cuboidal	Thyroid, choroid plexus, ducts of many glands, inner surface of the capsule of the lens, covering surface of ovary	
Simple columnar	Surface epithelium of stomach	
	Small and large intestine	Striated border
	Proximal convoluted tubule of kidney	Brush border
	Distal convoluted tubule of kidney	Basal striations
	Gallbladder, excretory ducts of glands	
	Uterus, oviducts	Cilia
	Small bronchi of lungs	Cilia
	Some paranasal sinuses	Cilia
Pseudostratified columnar	Large excretory ducts of glands, portions of male urethra	
	Epididymis	Sterocilia
	Trachea, bronchi	Cilia
	Eustachian tube	Cilia
	Portions of tympanic cavity	Cilia
Stratified squamous	Buccal surface, esophagus, epiglottis, conjunctiva, cornea, vagina	
	Epidermis of skin	Keratin
	Gingiva, hard palate	Keratin
Stratified cuboidal	Ducts of sweat glands	
Stratified columnar	Cavernous urethra, fornix of conjunctiva, large excretory ducts of glands	
Transitional	Urinary system; renal calyces to urethra	
Germinal	Seminiferous tubules of adult testes	

called the junctional complex, which consists of three distinct regions (see atlas figure 2-22). Near the free surface, the external laminae of adjacent plasma membranes fuse and the intercellular space is obliterated. This region is the **zonula occludens (tight junction),** an area of specialization that forms a zone or belt around the perimeter of each cell to create an occluding seal between the apices of adjacent epithelial cells. Materials that pass through the epithelial sheet must cross the plasma membranes and cannot pass between cells through the intercellular spaces. The zonula occludens junction is important in separating apical from basolateral cell membrane domains by preventing the lateral migration of specialized membrane proteins (e.g., receptors, transport proteins) in the plasmalemma. In most cases, membrane proteins in the apical plasmalemma function quite differently from those occupying the basolateral regions. Tight junctions also have been reported in simple squamous epithelia and in the superficial layers of stratified squamous epithelia.

The second part of the junctional complex, the **zonula adherens,** also forms an adhering belt or zone that surrounds the apex of an epithelial cell, immediately below the zonula occludens. Adjacent plasma membranes are separated by an intercellular space 15 to 20 nm wide, and in this region plaques along the internal laminae of the plasma membranes often are associated with an actin filament network. The plaques contain α-actinin and vinculin, two actin-binding proteins. Actin is linked to a transmembrane glycoprotein (calherin) that holds cells together in this region in the presence of calcium ions.

The third element of the junction is the **macula adherens,** also called the **desmosome.** These small, elliptical discs form spotlike points of attachment between cells that function to link the intermediate filament network of adjacent cells. The internal laminae of the adjacent plasma membranes appear dense and thick due to the presence of an amorphous material called a **plaque.** Intermediate filaments (usually cytokeratins) extend into the plaque, where they appear to form hairpin loops. A thin, moderately dense

lamina often is seen in the intercellular space of each desmosome. These are thought to contain transmembrane linking proteins (desmogleins) that hold adjacent cell membranes in close apposition. Desmosomes are scattered along epithelial surfaces and are not restricted to regions of tight junctions (see atlas figures 2-23 and 2-24). They are especially abundant in stratified squamous epithelia, where they are associated with numerous **tonofilaments** — intermediate filaments of the keratin type. Desmosome-like junctions that lack attachment plaques and associated tonofilaments also occur between epithelial cells. This type of cell junction has been called a **punctum adherens.**

The basal plasma membrane, although not immediately adjacent to another cell, also shows an attachment, the **hemidesmosome,** which closely resembles one-half of a desmosome. Hemidesmosomes act as points of adhesion between the basal plasma membrane and the underlying basal lamina and link the intermediate filament network of the epithelial cells to the extracellular matrix via transmembrane anchoring proteins (see atlas figure 2-24). The integrity of desmosomes and hemidesmosomes appears to depend on the presence of calcium ions. Heparan sulfate–rich proteoglycans in the basal lamina give its surface a strong ionic charge that, acting with calcium ions, aids in attaching the epithelium to the basal lamina. Fibronectin on the connective tissue surface of the basal lamina binds it to the underlying connective tissue.

Nexus Junction

KEY WORDS: **nexus (gap junction), connexon, connexin, communicating junction**

The **nexus** or **gap junction,** like tight junctions and desmosomes, forms a relatively firm point of attachment between adjacent cells (see atlas figures 2-25 and 2-26). At a nexus, the plasma membranes are separated by a gap 2 nm wide that is bridged by particles 8 nm in diameter. These particles, the **connexons,** mainly consist of the protein **connexin.** Connexon units are thought to extend through the plasmalemma and cross the intercellular gap to join a corresponding unit from the opposing cell membrane. A hydrophilic channel within the center of each connexon permits intercellular passage of ions, amino acids, and nucleotides. The nexus also provides an avenue whereby cyclic adenosine monophosphate (AMP), released by one cell, can pass to adjacent cells. Thus, the response of a number of cells to a specific hormonal stimulus can be coordinated. Because nexus junctions seem to act as sites of communication between epithelial cells, they often are called **communication junctions.** Nexus junctions also appear to be capable of changing from low to high resistance and thereby inhibit cell communication.

Adjacent lateral cell membranes often do not run parallel to one another but show numerous interdigitations. Such interlocking of cell membranes also is thought to aid in maintaining cell-to-cell adhesion in an epithelial sheet.

Specializations of Epithelial Membranes

The cells in an epithelial sheet often show special adaptations of apical or basal-lateral surfaces that may increase the surface area of the cell, constitute motile "appendages" that move material across the surface, or have receptor functions. The surface specializations include microvilli, cilia, and basal-lateral infoldings.

Microvilli

KEY WORDS: **striated border, brush border, stereocilia**

Microvilli are minute, fingerlike evaginations of the apical plasma membrane that enclose cores of cytoplasm. Scattered microvilli occur on the surfaces of most cells of simple epithelia, but individually they are usually too small to be seen with the light microscope (see atlas figure 2-18). In epithelia such as that lining the small intestine, however, microvilli are so numerous, uniform, and closely packed that they form a **striated border** that is visible by light microscopy (see

atlas figures 2-15 through 2-17). Microvilli also are numerous on the cells of the proximal convoluted tubules of the kidney, where they are somewhat longer and less uniform than those in the small intestine and appear as tufts on the cell apices. Because of this appearance, they are called a **brush border.** Microvilli increase the surface area enormously, thereby enhancing the absorptive capacity of epithelial cells.

Epithelial cells that line the epididymis show unusually long, slender, branching microvilli that have been called **stereocilia** (see atlas figure 2-20). However, stereocilia are not cilia but are true microvilli and also serve to increase the surface area of a cell.

Cilia

KEY WORDS: **microtubule, doublet, central pair, (9 + 2), dynein, basal body, triplet, (9 + 0), ciliated simple columnar epithelium, ciliated pseudostratified columnar epithelium**

Like microvilli, cilia represent appendages of the apical cell membrane but are relatively large and often are motile. They may be single or occur in large numbers and are seen readily with the light microscope (see atlas figure 2-9). The limiting plasmalemma of the cilium is continuous with that of the cell and encloses a core of cytoplasm containing 20 **microtubules.** Nine pairs of fused microtubules, the **doublets,** form a ring at the periphery of the cilium and surround a **central pair** of individual microtubules (see atlas figures 2-14 and 2-19). This arrangement has been called the **(9 + 2)** configuration (Fig. 2-1). Within each doublet, the microtubules are named the A and B microtubules. Microtubule A has two short, divergent arms that project toward tubule B of the adjacent doublet. The arms consist of the protein **dynein,** which has activity like adenosinetriphosphatase (ATPase). Radial spokes project from the doublets to the central air of microtubules.

The microtubules of a cilium originate from a **basal body** in the apical cytoplasm of the cell (see atlas figure 2-14). The basal body is similar in structure to the centriole and appears as a hollow

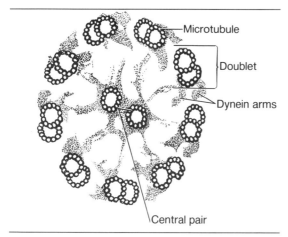

Labels on figure: Microtubule, Doublet, Dynein arms, Central pair

Fig. 2-1. Diagrammatic representation of a cilium in cross section.

cylinder, the wall of which consists of nine **triplet** microtubules. Since there are no central microtubules in a basal body, the arrangement of microtubules is expressed as **(9+0).** Each of the nine doublets in the cilium is continuous with the two innermost microtubules of the triplets in the basal body. The two central microtubules of the ciliary shaft terminate as they reach the basal body and do not join with it. Ciliary motion is thought to involve a sliding tubule mechanism, dependent on the ability of the dynein protein to generate energy through its ATPase-like activity.

Cilia are numerous on epithelial cells that line much of the respiratory tract and parts of the female reproductive tract (see atlas figure 2-13). Groups of cilia beat in a coordinated, rhythmic fashion to move a thin layer of fluid in one direction across the epithelial surface. In regions such as the distal tubules of the kidney, where each cell bears a single cilium, or in the olfactory epithelium, where they occur in small groups on cells, the cilia are nonmotile and are believed to act as chemoreceptors. Cilia also are found in the maculae and cristae of the inner ear and act as mechanoreceptors. The most extreme modification of cilia is seen in the formation of the outer segments of the rods and cones of the retina, where the modified cilia serve as photoreceptors.

The presence of cilia contributes to the classification of epithelia. Where cilia are present on simple columnar epithelial cells, as in the oviduct, the epithelium is called a **ciliated simple columnar epithelium.** When cilia are associated with pseudostratified epithelium, as in the trachea, the epithelium forms a **ciliated pseudostratified columnar epithelium.**

Basal Lateral Infoldings

KEY WORDS: basal-lateral plasmalemma, fluid transport, basal striations

In addition to the apical specializations, some epithelial cells show elaborate infoldings of the **basal-lateral plasmalemma** (see atlas figure 2-21). These are called basal-lateral infoldings and usually are prominent in epithelia active in **fluid transport,** such as in the proximal and distal convoluted tubules of the kidneys and in some ducts of salivary glands. Like microvilli, they greatly increase the surface area of the cell membrane. Mitochondria, which often are numerous in this area of the cell, tend to lie parallel to the infoldings of the plasma membrane. Because of this association, the infoldings are visible with the light microscope and appear as **basal striations.**

Glandular Epithelium

In addition to performing functions such as protection and absorption, the cells of an epithelial sheet may secrete materials also. Epithelial cells adapted specifically for secretion constitute the glands.

Classification of Glands

KEY WORDS: unicellular, multicellular, exocrine, endocrine, type and mode of secretion

Glands can be classified according to their histologic organization, possession of ducts, type of material secreted, and manner in which material is secreted. Glands that consist of only a single cell are called **unicellular;** aggregates of secreting cells form **multicellular** glands. The latter can be divided into **exocrine** and **endocrine** types according to whether or not they secrete onto a surface. Exocrine glands can be subdivided on the basis of the branching of their ducts, the configuration of the secretory end piece, and the **type and mode of secretion.** A classification of glands is shown in Table 2-2.

Unicellular Glands

KEY WORDS: goblet cell, mucin, mucus

The classic example of a unicellular gland is the **goblet cell,** found scattered among columnar epithelial cells as in the trachea, small intestine, and colon (see atlas figures 2-27 and 2-29). The cell has a narrow base and an expanded apex filled with secretory droplets. Goblet cells elaborate **mucin,** which, on hydration, produces a viscous lubricating fluid called **mucus.** Hence, a goblet cell can be classified as a unicellular, exocrine gland. Unicellular, endocrine cells (glands) also occur.

Table 2-2. Classification of Glands

Type	Example
Unicellular glands	
Exocrine	Goblet cells
Endocrine	Gastrin-cell and other endocrine cells of the gastrointestinal mucosa
Multicellular exocrine glands	
Secretory sheet	Surface epithelium of gastric mucosa
Intraepithelial glands	Urethral (Littre's) glands
Simple tubular glands	Intestinal glands
Simple coiled tubular glands	Apocrine sweat glands
Simple branched tubular glands	Esophageal glands
Simple branched acinar glands	Meibomian glands
Compound tubular glands	Glands of gastric cardia
Compound tubuloacinar glands	Pancreas
Compound saccular glands	Prostate

Multicellular Glands

KEY WORDS: secretory sheet, intraepithelial gland

The simplest form of multicellular gland is the **secretory sheet,** exemplified by the gastric lining epithelium, in which the secreting cells form a continuous epithelial layer. **Intraepithelial glands** are small clusters of secretory cells that lie wholly within an epithelial sheet, clustered about a small lumen.

Exocrine Glands

KEY WORDS: compound, simple, tubule, acinus, alveolus, saccule

Exocrine glands secrete onto an epithelial surface either directly, as in secretory sheets and intraepithelial glands, or by a ductal system. If the duct branches the gland is said to be **compound;** if it does not branch, the gland is **simple** (Fig. 2-2).

The secretory cells may form **tubules, acini, alveolae,** (berrylike end pieces), or saccules (dilated, flasklike end pieces). Simple and compound glands can be named from the shape of the secretory portion. Thus, simple glands can be classed as simple tubular, simple coiled tubular, simple branched tubular, or simple branched acinar (see atlas figures 2-29 through 2-32). Similarly, compound glands are subdivided into compound tubular, compound saccular, and compound tubuloacinar (tubuloalveolar) (see atlas figures 2-33 through 2-35). The initial subdivision into simple and compound is made according to whether or not the ducts branch. Subsequent classification depends on the shape and configuration of the secreting portion.

Endocrine Glands

KEY WORDS: lack ducts, hormone

Like exocrine glands, the endocrine glands arise from an epithelial sheet, but during their formation, endocrine glands lose their connections with the surface and thus **lack ducts** (Fig. 2-3). Cells of endocrine glands secrete regulatory material — **hormones** — directly into the bloodstream, lymphatics, or intercellular spaces

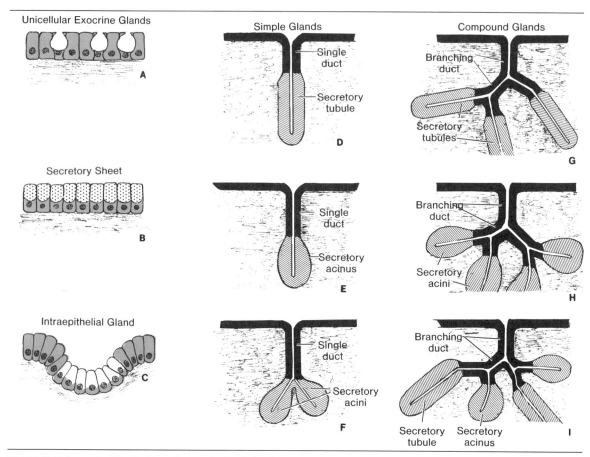

Fig. 2-2. Schematic illustration of several glandular forms. *A.* Unicellular glands. *B.* Secretory sheet. *C.* Intraepithelial gland. *D.* Simple tubular gland. *E.* Simple acinar gland. *F.* Simple branched gland. *G.* Compound tubular gland. *H.* Compound acinar gland. *I.* Compound tubuloacinar gland.

(paracrine and/or autocrine secretion). Scattered, solitary endocrine cells occur in the gastrointestinal tract and along the conducting portion of the respiratory tract (see atlas figure 2-28).

The structure of the large endocrine glands is so diverse that the organs do not readily lend themselves to histologic classification. However, some overall structural patterns can be made out, and the cells may be arranged as clumps, cords, or hollow spheroidal structures called follicles.

Type and Mode of Secretion

KEY WORDS: mucous, serous, mixed gland, merocrine, holocrine

Glands can be classified as mucous, serous, or mixed according to the type of material secreted. Cells of **mucous** glands have pale, vacuolated cytoplasm and flattened, dense nuclei oriented toward the base of the cell (see atlas figures 2-34 and 2-35). **Serous** cells show spheroidal nuclei

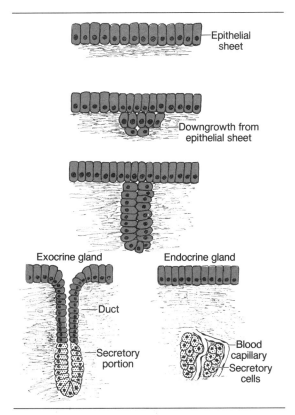

Fig. 2-3. Formation of exocrine and endocrine glands. All glands form as an invagination from an epithelial sheet. Glands that retain a connection (duct) to the epithelial sheet of origin are classed as exocrine glands. Those that lose their connection are called endocrine glands and secrete into the blood vasculature.

surrounded by a basophilic cytoplasm that contains discrete secretory granules. **Mixed glands** contain variable proportions of serous and mucous cells (see atlas figure 2-35).

From the mode of secretion, two types of glands can be distinguished. **Merocrine** secretion refers to release of the product through fusion of secretory vesicles with the apical plasmalemma (see atlas figures 2-37 and 2-38). This is the process identified as exocytosis by electron microscopy, and most exocrine secretion is of this type. **Holocrine** secretion involves release of whole cells (such as sperm from the testes) or the breakdown of an entire cell to form the secretion (e.g., sebum in sebaceous glands). A third type of secretion, apocrine, has been described in which a portion of the apical cytoplasm was said to be lost along with the secretory material. Electron microscopy has failed to support this mode of secretion except perhaps for the mammary glands. Even here, however, the existence of an apocrine secretion is dubious.

Myoepithelial Cells

The secretory units of some glands are associated with myoepithelial cells, which are specialized cells located between the glandular cells and the basal lamina (see atlas figure 2-36). The cells are contractile and their cytoplasm contains numerous actin filaments. Long cytoplasmic processes extend from the body of the cell to course around the secretory unit. The processes, by their contraction, aid in expressing products from the secretory units into the ductal system. Myoepithelial cells occur in sweat, mammary and salivary glands, and glands along the bronchi and esophagus.

Development of Epithelium

Epithelium can arise from ectoderm, endoderm, or mesoderm. Sheets of epithelium derived from the germ layers cover the surface of the developing embryo and line the forming body cavities and tubular structures. Glands form as outpockets of epithelial sheets from which ductal systems and secretory units develop as the epithelial outgrowth expands. If ductal connections are maintained with the epithelial sheet of origin, an exocrine gland is formed. If the connection is lost, an endocrine gland may result (see Fig. 2-3). A summary of epithelial origins is shown in Table 2-3.

Functional Summary

Epithelium covers the entire body surface and lines the digestive, respiratory, cardiovascular, and urogenital systems. Any substance that enters or leaves the body must pass through an epithelial layer. Epithelia protect the organism from mechanical trauma and invasion by small organisms. They also limit fluid loss from underlying connective tissues and thus aid in preventing dehydration. Other functions they contribute to are absorption, transport of useful materials, and excretion of wastes. In the form of glands, they secrete products such as hormones, which regulate and integrate the activities of many tissues and organs.

Surface specializations — microvilli, stereocilia, and basal-lateral infoldings — provide a greatly increased cell surface for the absorption and transport of materials into or out of the cells. Cilia move materials across the surface of an epithelium. The nonmotile cilia of olfactory epithelia and kidney tubules serve as chemoreceptors, the cilia of the inner ear act as mechanoreceptors, and the modified cilia of retinal rods and cones are involved in photoreception.

The junctions between adjacent epithelial cells hold the cells together to form a continuous sheet. Desmosomes help maintain these cell-to-cell adhesions and also act as sites where tonofilaments of the cytoskeleton are anchored. The zonula occludens provides a tight seal between cells so that material crossing an epithelium must pass through the cell membrane and not through intercellular spaces between cells. Thus, the ultimate barrier between the external world and the interior of the body is the plasmalemma. Nexus junctions provide an avenue for intercellular communication and exchange of materials and coordinate responses to stimuli throughout a mass of cells.

All epithelia lie on a basal lamina that provides physical support and serves as a surface for attachment and migration of cells. It also acts as a barrier for some molecules, depending on their size, charge, and shape, and plays an important inductive role in differentiation. It is important in repair processes after injury.

Clinical Correlations

Healing of small surface wounds, whether caused by trauma, infection, or toxins, occurs quickly if the basement membrane beneath the epithelium is not destroyed and if the damaged epithelium is capable of regeneration. Initially there is little mitotic activity, and epithelial continuity is restored by migration of cells from the surrounding epithelium. Guided by the persisting basement membrane, the migrating cells flatten and spread over the denuded area to form a cover. Later, cells at the margins of the lesion divide to provide new cells that rapidly fill the gap. Once the area is covered, the epithelial cells assume their normal morphology. More extensive wounds that destroy the basement membrane and penetrate underlying connective tissue heal more slowly, and

much of the defect is filled by connective tissue, forming a scar. Depending on the size of the area involved, the scar may be covered by new epithelium and a resynthesized basement membrane.

Damage to desmosomes by a combination of antibodies and complement acting on intercellular material occurs in pemphigus. Cell junctions in the skin and mucous membranes disappear, resulting in formation of large intraepithelial blisters.

Uncoordinated or an absence of ciliary beating can occur in ciliated epithelium, a condition referred to as immotile ciliary syndrome. The structurally abnormal cilia are the result of a genetic defect. Infertility and failure of mucus clearance from the lungs are common conditions associated with this syndrome.

Epithelial tumors are by far the most common

Table 2-3. Epithelial Derivatives

Epithelial sheets

Ectoderm	Epidermis; corneal covering; lining of nasal cavities, nasal sinuses, mouth, and anal canal; nails, hair
Endoderm	Covering of posterior one-third of tongue; lining of pharynx, Eustachian tube, larynx, trachea, lungs, gastrointestinal tract, urinary bladder, urethra
Mesoderm	Lining of blood vessels, lymphatics, body cavities; joint cavities, ureter, genital ducts

Glands

Ectoderm	Sweat, sebaceous, mammary, salivary glands; adenohypophysis
Endoderm	Thymus, thyroid, parathyroids; esophageal, duodenal, and intestinal glands; pancreas, liver
Mesoderm	Kidneys, gonads, adrenal cortex

tumor type, possibly because epithelia occur as surface coverings through which everything must pass to enter the body. Consequently, epithelia have greater exposure to carcinogens. Certain characteristics of epithelia — their tendency to form sheets or groups of cells with little intervening intercellular substance, the lack of blood supply, and the need for a stroma of connective tissue to supply nourishment and support — are seen in its tumors also. Adherence of cells in small or large groups indicates an epithelial origin, even in tumors that have lost all other distinctive features of the tissue or organ in which they arose.

The organization of an epithelium also affects the structure of its tumors, especially in the slow-growing, well-differentiated, benign tumors. Surface epithelia usually give rise to papillomata, irregular, branching, frondlike masses in which each frond contains a core of connective tissue. The epithelial covering corresponds to the type of epithelium from which the tumor arose. Papillomata arising in stratified squamous epithelium (e.g., skin) are covered with stratified squamous epithelium; those arising in transitional epithelium (urinary tract tumors) are covered by transitional epithelium. Columnar epithelia also can give rise to papillomas, as in the large intestine, but the picture may be complicated by the relationship to glands.

The epithelia of glands, exocrine or endocrine, give rise to adenomata. Those arising from exocrine glands vary in the details of their structure but tend to follow a common plan. As the tumor cells multiply, they form small clusters into the centers of which the cells secrete, thus forming a lumen surrounded by one or two layers of tumor cells. These secreting units (tumor acini) have no ductal connections so the secretions accumulate. With substantial amounts of secretion, the tumor acini become distended and the epithelium stretched. Often the proliferative capacities of the cells are more pronounced than the secretory activities and the acini become more and more solid. While an adenoma may retain a glandular appearance, the epithelium may change to a relatively simple, nondescript or mucus-secreting type and show none of the characteristics associated with the gland of origin.

Benign tumors usually are slow growing and do not invade other tissues or metastasize (seed to distant sites), but they do expand locally and may compress other organs and tissues and mechanically interfere with blood supply, innervation, or function of these organs.

Malignant epithelial tumors are called carcinomas and may arise from preexisting benign tumors or arise directly from nontumorous tissue. They also retain the main features of epithelium and form sheets or masses of cells that are supported by connective tissue. The epithelial element may retain some semblance of the tissue from which the tumor arose but may be poorly organized with only vague resemblances to the tissue of origin. Most malignant tumors exist as squamous cell carcinoma and adenocarcinoma, reflecting malignant tumors of surface epithelia and glands, respectively.

In addition to forming at obvious sites where squamous epithelia exist, squamous carcinomas may arise in organs that normally contain no squamous epithelium, as in the bronchi, urinary tract, and gallbladder, and it is believed that the carcinomas arising in these sites do so in areas of squamous metaplasia. Malignant tumors are characterized by their ability to invade local tissues and replace them and to enter lymphatics and blood vessels to seed remote parts of the body and set up new tumors — that is, to metastasize.

Atlas and Table of Key Features

Key Features in Epithelial Classification

Number of layers	Cell shape	Epithelial classification*
One	Flat, platelike	Simple squamous
One	Cuboidal, height equals width	Simple cuboidal
One	Columnar, height greater than width	Simple columnar
Cells staggered suggest stratification but all in contact with basement membrane	Majority columnar, cuboidal cells present at base	Pseudostratified columnar
Two or more, superficial cells not in contact with basement membrane	Surface layer squamous	Stratified squamous
Two or more, superficial cell not in contact with basement membrane	Surface layer cuboidal	Stratified cuboidal
Two or more, superficial cells not in contact with basement membrane	Surface layer columnar, deep layer(s) cuboidal	Stratified columnar
Multiple	Variable, surface cells, dome-shaped; in distended organs surface cells may be squamous	Transitional
Multiple	Columnar supporting (Sertoli) cells, round (or polyhedral) spermatogenic cells	Germinal (of male).

*Prefixes such as ciliated, keratinized, or non-keratinized may be added to the classification.

Simple Epithelia

Cell
boundary

Nuclei

Collagen
fiber

Fig. 2-4. A portion of mesentery treated with silver nitrate to demonstrate cell boundaries. The intercellular cement has become impregnated with silver. Note the collagen fibers showing through the translucent cytoplasm of the simple squamous mesothelial cells. (LM, ×400.)

Cell
boundary

Nucleus

Fig. 2-5. Simple squamous epithelial cells (periderm) covering the forming skin of an embryo. Note the distinct cell boundaries and nuclear profiles. (SEM, ×400.)

Fig. 2-6. An example of simple cuboidal epithelium taken from a human thyroid. Note that several thyroid follicles lie immediately adjacent to one another. (LM, ×300.)

Fig. 2-7. A region of simple columnar epithelium taken from the lining of a human stomach. Note that the epithelium lies on a distinct basement membrane and that the apical region of each cell is filled with secretory granules. (LM, ×500.)

Epithelium
(columnar)

Capillary
endothelium
(squamous)

Epithelium
(squamous)

Epithelium
(cuboidal)

Fig. 2-8. A region of the medulla from a human kidney illustrates tubules formed by the three types of simple epithelia: squamous, cuboidal, and columnar. (LM, ×250.)

Epithelium

Connective
tissue

Cilia

Nuclei

Fig. 2-9. A demonstration of ciliated pseudostratified columnar epithelium taken from the trachea. Nuclei are found at different levels within this simple epithelium — hence its name. (LM, ×400.)

Stratified Epithelia

Epithelium

Connective
tissue

Nuclei in
surface
cells

Fig. 2-10. An example of non-keratinized stratified squamous epithelium from the lining of the esophagus. Note that the surface cells retain their nuclei. (LM, ×300.)

Epithelium

Keratin

Connective
tissue

Fig. 2-11. Keratinized stratified squamous epithelium taken from the skin covering a human thigh. Note the layer of keratin and that cells forming the surface-most layer have lost their nuclei. (LM, ×250.)

Binucleate cell

Epithelium

Connective tissue

Fig. 2-12. Transitional epithelium lining the urinary bladder is of considerable depth. The surface-most cells often appear dome-shaped in the nondistended condition, and many surface cells are binucleate. (LM, ×300.)

Specializations of Plasmalemma

Microvilli

Cilia

Fig. 2-13. Surface specializations (cilia, microvilli) of the ciliated simple columnar epithelium lining the oviduct. (SEM, ×5,000.)

Fig. 2-14. Surface specializations (cilia, microvilli) as seen cut in longitudinal profile. Note the difference in size and that a basal body gives rise to microtubules within individual cilia. (Sample from the ciliated pseudostratified columnar epithelium lining the trachea.) (TEM, ×20,000.)

Fig. 2-15. The apical plasmalemma of simple columnar epithelial cells lining the small intestine is in the form of a striated (microvillus) border. (LM, ×400.)

Microvilli

Vacuoles

Mitochondrion

Fig. 2-16. The microvillus border of an intestinal lining epithelial cell. Individual microvilli can be visualized. (TEM, ×20,000.)

Fig. 2-17. Surface features of the striated (microvillus) border as seen by scanning electron microscopy. (Intestinal lining epithelial cell.) (×17,000.)

Fig. 2-18. Scattered, small microvilli on mesothelial cells forming the visceral pleura covering the lung. (SEM, ×5,000.)

Fig. 2-19. Cilia and microvilli from epithelial cells lining the trachea as seen in cross section. Compare the diameters and note the central axoneme of microtubules within each cilium. Basal bodies are seen in the apical cell cytoplasm. (TEM, ×4,000. Inset, ×80,000.)

Clump of stereocilia

Branched stereocilium

Fig. 2-20. The apical plasmalemma of cells lining the epididymis is in the form of a branched, elongated microvillus termed a stereocilium. (TEM, ×4,000.)

Nucleus

Mitochondria

Cell membranes

Basal lamina

Fig. 2-21. Basal-lateral infoldings of the cell membrane from a cell within the proximal tubule of the kidney. Note the parallel alignment of associated mitochondria. (TEM, ×2,000.)

Cell Attachments

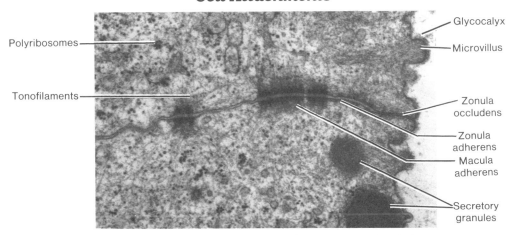

Polyribosomes

Tonofilaments

Glycocalyx

Microvillus

Zonula occludens

Zonula adherens

Macula adherens

Secretory granules

Fig. 2-22. A tripart junctional complex between two gastric lining epithelial cells of a human stomach. This complex is formed by a zonula occludens, a zonula adherens, and a macula adherens. (TEM, ×22,500.)

Desmosomes

Crista

Inner mitochondrial membrane

Outer mitochondrial membrane

Nucleus

Mitochondrion

Fig. 2-23. Desmosomes (maculae adherens) between two adjacent human intestinal epithelial cells. (TEM, ×30,000.)

Ribosomes

Hemidesmosome

Basal lamina

Tonofilaments

Reticular fibers

Desmosomes

Fig. 2-24. Hemidesmosomes along the basal cell membrane of cells from the stratum basale of the epidermis. Note the abundance of tonofilaments (keratin filaments) associated with the hemidesmosomes. (TEM, ×12,000.)

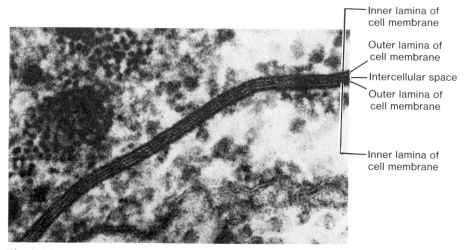

Inner lamina of cell membrane

Outer lamina of cell membrane

Intercellular space

Outer lamina of cell membrane

Inner lamina of cell membrane

Fig. 2-25. Subcomponents of a nexus (gap) junction between two adjacent epithelial cells. (TEM, ×206,000.)

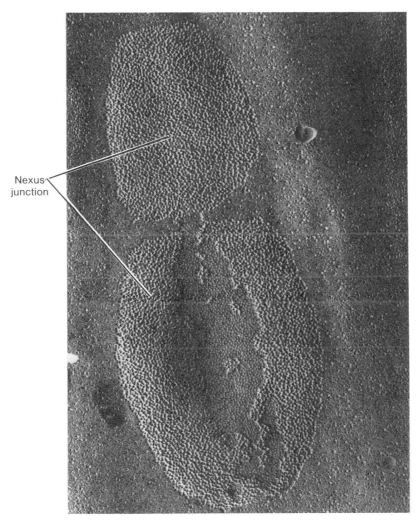

Nexus-
junction

Fig. 2-26. A nexus (gap) junction between adjacent cells as seen
using the freeze-fracture technique. ($\times 80,000$.)

Unicellular Glands

Villus

Goblet
cells

Fig. 2-27. Goblet cells (unicellular exocrine glands) within the intestinal lining epithelium of the duodenum. (LM, ×250.)

Lysosome

Gastrin
(G) cell

Secretory
granules

Fig. 2-28. A gastrin (G) cell from the human stomach is an example of a unicellular endocrine gland. (TEM, ×5,000.)

Multicellular Glands

Villus

Goblet cells

Intestinal gland

Fig. 2-29. Intestinal glands within the mucosa of the human jejunum are simple tubular glands. (LM, ×250.)

Ducts

Secretory tubule

Connective tissue

Fig. 2-30. A sweat gland is a simple coiled tubular gland. (Sample from human skin.) (LM, ×250.)

Secretory tubules

Duct

Diffuse lymphatic tissue

Fig. 2-31. The human duodenal gland shown is an example of a simple branched tubular gland. (LM, ×200.)

Acini

Duct

Fat cells

Fig. 2-32. A meibomian gland from a human eyelid is an example of a simple branched acinar gland. (LM, ×100.)

Intralobular
ducts

Fat cells

Serous
acinus

Fig. 2-33. The parotid is a compound tubuloacinar gland that is serous. (LM, ×100.)

Nuclei

Cross sections
of cells

Connective
tissue

Mucous
tubule

Fig. 2-34. The secretory units of the human esophageal glands consist of mucous cells. (LM, ×300.)

Mucous cells

Serous cells

Serous demilune

Fig. 2-35. The human submandibular gland is a mixed compound tubuloacinar gland. (LM, ×300.)

Capillary

Nucleus of serous cell

Processes of myoepithelial cell

Serous cell

Fig. 2-36. A myoepithelial cell enveloping a serous cell of a bronchial gland in an opossum lung. (TEM, ×4,500.)

Secretory granule fusing with cell membrane

Secretory material

Discharging secretory granule

Fig. 2-37. Exocytosis (merocrine secretion) by a human gastric lining epithelial cell. (TEM, ×5,000.)

Discharging granule

Secretion material

Microvilli

Lumen of gland

Secretory granule in lumen

Zonula occludens

Fig. 2-38. Merocrine secretion by cells comprising secretory units of a human duodenal gland. (TEM, ×25,000.)

Review Questions and Answers

Questions

8. How are sheet or lining epithelia classified?
9. List three specializations of epithelial cell membranes and briefly discuss their functional significance.
10. List three cell attachments and comment on their function.
11. Briefly discuss how exocrine glands may be classified.

Answers

8. The lining or sheet form of epithelia is classified according to the number of layers of cells and the geometric shape of component cells (squamous, cuboidal, columnar). If an epithelia sheet consists of a single layer of cells, it is simple; if more than one layer of cells is present and the superficial cells are not in contact with the basement membrane, the epithelium is termed stratified. In cases where more than one cell type is present and in which not all of the cells reach the surface but all are in contact with the basement membrane, this form of epithelium is termed pseudostratified. The stratified forms of epithelia are classified further by the geometric shape of the most superficial cells (e.g., stratified squamous, stratified columnar). If cells of an epithelial sheet exhibit adaptations or specializations (keratinization, cilia), the specialization is often included in the classification: keratinized or nonkeratinized stratified squamous epithelium; ciliated simple columnar or ciliated pseudostratified columnar epithelium.

9.a. Microvilli are fingerlike evaginations of the apical cell membrane. In regions of high concentration (small intestine, proximal convoluted tubule of the kidney), they form a microvillus border that greatly increases the surface area and absorptive capacity of the cell.

   b. Cilia are large, elongated evaginations of the apical cell membrane that contain two central and nine peripheral pairs of microtubules associated with an underlying basal body. In some regions they are numerous, motile, and beat in a coordinated manner to move a thin fluid film in a single direction (oviduct, trachea). In other locations where they occur singly or in small groups (olfactory epithelium, collecting tubules), cilia may function as chemoreceptors.

   c. Basal-lateral infoldings are elaborate infoldings of the basal and lateral cell membrane found in the proximal and distal tubules of the kidney and the striated ducts of salivary glands. They greatly increase the surface area of the plasmalemma at the base of the cell and are associated with numerous mitochondria. They are observed in regions of high fluid/ion transport.

10.a. The zonula occludens is a fusion of the external laminae of adjacent epithelial cell membranes bordering a lumen. It forms an impermeable seal around the perimeter of each cell, uniting them in an epithelial sheet. The zonula occludens junction also is important in separating apical from basal-lateral cell membrane domains by preventing the migration of specialized membrane proteins (receptors, transport proteins) in the plasmalemma.

   b. A nexus is a firm attachment point between adjacent cells. The intercellular space of this junction measures about 2 nm, and it is here that exchange of ions and small molecules may occur, allowing direct intercellular communication.

   c. The macula adherens (desmosome) acts as a firm attachment point between adjacent-cell membranes and also as an anchoring point for numerous keratin filaments in the cytoplasm.

11. Exocrine glands may be classified as either (1) unicellular or multicellular; (2) by the nature of the duct; simple (unbranched) or compound (branched); (3) by the shape of the secretory unit (acinus, tubule, saccule); (4) by the type of secretory cell (serous, mucous, or, where both are present, a mixed gland); or (5) by the mode of secretion (merocrine, apocrine, holocrine).

3 General Connective Tissue

Connective tissues form a diverse group of tissues derived from mesenchyme and in keeping with the diversity of types, have a number of different functions. They provide structural elements; serve as a foundation for the support of organs; form a packing material for otherwise unoccupied space; provide an insulating layer (fat) that also acts as a storage depot that can be used to provide energy; and play a vital role in the defense mechanisms of the body and in repair after injury. Some are functions of ordinary (general) connective tissues; others are functions of specialized connective tissues. In organs, connective tissues form the *stroma* and epithelial components make up the *parenchyma*.

Organization

KEY WORDS: cell, intercellular substance, fiber, ground substance, matrix

Like all basic tissues, connective tissues are made up of **cells** and **intercellular substances.** The latter consist of **fibers, ground substance,** and tissue fluid. Unlike epithelium, where the cells are closely apposed with little intercellular material, connective tissue cells are widely separated by the intercellular fibers and ground substance that form the bulk of these tissues. Together, the fibers and ground substance form the **matrix.** With some exceptions, connective tissue is generally well vascularized.

Classification

KEY WORDS: extracellular material, general, loose, dense, regular, irregular

Classification of connective tissues into various subgroups is largely descriptive of **extracellular materials** rather than features of the cellular components. Two large categories can be defined — general and special — from which further subdivisions are made. **General** connective tissues are distinguished as loose or dense according to whether the fibers are loosely or tightly packed. **Loose** connective tissues can be subdivided on the basis of some special properties of their constituents, such as adipose (fatty) tissue, reticular tissue, and so forth. **Dense** connective tissues can be divided according to whether the fibers are randomly distributed or show an orderly arrangement. Thus, dense connective tissues are classed as dense **irregular** or dense **regular** connective tissues. A classification of connective tissues is given in Table 3-1.

Loose Connective Tissue

Loose connective tissue is a common and simple form of connective tissue and can be considered the prototype of connective tissue. Essentially, all other types of connective tissues are variants of loose connective tissue in which one or more components have been emphasized to serve specific functions.

Table 3-1. Subdivisions of connective tissue

Type	Locations
General connective tissues	
Loose connective tissue	
Mesenchyme	Primarily in the embryo and developing fetus
Mucoid	Umbilical cord
Areolar	Most organs and tissues
Adipose	Omentum, subcutaneous tissue
Reticular	Lymph nodes, bone marrow
Dense connective tissue	
Irregular	Dermis, capsules of organs, periosteum, perichondrium
Regular	
Collagenous	Tendon, ligaments, aponeurosis, cornea
Elastic	Ligamentum nuchae, ligamenta flava
Special connective tissues	
Cartilage	
Hyaline	Costal cartilages, trachea
Fibrous	Symphysis pubis, intervertebral disk
Elastic	External ear, epiglottis
Bone	Skeleton
Blood	Cardiovascular system
Hemopoietic	Bone marrow, lymphatic tissue and organs

Fibers of Connective Tissue

KEY WORDS: collagen fiber, unit fibril, tropocollagen, alpha unit, reticular fiber, elastic fiber, microfibril, elastin

The fibrous intercellular substances in connective tissue consist of collagenous, reticular, and elastic fibers. **Collagen fibers** are present in all connective tissues and run an irregular course with much branching (see atlas figures 3-2 through 3-4). The fibers vary in thickness from 1 to 10 μm and are of undefined length. Although flexible, collagenous fibers have extremely high tensile strength. Ultrastructurally, the fibers consist of parallel fibrils, each of which represents a structural unit (see atlas figures 3-5 and 3-8). These **unit fibrils** show repeating transverse bands spaced at 64-nm intervals along their length and are composed of macromolecules of **tropocollagen** that measure about 260 nm long by 1.5 nm wide. The tropocollagen molecules lie parallel to each other, overlapping by about one-fourth of their lengths; the overlap is responsible for the banding pattern. Each molecule of tropocollagen consists of three polypeptide chains called **alpha units** arranged in a helix and linked by hydrogen bonds. The polypeptides are rich in glycine and proline and also contain hydroxyproline and hydroxylysine. However, alpha units isolated from collagens taken from different sites vary somewhat in the composition and sequence of amino acids. Several distinct molecular types of collagen have been identified, all of which consist of three alpha units arranged in a righthand helix and differ mainly in the amino acid constituents of the alpha chain (Table 3-2). Various types of collagen can be made by cells other than fibroblasts, and collagen is synthesized by chondroblasts, osteoblasts, odontoblasts, epithelial cells, and smooth muscle cells. Collagen molecules are important components of basement membranes.

Reticular fibers do not gather into bundles as do collagenous fibers but tend to form delicate networks. They are not seen in routinely prepared sections but can be shown with silver stains or

Table 3-2. Types of collagen*

Type	Morphologic features	Distribution
I	Broad, banded fibrils	Widespread; tendon, bone, dermis, dentin, fascia
II	Small diameter, banded fibrils	Hyaline cartilage, vitreous body, nucleus pulposus, notochord
III	Small diameter, banded fibrils	Corresponds to reticular fibers; prominent in organs with a major smooth muscle component; uterus, blood vessels
IV	Feltwork of nonbanded fibrils	Basal laminae of epithelial cells, glomerular epithelium
V	Thin, nonbanded fibrils	Widespread; pericellular laminae of smooth and striated muscle cells, tendon sheaths

*Various types of collagen can be elaborated by cells other than fibroblasts. Collagen is known to be synthesized by chondroblasts, osteoblasts, odontoblasts, and smooth muscle cells.

by the periodic acid-Schiff reagent, which reacts with proteoglycans that bind reticular fibers together (see atlas figure 3-7). In electron micrographs, reticular fibers show the same banding pattern as collagen. They differ principally in the number, diameter, and arrangement of the unit fibrils (see atlas figure 3-8).

Elastic fibers appear as thin, homogeneous strands that are similar and of more uniform size than collagen fibers. They cannot be distinguished in routine sections and require special stains to make them visible (see atlas figure 3-6). In electron micrographs, elastic fibers are seen to consist of bundles of **microfibrils** embedded around an amorphous component called **elastin** (see atlas figure 3-8). The microfibrils are about 11 nm in diameter and lack crossbanding. During formation of elastic fibers, microfibrils are laid down first and elastin is added secondarily but soon forms the bulk of the fiber. A precursor molecule, tropoelastin, is released by cells and polymerizes extracellularly to form elastin. The microfibrillar component tends to be peripherally located on the fiber. Elastin, like collagen, contains glycine and proline but has little hydroxyproline and lacks hydroxylysine. It has a high content of valine and contains two amino acids, desmosine and isodesmosine, that are specific to

elastin. The microfibrillar protein differs from elastin; it contains less glycine and has no hydroxyproline, desmosine, or isodesmosine.

Elastic fibers can stretch more than 130 percent of their original length, and their presence permits connective tissues to undergo considerable expansion or stretching with return to the original shape or size when the deforming force is removed. In addition to forming fibers, elastin may be present in fenestrated sheets as in some arterial walls.

Ground Substance

KEY WORDS: gel, proteoglycan, glycosaminoglycan, bound water, fibronectin, laminin

The fibers and cells of connective tissue are embedded in an amorphous material called ground substance that is present as a transparent **gel** of variable viscosity. Ground substance consists of glycoproteins, glycosaminoglycans, and proteoglycans that differ in amount and type in different connective tissues (Table 3-3). **Proteoglycans** have a bottle brush configuration with long protein cores bound covalently to numerous glycosaminoglycan side chains. **Glycosaminoglycans** are linear polymers of repeating

Table 3-3. Types of glycosaminoglycans

Types of glycosaminoglycans	Some locations
Hyaluronic acid	Umbilical cord, vitreous humor, synovial fluid, loose connective tissue
Chondroitin	Cornea
Chondroitin-4-sulfate	Aorta, bone, cartilage, cornea
Chondroitin-6-sulfate	Cartilage, nucleus pulposus, sclera, tendon, umbilical cord
Dermatan sulfate	Aorta, heart valves, ligamentum nuchae, sclera, skin, tendon
Keratan sulfate	Bone, cartilage, cornea, nucleus pulposus

disaccharide units that contain hexosamine, D-glucosamine, or D-galactosamine as their most constant feature. Tropocollagen has been extracted from ground substance but cannot be demonstrated histologically.

Ground substance contains a high proportion of water, which is bound to long-chain carbohydrates and proteoglycans; most of the extravascular fluid is in this state. This **bound water** acts as a medium by which nutrients, gases, and metabolites can be exchanged between blood and tissue cells. Hyaluronic acid is the chief glycosaminoglycan of loose connective tissue, and because of its ability to bind water, it is primarily responsible for changes in the permeability and viscosity of loose connective tissue. Proteoglycans have an important role in maintaining the structural organization of the fibrous constituents in the matrix and basal laminae and aid in preventing or retarding the spread of microorganisms and their toxic materials from the site of an infection.

The main glycoproteins of the matrix are fibronectin and laminin. **Fibronectin** occurs in the basal laminae of epithelia, in the external laminae of muscle cells and Schwann's cells, and on the surfaces of other cells. Fibronectin is thought to mediate adhesion between cells and between cells and substrates in the matrix. It may be involved in cell spreading and locomotion. **Laminin** is found mainly in basal laminae and is implicated in the attachment of epithelia to type IV collagen in this supporting layer.

Cells of Connective Tissue

KEY WORDS: fibroblast, myofibroblast, macrophage, system of mononuclear phagocytes, mast cell, heparin, histamine, fat cell, plasma cell, leukocyte, neutrophil, eosinophil, lymphocyte, monocyte

Connective tissue contains several different cell types. Some are indigenous to the tissues, others are transients derived from blood. The most common connective tissue cells are **fibroblasts** — large, flattened cells with elliptical nuclei that contain one or two nucleoli (see atlas figures 3-2, 3-4, and 3-9). The cell body is irregular and often appears stellate with long cytoplasmic processes extending along the connective tissue fibers. The boundaries of the cell are not seen in most preparations, and the morphology varies with the state of activity. In active cells the nuclei are plump and stain lightly, whereas the nuclei of inactive cells appear slender and dense. Ultrastructurally, active cells show increased amounts of granular endoplasmic reticulum (GER). Fibroblasts elaborate the precursors of collagen and reticular and elastic fibers, produce the ground substance, and maintain the extracellular materials that are constantly being removed and renewed.

The peptides of collagen are formed on the ribosomes of the GER, from which they are transported to the Golgi complex. Procollagen, a molecular form of collagen, is released at the maturing face of the Golgi body into the surrounding cytoplasm and then released from the cell (Fig. 3-1). An enzyme called procollagen peptidase converts

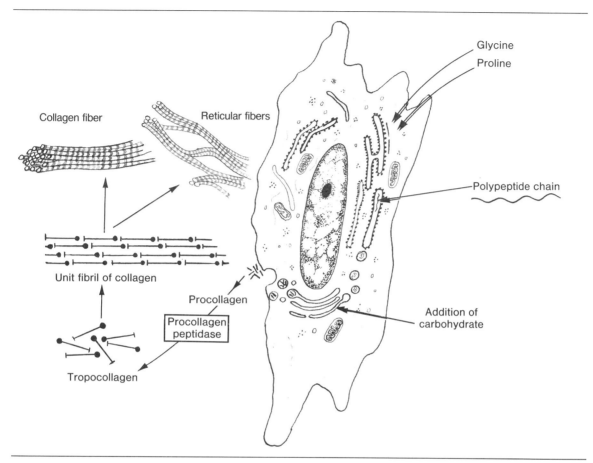

Fig. 3-1. Formation of collagen by fibroblasts.

the procollagen molecule into tropocollagen, which then polymerizes to form the unit fibril of collagen.

Myofibroblasts resemble fibroblasts but contain aggregates of actin microfilaments and myosin. Normally found only in small numbers, they increase following tissue injury. Myofibroblasts produce collagen, and their contractile activity contributes to the retraction and shrinkage of early scar tissue.

Macrophages (histiocytes) are almost as abundant as fibroblasts in connective tissue. They are actively phagocytic, ingesting a variety of materials from particulate matter to bacteria, tissue

debris, and whole dead cells (see atlas figure 3-10). The material ingested is broken down by lysosomal digestion. Macrophages commonly are described as irregularly shaped cells with blunt cytoplasmic processes and ovoid or indented nuclei that are smaller and stain more deeply than those of fibroblasts. In fact, macrophages are difficult to distinguish from fibroblasts, especially active fibroblasts, unless the macrophages show evidence of phagocytosis.

The macrophages of loose connective tissue are part of a widespread **system of mononuclear phagocytes** that includes phagocytes of the liver (Kuppfer's cells), lung (alveolar macrophages), serous cavities (pleural and peritoneal macrophages), nervous system (microglia), lymphatic tissue, and bone marrow. Regardless of where they are found, macrophages have a common origin from precursors in the bone marrow, and the monocytes of blood represent a transit form of immature macrophages.

Mast cells are present in variable numbers in loose connective tissue and often collect along small blood vessels. They are large, ovoid cells 20 to 30 μm in diameter with large granules that fill the cytoplasm (see atlas figures 3-9 and 3-11). Two populations of mast cells are known to exist: connective tissue mast cells and mucosal mast cells. In humans, the granules of connective tissue mast cells are membrane bound and in electron micrographs show a characteristic tubular pattern (see atlas figures 3-11 and 3-12). The granules contain **heparin,** a potent anticoagulant; **histamine,** an agent that causes vasodilation and increased permeability of capillaries and venules; and a vasoactive peptide. The granules of mucosal mast cells contain chondroitin sulfate rather than heparin. Both mast cell types arise from bone marrow stem cells. Mast cells promote immediate hypersensitivity reactions following their release of secretory granules, which act as chemical mediators.

Fat cells are specialized for synthesis and storage of lipid. Individual fat cells may be scattered throughout loose connective tissue or may accumulate to such an exent that other cells are crowded out and an adipose tissue is formed. Each fat cell acquires so much lipid that the nucleus is flattened to one side of the cell and the cytoplasm forms only a thin rim around a large droplet of fat (see atlas figure 3-15). In ordinary sections, fat cells appear empty due to the loss of lipid during tissue preparation, and groups of fat cells have the appearance of chicken wire.

Plasma cells are not common in most connective tissues but may be numerous in the lamina propria of the gastrointestinal tract and are present in lymphatic tissues. Plasma cells appear somewhat ovoid, with small eccentrically placed nuclei in which the chromatin is arranged in coarse blocks to form a "clock face" pattern. The cytoplasm is deeply basophilic due to the abundance of GER (see atlas figure 3-14). A weakly staining area of cytoplasm often appears adjacent to one side of the nucleus and corresponds to the site of the Golgi complex (see atlas figure 3-13). Plasma cells produce immunoglobulins (antibodies) that form an important defense against infections. Various acidophilic inclusions may be found in the cytoplasm of some plasma cells. Plasma cells are a differentiated form of the B-lymphocyte.

Variable numbers of **leukocytes** constantly migrate into the connective tissues from the blood (diapedesis). **Neutrophils** are one type of leukocyte characterized by a lobed nucleus. In this cell type, the granules are said to be neutrophilic although in sections they stain faintly pink (i.e., acidophilic). The cells are avidly phagocytic for small particles and are especially numerous at sites of infections. They are the major cellular component of pus. **Eosinophils** also are characterized by lobed nuclei, but their cytoplasmic granules are larger, more spherical, and more discretely visible than those of neutrophils. The granules stain intensely with acid dyes such as eosin. These cells are phagocytic and have a special avidity for antigen-antibody complexes. They increase in number as a result of allergic or parasitic types of disease. **Lymphocytes** belong to the class of leukocytes called mononuclear leukocytes and are characterized by a single, round, nonlobed nucleus. They are the smallest of the cells that migrate into connective tissues and measure about 7 μm in diameter. These cells form part of the immunological defense system and may give rise to antibody-producing cells or elaborate nonspecific factors that destroy foreign cells. They are few in number in normal connective tissue but increase markedly in areas of chronic inflammation. **Monocytes** are the blood-borne forerunners of tissue macrophages. Once the cells have entered connective tissue it is difficult, if not impossible, to distinguish them from macrophages. Monocytes can fuse with one another to form multinucleated giant cells in an attempt to engulf or wall off objects that are too large or resistant to phagocytosis by a single cell (see atlas figure 3-16).

Subtypes of Loose Connective Tissue

KEY WORDS: mesenchyme, mucoid tissue, areolar connective tissue

Mesenchyme is loose, spongy tissue that serves as packing between the developing structures of the embryo (see atlas figure 3-17). It consists of a loose network of stellate and spindle-shaped cells embedded in an amorphous ground substance with thin, sparse fibers. The cells have multiple developmental potentials and can give rise to any of the connective tissues. The presence of mesenchymal cells in the adult often has been proposed to explain the expansion of adult connective tissue. However, fibroblasts, too, are capable of sequential divisions, and the idea of mesenchymal rests can well be discarded.

Mucoid tissue occurs in many parts of the embryo but is particularly prominent in the umbilical cord, where it is called Wharton's jelly. It resembles mesenchyme in that the constituent cells are stellate fibroblasts with long processes that often make contact with those of neighboring cells, and the intercellular substance is soft and jellylike and contains thin collagen fibers. The fiber content increases with the age of the fetus. Mucoid tissue does not have the developmental potential of mesenchyme.

Areolar connective tissue is a loosely arranged connective tissue that is widely distributed in the body. It contains collagen fibers and a few elastic fibers embedded in a thin, almost fluidlike ground substance. This kind of connective tissue forms the fascia that binds organs and organ components together. It forms helices about the long axes of expandable tubular structures such as the ducts of glands, the gastrointestinal tract, and blood vessels.

Adipose Tissue

KEY WORDS: white fat, unilocular, brown fat, multilocular

Adipose tissue differs in two respects from other connective tissue: Fat cells and not the intercellular substances predominate, and unlike other connective tissue cells, each fat cell is surrounded by its own basal lamina. Reticular and collagenous fibers also extend around each fat cell to provide a delicate supporting framework that contains numerous capillaries.

Adipose tissue can be subdivided into white and brown fat. **White fat** is the more plentiful and is found mainly in the subcutaneous tissue (where it forms the panniculus adiposus), omenta, mesenteries, pararenal tissue, and bone marrow. White fat is an extremely vascular tissue and also contains many nerve fibers. In white fat, the cells are filled by a single, large droplet of lipid; thus, it is often referred to as **unilocular** fat (see atlas figure 3-15). The lipid droplet is composed of glycerol esters and fatty acids. The materials within the fat droplet are in a constant state of flux and are not permanent entities. White fat serves as a storage depot for calories taken in excess of the body's needs and can be used for production of energy as required or as a source of material for steroid hormone synthesis. It also acts as an insulating layer to conserve body heat, acts mechanically as a packing material, and forms shock-absorbing pads in the palms of the hands, on the soles of the feet, and around the eyeballs.

Brown fat is present in many species, including humans, and is prominent in hibernating animals and newborns. Brown fat has a restricted distribution, occurring mainly in the interscapular and inguinal regions. The brown or tan color is due to the high content of cytochrome enzymes. The cells show round nuclei, and the cytoplasm is filled with multiple small droplets of lipid; hence, this type of fat is called **multilocular** fat. Mitochondria here are more numerous and larger than those in the cells of white fat. Each cell of brown fat receives direct sympathetic innervation. During arousal from hibernation, the lipid within the brown fat is rapidly oxidized to produce heat and release substances such as glycerol that are used by other tissues. Because brown fat is even more vascular than white fat, it raises the temperature of the blood significantly, thus increasing the general body temperature.

Reticular Connective Tissue

KEY WORDS: reticular cell, reticular fiber, fibroblast

Reticular connective tissue is characterized by a cellular framework as seen in lymphatic tissues and bone marrow. **Reticular cells** are stellate, with processes extending along the **reticular fibers** to make contact with neighboring cells. The cytoplasm stains lightly and is attenuated, and the large nucleus stains weakly. The reticular cell is equivalent to the **fibroblast** of other connective tissues and is responsible for the production and maintenance of the reticular fibers, which are identical to those found in loose connective tissue.

Dense Connective Tissue

KEY WORDS: dense irregular, dense regular

Dense connective tissue differs from the loose variety chiefly in the concentration of fibers and reduction of the cellular and amorphous constituents. Two types, dense irregular and dense regular, are identified.

Dense irregular connective tissue contains abundant, thick, collagenous bundles that are woven into a compact network. Among the collagen fibers is an extensive network of elastic fibers. An example of dense irregular connective tissue is the dermis of the skin (see atlas figure 3-3).

Dense regular connective tissue also contains a predominance of collagen fibers arranged in bundles, but these have a regular, precise arrangement (see atlas figure 3-4). The organiza-tion of the collagen bundles reflects the mechanical needs of the tissue. In tendons and ligaments, for example, they are oriented in the direction of pull. Fibroblasts are the primary cells present and occur in rows parallel to the bundles of collagen fibers.

Special Connective Tissue

Special connective tissues have functions and a histologic organization sufficiently unique to warrant their consideration as distinct and special forms of connective tissue. They are considered individually in succeeding chapters.

Development of Connective Tissues

All connective tissues originate from mesoderm, the middle of the three primary germ layers of the early embryo. Mesoderm consists mainly of large, stellate mesenchymal cells whose numerous processes are in contact with those of adjacent cells. Initially, only mesenchymal cells and a thin ground substance are present, but as development proceeds, an interlacing network of fine collagenous fibers appears. Very early in development the mesodermal layer is transformed into a mesenchymal compartment separated from surrounding epithelium by a basal lamina. Collagen molecules form a major component of such laminae, which are important in determining what substances enter or leave the connective tissue compartment. With further development, the mesenchymal compartment becomes transformed into numerous irregularly shaped connective tissue passageways that surround neural and muscular tissues or lie between epithelial tissues. Glands and organs develop from invaginations of epithelium that extend into the mesenchymal compartments. Interaction between epithelium and mesenchyme is essential for normal development to occur.

Functional Summary

The functions of connective tissue are mainly passive, but mechanically they are indispensable. They provide the supporting framework for organs and for the body itself and serve to connect distant structures as, for example, in the connection of muscle to bone by tendons. Connective tissues bind organs and unite the organ components into a functioning unit. Adipose tissue forms an insulating blanket to limit heat loss and forms mechanically protective cushions in the hands and feet and about the eyeball. It also stores excess calories in the form of fat that can be called on and used as needed.

Collagenous fibers provide tissues with flexibility and tensile strength; elastic fibers allow considerable deformity of an organ with recovery of the shape and size when the force is removed. Collagen molecules form a major component of basal laminae, which determine vascular and epithelium permeability.

Connective tissue also contributes significantly to the defense of the body. This is the function of cellular components mainly, as in the phagocytic activity of macrophages and granular leukocytes and the antibodies and cytotoxic agents elaborated by plasma cells and lymphocytes. The matrix also plays an important role in the body's defenses by preventing or slowing the spread of microorganisms and their toxic products from sites of infection.

The various connective tissues together form a single vast compartment limited by sheets of epithelia. It is through this compartment that tissue fluid must pass during exchange of nutrients and waste products between cells and tissue and the blood vasculature. Most immune reactions take place in this compartment. Because the ground substance of loose connective tissue binds water, it can act as the medium by which these exchanges are effected.

Clinical Correlations

Whenever an epithelial barrier is breached by chemical, physical, or infective agents, toxins, or trauma, the connective tissue responds with an inflammatory process, a major defense mechanism of the body that accounts for many of the signs and symptoms of disease. The intensity and duration of the response generally corresponds to the severity of the injury and to the persistence of the injurious agent. The local features of acute inflammation are reddening, swelling, warmth, and pain; depending on location, there also may be partial immobilization.

One of the first events of inflammation is local dilatation of and increased blood flow through small blood vessels in the area, accounting for the redness and warmth. Fluid leaks from the dilated vessels into the surrounding tissue, resulting in swelling and pain. The latter is thought to be due to stimulation of nerve endings by the pressure of the increased fluid volume, but chemical mediators released during injury and the subsequent inflammatory response also may be involved. The vascular events, especially increased permeability, appear to be mediated by histamine released from mast cells in response to the original tissue damage. Within a few hours, neutrophil granular leukocytes and monocytes make their way out of damaged vessels and spread through the injured tissue, forming an exudate. Neutrophil granulocytes migrate earlier and more rapidly than monocytes so that in a short-lived, acute inflammation, the major neutrophil response is over before monocytes appear in any number. In prolonged inflammation (e.g., pyogenic bacteria), migration of neutrophils continues until most of the organisms have been destroyed, after which macrophages appear to clear up tissue debris, dead leukocytes, and any remaining organisms.

Acute inflammation may subside and the tissues return to normal, or it may progress to suppuration or chronic inflammation. Suppuration results from infection with pyogenic bacteria from local injury severe enough to cause death of tissue in the center of the lesion and an intense migration of granular leukocytes. The necrotic tissue is digested by lysosomal enzymes released by the leukocytes, leaving a cavity that becomes filled with an exudate rich in granulocytes but also containing bacteria, dead tissue, and cell debris. The cavity forms an abscess; its contents form pus. Abscesses may heal with formation of scars.

Prolonged tissue injury results in chronic inflammation characterized by formation of new fibrous tissue. At first this is very cellular and vascular; the fibroblasts are plump and have pale, vesicular nuclei, and the newly formed collagen fibers are fine and scanty. The fibrous tissue becomes more dense and less cellular, collagenous fibers thicken, fibroblasts appear less active and are reduced in number, and the tissue becomes less vascular. Plasma cells, lymphocytes, and macrophages usually are the predominate cells, although some granulocytes may be present also. Macrophages may fuse to form multinucleated giant cells, as in tuberculosis or the response to nondigestible material (slivers of wood, silica, asbestos), in an attempt to engulf the particles. If an organism cannot be ingested or otherwise destroyed, it may become enclosed in a dense capsule of collagenous fibers; in tuberculosis, the capsule may even calcify.

Connective tissue is important in healing processes, and the ability of fibroblasts to proliferate and synthesize collagen in response to injury makes these cells the chief agent in tissue repair. Myofibroblasts proliferate into the damaged area following injury, secrete collagens, and contract to reduce the size of the wound (wound contraction). Type I collagen is the main collagen synthesized during normal wound healing although initially, type III collagen is deposited but later replaced. Hyaluronic acid is the chief glycosaminoglycan found during the first week of the healing process. By the end of the third week, dermatan sulfate and chondroitin-4-sulfate have become predominant and thereafter decline. The glycosaminoglycans are thought to influence the extracellular arrangement of the collagen molecules. Crosslinking of collagen molecules and replacement and resynthesis of collagen may continue for a year or more before wound healing or scar formation is complete. Keloids are grossly exaggerated scars in which excessive, disfiguring masses of poorly cellular fibrous tissue is formed in response to even minor injuries. Disordered matrix production and random arrangement of collagen with reduced crosslinking are the main features of keloids.

Collagen metabolism is affected by nutrition, aging, and other factors. For example, scurvy results from deficiency of vitamin C, which is important for conversion of proline to hydroxyproline during collagen synthesis. Absence of vitamin C results in defective production and deposition of collagen by fibroblasts in bones and teeth and during the healing of wounds.

Cells of general connective tissue may form tumors, which may be either malignant (sarcomas) or benign. In general, cells of such tumors resemble the cells of origin. For example, tumors resulting from a proliferation of fibroblasts may be either malignant (fibrosarcoma) or benign (fibroma). Tumors of unilocular (white) fat cells also occur and are classified as malignant (liposarcoma) or benign (lipoma). Tumors of multilocular (brown) fat cells also occur and are termed hibernomas.

Atlas and Tables of Key Features

Key Features of Connective Tissue Cells

Cell types	Nuclear characteristics	Cytoplasmic characteristics	Primary activity
Resident			
Fibroblasts	Oval, centrally placed, staining variable depending on activity	Elongate, spindle- or stellate-shaped cell; usually not visible in sectioned material	Produce fibers and proteoglycans
Myofibroblasts	Same as above	Same as above; bundles of actin filaments at electron microscopic level	Produce collagen fibers, contract
Adipose cells			
Unilocular fat cells	Usually compressed at edge of cell (signet ring–like), staining variable	Forms a thin rim around single central lipid droplet	Store lipid
Multilocular fat cells	Central, spheroid, light staining	Numerous lipid droplets, abundant mitochondria	Store lipid
Mast cells	Central, spheroid to ovoid, may show abundant heterochromatin	Filled with granules	Store and release histamine, heparin, vasoactive peptide
Macrophages	Large, ovoid, most frequently indented	Light staining; contains phagocytosed material	Phagocytic for a variety of materials
Plasma cell	Usually eccentric, spheroid; heterochromatin clumps may form "clock face"	Basophilic, slate gray in color; may show negative Golgi image	Antibody production
Migratory			
Neutrophils	Polymorphonuclear, 3–5 lobes common, chromatin dense	Lilac staining	Phagocytic for small particles

Key Features of Connective Tissue Cells (continued)

Cell types	Nuclear characteristics	Cytoplasmic characteristics	Primary activity
Eosinophils	Polymorphonuclear, 2–4 lobes common, chromatin dense	Red-orange granules fill cytoplasm	Phagocytic for antigen-antibody complexes
Lymphocytes	Single, spheroid, abundant heterochromatin	Thin rim, light blue staining	Antibody production, cytotoxic agents

Key features of connective tissue fibers

Fiber type	Light microscopic appearance	Electron microscopic appearance	Primary locations
Collagen fiber (type I collagen)	Coarse fibers 0.5–10.0 μm in diameter; indefinite length; stain with protein dyes	Unit fibrils 50–150 nm in diameter; repeating transverse bands every 64 nm; organized into large fibers	Tendon, ligament, dermis, fascia, capsules, sclera, bone, dentin
Reticular fiber (type III collagen)	Delicate network of fine fibers; must be stained specifically to demonstrate, usually by reduction of silver	Banded unit fibrils 50 nm or less in diameter, organized into tiny fibers	Stroma of lymphatic organs, bone marrow, glands
Elastic fiber	Smooth, homogeneous fibers; varying diameter; must be stained specifically to demonstrate (orcein, Verhoeff's stain)	Amorphous core of elastin; microfibrils 11 nm in diameter; periphery of fiber	Dermis, lung, arteries, organs that expand

General Connective Tissue

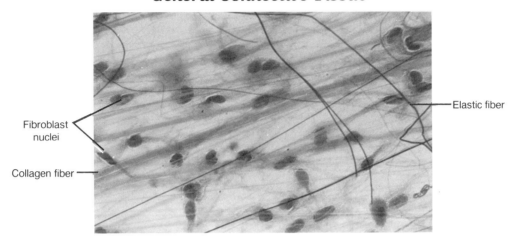

Fibroblast
nuclei

Elastic fiber

Collagen fiber

Fig. 3-2. A spread preparation of loose areolar connective tissue stained with orcein, which selectively stains elastic fibers. Note that collagen fibers and numerous fibroblasts also are shown. (LM, ×400.)

Collagen
bundle

Capillary

Collagen
fiber

Arteriole

Fibroblast
nuclei

Fig. 3-3. The dermis of human skin is a classic example of dense irregular connective tissue. (LM, ×250.)

Collagen–
bundle

Collagen–
bundle

Fibroblast
nuclei

Fig. 3-4. Dense regular connective tissue from a human tendon.
(LM, ×400.)

Collagen–
fiber

Fibroblast
cytoplasm

Elastin

Cross sections
of unit
fibrils

Unit
fibrils

Fig. 3-5. Elastic and collagen fibers from the connective tissue
component of the pleura as seen in the electron microscope. Note
that each collagen fiber is made up of several unit fibrils that show
cross striations. (TEM, ×11,000.)

Elastic
laminae

Elastic
laminae

Fig. 3-6. A region of the human aorta stained with orcein to demonstrate elastic laminae. (LM, ×150.)

Reticular
fibers

Reticular
fibers

Fig. 3-7. A portion of liver stained with silver, which is selective for demonstrating reticular fibers. (LM, ×200.)

Reticular fibers

Elastin

Collagen unit fibrils

Fibroblast plasmalemma

Fibroblast cytoplasm

Fig. 3-8. A region of the visceral pleura contains the three fiber types of connective tissue: reticular, collagen, and elastic. (TEM, ×18,000.)

Mast cell

Fibroblast

Collagen
fibers

Space occupied
by ground
substance

Fibroblast
nucleus

Fibroblast
cytoplasm

Fig. 3-9. A region of dermis demonstrates the association between cells (fibroblasts, mast cells), collagen fibers, and the ground substance of dense connective tissue. (TEM, ×2,000.)

Nucleus ————

Mitochondria

Lysosomes

Phagosome

Fig. 3-10. An active macrophage that has recently phagocytosed foreign material. (TEM, ×4,000.)

Fig. 3-11. Human mast cells. (LM, ×1,100.) Note the tubular patterns of the mast cell granules, which identify this mast cell as being human. (TEM, ×50,000.)

Pseudopod

Mitochondria

Fibroblast nucleus

Granules

Nucleus

Fig. 3-12. A human mast cell from the lamina propria of the stomach. (TEM, ×4,000.)

Plasma cell

Negative Golgi image

Plasma cell

Fig. 3-13. Several plasma cells taken from the loose connective tissue of a human lactating breast. (LM, ×400.)

Granular endoplasmic reticulum

Heterochromatin

Euchromatin

Mitochondria

Fig. 3-14. A human plasma cell taken from the lamina propria of the stomach. (TEM, ×5,000.)

Cytoplasmi rim of fat cell

Space of fat droplet

Fat cell

Nucleolus

Fat cell nucleus

Fibroblast nucleus

Fig. 3-15. White (unilocular) fat cells taken from a region of adipose tissue. (LM, ×350.)

Lymphocytes

Foreign body
giant cell

Fig. 3-16. Numerous lymphocytes and a foreign body giant cell
from a site of infection in a human eyelid. (LM, ×250.)

Development

Mesenchymal cell

Mesenchymal cell

Fig. 3-17. Numerous mesenchymal cells that form the mesenchyme of an early embryo. (SEM, ×1,000.)

Review Questions and Answers

Questions

12. How do connective tissues differ from epithelia?
13. What is the difference between collagen and reticular fibers?
14. What conclusions would you draw from the appearance by light and electron microscopy of the plasma cell?
15. In what ways does adipose tissue differ from other loose connective tissues?
16. Briefly define "ground substance" and discuss its role in connective tissue.
17. What role does the fibroblast play in the connective tissues?

Answers

12. Connective tissues differ from epithelia in the proportion of cells and intercellular substances. In epithelia, the cellular component predominates, the cells are closely apposed, and there is little intercellular material between them. Connective tissues, on the other hand, are characterized by a preponderance of intercellular materials, and the cells are widely separated by the ground substance and fibers. With rare exceptions, connective tissues are well vascularized, whereas epithelia are avascular.

13. Collagen and reticular fibers differ in the number and arrangement of the unit fibrils of which the fibers are composed. From electron microscopic observations, reticular fibers show the same banding pattern and consist of the same unit fibrils that are present in collagen. Typical banded collagen fibers consist of type I collagen, whereas reticular fibers consist primarily of type III collagen.

14. The deeply basophilic cytoplasm indicates the presence of a large amount of granular endoplasmic reticulum, and the clear area of the cytoplasm corresponds to a prominent Golgi complex. These are consistent with a cell that is actively engaged in protein (glycoprotein) synthesis. Plasma cells produce immunoglobulins (antibodies).

15. Adipose tissue differs from other connective tissues in the predominance of fat cells over intercellular substances, and, unlike other connective tissues, the fat cells of adipose tissue are each surrounded only by their own basal laminae.

16. The ground substance is best defined as that amorphous component of connective tissue in which the cells and extracellular fibers are embedded. The ground substance together with extracellular fibers constitute the matrix of connective tissue. Ground substance usually occurs as a transparent gel and is of variable viscosity. It is made up of a number of proteoglycans, glycosaminoglycans, and glycoproteins that differ in type, amount, and consistency depending on the kind of connective tissue. Most extravascular fluid is bound within the ground substance and serves as a medium in which metabolites, nutrients, and gases can be exchanged between tissue cells and the surrounding vasculature. Ground substance also plays an important role in retarding the spread of microorganisms and toxic materials from the sites of infections.

17. Fibroblasts are the most common and widespread of the connective tissue cells. They elaborate and maintain the extracellular fibers of connective tissue (collagenous, reticular, and elastic fibers) as well as the amorphous ground substance.

4 Special Connective Tissue: Cartilage, Bone, and Joints

Cartilage

Although adapted to provide support, cartilage contains only the usual elements of connective tissue — cells, fibers, and ground substance. It is the ground substance that gives cartilage its firm consistency and ability to withstand compression and shearing forces. Collagen and elastic fibers embedded in the ground substance impart tensile strength and elasticity. Together, the fibers and ground substance form the matrix. Cartilage differs from other connective tissues in that it lacks nerves, a blood supply, and lymphatics and is nourished entirely by diffusion of materials from blood vessels in adjacent tissues. Although relatively rigid, the cartilage matrix has a high water content and is freely permeable, even to fairly large particles.

Classification of cartilage into hyaline, elastic, and fibrous types is based on differences in the abundance and type of fibers in the matrix.

Hyaline Cartilage

KEY WORDS: **chondrocyte, lacuna, isogenous group, proteoglycan, territorial matrix, interterritorial matrix, perichondrium**

Hyaline cartilage is the most common type of cartilage and forms the costal cartilages, articular cartilages of joints, and cartilages of the nose, larynx, trachea, and bronchi. It is present in the growing ends of long bones. In the fetus, most of the skeleton is first laid down as hyaline cartilage.

The cells of cartilage are called **chondrocytes** and reside in small spaces called **lacunae** scattered throughout the matrix (see atlas figures 4-7 and 4-9). The cells generally conform to the shape of the lacunae in which they are contained. Deep in the cartilage the cells and their lacunae usually appear rounded in profile, whereas at the surface, they are elliptical, with the long axis parallel to the surface. Chondrocytes often occur in small clusters called **isogenous groups** that represent the offspring of a single cell.

In the usual preparations, the cells show an irregular outline and appear shrunken and pulled away from the walls of the lacunae. Electron microscopy reveals that each cell completely fills the lacunar space and sends short processes into the surrounding matrix, but neighboring cells do not communicate with each other. The nucleus is round or oval and contains one or more nucleoli. The cytoplasm shows the usual organelles as well as lipid and glycogen inclusions (see atlas figure 4-6). In growing chondrocytes the Golgi body and endoplasmic reticulum are well developed.

In fresh cartilage and in routine histologic sections, the matrix appears homogeneous since the ground substance and the collagen fibers embedded in it have the same refractive index (see atlas figures 4-5 and 4-7). The collagen in hyaline cartilage rarely forms bundles but is present as a feltwork of slender fibrils in which the banding pattern shows variable periodicities or even is lacking. Collagen in cartilage appears to be less polymerized than in other tissues; cartilage is unique in that only type II collagen is present. Chondronectin, a glycoprotein, mediates the adhesion of type II collagen to chondroycytes. The ground substance consists mainly of **proteoglycans,** the specific glycosaminoglycans of cartilage being chondroitin-4- and chondroitin-6-sulfate, keratan sulfate, and a small amount of hyaluronic acid. The proteoglycans are responsible for the basophilic properties of the ground substance. The matrix around each isogenous group stains more deeply than elsewhere, forming the **territorial matrix.** The less densely stained intervening areas form the **interterritorial matrix.**

Except for the free surfaces of articular cartilages, hyaline cartilage is enclosed by a specialized sheath of connective tissue called the **perichondrium** (see atlas figures 4-7 and 4-8). The outer layers of the perichondrium consist of well vascularized, dense, irregular connective tissue that contains elastic and collagen fibers and fibroblasts. Where it lies against cartilage, the perichondrium is more cellular and passes imperceptibly into cartilage. The slender collagen fibers of the cartilage matrix blend with the wider, banded fibers of the perichondrium. Perichondrial cells adjacent to the cartilage retain the capacity to form new cartilage.

Elastic Cartilage

KEY WORDS: elastic fibers

Elastic cartilage is a variant of hyaline cartilage, differing chiefly in that it contains branched elastic fibers in the matrix (see atlas figure 4-10). Collagen fibers of the type found in hyaline cartilage also are present but are masked. Deep in the cartilage, **elastic fibers** form a dense, closely packed mesh that obscures the ground substance, but beneath the perichondrium, the fibers form a looser network and are continuous with those of the perichondrium. The chondrocytes are similar to those of hyaline cartilage and elaborate the elastic and collagen fibers. Elastic cartilage is more flexible than hyaline cartilage and is found in the external ear, auditory tube, epiglottis, and some of the smaller laryngeal cartilages.

Fibrous Cartilage

Fibrous (or fibro-) cartilage represents a transition between dense connective tissue and cartilage. It consists of typical cartilage cells enclosed in lacunae, but only a small amount of ground substance is present in the immediate vicinity of the cells (see atlas figure 4-11). The chondrocytes lie singly, in pairs, or in short rows between bundles of dense collagen fibers that show the 64-nm banding. Fibrous cartilage always lacks a perichondrium and merges into hyaline cartilage, bone, or dense fibrous tissue. It occurs in the intervertebral discs, in some articular cartilages, in the symphysis pubis, and at sites of attachment of certain tendons to bone.

Bone

Bone is a connective tissue specialized for support. However, in bone the matrix is mineralized and forms a dense, hard, unyielding substance with high tensile, weight-bearing, and compression strength. Despite its strength and rigidity, bone is a dynamic, living tissue constantly turning over, constantly being renewed and reformed throughout life.

Macroscopic Structure

KEY WORDS: cancellous (spongy) bone, trabecula, compact (dense) bone, diaphysis, epiphysis, periosteum, endosteum, diploë

Grossly, cancellous and compact forms of bone can be identified. **Cancellous (spongy) bone** consists of irregular bars or **trabeculae** of bone that branch and unite to form a three-dimensional, interlacing network of boney rods, delimiting a vast system of small communicating spaces that in life, are filled with bone marrow (see atlas figures 4-12 and 4-13). **Compact (dense) bone** appears as a solid, continuous mass in which spaces cannot be seen with the naked eye. The two types of bone are not sharply delimited and merge into one another (see atlas figure 4-12).

In a typical long bone the shaft or **diaphysis** appears as a hollow cylinder of compact bone enclosing a large central space called the marrow cavity. The ends of the long bones, the **epiphyses,** consist mainly of cancellous bone covered by a thin layer of compact bone. The small intercommunicating spaces in the spongy bone are continuous with the marrow cavity of the shaft.

Except over articular surfaces and where tendons and ligaments insert, bone is covered by a fibroelastic connective tissue called the **periosteum.** The marrow cavity of the diaphysis and the spaces within spongy bone are lined by **endosteum,** which is similar to periosteum but is thinner and not as fibrous. Periosteum and endosteum have the ability to form bone under appropriate stimulation.

Flat bones, such as those of the skull, also consist of compact and spongy bone. The inner and outer plates (often called tables) consist of thick layers of compact bone, while the space between the plates is bridged by spongy bone called the **diploë.**

Microscopic Structure

KEY WORDS: lamella, lacuna, osteocyte, canaliculus, osteon (haversian system), interstitial lamella, cement line, circumferential lamella, haversian canal, Volkmann's canal

A fundamental characteristic of bone is the arrangement of its mineralized matrix into layers or plates called **lamellae.** Small, ovoid spaces, the **lacunae,** occur rather uniformly within and between the lamellae, each occupied by a single bone cell or **osteocyte.** Slender tubules called **canaliculi** radiate from each lacuna and penetrate the lamellae to link up with the canaliculi of adjacent lacunae (see atlas figure 4-15). Thus, lacunae are interconnected by an extensive system of fine canals.

In compact bone, the lamellae show three arrangements (see atlas figure 4-14). Most are arranged concentrically around a longitudinal space to form cylindrical units that run parallel to the long axis of the bone. These are **osteons** or **haversian systems** that make up the structural units of bone (see atlas figure 4-14). Osteons

vary in size and consist of 8 to 15 concentric lamellae that surround a wide space occupied by blood vessels. In longitudinal sections, an osteon appears as plates of boney matrix running parallel to the slitlike space of the vascular channel. Throughout its thickness, compact bone contains a number of osteons running side by side. Osteons take an irregular course through the length of the bone and may branch.

Other lamellae appear as angular, irregular bundles of lamellar bone that fill the spaces between osteons. These are called **interstitial lamellae** (see atlas figure 4-14). Osteons and interstitial lamellae are outlined by a refractile line, the **cement line,** which consists of modified matrix. Cement lines are not traversed by canaliculi.

At the external surface of the bone, immediately beneath the periosteum, several lamellae run around the circumference of the bone (see atlas figure 4-14). A similar but less well-developed system of lamellae is present on the inner surface, just beneath the endosteum. These two systems of lamellae are the outer and inner **circumferential lamellae,** respectively. The lamellar arrangement of bone is shown in Figure 4-1.

The longitudinally oriented channels at the center of osteons are the **haversian canals** (see atlas figures 4-14 through 4-16). These communicate with one another by oblique branches and by transverse connections called **Volkmann's canals** that penetrate the bone from the endosteal and periosteal surfaces. Unlike haversian canals, Volkmann's canals are not surrounded by concentric lamellae. Volkmann's canals unite the blood vessels within the haversian canals with vessels of the marrow cavity and periosteum. Thus, the nutritional needs of compact bone are met by a vast, continuous network of vascular channels. Canaliculi adjacent to an haversian canal open into the perivascular space, and the canalicular system brings all of the lacunae into communication with the canal.

Spongy bone shows a lamellar structure also but differs from compact bone in that its trabeculae are thin and not usually traversed by blood vessels. Therefore, osteons are rare or lack-

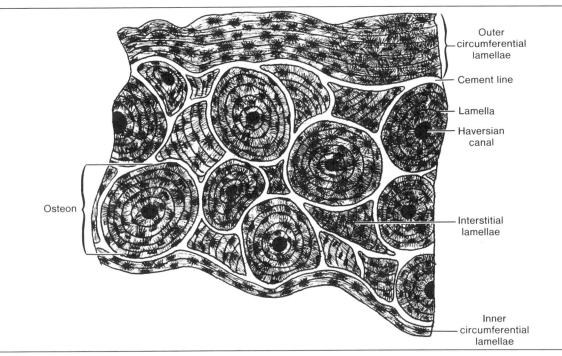

Outer circumferential lamellae

Cement line

Lamella

Haversian canal

Osteon

Interstitial lamellae

Inner circumferential lamellae

Fig. 4-1. Diagrammatic representation of a cross section of ground bone.

ing in the irregular rods of lamellar bone that comprise spongy bone.

Periosteum and Endosteum

KEY WORDS: dense irregular connective tissue, Sharpey's fibers

The outermost layer of the periosteum is a relatively acellular **dense irregular connective tissue** with abundant collagen fibers, a few elastic fibers, and a network of blood vessels, branches of which enter Volkmann's canals. The deeper layers of periosteum (those closest to the bone) are more cellular (osteogenetic layer) and consist of more loosely arranged connective tissue. During development of bone, collagen fibers of the periosteum are trapped in the circumferential lamellae and form **Sharpey's fibers,** which anchor the periosteum to the underlying bone (see atlas figure 4-17).

Endosteum lines all the cavities of bone, including the marrow spaces of the diaphysis and epiphysis and the haversian and Volkmann's canals. It consists of a single layer of squamous to cuboidal cells with a small and variable content of reticular and collagen fibers. As do the cells of the inner layer of the periosteum, the cells of the endosteum retain osteogenic potential.

Cells of Bone

KEY WORDS: osteocyte, osteoblast, osteoclast, Howship's lacunae, ruffled border

Osteocytes are the chief cells found in mature bone and take the shape of the lacunae in which they are housed (see atlas figure 4-18). They differ from **osteoblasts,** which are bone-forming cells. Osteocytes are not isolated in their lacunae but maintain extensive communication with nearby osteocytes. Delicate cytoplasmic processes extend from the cell bodies and traverse the canaliculi to contact processes from neighboring cells. At the points of contact, apposed cells form nexus (communicating) junctions. A thin layer of unmineralized matrix separates the cell and its processes from the walls of the lacunae and canaliculi and provides the means for diffusion of materials throughout the bony matrix.

Osteocytes contain the usual cell organelles, but the Golgi apparatus is relatively inconspicuous, and ribosomes, mitochondria, and endoplasmic reticulum are scarce (see atlas figure 4-25). Although the osteocyte appears to be not actively elaborating protein, it is not metabolically inert. It is responsible for maintaining bone, plays an active role in regulating calcium concentration in the body fluids, and is implicated in the resorption of bone.

In areas where bone is being resorbed, large multinucleate giant cells are present. These are **osteoclasts** that often lie within shallow depressions scooped into the surface of the bone, most frequently along an endosteal surface (see atlas figure 4-26). These cavities are called **Howship's lacunae.** Although the cell may contain as many as 30 nuclei, the individual nuclei show no unusual features and usually are located in the part of the cell farthest from the bone. The cytoplasm, usually weakly to moderately acidophilic, contains multiple Golgi bodies and centriole pairs and numerous mitochondria and lysosomes. The cell surface adjacent to the bone shows a **ruffled border,** a surface modification unique to osteoclasts; osteoclasts that lack a ruffled border do not participate in bone resorption. The border consists of elaborate folds and clefts that abut the surface of the bone; the plasmalemma on the ruffled border is covered by small, bristlelike projections. A clear zone containing many actin filaments lies adjacent to the ruffled border, and mitochondria tend to accumulate nearby. The cell surface farthest from the bone shows a smooth contour. The cytoplasm of active osteoclasts has a frothy appearance due to numerous vacuoles that contain fragments of collagen and crystals of matrix. Osteoclasts arise by fusion of monocytes that have emigrated from the blood.

Osteoclasts are stimulated by parathyroid hormone.

Matrix of Bone

KEY WORDS: ground substance, collagen fiber, inorganic component

Bone matrix forms the bulk of bone and consists of collagen, ground substance, and inorganic components. The **ground substance** contains proteoglycans similar to those of cartilage but in a lesser concentration. Most of the proteoglycans of bone lack acidic sulfate groups.

Collagen fibers are the major organic constituent of bone and are striated fibers whose cross-linked molecules form a network on which bone mineral is deposited. The collagen is present in a highly organized arrangement: In any one lamella the fibers are parallel to each other but run a helical course. The pitch of the helix differs in adjacent lamellae such that the fibers are at right angles to those in the next lamellae. The collagen of bone is exclusively type I.

The **inorganic component** is responsible for the rigidity of bone and consists of calcium phosphate and carbonate with small amounts of calcium and magnesium fluoride. The minerals are present as crystals with a hydroxyapatite structure and are present on and within the collagen at regular intervals along the fibers.

Joints

Adjacent bones are united at joints, which show considerable variation in their structure and function. At some joints, the articulating bones are so interlocked they are immovable, while at others, the joint structure permits a wide range of motion. Based on their structure, joints can be classified as fibrous, cartilaginous, or synovial.

Fibrous joints

KEY WORDS: suture, syndesmosis, gomphosis

Fibrous joints are formed by dense fibrous connective tissue and permit little or no movement.

Sutures are immovable fibrous joints found only in the skull. The gap between the articulating bones is filled by a fibrovascular connective tissue and is bridged at the surfaces by periosteum. Sutures are sites of osteogenic activity and allow for growth of the skull. They are temporary joints; with aging the fibrous connective tissue gradually is replaced by bone to form a permanent boney union (synostosis). The adjoining edges of the bones are highly irregular and interlock to create a firm union. A **syndesmosis,** such as occurs at the inferior tibiofibular joint, contains much more connective tissue than does a suture, allowing somewhat more movement. A third type of fibrous joint is the **gomphosis,** a peg-and-socket joint restricted to the fixation of the teeth into the jaws.

Cartilaginous Joints

KEY WORDS: **epiphyseal plate, synchondrosis, symphysis, amphiarthrosis, intervertebral disc, annulus fibrosus, nucleus pulposus**

Cartilaginous joints are present when bones are united by a continuous plate of hyaline cartilage or a disc of fibrocartilage. The hyaline cartilage of an **epiphyseal plate** forms a temporary joint uniting the shaft and epiphysis of a long bone during its development. This type of immovable joint, a **synchondrosis,** sometimes is classed as a primary cartilaginous joint. Permanent or secondary cartilaginous joints are represented by **symphyses,** which include unions such as those between the pubic bones (pubic symphysis) and between the vertebral bodies. The articulating surfaces are covered by thin layers of hyaline cartilage that in turn are joined to a central disc of fibrous cartilage. The bone, hyaline cartilage, and fibrous cartilage are intimately united, and the joint allows only limited movement (**amphiarthrosis**). The degree of movement possible depends on the thickness of the fibrous cartilage. A slitlike cavity may appear in the fibrous cartilage of some symphyses (e.g., symphysis pubis), but the specialized sliding surfaces of a synovial joint are absent.

In the spine, specialized discs of fibrous car-

tilage form the **intervertebral discs** that make up the major connections between adjacent vertebral bodies. The outer part of the disc, the **annulus fibrosus,** consists of a peripheral zone of collagen fibers and an inner zone of fibrous cartilage that is especially rich in collagen. The central part of the disc, the **nucleus pulposus,** is soft and gelatinous in the young but with aging is gradually replaced by fibrous cartilage. The articular surfaces of each vertebra are covered by thin plates of hyaline cartilage. The annulus fibrosus is firmly attached to the vertebral body by collagen fibers that pierce the cartilaginous end plates and enter the compact bone of the vertebral body as Sharpey's fibers.

Synovial Joints

KEY WORDS: **diarthrosis, capsule, articular disc, meniscus, articular cartilage, tangential zone, transitional zone, radial zone, calcified zone, lamina splendens**

Synovial joints, also called **diarthroses,** are complex, freely mobile joints capable of a wide range of motion. Most of the joints of the limbs fall into this category. The bones involved in the joint are contained within and linked by a **capsule** of dense irregular connective tissue that is continuous with the periosteum over the articulating bones. Additional stability may be provided by intra- and extracapsular ligaments that also are dense irregular connective tissue. The opposing boney surfaces are covered by articular cartilages that provide low-friction gliding surfaces. Although it appears smooth to the naked eye, the free surface of the cartilage is beset with various undulations, troughs, and valleys.

The inner surface of the capsule is lined by a synovial membrane that elaborates the lubricating synovial fluid. An **articular disc** may be interposed completely or partially between the articular surfaces; a partial disc is called a **meniscus.** Discs and menisci consist of fibrous cartilage with an abundance of collagen fibers: at the periphery, they are connected to the capsule. The general structure of a synovial joint is shown in Figure 4-2.

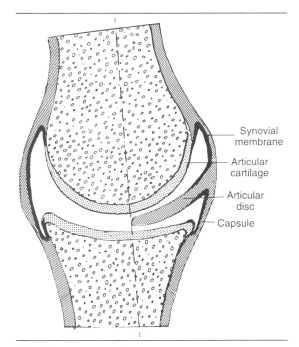

Fig. 4-2. The synovial joint.

The **articular cartilages** of most joints are hyaline in type but show a greater content of collagen than usual. In some joints (e.g., temporomandibular), frank fibrous cartilage is present. Articular cartilage lacks a periosteum, and joint contact is made between the free, uncovered surfaces of the opposing cartilages.

The collagen fibers of articular cartilage have a unique arrangement. At the surface, the fibers are organized into tight bundles that tend to run at right angles to one another and are parallel to the surface. This forms the **tangential zone.** In the deeper **transitional** and **radial zones,** the collagen fibers are randomly arranged. Where it abuts the underlying bone, the articular cartilage becomes calcified and fuses with the bone, thus forming the **calcified zone** in which the collagen fibers are perpendicular to the surface. The diameters of the fibers increase progressively as they pass from the tangential zone to the calcified zone. The fibers of the calcified layer penetrate the subchondral bone, where they are firmly embedded like Sharpey's fibers. Overlying the tangential zone is the **lamina splendens,** a layer of randomly arranged fine fibrils.

The junction between bone and calcified cartilage is irregular and shows fine ridges, grooves, and interdigitations that help unite the subchondral bone and articular cartilage. The junction between the calcified and radial zones appears, in sections, as a basophilic "tide line" that represents the advancing front of the calcification process.

The cells of the articular cartilage also show zonal differences. The tangential zone contains several layers of flattened, fibroblastlike cells whose long axes, like those of the fibers, are parallel to the surface. Their oval or elongated nuclei usually have smooth outlines, but some are irregular and show a variety of undulations, deep indentations, or clefts; the patchy, clumped chromatin stains deeply. The cytoplasm contains short cisternae of granular endoplasmic reticulum (GER), a small Golgi body, and small, round mitochondria. Inclusions such as lipids and glycogen are rare, but pinocytotic vesicles are plentiful.

In the transitional zone, the cells are rounded and show many long cytoplasmic processes that often bifurcate at their tips. The round, usually eccentric nuclei contain finely granular chromatin and frequently show one or more nucleoli. Granular endoplasmic reticulum is abundant, the Golgi apparatus is well developed, and secretory granules are prominent. The cells are scattered randomly throughout the transitional zone.

The cells of the radial zone also are rounded but tend to form short columns or isogenous groups. The endoplasmic reticulum is less developed, the Golgi body is sparse, and mitochondria are small and dense. Intracellular filaments are increased in number, and lipid droplets and glycogen granules are common.

The calcified zone is characterized by short columns of enlarged, pale-staining cells that are in the advanced state of degeneration. The nuclei are dense and pyknotic, the nuclear envelope is fragmented, and cytoplasmic organelles are lacking.

The organization of the chondrocytes of articular cartilage into successive zones is reminiscent of the arrangement of cells in an epiphyseal plate during endochondral bone formation. Indeed, during growth, articular cartilage does serve as a growth zone for the subchondral bone. When epiphyseal growth is complete, the deep zones of chondrocytes in the articular cartilage are converted to compact bone and incorporated into the subchondral bone layer.

Like other cartilage, articular cartilage is avascular and aneural. The central regions of the cartilage receive their nutrition by diffusion from the synovial fluid, which bathes the cartilages, and, to a lesser extent, from vessels in the subchondral bone. At their edges, the articular cartilages are well nourished from blood vessels in the nearby synovial membrane.

Synovial Membrane

KEY WORDS: synovial cell, A-cell, B-cell, areolar synovial membrane, adipose synovial membrane, fibrous synovial membrane, synovial fluid

The synovial membrane is one of the characteristic features of a synovial joint. It is a loose-textured, highly vascular connective tissue that lines the fibrous capsule and extends onto all intra-articular surfaces except those subjected to compression during movement of a joint. Thus, articular cartilages, articular discs, and menisci are not covered by synovial membranes. Occasional fingerlike projections, the synovial villi, and coarser folds of the synovial membrane project into the joint cavity.

The free surface (synovial intima) of the synovial membrane consists of one to three layers of flattened **synovial cells** embedded in a granular, fiber-free matrix. The surface cells do not form a continuous layer, and in places, neighboring cells are separated by gaps through which the synovial cavity communicates with tissue spaces in the synovial membrane. Where the cells do make contact, their surfaces may be complex and interdigitated. Desmosomal junctions have been described in rat synovial membranes, but their presence in humans has not been confirmed.

Ultrastructurally, two types of synovial cells have been described. **A-cells** are predominant and resemble macrophages (hence their alternate name, M-cells). The cell membrane shows numerous invaginations, filopodia, and micropinocytotic vesicles while the cytoplasm contains large Golgi bodies and numerous mitochondria and lysosomes, but only scant profiles of GER. **B-cells** resemble fibroblasts and sometimes are called F-cells. They have a smooth outline and contain abundant GER and scattered free ribosomes. Both cell types contain much glycogen but only a few lipid inclusions. The relationship between A- and B-cells is unknown, but the existence of intermediate forms (AB-cells) suggests that the two may be merely different functional forms of a single type.

The subintimal tissue varies from place to place within the same joint, and based on the structure of this tissue, the synovial membrane is classified as areolar, adipose, or fibrous. In **areolar synovial membranes,** the underlying tissue is a loose connective tissue with relatively few collagen fibers and an abundant matrix. Cellular constituents include fibroblasts, mast cells, macrophages, and lymphocytes. **Adipose synovial membranes** line the articular fat pads, and the subintimal tissue mainly consists of fat cells. In **fibrous synovial membranes,** the underlying tissue is a dense irregular connective tissue and is found in regions subjected to tension; where such forces are extremely high, fibrous cartilage may be present.

Synovial fluid is a clear or slightly yellow viscous fluid that bathes the joint surfaces. Normally, the volume of fluid is sufficient only to form a thin film over all of the surfaces within a joint. In composition, synovial fluid is an ultrafiltrate of plasma to which mucin has been added. Mucin is a product of the surface synovial cells and consists mainly of highly polymerized hyaluronic acid, which gives the viscosity to synovial fluid. Normal synovial fluid contains only 50 to 100 cells per ml, and these consist of macrophages, free synovial cells, and an occasional leukocyte. Amorphous particles and fragments of cells and fibrous tissue may be present and are believed to result from slow wearing of the joint surface.

Development of Cartilage, Bone, and Joints

Cartilage

KEY WORDS: chondroblast, chondrocyte, interstitial growth, appositional growth

All cartilage arises from mesenchyme, and at sites where cartilage is to form, the mesenchymal cells lose their processes, round up, proliferate, and crowd together in a dense aggregate (center of chondrification). The cells in the interior of the mass are **chondroblasts,** which lay down fibers and ground substance. As the amount of intercellular material increases, the cells become isolated in individual compartments (lacunae) and take on the characteristics of **chondrocytes.** New chondroblasts are recruited from the more peripherally placed immature cells. The perichondrium is derived by condensation of the mesenchyme that surrounds the developing cartilage. Further growth occurs by expansion of the mass of cartilage from within (interstitial growth) and by formation of new cartilage at the surface (appositional growth).

Interstitial growth results from proliferation of young chondrocytes that divide and lay down a new matrix to produce an internal expansion of cartilage (see atlas figure 4-6). Such growth occurs only in young cartilage that is plastic enough to allow daughter cells to move away from each other after division. **Appositional growth** occurs as a result of perichondrial chondrogenic activity. The cells immediately adjacent to the cartilage (chondrogenic layer) divide and differentiate into chondrocytes, secrete matrix about themselves, and add new cartilage to the surface. Although adult perichondrium retains some potential to form new cartilage, the capacity for growth and repair is limited by its avascularity. Adult cartilage has the lowest mitotic rate of any skeletal tissue.

Where elastic cartilage forms, chondroblasts at first elaborate fibers that are neither elastic nor collagen in character. These indifferent fibers subsequently mature into elastic fibers. Fibrous cartilage develops much as does ordinary connective tissue, but some fibroblasts transform into chondroblasts and secrete a small amount of cartilage matrix about themselves.

Bone

Bone is mesenchymal in origin and develops by replacement of a pre-existing tissue. If bone is formed directly in a primitive connective tissue, the process is called intramembranous ossification; when replacement of a preformed cartilaginous model is involved, the process is known as endochondral ossification. The essential process of bone formation is the same in both, however.

Intramembranous Ossification

KEY WORDS: osteoprogenitor cell, osteoblast, osteocyte, osteoid, woven bone

The flat bones of the cranium and part of the mandible develop by intramembranous ossification; these bones frequently are called membrane bones. In the areas where bone is to form, the mesenchyme becomes richly vascularized and the cells proliferate actively. Some cells undergo changes that subsequently lead to bone formation and are regarded as **osteoprogenitor cells.** Structurally they closely resemble the mesenchymal cells from which they arise, and their identification depends mostly on their proximity to forming bone.

The osteoprogenitor cells enlarge and transform into **osteoblasts** that lay down bars of matrix. The osteoblasts remain in contact with one another by long tapering processes, and as more and more matrix is deposited, the cells and their processes become entrapped in the matrix (see atlas figure 4-18). The cells then are called **osteocytes.** Ultimately the cells and cell processes are completely enclosed in the matrix, thus forming the lacunae and canaliculi. The first matrix consists of ground substance and collagen fibers and, being unmineralized, is soft. At this stage, the matrix is called **osteoid**; after a short lag period, it becomes mineralized to form true bone. As osteoblasts become trapped in the newly deposited matrix and become osteocytes, new osteoblasts are recruited from differentiation of osteoprogenitor cells.

Bone development by intramembranous ossification occurs in several foci throughout the mesenchymal field and results in the formation of scattered, irregular trabeculae of bone that increase in size by apposition of new bone to their surfaces (see atlas figure 4-24). The resulting bone is of the spongy type. In the first formed bone, collagen fibers run in every direction; the bone is called **woven bone** and has randomly scattered osteocytes and lacks a lamellar arrangement. Woven bone is gradually replaced by lamellar bone.

In areas that become compact bone, such as the inner and outer tables of the skull, the trabeculae continue to thicken by appositional growth and the spaces between them are gradually obliterated. As bone encroaches on vascular spaces, the matrix is laid down in irregular, concentric layers that surround blood vessels and come to resemble osteons, except that the collagen fibers in the lamellae are randomly arranged. These are called primary osteons. Between the plates of compact bone, where spongy bone persists, thickening of the trabeculae ceases and the intervening connective tissue becomes the blood-forming marrow.

The connective tissue surrounding the developing bone condenses to form the periosteum. The osteoblasts on the outer surface of the bone assume a fibroblastlike appearance and are incorporated into the inner layer (cambium) of the periosteum, where they persist as potential bone-forming cells. Similarly, osteoblasts on the inner surface and those covering the trabeculae of spongy bone are incorporated into the endosteum and also retain their potential for producing bone.

Endochondral Bone Formation

KEY WORDS: primary ossification center, periosteal collar, periosteal bud, zone of reserve cartilage, zone of proliferation, zone of maturation and hypertrophy, zone of calcification and cell death, zone of ossification, zone of resorption, epiphyseal (secondary) ossification center, epiphyseal plate, primitive osteon, definitive osteon

The bones of the vertebral column, pelvis, extremities, face, and base of the skull develop by formation of bone in a cartilage model or precursor that must be removed before bone can be laid down. Endochondral bone formation involves simultaneous formation of the bone matrix and removal of the cartilage model. The cartilage does not contribute directly to the formation of bone, and much of the complex process involved in endochondral bone formation is concerned with removal of cartilage.

The first indications of ossification of a long bone appear in the center of the cartilage model in the region destined to become the shaft or diaphysis. In this area, called the **primary ossification center,** the chondrocytes hypertrophy and their cytoplasm becomes vacuolated. Lacunae enlarge at the expense of the surrounding matrix, and the cartilage between adjacent lacunae is reduced to thin, fenestrated partitions. The matrix in the vicinity of the hypertrophied chondrocytes becomes calcified by deposition of calcium phosphate. Diffusion of nutrients through the calcified matrix is reduced and the cells undergo degenerative changes leading to their death.

While these events take place in the cartilage, the vascular perichondrium in this area assumes an osteogenic function. A layer of bone, the **periosteal collar,** forms around the altered cartilage and provides a splint that helps maintain the strength of the shaft. The osteoblasts responsible for development of the bone are derived from perichondrial cells immediately adjacent to the cartilage. In the region of the boney collar the perichondrium now has become a periosteum. Blood vessels from the periosteum invade the altered cartilage forming the **periosteal bud** (see atlas figure 4-19). Contained within the connective tissue sheath that accompanies the blood vessels are cells with osteogenic properties.

With death of the chondrocytes there is no longer a means of maintaining the matrix, which softens. With the aid of the erosive action of invading blood vessels, the thin plates of matrix between lacunae break down. As the adjoining lacunar spaces are opened up, narrow tunnels are formed that are separated by thin bars of calcified cartilage. Blood vessels grow into the tunnels, bringing in osteogenic cells that align themselves on the surface of the cartilaginous trabeculae, differentiate into osteoblasts, and begin to elaborate bone matrix. At first the matrix is laid down as osteoid, but it soon becomes mineralized to form true bone. The early trabeculae thus consist of a core of calcified cartilage with a shell of bone. These primitive trabeculae soon are removed both by continued resorption of the calcified cartilage and through the activity of osteoclasts that appear on the boney shell. An expanding cavity is opened up within the developing shaft. Support for the bone is provided by extension of the periosteal collar, which also becomes thicker as the periosteum lays down new bone at the surface.

This entire process continues as an orderly progression of activity that extends toward both ends of the developing bone. Several areas or zones of activity can be distinguished in the cartilage. Beginning at the ends farthest from the primary ossification center, these are the following:

Zone of reserve cartilage.
This area consists of hyaline cartilage and initially is a long zone but shortens as the process of ossification encroaches on it (see atlas figure 4-20). The cells and their lacunae are randomly arranged throughout the matrix, and there is slow growth in all directions.

Zone of proliferation.
In this region the chondrocytes actively proliferate, and as the cells divide, the daughter cells become aligned in rows separated by a small amount of matrix (see atlas figures 4-20, 4-21, and 4-23). Within the rows, the cells are separated only by thin plates of matrix. Growth occurs mainly in the regions farthest from the reserve cartilage, and the length is increased more than the diameter.

Zone of maturation and hypertrophy.
Cell division ceases and the cells mature and enlarge, further increasing the length of the cartilage (see atlas figures 4-20, 4-21, and 4-23). Lacunae expand at the expense of the intervening matrix, and the cartilage between adjacent cells in the rows becomes even thinner.

Zone of calcification and cell death.
The matrix between the rows of chondrocytes becomes calcified and the cells die, degenerate, and leave empty spaces (see atlas figures 4-21 and 4-22). The thin plates between the cells break down and the lacunar spaces are opened up to form irregular tunnels bounded by the remains of calcified cartilage that had been present between the rows of cells.

Zone of ossification.
Vascular connective tissue invades the tunnellike spaces and provides osteogenic cells that differentiate into osteoblasts. These gather on the surface of the calcified matrix and lay down bone.

Zone of resorption.
Osteoclasts appear on the trabeculae and begin to resorb the bone. Ultimately all the calcified cartilages and their boney coverings are resorbed and the marrow cavity increases in size.

As these changes occur within the cartilage, the periosteal collar increases in length and thickness, gradually extending toward the ends of the developing bone to provide a continuous splint around the area of changing and weakening cartilage.

At about the time of birth, new centers of ossification, **epiphyseal** or **secondary ossification centers,** appear at the ends of long bones. The cartilage of the epiphyses passes through the same sequences as in the diaphysis, but cartilage growth and subsequent ossification spread in all directions and result in a mass of spongy bone. Ultimately, all the cartilage of the epiphysis is replaced by bone except for that at the free end, which remains as articular cartilage. Cartilage also persists between the epiphysis and diaphysis and forms the **epiphyseal plate,** whose continued growth permits further elongation of the bone.

Ossification occurs at the diaphyseal side, and for a time formation of new cartilage and its replacement by bone take place at the same rate so that the thickness of the epiphyseal plate remains constant. Eventually, growth in the plate ceases, the cartilage is replaced by bone (closure of the epiphysis), and further increase in length of the bone is no longer possible. Increase in diameter of the bone results from deposition of bone at the outer surface as a result of the activity of the periosteum, while at the same time, osteoclasts resorb lesser amounts of bone at the endosteal surface. Thus, not only is the gross diameter increased, the thickness of the compact bone and the size of the marrow cavity also increase.

Bone formed by the periosteum represents intramembranous bone and results in a lattice of irregular, boney trabeculae. This is converted to compact bone by a gradual filling of the spaces between trabeculae. Bone is laid down in ill-defined layers, and where they surround and enclose blood vessels, the first haversian systems or **primitive osteons** are formed, in the same way that they form during development of membranous bone. In the primitive osteons the collagen is laid down at random in each lamella. Constant remodeling and reconstruction of bone occurs throughout life, with the primitive osteons being replaced by **definitive osteons;** these in turn are replaced by successive generations of osteons.

Replacement of osteons begins with formation of tunnels within the compact bone as a result of the osteolytic activity of osteocytes and osteoclasts. The cavities widen and enlarge to reach considerable lengths. Osteolytic activity ceases, osteoblasts become active, and bone is deposited on the walls of the cavity until it is refilled as a definitive osteon. The process continues throughout life; resorption cavities continue to form and to be filled with third, fourth, and higher generations of osteons. The resorption cavities do not always coincide with the osteon being replaced, and fragments of older osteons remain as interstitial lamellae. Replacement of osteons and the remodeling of bone is shown in Figure 4-3.

The successive changes occurring during de-

velopment of a long bone are summarized in Figure 4-4. The cartilage model (A) becomes encircled by a periosteal collar in the region that will become the shaft (B), and the cartilage in this area calcifies and degenerates (C). A vascular bud of connective tissue and blood vessels penetrates the altered cartilage, which is resorbed, and the cartilage remnants become covered by bone to form irregular trabeculae. These in turn are soon resorbed and an expanding marrow-filled cavity develops as the process extends toward each end (D). Secondary ossification centers appear in the epiphyses, gradually expanding in all directions (E). Cartilage persists at the ends of the bone and, for a time, as the epiphyseal plate from which all further lengthening will occur (F). Cartilage in the epiphyseal plate ceases its growth and is replaced by bone. The marrow cavity then becomes continuous throughout the length of the bone (G).

Joints

Fibrous Joints

Fibrous joints form simply by the condensation and differentiation of the mesenchyme that persists between developing bones, resulting in formation of a dense irregular connective tissue that binds the bones together.

Cartilaginous Joints

In the early stages of development, a symphysis is represented by a plate of mesenchyme between separate cartilaginous rudiments of bone; the mesenchyme differentiates into fibrous cartilage. When the adjacent cartilaginous bone models have ossified, thin layers of hyaline cartilage are left unossified and persist as laminae of hyaline cartilage between the bone and fibrous cartilage.

The nucleus pulposus of an intervertebral disc develops from the notochord. Early in embryonic life, notochordal cells in the regions between future vertebrae proliferate rapidly but later undergo mucoid degeneration to give rise to the gelatinous nucleus pulposus. The surrounding fibrocartilage of the annulus fibrosus is derived

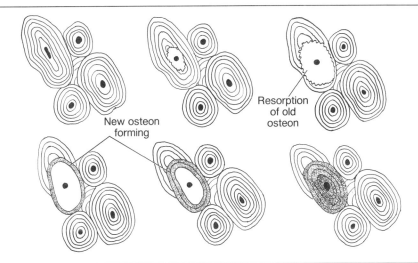

Fig. 4-3. Replacement of osteons during remodeling of bone.

from the mesenchyme between adjacent vertebrae.

Synovial Joints

The formation of appendicular bones is heralded by development of cartilage in the center of each future skeletal element. As the cartilage models expand, their ends approach one another, and the intervening undifferentiated tissue condenses to form the interzonal mesenchyme or midzone from which the joint will form. Simultaneously, the outer layer of mesenchyme also condenses to form the primitive joint capsule, which is continuous with the mesenchyme that gave rise to the perichondrium over the adjacent cartilage model. The mesenchyme enclosed by the primitive joint capsule forms three distinct zones: a central, loose layer of randomly arranged cells lying between two dense layers in which the cells are parallel to the surface of the underlying cartilage. The dense zones give rise to the articular cartilages.

Development of the joint cavity begins in the loose, central region of the interzone with the appearance of small, fluid-filled spaces between the mesenchymal cells. The spaces coalesce and come to form a continuous cavity separating the dense chondrogenic layers and extending along the margins at the ends of the cartilage models. As the spaces unite, the primitive joint capsule completes its differentiation and forms two layers. The outer layer becomes the dense irregular connective tissue of the joint capsule proper, while the inner layer becomes cellular and gives rise to the synovial membrane. Menisci and articular discs develop from the mesenchyme that gave rise to the fibrous joint capsule.

Repair of Cartilage and Bone
Cartilage

Because of its avascularity, mammalian cartilage has a limited capacity to restore itself after injury. Damaged regions of cartilage become necrotic, and these areas then are filled in by connective tissue from the perichondrium. Some of the connective tissue may slowly differentiate into cartilage, but most remains as dense irregular connective tissue that may later calcify or even ossify.

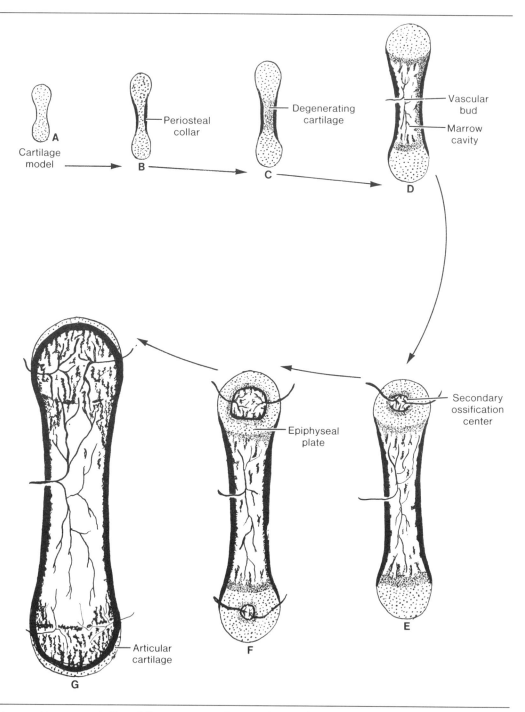

Fig. 4-4. Diagrammatic representation of the successive changes during the development of a long bone.

Bone

Repair of a broken bone is influenced by the size of the bone, the thickness of its compact bone, and the complexity of the fracture. However, the underlying process of repair remains the same and in general recalls the events of bone formation.

A fracture ruptures blood vessels in the marrow, periosteum, and bone itself, and bleeding may be extensive. As a result of the vascular damage, bone dies for some distance back from the fracture site, as do the periosteum and marrow. However, the latter have a greater blood supply than bone tissue itself, so the area of cell death in these tissues is not as great. The blood clot that forms is removed by lysis and phagocytosis. Fibrovascular invasion of the clot immediately around and within the fracture and its conversion to a fibroconnective tissue is not a prominent phenomenon in humans. Repair occurs by activation of osteogenic cells in the viable endosteum and periosteum near the fracture site. The cells proliferate and form new trabeculae of bone within the marrow cavity and beneath the periosteum.

Repair occurring within the marrow cavity can be very important in human fractures. Medullary healing begins as foci of vascular and fibroblastic proliferations in the viable tissue that borders the damaged marrow, followed by osteogenic activity and bone formation. Ultimately, a network of fine bony trabeculae extends across the marrow cavity from cortex to cortex on either side of the fracture and finally across the fracture line, providing an internal scaffold until union of the fractured ends can be effected. All of this new bone arises by intramembranous bone formation and is woven bone. Medullary bone healing is particularly important for the union of fractures in cancellous bones such as the spinal bodies and lower end of the radius and fractures through the metaphysis of long bones.

On the periosteal surface, the repair process arises from the inner osteoblastic layer of the periosteum (osteogenetic layer) beginning a short distance from the fracture zone. Periosteal proliferation occurs on both sides of the fracture gap, resulting in collars of bony trabeculae that grow outward and toward each other, ultimately fusing to span the gap in a continuous arch. The new trabeculae are firmly attached to the old bone surface, including the dead bone. Growth of the osteogenic cells outstrips their vascular supply, so that in the midzone of the fracture site, the cells differentiate into chondroblasts rather than osteoblasts and lay down a callus of hyaline cartilage. This also bridges the fracture gap to form a stabilizing splint around the fracture. The cartilage is converted to bone by endochondral bone formation, but the process is self-limiting and all the cartilage disappears without continuous formation of new cartilage as in an epiphyseal plate. Cartilage always appears during the repair of long bones, whereas flat bones heal without cartilage formation.

Union of the compact cortical bone occurs from sources arising in the medullary cavity or from the periosteum. Since the ends of the bone at the fracture line consist of dead bone, direct union of the fractured ends is very rare if it occurs at all. Occasionally the gap is filled by formation of hyaline cartilage, which then undergoes endochondral ossification to achieve cortical union. More frequently, the bone that initially unites the broken ends is a network of woven bone formed by intramembranous bone formation. The last act in repair is the resorption of excess bone and the remodeling of newly formed and dead bone that is replaced by lamellar bone.

Functional Summary

Cartilage serves as a rigid yet lightweight and flexible supporting tissue. It forms the framework for the respiratory passages to prevent their collapse, provides smooth "bearings" at joints, and forms a cushion between the vertebrae, acting as a shock absorber for the spine. Cartilage is important in determining the size and shape of bones and provides the growing areas in many bones. Its capacity for rapid growth while maintaining stiffness makes cartilage suitable for the embryonic skeleton. About 75 percent of the water in cartilage is bound to proteoglycans, and these compounds are important in the transport of fluids, electrolytes, and nutrients throughout the cartilage matrix.

Bone forms the principal tissue of support and is capable of bearing great weight. It provides attachment for muscles of locomotion, carries the joints, serves as a covering to protect vital organs, and houses the hemopoietic tissue. Bone is the major storehouse of calcium and phosphorus in the body.

Osteocytes are the dominant cells of mature bones and are responsible for maintaining the matrix. They also aid in regulating the calcium and phosphorus levels of the body and play a role in the resorption of bone. Osteoclasts are specifically implicated in bone resorption. They destroy the ground substance and collagen and release minerals from the matrix. These cells elaborate lysosomal enzymes and contain high concentrations of citrate, which is involved in mobilizing calcium from bone. The initial stages of bone resorption by osteoclasts is extracellular; glycosaminoglycans of the matrix are degraded, permitting fragmentation of the bone. The fragments are phagocytosed by osteoclasts and digested intracellularly. The ruffled border of the osteoclasts increases the surface area and may seal off the area of resorption and allow a local environment conducive to the digestion of bone.

Longitudinal growth of a developing bone depends on the interstitial growth of cartilage in the zone of proliferation of the epiphyseal plate and on the enlargement of chondrocytes in the zone of maturation and hypertrophy nearby. Cartilage of the epiphyseal plate is under the influence of growth hormone secreted by cells in the anterior pituitary gland. Increased width of the bone is achieved by appositional growth and the deposition of bone at the boney collar. The first primitive trabeculae consist of cores of cartilage covered by bone. They are formed in the region where the boney collar is thinnest and serve as internal struts to support the developing bone until the collar is thick enough to provide support. As the collar increases in thickness, osteoclasts remove bone at the endosteal surface, thereby enlarging the marrow cavity.

Although most joints serve to allow movement, sutures are immobile and act only to unite bones. Sutures in the young provide areas where bone can grow, and it is only after they have been replaced by boney unions that their uniting functions become paramount. Even the articular cartilages of synovial joints serve as areas of growth for subchondral bone during development. The cartilaginous joints of the spine, although permitting some degree of motion, serve primarily as shock absorbers to dampen and distribute mechanical forces acting on the spine. This is mainly the function of the nucleus pulposus, which, because of its high water content, can act as a water cushion.

The joints specifically designed for movement are the synovial joints. The fibrous capsule and ligaments provide a tough, unyielding binding for the articulating bones yet remain flexible enough to allow movement of the joint. The synovial membrane mainly produces the lubricant of the joint, the synovial fluid, but may also participate in removing particulate matter from the joint cavity. Synovial villi increase the surface area for secretion and absorption, while the larger folds serve as flexible pads that can accommodate to the changing shape and size of the joint space and its recesses during movement. The function of the articular discs and menisci is uncertain, but they may act as shock absorbers, improve the fit between the joint surfaces, spread lubricant, distribute weight over a larger area, or protect the edges of the articular cartilages.

Cartilages form the bearings on which the articulating surfaces of the joint move and offer a wear-resistant surface of low friction — about half that of Teflon, the most slippery of synthetic materials. The arrangement of fibers in the tangential zone places a dense mat of collagen fibers right at the articulating surface. The cartilage is anchored to the underlying bone by collagen fibers (Sharpey's fibers) that are embedded in subchondral bone. The irregular and interlocking margin between the calcified zone and bone further stabilizes the cartilage. The calcified zone also may help regulate diffusion of materials between bone and cartilage.

Synovial fluid provides for the nutrition of articular cartilages, menisci, and articular discs and also lubricates the joint surfaces. Exactly how the synovial fluid performs its lubricating function is unknown. It has been suggested that the fluid forms a thin film between the bearing surfaces and that the lubricating activity depends on internal properties of the fluid such as cohesiveness, shear rate, and flow rate. Another mechanism, "weeping lubrication," has been proposed as a method of joint lubrication. Because of the content of proteoglycans, articular cartilage avidly binds water that, during compression, exudes ("weeps") from the cartilage to lubricate the surface. When compression is removed, fluid is reabsorbed into the cartilage. Thus, weeping lubrication could also serve as a method for pumping nutrients and wastes into and out of the cartilage. A mechanism of "boosted lubrication" takes into account the irregularities normally seen on the surface of articular cartilage. As the cartilage is compressed, pools of synovial fluid are trapped in the furrows and valleys of the articular surfaces. As compression increases, a mobile component of the fluid containing small molecules is forced into the cartilage at the areas of pressure. The fluid in the valleys thus becomes increasingly rich in hyaluronidate and more viscous so that as the pressure increases, the synovial fluid progressively becomes more effective as a lubricant.

Clinical Correlations

Cartilage and Bone

A rare condition of hyaline cartilage is the production of soft, silky fibers that degenerate, leaving variously sized cavities. With aging, extensive degenerative changes occur with loss of chondrocytes and calcification, leaving hard, brittle cartilage.

Osteoporosis is the most common metabolic bone disease. With advancing age, a net loss of bone from the skeleton occurs, apparently progressing more rapidly in women than in men. The condition is asymptomatic until bone fragility leads to pain, disability, and, ultimately, fracture after mild trauma. In osteoporosis, reformation of bone does not keep up with or fully replace the bone resorbed. Mineralization mechanisms are mostly intact, but osteoblastic function is reduced. Microscopically, the spongy bone becomes less dense, marrow spaces are widened, and the cortex is thinned. Haversian canals are enlarged, giving a spongy appearance to the cortical bone. Only scattered osteoblasts are present at the edges of the bone trabeculae. The bone changes occur early in the metaphysis and subchondral regions, where the bone turnover rate is higher.

Scurvy (caused by lack of vitamin C) in the young can produce significant changes in skeletal growth due to depression of normal cellular activity. Reduced osteoblastic activity leads to decreased formation of the bone matrix. Proliferation of chondrocytes in the epiphyseal cartilage is diminished, and the chondrocytes, rather than forming longitudinal columns, show a disorderly arrangement. The zone of calcification is thickened and extended laterally, lifting the periosteum and stimulating the production of periosteal bone at the metaphysis. The trabeculae at this junction of the developing shaft and epiphysis consist of calcified cartilage and lack the borders of osseous tissue; hence they are brittle. Extensive resorption of bone contributes to the tendency to fracture at this region. The epiphyseal plate may separate from the shaft partly or completely, but permanent growth disturbances because of this are unusual.

Osteogenesis imperfecta is a generalized disorder of the connective tissues characterized by abnormal maturation of collagen. Skeletal changes are referable chiefly to defects in the bone matrix. Periosteal bone formation is decreased, resulting in faulty growth in the circumference of long bones. The failure to replace primitive fetal bone by normal lamellar bone leaves a thinned and weakened cortex. The immature collagen in the matrix calcifies poorly and results in irregular, granular areas of calcification. Another collagen disorder, *fibrosis imperfecta ossium*, is characterized by abnormal collagen deposition in lamellar bone, resulting in incomplete mineralization and deposition of abnormally wide bands of osteoid.

Achondroplasia is a genetic disease resulting from failure of endochondral bone formation. All the bones developing in this manner are small, while membranous ossification is normal. At the epiphyseal line, the cartilage cells form only short rows and are irregularly arranged, and little ossification develops. If death does not occur, the child survives as a dwarf with short, thick limbs.

Cells of cartilage or bone may occasionally form benign or malignant tumors (sarcomas). These are classified as either a chondroma, osteoma, chondrosarcoma, or osteosarcoma.

Joints

All joints change with age, and though not necessarily a degenerative change as such, even the simply constructed fibrous sutures become boney unions. In the spine, intervertebral discs undergo progressive alterations and after the third decade of life are likely to show degenerative changes. The nucleus pulposus slowly is replaced by fibrous cartilage and loses water, thereby becoming less resilient and less able to accommodate to changes in pressure. At the same time, the annulus fibrosus becomes softened and weakened and localized fissures or tears may develop. At this stage, a comparatively minor strain on such a joint may cause the nucleus pulposus to bulge into or actually burst through the annulus fibrosus — a so-called slipped disc.

All components of a synovial joint are subject to aging changes. The synovial villi, for example, increase in number and may become very prominent. It is the joint capsules that show the greatest changes. The collagen fibrils of the articular cartilage increase significantly in diameter, and although they retain their normal orientation, the fibrils of the tangential zone becomes less organized, are no longer arranged in tight bundles, and appear fragmented. Gaps occur in the lamina splendens, exposing bundles of collagen to the free surface. Chondrocytes hypertrophy greatly and show extensive development of the GER and Golgi bodies; mitochondria are numerous. Glycogen and lipid inclusions are increased, and myelin figures, derived from lysosomal activity, are common.

Changes also occur at the osteochondral junction, and areas of new bone formation occur in the calcified zone of the articular cartilage and in the adjacent bone. Reduplication of the tide line attests to progressive remodeling of the deep layers of the articular cartilage and indicates advancement of the mineralizing front.

Osteoarthritis is a degenerative disease of synovial joints and appears to be a severe continuation and extension of the degenerative changes associated with aging. The surface of the articular cartilages become roughened, tears that extend into the radial zone appear, and portions of cartilage shear off. The cartilage gradually decreases in thickness, and ultimately, disintegration of the cartilage progresses to where it is worn through to the bone. Microfractures occur in the subchondral bone, and in load-bearing areas, cystic cavities may appear. In advanced osteoarthritis the cavities may communicate with the marrow space.

Spurs or lips of bone (osteophytes) form at the margins of the joint surfaces where the articular cartilage, bone, and capsular tissues meet. This zone is well nourished by the synovial vessels, whereas the central area of the cartilage is less well favored and is prone to degenerative rather than proliferative changes. The spurs are mixtures of woven bone, calcified cartilage, and fibrous tissue. Articular cartilage has the lowest mitotic rate of any skeletal tissue, and repair and growth of articular cartilage is rare if it occurs at all. Osteophyte formation might be regarded as an attempt at repair.

Rheumatoid arthritis is an inflammatory arthritis of unknown cause, but immunologic sequences are involved. Antigen-antibody complexes within the joint appear to initiate and propagate an inflammatory reaction, and the synovial fluid contains excessive numbers of leukocytes including lymphocytes and plasma cells. The main target of the disease is the synovial membrane, which becomes swollen, edematous, highly vascular, and hypercellular. It is densely infiltrated by granular leukocytes, plasma cells, and lymphocytes; multinucleate giant cells also may be present. Proliferation of synovial cells contributes to the thickening of the membrane, which grows out from the articular margins and extends toward the cartilages, eventually covering them. This membrane (pannus) leads to the destruction of the cartilage either through enzyme activity, interruption of the nutrient supply, or both. Beginning at the articular margins, the cartilage becomes disorganized, loses the intercellular matrix, and gradually is destroyed. The characteristic joint deformities that develop reflect the loss of cartilage and subchondral bone and the involvement of the capsule and ligaments in the inflammatory process. The synovial villi increase in size and come to form frond-like structures 1 to 2 mm in diameter. Increased amounts of a low-viscosity synovial fluid are produced.

Gout represents a disease with an underlying metabolic deficiency associated with deposition of crystals in joints, resulting in joint disease. During acute gouty arthritis the synovial fluid may contain numerous white blood cells, most of which are granular leukocytes. The joint cavity contains phagocytosed, needle-shaped crystals of uric acid that damage and kill the leukocytes. Cell necrosis with release of lysosomal enzymes, cell debris, and crystals induces an inflammatory response in the synovial membrane. Thinly encapsulated deposits of uric acid crystals form in the superficial part of the membrane and also may be involved in evoking the inflammation. With repeated attacks, urate deposition occurs in the articular cartilage, synovial membranes, and capsular tissues. Urates penetrate the thickness of the cartilage and collect in the subchondral tissues, resulting in degenerative changes and fragmentation of the cartilage, portions of which are sloughed. Synovial villi are thickened and fragments of cartilage become embedded in or on the surface, producing local irritations. Bone erosion is very common in chronic gouty arthritis and may produce joint deformities similar to those seen in rheumatoid arthritis.

Atlas and Table of Key Features

Key Features in Identifying Cartilage, Bone, and Tendon

Type	Arrangement of cells and lacunae	Other features
Hyaline cartilage	Glasslike matrix; lacunae randomly arranged, slitlike in appearance near perichondrium	Isogenous groups; territorial matrix
Elastic cartilage	Matrix more fibrous in appearance; elastic fibers (need to be stained selectively)	Large isogenous groups
Decalcified bone	Lacunae show organization within lamellae of osteons; haversian canals	Tide marks; bone marrow
Ground bone	Haversian systems; interstitial and circumferential lamellae	Canaliculi between lacunae
Fibrous cartilage	Dense fibrous connective tissue a dominant feature with a small amount of ground substance; lacunae few in number and scattered between fibers	Round-shaped chondrocytes
Tendon	Fibroblast nuclei; dense staining and elongate; lie in parallel rows between collagen fibers	Lacunae absent

Cartilage

Chondrocytes

Matrix

Territorial matrix

Fig. 4-5. Developing hyaline cartilage from the wall of a trachea. (LM, ×250.)

Fig. 4-6. Chondrocytes in growing hyaline cartilage from the trachea. Note the fibrils in the matrix surrounding the chondrocytes. (TEM, ×2,500.)

Chondrocytes

Lacunae

Matrix

Perichondrium

Fig. 4-7. A region of mature hyaline cartilage from the trachea that illustrates the perichondrium. (LM, ×400.)

Fig. 4-8. A region of perichondrium of hyaline cartilage shows the progressive differentiation of fibroblastlike cells to chondroblasts (appositional growth). When surrounded by matrix these cells are termed chondrocytes. (TEM, ×2,500.)

Chondrocytes

Matrix

Lacuna

Fig. 4-9. An example of tracheal hyaline cartilage when examined by scanning electron microscopy. (× 1,000.)

Chondrocytes

Perichondrium

Elastic fibers

Fig. 4-10. An example of elastic cartilage taken from the external ear (pinna). Elastic fibers have been stained specifically by orcein. (LM, × 250.)

Chondrocytes in lacunae

Chondrocytes in lacunae

Collagen bundles

Fig. 4-11. Fibrous cartilage taken from a human symphysis pubis. Note that collagen bundles dominate the field of view and that chondrocytes in lacunae appear only as scattered entities. (LM, ×300.)

Bone

Compact bone

Trabeculae of spongy bone

Fig. 4-12. A cut through the shaft of a human ulna illustrates both compact and spongy bone. (×5.)

Fig. 4-13. A scanning electron micrograph illustrates in greater detail the trabeculae of spongy bone (compare with 4-12). (×50.)

Fig. 4-14. A region of ground, compact bone taken from the peripheral edge of a human ulna illustrates its substructure. (LM, ×250.)

Fig. 4-15. An osteon and its subcomponents taken from a region of compact bone in a human ulna. (LM, ×400.)

Fig. 4-16. A haversian canal in compact bone. (SEM, ×500.)

Fig. 4-17. Sharpey's fibers unite compact bone to the surrounding periosteum (not shown). (LM, ×250.)

Bone Formation

Fig. 4-18. A region of compact bone adjacent to the marrow cavity. Note the presence of osteoblasts. (LM, ×400.)

Periosteum

Osteocyte in lacuna

Layer of osteoblasts

Periosteal collar

Invading connective tissue

Hypertrophied chondrocytes

Fig. 4-19. Invasion of the osteogenic bud into the hyaline cartilage model of a human radius initiates endochondral bone formation. (LM, ×250.)

Osteocytes

Osteoblasts

Osteoclast

Spicule of bone

Zone of reserve cartilage

Zone of proliferation

Hemopoietic tissue

Zone of hypertrophy

Fig. 4-20. Endochondral bone formation in a human fetal finger. (LM, ×100.)

Zones of
calcification
and hypertrophy

Zone of
proliferation

Calcified
cartilage

Fig. 4-21. A region of epiphyseal plate during endochondral bone formation demonstrates several regions of activity. (Sample from fetal human finger.) (LM, ×250.)

Bone

Osteocytes

Hemopoietic
tissue

Zone of
calcification

Calcified
cartilage

Fig. 4-22. A region of epiphyseal plate during endochondral bone formation clearly demonstrates formed bone and the penetration of calcium resulting in the zone of calcification. (Sample from fetal human finger.) (LM, ×250.)

Osteoblasts

Periosteal bone

Osteoblasts

Osteoclast

Hemopoietic tissue

Zone of proliferation

Zone of hypertrophy

Fig. 4-23. A region of endochondral bone formation near the periosteal collar. (Sample from fetal human finger.) (LM, ×300.)

Bone

Mesenchyme

Fig. 4-24. An example of intramembranous bone taken from a human skull. (LM, ×100.)

Fig. 4-25. A pre-osteocyte nearly enveloped by mineralized crystals in the bone matrix. (TEM, ×9,500.)

Fig. 4-26. An osteoclast from a developing human radius. (LM, ×500.)

——————— *Review Questions and Answers* ———————

Questions

18. What would be the advantages and disadvantages of entering the thoracic cavity by an incision made through the costal cartilages? (Ignore the structures in the intercostal spaces.)

19. In what ways are bone and cartilage similar? How do they differ? What do these similarities and differences tell you about possible reparative processes in bone and cartilage?

20. What contributes to lengthening of a bone during endochondral ossification?

21. In which dimension will activity in the secondary ossification center result in an increase in bone size? Growth from the epiphyseal plate increases bone size in which dimension and of which part of the bone?

22. Describe the unit structure of compact bone.

23. What are interstitial lamellae and what is their origin?

Answers

18. Being cartilaginous, the costal cartilages are without a nerve or blood supply of their own. Section through the cartilages therefore would be bloodless and would not sacrifice nerves. However, because cartilage has no blood supply, healing is poor.

19. Bone and cartilage are similar in that the intercellular substance forms the bulk of the tissues, and their constituent cells reside in spaces (lacunae) within the intercellular substance. They are also similar in that both bone and cartilage (except for fibrous cartilage and articular cartilage) are covered by connective tissue membranes (periosteum and perichondrium, respectively) that are able to lay down new bone or cartilage by the process of appositional growth. The tissues differ in that the cartilage cells are isolated and do not communicate, whereas bone cells contact neighboring cells by means of cytoplasmic processes that traverse the bone matrix through the canaliculi. In bone the matrix becomes calcified, whereas under normal conditions cartilage does not calcify; if it does the chondrocytes degenerate. Cartilage is avascular and nutrition is supplied totally by diffusion through the matrix; (compact) bone is a relatively vascular tissue, and diffusion throughout the tissue is accomplished through the canaliculi. Because of its rich vascular supply, bone heals readily following injury, whereas cartilage rarely heals once fractured due to its poor vascularization.

20. Lengthening of bone during its development results from events occurring within the cartilage. Increase in size occurs as a result of interstitial growth in the zone of cell proliferation, with increase in length occurring since the cells tend to align themselves in rows oriented in the long axis. Further increase in length occurs in the region of cell hypertrophy as the cells enlarge.

21. Since bone formation in the secondary centers occurs in all directions, increase in bone size (epiphysis) will likewise be in all directions. Replacement of cartilage by bone occurs at the diaphyseal side of the epiphyseal plate and therefore will result in lengthening of the shaft. It will not contribute to an increase in size of the epiphysis.

22. The unit structure of compact bone is the osteon (or haversian system), which consists of 8 to 12 concentric lamellae of bone arranged about a central canal called the haversian canal. In life the haversian canal is occupied by blood vessels. Arranged

rather uniformly within and between lamellae are lacunae that contain the osteocytes. Extending from each lacunae are fine channels or canaliculi, which join similar structures from adjacent lacunae; the canaliculi that border on a haversian canal make contact with the space of the canal. Thus, all the lacunae are continuous with each other and ultimately with the haversian canal by means of the canalicular system. Osteons are separated from neighboring osteons or other lamellar structures by the cement line. Canaliculi do not penetrate the cement line, so each osteon represents a discrete unit.

23. Interstitial lamellae are angular or irregular groups of lamellae that fill in the spaces between osteons. They represent the remnants of earlier osteons that have been replaced during remodeling of bone.

5 Special Connective Tissue: Blood

Blood often is defined as a special connective tissue in which the intercellular substance is a fluid. Unlike other connective tissues, however, the intercellular substance of blood lacks a fibrous component, and most of the intercellular protein is produced by cells in other tissues (chiefly the liver) and not by the blood cells. In mammals, many of the formed elements of blood consist of anucleate elements (erythrocytes) and bits of cytoplasm (platelets). True cells — leukocytes — make up only a small part of the formed elements and are present only as transients that use the blood for transportation to other organs and tissues into which they migrate to carry out their functions. Only erythrocytes and platelets function while in the bloodstream. None of the formed elements normally replicate within the blood; as they are lost, new elements are added from special blood-forming tissues outside the circulation. Thus, blood can be considered the secretory product of several organs and tissues, rather than a tissue per se.

Regardless of species, the total quantity of blood forms a rather constant proportion of the body mass, generally accounting for 6 to 8 percent of the body weight. In humans the volume is about 5 liters or approximately 7.5 percent of body weight.

Components of Blood

KEY WORDS: formed elements, erythrocyte, platelet, leukocyte, plasma, albumin, fibrinogen, globulin, serum

Blood consists of **formed elements** that include erythrocytes, platelets, leukocytes, and a fluid intercellular material called plasma. These elements can be separated by centrifugation, and when done in calibrated tubes, the result (hematocrit) gives an estimate of the volume of the formed elements. The heaviest components, **erythrocytes,** form the lower layer and in humans make up about 45 percent of the blood volume. **Platelets** and **leukocytes** are present in the buffy coat, a grayish-white layer immediately above the erythrocytes, and form about 1 percent of the total blood volume. The uppermost layer consists of **plasma,** which contains three main types of protein: albumin, globulin, and fibrinogen. **Albumin,** the most abundant and smallest of the plasma proteins, is formed in the liver as is **fibrinogen,** an essential component for blood clotting. The **globulins** (alpha, beta, and gamma) include several proteins of different sizes. The gamma globulins are immunoglobulins (antibodies) synthesized by cells of the lymphatic organs and tissues.

Plasma is obtained from blood after treatment with an anticoagulant and contains all the components of the fluid portion of the blood. **Serum** is obtained from clotted or defibrinated blood and does not contain fibrinogen; it does contain other components elaborated during the process of blood clotting.

Erythrocytes

At rest the average human uses about 250 ml of oxygen and produces almost 200 ml of carbon dioxide per minute. With activity, these quantities can increase 10- to 20-fold. Oxygen and carbon dioxide are carried by the erythrocytes, which transport the gases with great efficiency. Exchange of gases occurs in the blood capillaries of the lung, through which the erythrocytes pass in less than 1 second, yet gaseous exchange is complete in approximately the first third of this time.

Structure

KEY WORDS: anucleate, hemoglobin, absence of organelles

In blood smears and tissue sections, mammalian erythrocytes appear as **anucleate**, uniformly acidophilic bodies devoid of any internal structure. The pigment, **hemoglobin**, makes up about 95 percent of the dry weight. "Erythroplastid" more aptly describes these elements, but custom and common use have given the terms *erythrocyte* and *red cell* the status of proper terminology. Electron microscopy confirms the **absence of organelles** in the interior of mature mammalian red cells, which are unable to synthesize protein or renew constituents of their cell membrane. The cholesterol of the plasmalemma, important for the flexibility of the cell, is controlled by the plasma concentration of cholesterol, not by cell metabolism.

In fish, amphibians, reptiles, and birds, the red cells retain a nucleus and some also show mitochondria, a Golgi complex, and vestiges of endoplasmic reticulum. The purpose of the organelles and nuclei in these red cells is uncertain since they are not known to contribute to the functioning of the cells. At the other extreme is the icefish, which has no erythrocytes. It inhabits the cold waters of the Antarctic, has a slug-

gish existence, and transports gases in the plasma.

Shape and Size

KEY WORDS: biconcave disc, central depression, cell membrane, spectrin, ankyrin

The mammalian red cell usually is described as a **biconcave disc**, but while this shape is typical in humans and some other mammals, it is less obvious in many other species, whose cells appear as flat discs. Face on, the normal erythrocyte presents a smooth rounded contour with a **central depression** in the biconcave forms (see atlas figures 5-1 through 5-3). Elliptical or cigar-shaped red cells are characteristic of the camel, alpaca, and llama, and small spherocytes are present in the chevrotain (mouse deer).

The diameter of red cells varies widely between species but is maintained within close limits within a species and in the individuals of a species. In smears human erythrocytes average 7.6 μm in diameter, are slightly smaller in tissue sections (6.5–7.0 μm), and are slightly larger (about 8 μm) in fresh blood. The largest of all red cells are those of *Amphiuma* and measure 70 μm in their greatest diameter and 37 μm in their least diameter. Among mammals, the smallest red cells are found in the chevrotain while the largest occur in the Indian elephant. Despite the wide variations in diameter, the thickness of the red cell, about 2 μm, is remarkably consistent in all species. Apparently this thickness allows hemoglobin to maintain a distance from the cell surface that is optimum for its function.

Erythrocytes are enclosed in a typical **cell membrane**, whose flexibility and elasticity allow the red cell to accommodate its passage through the small capillaries. In vivo, the cells often assume a cup shape as they pass through blood vessels. A subplasmalemmal network of protein (spectrin) helps to maintain the biconcave shape and still allows flexibility. **Spectrin**, linked by actin, appears to form a web immediately beneath the plasmalemma and may act as a cytoskeleton. The network is attached to the cell membrane by the protein **ankyrin** so that the cytoskeleton and cell membrane are linked to act as a unit. Hemoglobin also might play a role in maintaining cell shape since marked changes in shape are associated with the abnormal hemoglobin of sickle cell anemia.

In fish, birds, reptiles, and amphibians, a bundle of microtubules encircles the perimeter of the flattened cell and serves as an element of the cytoskeleton. Similar structures are not found in mammalian erythrocytes.

Number and Survival

The number of circulating red cells varies among species, and while the correlation is not absolute, there appears to be an inverse relationship between cell size and their numbers. In *Amphiuma*, with its huge nucleated cells, the blood contains 20,000 to 30,000 red cells/mm³, while in the goat, whose red cells average only 4.5 μm in diameter, the same volume of blood contains 12,000,000 to 20,000,000 erythrocytes. Some mammals, including humans, show consistent sex differences in the number of red cells, with lower values occurring in the female. For humans, values of 4,500,000 to 6,000,000/mm³ in the male and 3,800,000 to 5,000,000/mm³ in the female are considered normal.

In general, the survival time of red cells is related to the metabolism of the species and is longer in animals with a low metabolic rate. Survival time increases during hibernation. In humans the survival time is about 120 days. Although red cells generally are removed as they age and wear out, a certain amount of random destruction also occurs; many red cells are destroyed in the marrow without ever being released. The presence of a nucleus does not appear to increase the life span of red cells since some of the shortest-lived erythrocytes are found in species with nucleated red blood cells.

As erythrocytes age, they use up most of the enzymes associated with adenosine triphosphate (ATP) and are unable to maintain themselves, synthesize protein, or renew their cell membranes. By the end of their life span, red cells have become rigid due to loss of cholesterol from the cell membrane and to degradation of protein and its cross-linkage with calcium. These aged red cells are trapped and destroyed by phagocytes mainly in the spleen but also in the liver and bone marrow. Iron in hemoglobin is recovered, stored, and recycled into new red cells.

Reticulocytes

KEY WORDS: polychromatophilic cell, ribonucleoprotein

Most erythrocytes stain an orange red with the usual blood stains, but a few take on a bluish or slate gray tint. These **polychromatophilic cells** are erythrocytes that are not fully mature and contain a small amount of **ribonucleoprotein** that, when stained with brilliant cresyl blue or new methylene blue, precipitates as a network or web. These cells are called reticulocytes (see atlas figure 5-4). Their numbers in peripheral blood provide a rough index of erythrocyte production. Normally, reticulocytes make up only 1 to 2 percent of the red cells in humans, about 1 percent in the dog, and 0.1 percent in cats. Reticulocytes are not found in normal equine blood.

Rouleaux

Mammalian erythrocytes tend to adhere to each other by their broad surfaces to form stacks called rouleaux (see atlas figure 5-1). The tendency is more pronounced in some species: Ruminants generally show little rouleaux formation, while the tendency may be extreme in equine species. Rouleaux depend on changes in the blood plasma rather than in the cell. Any condition that increases the net positive charge in the plasma produces changes in the surface charge of erythrocytes, allowing them to adhere to each other more readily. Rouleaux are temporary phenomena, may occur intravascularly, and appear to do no harm to the red cells. Increased rouleaux are reflected in an increase in the rate at which red cells settle out or sediment.

Abnormalities

KEY WORDS: anisocytosis, macrocyte, microcyte, poikilocytosis, crenated, sickling, hypochromia, target cell, Howell-Jolly bodies, siderocyte, basophilic stippling, spherocyte

Departures from normal size, shape, or staining properties of erythrocytes can be important indicators of disease, but to a much lesser degree, some of these abnormalities may be found in healthy individuals also. **Anisocytosis** describes abnormal variations in the size of red cells, which may be **macrocytes** (larger than normal) or **microcytes** (smaller than normal). In macrocytes the central pale area is less marked than in normal cells, but the concentration of hemoglobin is not increased.

Irregularity in shape is called **poikilocytosis;** the cells may show blunt, pointed, or hook-shaped projections from their surfaces. Under various conditions, red cells in vitro may become shrunken and show numerous projections on their surfaces; these cells are said to be **crenated** and are called echinocytes. Crenated cells can be produced by subjecting normal red cells to fatty acids, anionic compounds, elevated pH, or hypertonic media. The changes are reversible. One of the most severe changes in shape occurs during **sickling** of red cells in sickle cell anemia, in which erythrocytes appear as crescents, holly leaves, or even tubes (see atlas figure 5-5).

Hypochromia denotes cells that stain poorly due to a decrease in hemoglobin; it frequently accompanies microcytosis. In extreme forms, staining may consist simply of a narrow peripheral band. Cells that are thinner than normal (leptocytes) often appear as **target cells** in which the staining is disposed as a central disc and an external band separated by an unstained zone (see atlas figure 5-6).

Howell-Jolly bodies are nuclear fragments left over from the nucleated precursors of the red cell. They appear as one or two rounded or rod-shaped basophilic granules.

Siderocytes contain clusters of small, darkly stained granules that react positively for iron. They are rare in normal peripheral blood but are quite common in bone marrow. Normally the iron-containing granules are removed by the spleen without harming the cell.

Allied to polychromatophilia is **basophilic**

stippling, which appears as blue-black dots that may be coarse or fine and consists of precipitated ribonucleoprotein. It is found occasionally in leukemia and severe anemias but is of diagnostic importance in chronic lead poisoning.

In some pathologic conditions, globular rather than biconcave red cells are produced. These are called **spherocytes** and appear as small, deeply stained cells with a sharp, distinct outline.

Hemoglobin

Gas transport in mammals is carried out by hemoglobin, an iron-containing respiratory pigment that gives the red color to mammalian blood. Many invertebrates have respiratory pigments totally unlike hemoglobin: in crustaceans, for example, the pigment is a copper-containing hemocyanin that takes on a blue color when combined with molecular oxygen. Hemocyanin is not contained within corpuscular elements, however.

Structure

KEY WORDS: heme, globin, HbA, HbA2, HbF, sickle hemoglobin (HbS)

Hemoglobin is one of a group of catalytic compounds that has an iron porphyrin group, heme, attached to a protein, globulin. The **heme** group consists of four pyrrole rings combined with iron through their N groups. Structurally, hemoglobin is a symmetric molecule formed by two equal mirror image halves. Each half molecule contains two different peptide chains, each bearing a heme group around which the chain is coiled. The heme groups form the functional component, and the peptide chains make up the **globin** part of the molecule. The amino acid composition and sequences in the globin confer species specificity to the whole molecule and also determine the type of hemoglobin present. Humans synthesize four structurally different globin chains: alpha, beta, gamma, and delta. About 95 percent of normal adult hemoglobin is hemoglobin A **(HbA)** that contains two alpha and two beta chains; about 2 percent is **HbA2,** which consists of two alpha and two delta chains. The remainder, fetal hemoglobin **(HbF),** is composed of two alpha and two gamma chains. Fetal hemoglobin predominates in fetal life but is replaced by the adult type postnatally.

Even minor modifications of the peptide chain can result in gross changes in the entire hemoglobin molecule, as shown by the **sickle hemoglobin (HbS)** associated with sickle cell anemia. In this disease the only fault in the molecule is in the sixth position of the beta chain, where the glutamic acid of normal hemoglobin has been replaced by valine.

Platelets

Platelets are the second-most numerous of the formed elements of blood and are found only in mammals. In other vertebrates they are represented by thrombocytes. Platelets are not cells but merely fragments of cytoplasm derived from a large precursor cell (megakaryocyte) in the bone marrow.

Structure

KEY WORDS: granulomere (chromomere), hyalomere, actin, myosin, marginal bundle

Platelets are small, anucleate bodies 2 to 5 μm in diameter (see atlas figures 5-6 and 5-9). In stained smears, platelets show a granular part, the granulomere, and a pale, granule-free hyalomere. The **granulomere (chromomere)** often fills the central region of the platelet and may be so compact as to suggest a nucleus. Separation into two zones is not seen in circulating platelets nor in those fixed immediately by drawing blood into fixative. In these conditions, the granulomere remains evenly distributed. Electron micrographs show that the granulomere consists of lysosomes; mitochondria; dense-cored granules that contain serotonin, adenosine diphosphate (ADP), ATP, and calcium; and alpha particles that contain platelet-specific proteins, fibrinogen and other clotting factors, actin, myosin, adenosinetriphosphatase (ATPase), and agents that increase

vascular permeability (see atlas figure 5-7B). Mitochondria are small and few in number and have few cristae. Variable numbers of glycogen granules also are present.

The **hyalomere** represents the cytoplasmic matrix and appears as a homogeneous, finely granular background. A crisscross arrangement of **actin** and **myosin** filaments is present just beneath the plasmalemma. A narrow peripheral zone remains free of granulomere elements and is the site of a system of microtubules that forms the **marginal bundle.** This structure has been described as a single, coiled microtubule that acts as a stiffening element to help maintain the discoidal shape.

Each platelet is bounded by a typical cell membrane that invaginates the cytoplasm and becomes continuous with an elaborate system of channels.

Number

The number of platelets varies widely depending on the species and in individuals also. The variations reflect difficulties in obtaining accurate counts due to physiologic factors that affect the numbers and to inherent properties of the platelets, such as their tendency to stick to foreign surfaces or to each other to form clumps. When in contact with a foreign surface, platelets spread to cover an area several hundred times that of their initial surface. Although platelet levels in humans are given as 250,000 to 400,000/mm^3 of blood, some estimates extend the range to 900,000/mm^3. Transient fluctuations in platelets have been associated with variation in oxygen concentration, exposure to periods of cold, and food intake. Curiously, highly spiced foods have been reported to cause a significant reduction in circulating platelets. Emotional states such as fear and rage result in markedly elevated counts in some animals, especially the cat. A progressive decrease in the number of platelets occurs in women during the two weeks prior to menstruation, with a rapid return to normal values thereafter.

Thrombocytes

In birds, fish, amphibians, and reptiles, platelets are represented by nucleated cells called thrombocytes. Although their size varies somewhat, the general morphology of the thrombocytes is similar in different species. The nucleus conforms to the shape of the cell, which may be rounded, ovoid, or spindle-shaped, depending on the species. Specific granules, mitochondria, scattered ribosomes, and tubules and vesicles of endoplasmic reticulum are present. As in mammalian platelets, thrombocyte mitochondria are scarce, small, and simple in structure, containing only two to three cristae. Thrombocytes readily stick to each other and often appear in small clusters. The cells function in blood coagulation.

Leukocytes

Leukocytes (white blood cells; WBC) are true cells that have nuclei and cytoplasmic organelles and are capable of ameboid movement. They migrate from the blood into tissues, where they perform their functions.

Classification

KEY WORDS: granular, agranular, polymorphonuclear, mononuclear, neutrophil (heterophil), eosinophil, basophil, lymphocyte, monocyte

Leukocytes can be classed as **granular** or **agranular** on the basis of cytoplasmic granulation, or as **polymorphonuclear** or **mononuclear** according to the shape of the nucleus. Granular leukocytes contain multilobed nuclei and thus the terms *granular leukocyte* and *polymorphonuclear leukocyte* denote the same class of cell.

Granular leukocytes (or granulocytes) can be subdivided into **neutrophils (heterophils), eosinophils,** or **basophils** according to the color of their cytoplasmic granules after staining with standard blood stains. Heterophil granules do not stain the same in all species, so the term is used inclusively for this type of granular leukocyte, regardless of staining reaction or species. The term

neutrophil refers to the heterophil of humans. In fish and birds heterophil granules are rod-shaped and eosinophilic, while in rabbits and guinea pigs the homologue of the human neutrophil contains coarse, rounded eosinophilic granules. To distinguish from true eosinophils, the heterophils of rabbits and guinea pigs have been called pseudo-eosinophils.

Agranular leukocytes consist of **lymphocytes** and **monocytes,** which have inconspicuous or no granules and a single, nonlobed nucleus. Thus, the terms *mononuclear leukocytes* and *agranular leukocytes* are used to denote the same class of cells. The distinction between granular and agranular leukocytes is not absolute: Monocytes regularly show fine, dustlike granules that are barely resolvable by light microscopy, and lymphocytes may occasionally show a few coarse granules. The distinction is an old one based on appearances with less refined dyes but remains useful since the granules of granular leukocytes are specific, distinctive, and prominent.

Neutrophil (Heterophil) Leukocytes

KEY WORDS: lobe, filament, band form, drumstick, specific granule, lysozyme, lactoferrin, phagocytin, azurophil granule, lysosome

The neutrophil granulocyte varies from 12 to 15 μm in diameter and is characterized by the shape of the nucleus, which contains small **lobes** connected by fine **filaments** (see atlas figures 5-8A and 5-9). The nucleus stains deeply and the chromatin is aggregated into clumps that form a patchy network. Nucleoli are absent. The number of lobes varies, but in humans, two to four are usual. A single, elongated, nonlobed nucleus is seen in a small number of granulocytes; called **band forms,** they represent cells recently released from the bone marrow (see atlas figure 5-8B). Excessive lobation occurs in some diseases or as an inherited anomaly in humans, and several species normally show up to 7 or 8 lobes. In rats and mice the nucleus frequently forms a ring (annular nucleus) that may be twisted to assume the form of a figure 8. In other species lobation is not as prominent as in humans, and the thin filaments are replaced by coarse narrowings.

In addition to nuclear lobation, nuclear appendages in the shape of hooks, hand racquets, clubs, or **drumsticks** may be present (see atlas figure 5-9). Only the drumstick is significant: It represents the female sex chromatin and usually is found on a terminal lobe in about 2 to 3 percent of the neutrophils.

The cytoplasm of neutrophils contains two types of granules. Most numerous are the **specific granules** (secondary, type B granules), which are small and take on a pinkish hue. These granules contain **lysozyme,** an enzyme complex that acts against components of bacterial cell walls, collagenase, and **lactoferrin,** another antibacterial substance. Several other rather poorly characterized basic proteins (**phagocytins**) are present and also have antibacterial properties. **Azurophil granules** (primary, type A granules) are less numerous, somewhat larger, and stain a reddish purple. They contain lysozyme as well as a battery of acid hydrolases and are considered to be modified **lysosomes.** Azurophil granules are large and homogeneous, whereas the smaller, less dense-specific granules may contain a crystalloid body. A myeloperoxidase that complexes with peroxide to produce activated oxygen, a potent bactericide, also is present in the cytoplasm.

The granules are scattered throughout the cytoplasm except in a narrow peripheral zone that contains fine filaments and microtubules, which appear to function in cell movement (see atlas figure 5-13). A small Golgi complex and a pair of centrioles are located centrally in the cell. Rare profiles of endoplasmic reticulum, a few mitochondria, and ribosomes are present also.

Neutrophils produce a protein that converts plasminogen to plasmin, the proteolytic enzyme responsible for fibrinolysis. Whereas the release of granule-associated factors is associated with death of the cell, release of plasminogen-activating substance is a secretory activity directly related to cell viability.

Neutrophils are the chief leukocytes in humans, forming 55 to 70 percent of the circulating white blood cells. In other species (rats, mice) the heterophils may be less numerous and lymphocytes predominate.

Eosinophil Leukocytes

KEY WORDS: diurnal variation, nuclear lobation, crystalloid, lysosome, myeloperoxidase

Eosinophils form only a small proportion of the white cells and in humans normally make up 1 to 3 percent of the circulating leukocytes. Their numbers in blood bear some relation to the activity of the adrenal glands; a decrease in eosinophils is seen in the alarm reaction. This relationship may account for the wide range of values reported, even for the same animal. For example, the percentage of eosinophils reported in the blood of the cow has ranged from 0 to 30, and similar ranges have been recorded for monkeys and cats. Distinct **diurnal variations** related to activity cycles occur in many animals including humans.

The eosinophil is about the same size as the neutrophil and also is characterized by **nuclear lobation.** Although often described as having a bilobed nucleus, eosinophils with three or four lobes are not uncommon (see atlas figure 5-10A). Conditions that produce hypersegmentation in neutrophils also affect the eosinophil granulocyte. Annular nuclei are common in the eosinophils of rodents and opossums.

The distinctive feature of eosinophils is the closely packed, uniform, spherical granules that stain a brilliant red or orange-red. The granules are membrane-bound and show an internal structure called a **crystalloid** or internus (see atlas figures 5-16 and 5-17). In humans the crystalloid assumes various forms and may be multiple; in the cat the structures are cylindrical and show concentric lamellations. The crystalloid is embedded in a finely granular matrix.

Eosinophil granules are **lysosomes** and contain the usual lysosomal enzymes. They show a higher content of **myeloperoxidase** than do the azurophil granules of neutrophils and lack lysozyme and phagocytin. The granules also contain lipid and a major basic protein (MBP) that is responsible for the eosinophilia.

Basophil Leukocytes

KEY WORDS: nuclear lobe, filament, metachromatic

Basophil granulocytes rarely make up more than 1 percent of the leukocyte count, although an exception is the rabbit, in which values as high as 9 percent are not unusual. In humans basophils make up only about 0.5 percent of the total leukocytes. They are slightly smaller than neutrophil granulocytes and in blood smears measure 10 to 12 μm in diameter.

Nuclear lobes are less distinct than in the neutrophil or eosinophil, and nuclei with more than two or three lobes are rare. **Filaments** between lobes tend to be short and broad and rarely form the threadlike structures seen in neutrophils (see atlas figure 5-10B). Annular nuclei are sometimes seen in the rat, mouse, and opossum. The chromatin is relatively homogeneous and stains less deeply than in the other granulocyte types. Nucleoli are absent.

The cytoplasm of basophils contains prominent, rather coarse granules that stain a deep violet with the standard blood stains and **metachromatically** with toluidine blue or thionin. In the human, well-preserved granules are spherical and uniform but, being soluble in water or glycerin, frequently appear irregular in size and shape in fixed preparations. In the rat the granules are more ovoid, while in the guinea pig, they are distinctly oval and larger than in the human. The granules are scattered unevenly throughout the cytoplasms, often overlie and obscure the nucleus, and are neither as numerous nor as densely packed as the granules of eosinophil leukocytes. Electron microscopy shows an internal pattern of structure of the granules that varies depending on the species (see atlas figure 5-14). In humans a regular striation of the granule has been described, while in the mouse, the granules show a finely reticulated pattern. In the guinea pig a complex lamellation of the basophil granules gives them a honeycomb appearance. The granules contain myeloperoxidase, glycosami-

noglycans, eosinophilic chemotactic factors, prostaglandins, and a platelet-activating factor. The basophilia of the granules is due to the presence of heparin. There is no evidence that the granules have lysosomal activity.

Lymphocytes

KEY WORDS: agranulocyte, small lymphocyte, mononuclear leukocyte, B-lymphocyte (B-cell), humoral immunity, antibody, T-lymphocyte (T-cell), cell-mediated immunity, T-helper cell, T-suppressor cell, lymphokine, cytotoxic T-cell, null cell, large granular lymphocyte, natural killer cell, mitogen, blastogenic transformation, recirculation, memory cell, motility

Lymphocytes occur in all classes of vertebrates, and cells of superficially similar morphology are found in nonvertebrates also. In rats, mice, and guinea pigs, they are the dominant leukocyte, while in other animals they are second only to heterophils. Lymphocytes are the predominant **agranulocyte** in all species and in the adult human account for 20 to 35 percent of the circulating leukocytes.

Classification

Lymphocytes comprise a family of cells, each differing in functions, life span, background, and size. They are found in blood, lymph, lymphatic tissues, and organs. The most common type is the **small lymphocyte** (see atlas figure 5-11). In blood smears this cell has a diameter of 6 to 8 μm and appears to be little more than a nucleus surrounded by a thin rim of pale blue cytoplasm (see atlas figure 5-12A). At one aspect of the cell, the cytoplasm may be somewhat expanded. The round or slightly indented nucleus is heterochromatic and stains deeply. Except in living cells or in electron micrographs, nucleoli usually are not visible. Because of the round nucleus, lymphocytes are classified as **mononuclear leukocytes.** Electron micrographs reveal a small Golgi body and a few mitochondria and lysosomes; a small amount of smooth endoplasmic reticulum is present, but granular endoplasmic reticulum is very scarce. While lymphocytes are classified as agranular leukocytes, a few nonspecific azurophil granules may be present and represent lysosomes.

Although morphologically indistinguishable by ordinary means, small lymphocytes are a mixture of functional types that can be divided into two major classes, B- and T-lymphocytes, by means of distinctive surface markers. **B-lymphocytes (B-cells)** play a central role in **humoral immunity** and represent cells that have been conditioned to transform into plasma cells and secrete **antibody** when stimulated by foreign antigens. The antibody reacts specifically with the antigen that induced its formation. The organ responsible for conditioning B-cells in mammals appears to be the bone marrow. In aves, B-cells are processed in the bursa of Fabricius, a lymphoreticular, appendix-like diverticulum of the cloaca. B-cells form only 5 to 10 percent of the blood lymphocytes in humans.

T-lymphocytes (T-cells) have been processed by the thymus, where they acquire distinctive T-cell antigens and become immunologically competent. However, immunologic capacities are not fully developed until the cells are exported to peripheral lymphatic organs, especially the spleen. T-cells contribute to **cell-mediated immunity** and perform a variety of functions within the immune system. When appropriately stimulated, some T-cells interact with B-cells and, as **T-helper cells,** amplify the production of antibody; as **T-suppressor cells,** they dampen antibody formation. Other T-cells produce **lymphokines** that have important roles in body defenses. Of the many lymphokines described, the best characterized are agents that damage or destroy foreign cells or interfere with their replication, such as lymphotoxin, interleukin, interferon, and tumor necrosis factor; agents that inhibit migration of macrophages (MIF) and thus concentrate macrophages at the site of an antigen; macrophage-activating factor, which stimulates macrophage activity; lymphocyte blastogenic factor (LBF) that induces blastic transformation, growth, and differentiation of small lymphocytes; factors that attract neutrophil, eosinophil, or basophil granulocytes to the sites of antigens (i.e., chemotactic agents); and factors that increase vascular permeability. Thus, lymphokines represent a large class of lymphocyte-derived substances that have a role in controlling immunologic and inflammatory responses or have cytotoxic activities.

Some activated T-cells, the **cytotoxic T-cell** or killer (K) lymphocytes, take part in antibody-dependent, cell-to-cell interactions with foreign cells that result in lysis of the target cell. Only target cells that share antigens with the foreign cell originally inciting the appearance of cytotoxic cells are killed. Cytolysis of the foreign cell requires intimate contact between the effector and its target, the latter then undergoing a series of membrane changes that result in rupture of the cell. The K lymphocyte is unharmed by the interaction and remains free to react with other target cells.

A third class of small lymphocyte, the **null cell,** has been described. These cells lack B- or T-cell surface markers. Null cells also appear to be a diverse group among which may be circulating hemopoietic stem cells.

Larger forms of lymphocytes, 10 to 14 μm in diameter, also are present in peripheral blood in small numbers. These cells have been called **large granular lymphocytes.** The cytoplasm of these cells is more abundant and more basophilic than that of the small lymphocyte. Electron micrographs show an increased number of ribosomes and mitochondria, a greater amount of endoplasmic reticulum, and an increase in the size of the Golgi apparatus. Scattered azurophil granules are present. These cells are directly cytotoxic and also lyse target cells by contact, but they appear to function in the absence of antibody and without known prior exposure to antigen. Thus, they have been named **natural killer (NK) cells.** Commonly considered to be null cells, there is growing evidence that they are a subset of T-cells and may be related to immune-dependent, cytotoxic T-cells. The mechanism of NK cell activity is unknown, but it appears to involve the azurophil granules, which have been identified as lysosomes.

Stimulation by Antigens and Mitogens

Small lymphocytes are not simply terminal effector cells engaged in T- or B-cell activities; they also have the properties of "stem" cells and can propagate additional small lymphocytes when stimulated by antigens or nonspecific agents called **mitogens.** The best studied mitogens are plant extracts — phytohemagglutinin (PHA), concanavalin A (con A), pokeweed mitogen (PWM) — but other agents such as liposaccharide from *E. coli*, antilymphocyte serum, and various pollens also have mitogenic activity. These agents have a common ability to bind to surface groups on small lymphocytes, thereby triggering **blastogenic transformation.**

During transformation, small lymphocytes progressively enlarge; the nuclei increase in size and become euchromatic, nucleoli become visible, the Golgi body enlarges, and the cell synthesizes deoxyribonucleic acid (DNA) and ribonucleic acid (RNA). Within 36 to 48 hours, the small lymphocyte has assumed the appearance of a lymphoblast that divides and gives rise to new T- or B-cells. The new cells can produce lymphokines (T-cells) or become plasma cells and synthesize antibody (B-cells).

The reactions to mitogens show a degree of specificity: PHA and con A stimulate T-cells but not B-cells; *E. coli* lipopolysaccharide stimulates only B-cells; PWM activates both types of small lymphocyte. The mechanism of the reaction is not understood, but the reaction is specific to lymphocytes in that although these agents bind to the surface of other cells, they do not induce their transformation. The response of lymphocytes to mitogens resembles that after exposure to antigen or lymphoblastic lymphokine.

Lymphocytes **recirculate** repeatedly between the blood, lymphoid organs, and lymph. Only small lymphocytes recirculate, and most of these (80–85 percent) are long-lived cells of T-cell origin, with a life span measured in years. A small proportion (12–15 percent) of the circulating cells are short-lived B-cells with a life expectancy of several months. Until the lymphocytes make contact with an antigen, the cells continue to recirculate. A small number of long-lived cells, of T- and B-origin, are present as **memory cells.** These are small lymphocytes that have been stimulated by antigen but have not responded with production of antibody or lymphokines. They remain for years as conditioned cells that can react immediately to the same antigen on subsequent exposure to it.

Lymphocytes are highly **motile** cells that leave the bloodstream to enter lymphatic organs, migrate through connective tissues of the body, or penetrate into epithelia. They have little ability to adhere to or to spread on surfaces of any kind.

Monocytes

KEY WORDS: **mononuclear leukocyte, azurophil granule, primary lysosome, mononuclear phagocyte system**

Monocytes make up the second type of **mononuclear leukocyte** normally found in the blood. Their proportions are fairly consistent throughout most species, and they regularly form 3 to 8 percent of the circulating leukocytes. They vary in size from 12 to 20 μm in diameter and contain a fairly large nucleus that may be rounded, kidney-shaped, or horseshoe-shaped (see atlas figures 5-9 and 5-12B). Segmentation of the nucleus and formation of filaments never occur, but coarse constrictions with blunt, broad lobes may be present. The chromatin is more loosely dispersed than in lymphocytes and therefore stains much less densely. Two or three nucleoli may be seen. The blue-gray cytoplasm is abundant and contains numerous fine **azurophilic granules** that impart an opacity to the cytoplasm, giving it a "ground glass" or "dusty" appearance.

Ultrastructurally, the nucleus shows one or more nucleoli and the cytoplasm contains a small amount of granular endoplasmic reticulum, ribosomes, and polyribosomes. Small, enlongated mitochondria are present, and the Golgi apparatus is well formed. The azurophil granules represent **primary lysosomes** and in electron micrographs appear as dense, homogeneous structures.

Monocytes are part of the **mononuclear phagocyte system** and represent the cells of this system in transit. They serve little function while in the blood but migrate into various organs and tissues throughout the body, where they differentiate into macrophages. In addition to serving as tissue scavengers, monocytes also have a role in processing antigen in the immune response and are able to fuse with one another to form various phagocytic giant cells. Macrophages do not possess true storage granules for their enzymes as do granulocytes, and the cell behaves mostly as a secretory cell.

Abnormalities

KEY WORDS: leukocytosis, leukopenia, neutrophilia, neutropenia, lymphocytosis, lymphopenia, Döhle's bodies, toxic granulation, Alder's anomaly, hypersegmentation, macropolycyte, Pelger-Huët anomaly

As with erythrocytes, the total number of circulating leukocytes tends to fall within a relatively narrow range in normal individuals. In humans, this range is 5,000 to 12,000/mm³. An increase above normal is called a **leukocytosis** and may be due to disease or emotional or physical stress. In humans a leukocytosis with counts of 25,000 to 35,000/mm³ has been reported after severe exercise. The increase represents the flushing of leukocytes sequestered in capillary beds and marginated at the edges of the bloodstream. A decrease in leukocytes is called **leukopenia.** Diurnal variations of variable degree are associated with activity cycles in a number of animals, including humans. In some animals, higher white counts occur in males, but no significant sex differences in leukocyte counts have been recorded in humans.

Fluctuations in leukocyte numbers in humans usually involve neutrophil granulocytes and lymphocytes. If neutrophil granulocytes are in excess, a **neutrophilia** is said to be present; if decreased, a **neutropenia** is present. An increase or decrease in lymphocytes is a **lymphocytosis** or **lymphopenia,** respectively. Increases in eosinophils, basophils, and monocytes are referred to as an eosinophilia, basophilia, and monocytosis, respectively. Decreases in these cells are difficult to establish from smears because of their normally low numbers, but they do exist.

Various cytologic abnormalities may occur, especially among the granulocytes. **Döhle's bodies** are small, irregular blue clumps or patches, 0.5 to 2.0 μm in diameter, that may appear in the cytoplasm of neutrophils during some infections, after burns, in cancer, or after treatment with some oncolytic drugs. They appear to consist of altered ribonucleoprotein. **Toxic granulation** is seen as coarse, black or purple granules scattered in the cytoplasm of neutrophils and represents altered azurophil granules. Toxic granulation often accompanies Döhle's bodies and, with cytoplasmic vacuolation, may occur during severe bacterial infections. **Alder's anomaly** is a rare abnormality characterized by large, coarse granules in the cytoplasm of neutrophils. An apparently inherited anomaly, it has no pathologic significance.

Hypersegmentation of granulocyte nuclei occurs as an inherited anomaly of no significance and also accompanies anemia resulting from deficiency of vitamin B$_{12}$. In such anemia, the cells are abnormally large and have been called **macropolycytes.** At the other extreme, poorly segmented granulocytes are present in the **Pelger-Huët anomaly,** an inherited condition seen in humans and rabbits. All types of granulocyte are involved, and the mature cells rarely show more than two lobes; more frequently the cells have round nuclei with no filaments. In humans the anomaly is without significance.

Atypical lymphocytes may show vacuolated cytoplasm, folded (monocytoid) nuclei, nuclear vacuolation, or prominent nucleoli. Most of the atypical cells are medium lymphocytes. Dark, basophilic cytoplasmic granules have been reported in the cytoplasm of lymphocytes in cases of gargoylism (Hurler's syndrome), and inclusions similar to Alder's granules occur in the lymphocytes of children as a familial disorder.

Blood in Children

During infancy and childhood, the composition of blood differs significantly from that of adults. Hematologically, a child is not merely a small adult, and children and infants have their own specific blood pictures. In general, the younger the individual, the greater is the deviation from normal adult values and the greater the instability of the blood picture during disease. At birth, the hemoglobin content of red cells is higher than at any subsequent period, and compared to adult values, the number of red cells is increased (a polycythemia) and the cells are macrocytic. An increase in reticulocytes and the presence of nucleated red cells (normoblasts) are characteristic of the normal neonate. Within a few weeks after birth, macrocytes disappear and normal, adult-sized red cells are present. By about the third month of life, hemoglobin levels drop, accompanied by a small decrease in the number of red cells so that the red cells (as judged against adult standards) are hypochromic. This picture is maintained until about the second year, after which the values for red cells and hemoglobin gradually rise to reach adult levels at puberty. It is only after puberty that the sex differences in red cells and hemoglobin become apparent.

The number of leukocytes is much greater in the neonate than in the adult, and neutrophil granulocytes predominate. Most of these cells have only two lobes, many are band forms, and myelocytes and even premyelocytes (immature forms normally found only in bone marrow) may be present. The leukocyte count drops quickly and reaches adult levels by about the third month. From the second week to about the second year, lymphocytes dominate the blood picture rather than neutrophils as in the adult.

In disease states, a child's blood is apt to show far greater deviations and variations than occur in adult blood. An infection that in the adult would produce a mild leukocytosis and an increase in band form leukocytes, in a child may evoke a leukocytosis of leukemic proportions (leukemoid reaction) with the appearance of myelocytes and promyelocytes. Similarly, anemia in a child may be marked by the presence of nucleated red cells where in the adult only polychromatophilia would occur. Lymphocytosis develops much more readily in children, and platelets are apt to fluctuate wildly.

Functional Summary

Blood is important in the transport of materials throughout the body, maintaining the acid-base balance, and providing defense mechanisms. Transport functions include carriage of oxygen to all cells of the body, transport of nutrients, and removal of waste products of cell metabolism. It aids in regulating body temperature by dissipating heat formed during metabolism and distributes hormones, thus integrating the functions of the endocrine system. Through its buffering capacities, blood helps maintain the acid-base balance and ensures an environment in which cells may function normally.

Transport of oxygen and carbon dioxide is a function of erythrocytes and their hemoglobin. Packaging hemoglobin into a cell allows for a local environment in which hemoglobin can function most effectively and not be converted to useless forms. The red cell plasmalemma provides mechanical protection as well as enzymes, which prevent irreversible oxidation of hemoglobin. Retention of hemoglobin in a cell permits increased concentration of the pigment without increasing the viscosity of blood. The absence of a nucleus allows for a smaller cell and a more efficient distribution of hemoglobin within the cell; the anucleate cells of mammals are considerably more efficient in the transport of gases than are their nucleated counterparts. The biconcave shape of the anucleate forms gives hemoglobin optimum access to the surface for gas exchange and allows the cell to undergo considerable increase in volume without rupturing.

Platelets have several diverse functions concerned with maintaining the integrity of the blood vasculature. Because of their ability to stick to one another and to foreign surfaces, platelets can cover and temporarily plug small gaps in blood vessels. They play an important part in blood clotting, releasing factors that initiate the clotting process; they also contain fibrinolytic factors that dissolve clots and thus aid in maintaining the fluidity of blood. They are necessary for clot retraction, which results in a firm, dense clot and reduces its bulk to prevent obstruction of the vessel. Platelets also are important in maintaining the integrity of endothelium, which becomes more permeable when platelets are decreased. Although not synthesized by platelets, the vasoconstrictors epinephrine and 5-hydroxytryptamine (serotonin) are contained in platelets. While probably contributing little to the body's overall defenses, platelets can phagocytize small particles, viruses, and bacteria.

Neutrophils are avidly phagocytic and part of the first line of defense against bacterial infections. Azurophil granules are lysosomes, and phagocytosis by granulocytes is associated with fusion of the granules with the ingested material in the usual manner of lysosomal digestion. The cells also contain lysozyme, which hydrolyzes glycosides in bacterial cell walls, and peroxidase, which complexes with hydrogen peroxide to release activated oxygen, an antibacterial agent. Specific granules contain a number of antibacterial agents including lysozyme; lactoferrin, which binds iron (required by bacteria for growth); and cationic compounds with bactericidal properties.

Eosinophils have a special affinity for antigen-antibody complexes, which tend to bind complement and induce cell lysis. Phagocytosis of the complexes may suppress cell destruction in normal tissues. Enzymes such as histaminase released by eosinophils may dampen allergic responses by degrading histamine and histamine-like substances released from mast cells and basophils. Eosinophils also have a major role in controlling parasitic infections: Eosinophils selectively interact with the larvae of some helminthic parasites and damage them by oxidative mechanisms. A major basic protein (MBP) in the crystalloid core of the eosinophil granules enhances the antibody-mediated destruction of parasites.

Basophil granules have a high content of heparin (an anticoagulant), histamine, vasodilating agents, and slow-reacting substance (SRS). Histamine induces a prompt and transient vasodilation, whereas that induced by SRS is more sustained and occurs after a latent period. Both increase vascular permeability. Basophils play a role in acute systemic allergic reactions; antigens that bind to specific sites on the cell membrane cause degranulation with release of agents that cause smooth muscle spasm, mucous secretion, hives, itching, and rhinitis.

Lymphocytes are concerned primarily with the two major types of immune responses, humoral and cellular. The basis of humoral immunity is the production of antibodies and their diffusion throughout the body fluids. As an antigen enters the body, it is complexed on the surface of B-cells, whose surface antibodies fit determinants on the surface of the antigen. The antigen is internalized and triggers cell proliferation and the differentiation of the lymphocytes into antibody-producing cells. Some of the stimulated cells do not go on to produce immunoglobulins but remain as memory cells. The process of humoral immunity is highly specific: Only those antigens that fit receptors on the surface of B-cells elicit an immune response, and the antibody produced will react only with the antigen that induced its formation.

Cellular immunity depends on T-cells. In response to an antigen, T-cells proliferate and release a variety of lymphokines that may inhibit macrophage migration from the site of the antigen, increase the activity of macrophages, interfere with virus replication, or lyse bacterial walls. For most antigens that stimulate a humoral response, cooperation between T-cells and B-cells is essential, but the nature of this interaction is not known. T-cells may recognize the antigen as foreign and concentrate it on their surfaces before presenting it to the B-cell, or they may elaborate substances that activate the B-lymphocyte.

Monocytes leave the blood and differentiate into tissue macrophages. They not only serve as tissue scavengers, ingesting and removing particulate matter, tissue debris, and infective agents, they also play a role in the immune response. Their exact role in immune reactions is unknown, but macrophages may retain antigen on their surfaces to build up a critical amount that can stimulate B-cells, hold it long enough to stimulate B-cells, or in some way alter the antigen to expose antigenic determinants that are recognizable by lymphocytes. Macrophages also liberate antiviral agents and a number of enzymes that digest collagen, elastin, and fibrin.

Clinical Correlations

A decrease in the number of red cells and/or hemoglobin is called an anemia. Proportional decreases in the number of red cells and the amount of hemoglobin result in a normochromic normocytic anemia in which the red cells appear normal. This type of anemia is seen after acute blood loss, increased destruction of blood (hemolytic anemia), or decreased formation of blood (aplastic anemia).

Microcytic hypochromic anemias are characterized by small red cells that are poorly stained because of a lack of hemoglobin. In severe cases the microcytes show only a thin rim of staining. These anemias have in common defective production of hemoglobin, as in iron deficiency (because of chronic blood loss, or lactation), defective synthesis of heme as in lead poisoning, or defective production of globin as in excess of fetal hemoglobin seen in some thalassemias. In lead poisoning, basophilic stippling is an almost invariable finding.

Macrocytic anemias are most often due to deficiency of vitamin B_{12} or folic acid as occurs with defective absorption, increased demands, or presence of intestinal parasites (decreased absorption). Liver disease and leukemia also may result in a macrocytic anemia. The red cells in macrocytic anemia are large and well-filled with a smaller central area that is paler than normal, so that the cells appear hyperchromic. However, the amount of hemoglobin in the cell increases in proportion to its size, and the concentration of hemoglobin in the cell is normal.

Changes in the leukocytes of the peripheral blood may reflect alterations in the total numbers, the proportions of the different types, or both. A leukocytosis is more likely to be seen in acute than chronic infections, and a marked increase in neutrophil granulocytes (granulocytosis) with the appearance of young forms indicates a severe infection with good response. A normal or low number of granulocytes with the presence of young forms indicates either an early stage of infection or a poor response to infection. The presence of vacuoles and toxic granulation suggests a severe infection with extensive tissue destruction or a poor response to infection.

A localized infection, especially in a confined space such as the middle ear (otitis media) or appendix, tends to produce a greater granulocytosis than does a more generalized infection. Bacterial infections, especially coccal infections, are apt to elicit a neutrophilia. Viral infections are likely to be associated with low or normal counts and a lymphocytosis, as in syphilis, tuberculosis, and infectious mononucleosis. Allergic reactions, parasitic infections, skin diseases, and some neoplasms (e.g., Hodgkin's disease) are associated with an eosinophilia. An increase in monocytes is seen in typhoid fever and protozoal infections and during recovery from a coccal infection; a monocytosis in tuberculosis suggests progressive disease.

Decreased leukocyte counts (leukopenia) are found in acute viral infections, vitamin B_{12} and folic acid deficiencies (macrocytic anemias), and some types of leukemia.

Atlas and Table of Key Features

Key Features of Cells in Peripheral Blood

Cell	Diameter (mm)	Number	Cytoplasm	Nucleus	Nucleolus
Erythrocyte					
Male	7.6	4,500,000 to 6,000,000/mm³	Biconcave	—	—
Female	7.6	3,800,000 to 5,000,000/mm³	Disc eosinophilic	—	—
Platelet	2.1–5	200,000 to 400,000/mm³	Chromomere light blue Hyalomere pale	—	—
Neutrophil	10–15	55–70% of leukocytes	Numerous fine granules, lilac color	2–4 lobes connected by fine filament	—
Eosinophil	10–14	1–3% of leukocytes	Numerous round, red-orange granules	2 lobes connected by filament usual; 4–5 lobes may occur	—
Basophil	10–12	0.5% of leukocytes	Coarse, blue-black granules	Less distinct lobulation, broad nuclear filament	—
Lymphocytes					
Small	6–8	20–35% of leukocytes	Thin, blue rim	Round, deep staining	+
Large	10–14	Small number	Abundant, basophilic	Round, lighter staining than small form	+
Monocytes	10–12	3–8% of leukocytes	Abundant, bluish gray, opaque in appearance	Large, kidney or horseshoe shape	+

Peripheral Blood

Rouleaux

Fig. 5-1. Erythrocytes from human peripheral blood. (SEM, ×2,000.)

Fig. 5-2. Erythrocytes from human peripheral blood. (SEM, ×5,000.)

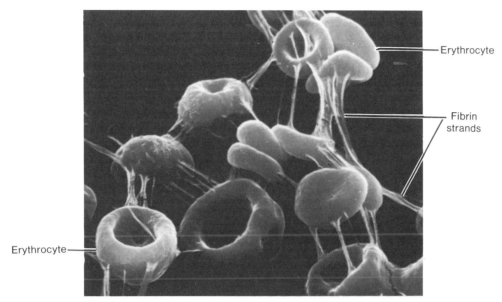

Fig. 5-3. Blood clot of human peripheral blood. (SEM, ×5,000.)

Fig. 5-4. Reticulocytes from human peripheral blood. (LM, ×1,000.)

Crenated erythrocytes

Sickle cell

Crenated sickle cell

Fig. 5-5. Erythrocytes of peripheral blood from a case of human sickle cell anemia. (SEM, ×5,000.)

Platelet

Target cells

Fig. 5-6. An example of human peripheral blood showing a number of erythrocytes that are thinner due to lessened amounts of hemoglobin. These are called target cells. (LM, ×1,000.)

Fig. 5-7. A. Human platelet from peripheral blood. (SEM, ×10,000.) B. Platelets of peripheral blood as seen in section. (TEM, ×8,000.)

Fig. 5-8. A. Neutrophil of human peripheral blood. (LM, ×1,500.) B. Neutrophil band form in human peripheral blood. (LM, ×1,500.)

Erythrocytes

Neutrophil

Platelet

Neutrophil Leukocyte

Monocyte

Drumstick

Fig. 5-9. Erythrocytes and leukocytes of human peripheral blood. (LM, × 1,000.)

Lobe of nucleus

Filament

Granules

Nuclear lobes

Granules

Fig. 5-10. A. Eosinophil from human peripheral blood. (LM, × 1,500.) B. Basophil from human peripheral blood. (LM, × 1,500.)

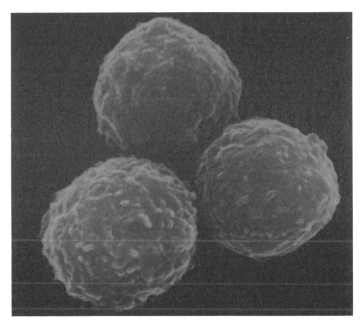

Fig. 5-11. Small lymphocytes from human peripheral blood. (SEM, ×10,000.)

Fig. 5-12. A. Lymphocyte from human peripheral blood. (LM, ×1,200.) B. Monocyte from human peripheral blood. (LM, ×1,200.)

Fig. 5-13. A neutrophil leukocyte within the vasculature of the human liver. (TEM, ×6,000.)

Fig. 5-14. Granules within the cytoplasm of a basophil leukocyte. Note the faint cross striations. (TEM, ×25,000.)

Fig. 5-15. Fibrin fibrils from purified human fibrinogen. (TEM, ×186,000.)

Fig. 5-16. An electron micrograph of a portion of a human eosinophil. The granules contain crystalloids. Note the nuclear filament. (TEM, ×15,000.)

Mitochondrion ——

Granules
with
crystalloids

Fig. 5-17. Granules within the rat eosinophil are characterized by crystalloids that give them a central banded appearance. (TEM, ×20,000.)

Review Questions and Answers

Questions

24. What comprises the complex fluid called blood?
25. How do serum and plasma differ?
26. What is the significance of the "drumstick" observed in polymorphonuclear leukocytes?
27. What is the functional significance of the two types of cytoplasmic granules found in neutrophil granulocytes?
28. Briefly discuss the two major functional types of small lymphocytes.

Answers

24. Most of the intercellular protein of blood is produced by cells in other tissues and not by blood cells. Albumin, the most abundant and smallest of the plasma proteins, is formed in the liver. Fibrinogen, an essential component for blood clotting, also is formed in the liver. Globulins, which include several proteins of different sizes, among which are the immunoglobulins (antibodies), are produced by cells of the lymphatic tissues and organs. The formed elements of blood consist of anucleate elements, erythrocytes, bits of cytoplasm, and the platelets, important in the blood clotting process. Leukocytes, the true cells, make up only a small part of the formed elements and are present as transients that use the blood for transportation to other organs. Only erythrocytes and platelets function while in the bloodstream.

25. Serum is obtained from defibrinated (clotted) blood and does not contain fibrinogen; it does contain other components formed during the clotting process. Plasma, on the other hand, is obtained from blood after treatment with an anticoagulant and contains all the components of the fluid portion of blood.

26. The drumstick of polymorphonuclear leukocytes usually is found on a terminal nuclear lobe and represents female sex chromatin.

27. The cytoplasm of neutrophilic granulocytes contains two types of granules: specific granules and azurophil granules. Specific granules contain lysozyme, collagenase, and lactoferrin. They also contain several other basic proteins called phagocytins that have antibacterial properties. Azurophil granules are considered to be modified lysosomes and contain numerous acid hydrolases as well as myeloperoxidase, a potent bactericide.

28. Lymphocytes are concerned primarily with the immune responses, of which there are two major types, humoral and cellular. The process of humoral antibody production is highly specific; only those antigens that fit receptors on the surface of B-lymphocytes elicit an immune response, and the antibody produced will react only with the antigen that induced its formation. The antigen is internalized and stimulates the proliferation and differentiation of B-lymphocytes into antibody-producing cells. For most antigens that stimulate a humoral response, cooperation between B-lymphocytes and T-lymphocytes is essential; however, the nature of this interaction is poorly understood. Cellular immunity depends on T-lymphocytes. In response to an antigen, T-cells proliferate and release a variety of lymphokines that may inhibit macrophage migration from the site of antigens, increase macrophage activity, lyse foreign cells, or interfere with virus replication. T-lymphocytes may concentrate antigen on their surfaces before presenting it to B-lymphocytes or they may release substances that activate B-lymphocytes. Some T-lymphocytes may suppress responses to foreign (or self) antigens; others may remain as memory cells.

6 Special Connective Tissue: Hemopoietic Tissue

The formed elements of blood are not self-replicating; their numbers in circulation are maintained by continuous replacement from specialized blood-forming (hemopoietic) tissues. In higher vertebrates these consist of bone marrow, spleen, lymph nodes, and thymus, but in lower animals, other organs may be involved. In fish, blood formation may occur in the kidney capsule, liver, wall of the digestive tract, heart, genital organs, or cranial capsule, depending on the species. Reptiles represent a class in which a transition to bone marrow as the major site of blood formation is occurring. In the horned toad, the chief blood-forming organ is the spleen, which produces erythrocytes, monocytes, lymphocytes, and thrombocytes, while the bone marrow is the organ for granulocyte production. In the turtle, the spleen and marrow share the task of hemopoiesis; in the lizard, bone marrow is the active site for production of granulocytes, erythrocytes, and thrombocytes.

Embryonic and Fetal Hemopoiesis

In adult mammals, blood formation is restricted to the bone marrow and lymphatic tissues, but in embryonic and fetal mammalian life, hemopoiesis occurs first in the yolk sac, then successively in the liver, spleen, and bone marrow. Some formation of red cells and platelets normally continues in the spleen in adult rodents and opos-

sums, and in some pathologic conditions, the human liver and spleen may resume a role in hemopoiesis.

Yolk Sac

KEY WORDS: blood island, primitive erythroblast

Blood development in the embryo is virtually the same for all mammals and begins soon after formation of the germ layers. It first occurs in the walls of the yolk sac with the appearance of **blood islands.** Discrete foci of mesenchymal cells of the yolk sac proliferate to form solid masses of cells that soon differentiate along two lines. The peripheral cells flatten and become primitive endothelial cells; the central cells round up, acquire a deeply basophilic cytoplasm, and detach from the peripheral cells to become the first hemopoietic precursors. Most of the first blood-forming cells differentiate into **primitive erythroblasts** that synthesize hemoglobin and become nucleated red cells characteristic of the embryo (see atlas figure 6-19). The isolated blood islands eventually coalesce to form a network of vessels that ultimately join with intraembryonic vessels. Few or no hemopoietic foci develop in the vessels of the embryo proper.

In the human, yolk sac hemopoiesis begins 19 days after fertilization and continues until the end of the twelfth week. Subsequent hemopoiesis in the liver, spleen, and bone marrow develops as the result of migration of stem cells from the yolk sac. The cells gain access to the embryonic circulation via vitelline and allantoic vessels.

Hepatic Hemopoiesis

KEY WORDS: erythropoiesis, definitive erythroblast

The liver is the second important blood-forming organ of the embryo. In humans hepatic hemopoiesis begins during the sixth week of gestation. At this time, hemopoietic cells already make up about 10 percent of the total cells present in the liver. Hemopoiesis reaches a peak at 7 to 8 weeks and remains steady until about the fifteenth week, after which it slowly declines. **Erythropoiesis** dominates throughout the entire period of hepatic hemopoiesis, and while there is significant production of macrophages (monocytes) and platelets during the first 2½ weeks, granulocyte formation is minor. Some neutrophils and eosinophils are produced, almost always in the connective tissue around portal spaces.

The liver remains the principal site of red cell formation from the third to sixth month of gestation; erythropoiesis continues, in decreasing amounts, until birth. Hemopoiesis in the liver resembles that in bone marrow, and the red cell precursors in the liver have been called **definitive erythroblasts** since they give rise to nonnucleated red cells. The developing cells form islands of hemopoietic tissue between the cords of developing hepatic cells, but there is no basement membrane between the hepatocytes and adjacent blood-forming cells (see atlas figures 6-4 through 6-6).

Splenic Hemopoiesis

A low level of splenic hemopoiesis overlaps that of the liver, contributing mainly to the production of erythrocytes, although some granulocytes and platelets are formed also. Erythroblastic islands and some megakaryocytes are present by the twelfth week of gestation. Splenic hemopoiesis wanes as the bone marrow becomes active, but the spleen produces lymphocytes throughout life. In some animals, red cells and megakaryocytes continue to be produced by the spleen even in the adult.

Myeloid Phase

The myeloid phase of hemopoiesis begins when ossification centers develop in the cartilaginous models of the long bones. A few hemopoietic cells can be found in the clavicle of the human fetus at 2½ months. Foci of erythropoietic cells are present in many bones by 4 months, and by 6 months the bone marrow is an important source of circulating blood cells. During the last 3 months of pregnancy, the bone marrow is the main blood-forming organ of the fetus.

Bone Marrow

In the adult mammal, bone marrow is the major organ for production of erythrocytes, platelets, granular leukocytes, and monocytes. Many lymphocytes also are produced in the marrow and reside in the lymphatic tissues secondarily. In toto, the bone marrow constitutes an organ that rivals the liver in weight and in humans is estimated to account for 4 to 5 percent of body weight.

Types

KEY WORDS: red marrow, active hemopoietic marrow, yellow (fatty) marrow, extramedullary hemopoiesis

Bone marrow is an extremely cellular connective tissue that fills the medullary cavities of bone (see atlas figures 6-7 through 6-9). On gross inspection, it may have a red or yellow color. **Red marrow** is actively engaged in the production of blood cells and represents the **active** or **hemopoietic marrow.** The red color is due to the content of red cells and their pigmented precursors. **Yellow (fatty) marrow** is inactive and its principal cellular components are fat cells. Fat cells also are scattered sparingly throughout the red marrow.

The amount and distribution of fatty marrow vary with age, the need for blood cells, and the species. All bones contain active marrow in the late fetus and neonate, but in large animals, including humans, active marrow gradually is replaced by fatty marrow during development and aging. Beginning in the shafts of long bones, fatty marrow gradually replaces red marrow until by adulthood, almost all the marrow in the limbs is the fatty type. Active marrow remains at the ends of the long bones and in the ribs, sternum, clavicles, vertebrae, pelvis, and skull. Gross areas of fatty marrow are not found in small animals, but fat cells are scattered throughout the red marrow. In these animals, fatty marrow makes up about 10 percent of the total marrow, whereas in humans it forms about 50 percent.

Fatty marrow is very labile and easily replaced by active marrow. In dogs that have been made anemic, transition from fatty to red marrow can occur within 48 hours. Yellow marrow serves as a reserve space for the expansion of active marrow to meet increased demands for blood. Active marrow first replaces the fat cells scattered within the red marrow itself, but if demands for blood remain high or are increased, red marrow gradually encroaches into the gross areas of fatty marrow. In animals with little yellow marrow, increased demands for blood are met by replacement of the scattered fat cells and by closer packing of hemopoietic cells. Prolonged or increased demands then are met by expansion of hemopoiesis into other organs or tissues such as the spleen, liver, or lymph nodes. Blood formation in tissues other than the bone marrow is called **extramedullary hemopoiesis** and occurs in humans in some pathologic states.

Structure

KEY WORDS: reticular connective tissue, reticular fiber, hemopoietic cell, free cell, reticular cell, fixed cell

Bone marrow is a specialized connective tissue that, on the basis of its fiber content, can be classed as a **reticular connective tissue.** A loose, spongy network of **reticular fibers** and associated cells fills the medullary cavities of bone and provides a framework for the **hemopoietic cells.** The network of fibers and cells is continuous with the endosteum of the bone and is intimately associated with blood vessels that pervade the marrow. Within the meshes of the reticular network are all of the cell types normally found in blood, their precursors, fat cells, plasma cells, and mast cells. These constitute the **free cells** of the marrow. The **reticular cells** are **fixed cells** that have no special phagocytic powers and do not give rise to precursors of hemopoietic cells. They are fibroblasts responsible for the formation of reticular fibers. Reticular cells have large, palely stained nuclei and irregularly branched cytoplasm that extend long slender processes along the reticular fibers.

Vasculature

KEY WORDS: nutrient artery, central nutrient (longitudinal) artery, sinusoid (venous sinus), adventitial reticular cell, central longitudinal vein

In long bones, the **nutrient artery** enters the marrow cavity through the nutrient canal and gives off **central nutrient (longitudinal)** branches that run centrally in the marrow cavity toward the ends of the bone (see atlas figure 6-8). These are supplemented by branches from epiphyseal and periosteal arteries. Along its course, the central nutrient artery provides numerous branches that pass toward the boney wall. Some of these branches enter the bone to supply osteons; others turn back to the marrow and join the venous system directly by uniting with sinusoids.

Sinusoids (venous sinuses) are thin-walled vessels, 15 to 100 μm in diameter, that form an extensive and complex network throughout the marrow (see atlas figures 6-8 and 6-9). They are lined by thin, flattened endothelial cells that are closely apposed and joined by zonula adherens and gap junctions. A basal lamina is absent or discontinuous, with only scattered patches present on the basal surface. The endothelium is incompletely wrapped by a loose coat of **adventitial reticular cells** whose broad, branching processes merge with the reticular mesh that supports the hemopoietic cells. The adventitial reticular cells contain ribosomes, granular endoplasmic reticulum, and bundles of microfilaments located just beneath the plasmalemma. The proportion of endothelium covered by these cells varies with the functional state of the marrow and may be reduced to one-third when there is heavy cell traffic across the sinusoidal wall.

Sinusoids are the first venous elements. They pass toward the center of the marrow cavity and join the **central longitudinal vein** either directly or after union with other sinusoids to form collecting sinusoids. Thus, in the marrow, blood flows from the center to the periphery and back to the center. The central longitudinal vein also is thin walled and consists of a low endothelium, a thin but complete basal lamina, and a thin outer layer of supporting reticular cells. The venous blood drains from the marrow by a main vein that exits through the nutrient canal, where it narrows abruptly. The blood supply appears to be "closed" — that is, there is endothelial continuity between venous and arterial components.

Distribution of Marrow Elements

KEY WORDS: hemopoietic compartment, vascular compartment, extravascular

The hemopoietic elements form irregular cords between the sinusoids, and collectively, these cords of blood-forming cells make up the **hemopoietic compartment**; the blood vascular components are referred to as the **vascular compartment.** In smears marrow cells appear to be randomly distributed, but in serial sections some ordering of the cells can be seen. Fat cells, though generally scattered, tend to concentrate toward the center of the marrow, where they cluster about the larger blood vessels. The vascular arrangement of the marrow results in a concentration of small vessels, especially sinusoids, at the periphery, and the hemopoietic cells are largely confined to the area near the vessels, close to the endosteum.

Erythrocytes develop in small islets close to the sinusoids with some ordering of the cells within a cluster according to their stage of development. The most mature cells occupy the outer rim of the islet. Macrophages are commonly associated with developing red cells and often lie in the center of an erythroblastic islet surrounded by several layers of red cells. Cells that give rise to platelets (megakaryocytes) are closely applied to the walls of sinusoids and frequently project small cytoplasmic processes through apertures in the sinusoidal wall. Developing granulocytes form nests of cells that tend to locate at some distance from the sinusoids.

Formation of blood cells occurs **extravascularly:** The cells form outside the blood vessels and enter the circulation through the sinusoids. The blood cells must penetrate the outer investment of reticular cells and cross the endothelial lining to gain access to the lumen. In areas of active passage of cells, the reticular sheath is much reduced and the vessel appears to consist only of an endothelium. Blood cells penetrate the endothelium through apertures in the cytoplasm and not by insinuating themselves between adjacent endothelial cells. The openings are relatively large, 1 to 3 μm in diameter. They are not permanent structures and develop only in relation to and during the actual passage of cells.

Stem Cells

KEY WORDS: pluripotent stem cell, spleen colony, colony forming unit (CFU), restricted stem cell, candidate stem cell

The hemopoietic cells of the marrow encompass various developmental stages, from a primitive stem cell to the mature circulating elements in the blood. A stem cell can be defined as a cell that can maintain itself through self-replication and can also differentiate into a more mature cell type. There is much evidence that bone marrow contains a **pluripotent stem cell** capable of giving rise to all the different types of blood cells. Mice given a lethal dose of irradiation soon die from loss of blood cells due to destruction of the hemopoietic organs. However, transfusion of bone marrow soon after exposure to radiation averts death, and both the marrow and the lymphatic tissues are reconstituted by functional cells derived from the transfused marrow. During recovery, macroscopic nodules appear in the spleen;

these **spleen colonies** represent islets of proliferating hemopoietic cells and contain undifferentiated and maturing blood cells. The cells in the marrow inoculum that give rise to the spleen colonies are called **colony-forming units (CFU).**

Some colonies consist only of cells of the erythrocyte line; others contain developing granulocytes or developing megakaryocytes, but many are mixed colonies that contain developing cells of all three lines. The unicellular origin of mixed colonies has been shown by transfusing donor cells that have been irradiated just sufficiently to form unique chromosome markers but not enough to destroy their abilities to replicate. When these cells form spleen colonies, all the constituent cells bear the same marker as the inoculated cells and therefore must have arisen from the same CFU. The unique chromosome marker also appears in cells that are repopulating the thymus and lymph nodes, indicating that the CFU has the potential for forming cells of lymphatic lineage as well. Cultures of cells from granulocytic and mixed colonies produce monocytes and macrophages that also carry the marker chromosome. The reconstituted marrow of these "rescued" animals, when injected into new recipient animals, produces spleen colonies that still carry the marker chromosomes.

Cells from spleen colonies give rise to new spleen colonies when injected into irradiated animals. Even colonies that are purely erythrocytic or granulocytic can give rise to colonies of all types. Thus, the CFU is not only capable of differentiation but also of self renewal, therefore fulfilling the definition of a stem cell. The bone marrow must contain pluripotent stem cells capable of feeding into the erythrocyte, granular leukocyte, megakaryocyte, monocyte, and lymphocyte lines.

In addition to pluripotent stem cells, bone marrow contains stem cells that have a more restricted capacity for development. These **restricted stem cells** are committed to the development of one specific cell line. Experimental evidence supports the existence of restricted stem cells for erythrocytes (CFU-E), granular leukocytes (CFU-G), and megakaryocytes (CFU-Meg).

Most studies suggest a common precursor for granulocytes and monocytes (CFU-GM). Restricted stem cells arise from pluripotent stem cells, are rapidly proliferative, but have limited capacity for self renewal. Pluripotent stem cells are capable of extensive replication but are only slowly proliferative and actually represent a reserve cell. It is the restricted stem cells that provide for the immediate, day-to-day replacement of blood cells.

Based on size, sedimentation velocities, and response to erythropoietin, three categories of restricted erythropoietic stem cells have been defined, and by their growth rates, size, and sedimentation characteristics, two CFU-GM are known. Within a given cell line, the various categories of committed stem cells represent progressions of development from more primitive, but restricted, stem cells to cells that are the immediate precursors of the classic, cytologically recognizable precursor cells.

While the existence of a pluripotent stem cell is certain, its morphology is in doubt; there is evidence, however, that it may be similar in appearance to a lymphocyte. Fractionation of bone marrow on sedimentation columns has shown that CFUs (stem cells) are contained in a fraction whose cells have a size and weight comparable to those of lymphocytes. The number of marrow stem cells can be increased by administering antimitotic drugs that destroy hemopoietic cells capable of division. Since pluripotent stem cells are only slowly proliferative, they are spared and their relative numbers in the marrow are greatly increased. Stem cells can be enriched further by density gradient centrifugation, and as shown by their ability to produce spleen colonies, stem cells increase in number in proportion to an increase in cells with lymphoid appearance. These lymphocyte-like cells have been called **candidate stem cells.** While the morphology generally is similar to that of a small lymphocyte, the nucleus is more irregular and less deeply indented than in most lymphocytes and the chromatin is more finely dispersed. Mitochondria are few in both types of cell but are smaller and more numerous in the candidate stem cell. Free ribosomes but no granular endoplasmic reticulum or lysosomes are present.

The earliest hemopoietic cells are those in the blood islands of the yolk sac, and there is evidence that undifferentiated cells from the yolk sac circulate in the fetus and successively seed the liver, spleen, and marrow. As hepatic hemopoiesis declines, the number of circulating stem cells increases, suggesting a large scale migration of stem cells into the marrow. Cells of blood islands do contain CFUs and can restore all the hemopoietic organs in an irradiated animal.

Development of Erythrocytes

KEY WORDS: erythropoiesis, proerythroblast, basophilic erythroblast, polychromatophilic erythroblast, acidophilic erythroblast (normoblast), reticulocyte

The process of red cell production is called **erythropoiesis,** during which the erythrocyte undergoes progressive changes that involve the cytoplasm and nucleus. The cell progressively becomes smaller, and the cytoplasm stains increasingly acidophilic as it accumulates hemoglobin and loses organelles. The nucleus shrinks and becomes more heterochromatic and condensed until ultimately it is lost from the cell.

Although it is possible to describe various "stages" in the developmental sequence, the process of erythropoiesis does not occur in stepwise fashion. The process is a continuous one in which, at several points, the cells show distinctive, recognizable features. Unfortunately, the nomenclature of the red cell precursors is confused by the multiplicity of names given by various investigators to stages in the maturational series. The terms used here are commonly used, but alternative nomenclature is provided.

The **proerythroblast** (pronormoblast, rubriblast) is the earliest recognizable precursor of the red cell line and is derived from the pluripotent stem cell through a series of restricted stem cells (see atlas figure 6-12). The proerythroblast is relatively large, with a diameter of 15 to 20 μm. The nongranular, basophilic cytoplasm frequently stains unevenly, showing patches that are rela-

tively poorly stained, especially in a zone close to the nucleus. The cytoplasmic basophilia is an important point in the identification of this early form of red cell. Synthesis of hemoglobin has begun, but its presence is obscured by the basophilia of the cytoplasm. The nucleus occupies almost three-fourths of the cell body, and its chromatin is finely and uniformly granular or stippled in appearance. Two or more nucleoli are present and may be prominent. In electron micrographs the endoplasmic reticulum and Golgi apparatus are poorly developed, but free ribosomes are abundant and polysomes are scattered throughout the cytoplasm. The proerythroblast undergoes several divisions to give rise to basophilic erythroblasts.

The **basophilic erythroblast** (basophilic normoblast, prorubricyte) generally is smaller than the proerythroblast, ranging from 12 to 16 μm in diameter. The nucleus still occupies a large part of the cell, but the chromatin is more coarsely clumped and deeply stained. Nucleoli usually are not visible. The cytoplasm is evenly and deeply basophilic, sometimes more so than in the proerythroblast (see atlas figure 6-15). Electron microscopy shows only a few or no profiles of endoplasmic reticulum, but free ribosomes and polyribosomes are abundant. Hemoglobin can be recognized as fine particles of low electron density but, as in the proerythroblast, is not always seen by light microscopy because of the intense cytoplasmic basophilia. The basophilic erythroblast also is capable of several mitotic divisions, its progeny forming the polychromatophilic erythroblasts.

The nucleus of the **polychromatophilic erythroblast** (polychromatophilic normoblast, rubricyte) occupies a smaller part of the cell and shows a dense chromatin network with scattered coarse clumps of chromatin. Nucleoli are absent and the cell is incapable of division. Cytoplasmic staining varies from bluish-gray to light slate gray, reflecting the changing proportions of ribosomes and hemoglobin (see atlas figures 6-13, 6-16A, and 6-21). When nucleoli disappear, no new ribosomes are formed and the change in staining characteristics is the result of a decrease in the concentration of ribosomes (which stain blue) and a progressive increase in hemoglobin (which stains red). Cell size varies considerably but generally is less than that of the basophilic erythroblast. The polychromatophilic erythroblasts encompass several generations of cells, the size reflecting the number of previous divisions that have occurred in the basophilic erythroblast. It is sometimes convenient to divide these cells into "early" and "late" stages on the basis of their size and on the intensity of the cytoplasmic basophilia.

Acidophilic erythroblasts (acidophilic normoblast, metarubricyte) are commonly called **normoblasts.** At this stage the cytoplasm is almost completely hemoglobinized and takes on a distinctly eosinophilic tint. Electron micrographs show a uniformly dense cytoplasm devoid of organelles except for a rare mitochondrion and widely scattered ribosomes. The nucleus is small, densely stained, and pyknotic and often is eccentrically located (see atlas figures 6-11, 6-12, 6-16B, 6-20, and 6-21). Ultimately, the nucleus is extruded from the cell along with a thin film of cytoplasm.

Reticulocytes are newly formed erythrocytes that contain a few ribosomes, but only in a few cells (less than 2 percent) are they in sufficient number to impart color to the cytoplasm. After the usual blood stains, these cells have a grayish tint instead of the clear pink of the more mature forms and hence are called polychromatophilic erythrocytes. When stained with brilliant cresyl blue, the residual ribosomal nucleoprotein appears as a web or reticulum that decreases as the cell matures and varies from a prominent network to a few granules or threads. Reticulocytes are about 20 percent larger in volume than normal mature red cells.

After loss of the nucleus the red cell is held in the marrow for 2 to 3 days until fully mature. Unless there are urgent demands for new erythrocytes, the reticulocytes are not released except in very small numbers. In humans, these young red cells form a marrow reserve equal to about 2 percent of the number of cells in circulation. Figure 6-1 illustrates the changes in cell morphology during formation of erythrocytes.

Proerythroblast. 15–20 μm diameter, basophilic cytoplasm, large nucleus, finely granular chromatin, prominent nucleoli.

Basophilic erythroblast. 12–16 μm diameter, deeply basophilic cytoplasm, nucleus smaller, with coarsely clumped chromatin, no nucleoli.

Polychromatophilic erythroblast. 10–12 μm diameter, cytoplasm varies from blue-grey to slate-grey. Nucleus small with a denser more compact chromatin structure.

Acidophilic erythroblast. 8–10 μm diameter, small pyknotic nucleus, acidophilic or slightly greyed cytoplasm.

Reticulocyte. Slightly larger than mature erythrocyte, acidophilic cytoplasm contains remnants of ribonucleoprotein stainable as a network or web.

Red blood corpuscle.

Fig. 6-1. Cytologic changes during development of erythrocytes.

Loss of Nucleus

Ordinarily, the nucleus assumes an eccentric position in the cell (late normoblast) and is lost just before the cell enters a marrow sinusoid. Active expulsion of the nucleus by the normoblast has been observed in vitro and may involve some contractile protein, possibly spectrin. Enucleation of erythrocytes also has been described as the cells pass through the pores in the sinusoidal endothelium. The flexible cytoplasm is able to squeeze through the pore, but the rigid pyknotic nucleus is held back and stripped from the cell along with a small amount of cytoplasm. Free nuclei are rapidly engulfed and destroyed by macrophages.

Development of Granular Leukocytes

KEY WORDS: granulocytopoiesis, myeloblast, promyelocyte, azurophil granule, myelocyte, specific granule, metamyelocyte, neutrophil band, eosinophil granulocyte, basophil granulocyte

The maturational process that leads to production of mature granular leukocytes is called **granulocytopoiesis**. During this process the cells accumulate granules and the nucleus becomes flattened and indented, finally assuming the lobulated form seen in the mature cell. During maturation, several stages can be identified, but, as in red cell development, the maturational changes form a continuum, and cells of intermediate morphology often can be found. The stages commonly identified are myeloblast, promyelocyte, myelocyte, metamyelocyte, band form, and polymorphonuclear or segmented granulocyte. An alternative nomenclature substitutes the stem "granulo" for "myelo" and the series of stages becomes granuloblast, progranulocyte, granulocyte, metagranulocyte, band form, and polymorphonuclear granulocyte.

Myeloblasts are the first recognizable precursors of granular leukocytes and represent a restricted stem cell committed to granulocyte and monocyte production. It is present in bone marrow only in low numbers. The myeloblast is relatively small, ranging from 10 to 13 μm in diameter. The cytoplasm is rather scant and distinctly basophilic, but much less so than in the proerythroblast, and lacks granules. Electron microscopy reveals abundant free ribosomes but relatively little granular endoplasmic reticulum; mitochondria are numerous and small. The round or oval nucleus occupies much of the cell, stains palely, and presents a somewhat vesicular appearance. Multiple nucleoli are present.

The **promyelocyte** is somewhat larger, measuring 15 to 20 μm in diameter. The nucleus may be slightly flattened, show a small indentation, or retain the round or oval shape. Chromatin is dispersed and lightly stained, and multiple nucleoli still are present. The basophilic cytoplasm contains purplish-red **azurophil granules,** which increase in number as the promyelocyte continues its development. Electron micrographs show abundant granular endoplasmic reticulum, free ribosomes, numerous mitochondria, and a well-developed Golgi apparatus. Azurophil granules are formed only during the promyelocyte stage and are produced at the inner (concave) face of the Golgi complex by fusion of dense-cored vacuoles.

Divergence of granulocytes into three distinct lines occurs at the **myelocyte** stage with the appearance of **specific granules.** Thus, neutrophil, eosinophil, and basophil myelocytes can be distinguished. Myelocytes are smaller than promyelocytes and measure 12 to 18 μm in diameter. The nucleus may be round or indented and the chromatin is more condensed. Some myelocytes still may show a nucleolus outlined by a condensation of chromatin, whereas in others the nucleolus is poorly defined. The myelocyte is the last stage capable of mitosis.

The cytoplasm of the neutrophil myelocyte contains two populations of granules: azurophil granules produced at the promyelocyte stage and smaller specific granules formed by the myelocyte (see atlas figures 6-10 through 6-12). Specific granules also arise by fusion of dense-cored vacuoles but are produced at the outer (convex) face of the Golgi body rather than the concave face. As the myelocyte undergoes successive divisions, the number of azurophil granules in each cell is progressively reduced, and specific granules soon outnumber the azurophil type. The cytoplasm becomes less basophilic, and free ribosomes and granular endoplasmic reticulum are decreased.

Specific neutrophil granules stain lightly in routine blood smears, taking up a delicate lilac-pink color, and are too small to be resolved individually with the light microscope. Azurophil granules are larger and stain purplish red with the usual blood stains, but are less numerous. With the electron microscope, azurophil granules appear more dense than neutrophil granules. The contents of the granules differ; azurophil granules are lysosomes and possess a complex of enzymes, among which aryl-sulfatase, acid phosphatase, β-galactosidase, β-glucuronidase, esterase, and nucleotidase have been identified. Specific neutrophil granules contain alkaline phosphatase and proteins with antibacterial properties.

Myelocytes eventually reach a state at which they no longer can divide and then mature into **metamyelocytes.** These cells show most of the features of the myelocyte except that the nucleus is deeply indented to form a horseshoe or kidney shape, nucleoli are lacking, and the chromatin forms a dense network with many well-defined masses of chromatin (see atlas figures 6-10 through 6-13). Specific granules make up more than 80 to 90 percent of the granules present; the remainder are azurophil.

The **neutrophil band** has the same general morphology as the mature polymorphonuclear cell except that the nucleus forms a variously curved or twisted band. It may be irregularly segmented but not to the degree that definite lobes and filaments have formed (see atlas figure 6-10).

The stages of maturation of **eosinophil granulocytes** are the same as for the neutrophil. Specific eosinophil granules appear at the myelocyte stage and usually are identifiable soon after they appear. Occasionally, the granules may have a slightly purple-blue color, becoming progressively more orange as the cell matures. A rare eosinophil granule may be present as early as the promyelocyte stage. The granules are much larger than the neutrophil type, stain brilliantly with eosin, and in electron micrographs are only slightly less dense and smaller than azurophil granules.

As the cells mature, the cytoplasm becomes less basophilic and the nucleus more and more indented to form lobes (see atlas figures 6-13 and 6-20). In the late myelocyte and the metamyelo-

cyte the contents of the eosinophil granules crystallizes. Some granules show a crystal of variable shape occupying the center of the granule, surrounded by a matrix of lower density; others remain dense and homogeneous. Eosinophil granules are lysosomes and contain the usual battery of lysosomal enzymes.

Basophil granulocytes also pass through the same maturational sequences. The definitive granules usually appear at the myelocyte stage and rarely are seen in the promyelocyte (see atlas figure 6-14). Initially, the granules are truly basophilic but become metachromatic and with toluidine blue or methylene blue stain violet rather than blue-black. In addition to chemotactic and platelet factors, the granules contain heparin, histamine, and several enzymes including diaphorase, dehydrogenases, peroxidases, and histidine carboxylase, which converts histidine to histamine.

The maturational changes and stages of development in granular leukocytes are depicted in Fig. 6-2.

Development of Platelets

KEY WORDS: **thrombopoiesis, megakaryocyte, demarcation membrane, megakaryoblast, endomitosis, polyploidy, promegakaryocyte**

Thrombopoiesis (thrombocytopoiesis) refers to the formation of mammalian platelets or, in other vertebrates, of thrombocytes. In mammals, platelets are derived from giant cells, the **megakaryocytes,** which measure 100 μm or more in diameter. In humans, as in most mammals, megakaryocytes are found only in bone marrow, but in small animals such as rodents, they are present in the spleen also, even in the adult. Those vertebrates that have thrombocytes in place of platelets do not have megakaryocytes.

The nucleus of the megakaryocyte is large and convoluted and contains multiple irregular lobes of variable size interconnected by constricted regions (see atlas figure 6-17). The coarsely patterned chromatin stains deeply. The cytoplasm is abundant and irregularly outlined and often has blunt pseudopods projecting from the sur-

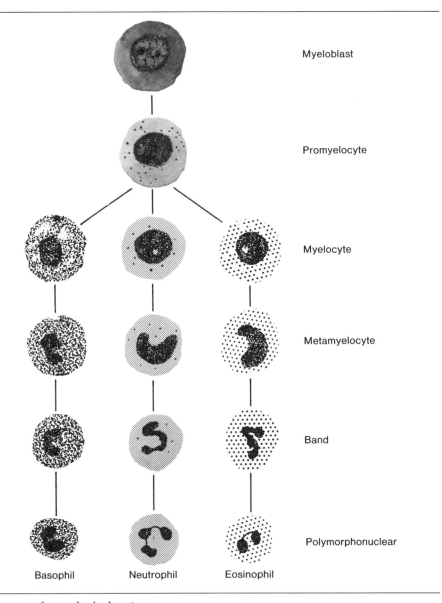

Myeloblast

Promyelocyte

Myelocyte

Metamyelocyte

Band

Polymorphonuclear

Basophil   Neutrophil   Eosinophil

Fig. 6-2. Maturational sequences of granular leukocytes.

face. In smears, the cytoplasm appears homogeneous and contains numerous azurophil granules. Ultrastructurally, a variable degree of zoning is apparent. Immediately around the nucleus a narrow perinuclear zone contains a few

mitochondria, the Golgi complex, granular endoplasmic reticulum, numerous polyribosomes, and some granules. A large intermediate zone is indistinctly separated from the perinuclear zone and contains granules, vesicles of different sizes and shapes, mitochondria, ribosomes, and components of the Golgi element. Depending on the degree of development of the megakaryocyte, the granules may be distributed uniformly or in small clusters outlined to a variable degree by a system of membranes. The outermost marginal zone is finely granular, varies in width, and lacks organelles; it does contain packets of microfilaments.

Platelets are formed by segmentation of the megakaryocyte cytoplasm via a system of **demarcation membranes** (see atlas figure 6-18). The azurophil granules form small clusters, and simultaneously, small vesicles appear that become aligned in rows between the groups of granules. The vesicles initially are discontinuous but subsequently elongate and fuse to create a three-dimensional system of paired membranes. The narrow spaces between the membranes form clefts that surround each future platelet; as they are shed, the platelets separate along the narrow clefts. Demarcation membranes are continuous with the plasmalemma, and thus each platelet is bounded by a typical cell membrane.

The megakaryocyte delivers platelets through openings in the walls of the sinusoids, either as individual platelets or as ribbons of platelets that separate into individual elements within the sinusoidal lumen. After shedding its platelets, the megakaryocyte consists only of a nucleus surrounded by a thin rim of cytoplasm with an intact cell membrane. It generally is assumed that such megakaryocytes are unable to restore their cytoplasm and degenerate, with new generations of megakaryocytes being formed to replace them. Degenerate megakaryocytes can be found in the circulation, especially in the capillaries of the lung, where they may remain for some time.

Megakaryocytes arise from stem cells, the first recognizable precursor being a large cell, 25 to 45 µm in diameter, with a single round or oval nucleus. The chromatin has a finely granular pattern and the basophilic cytoplasm is free of granules. These cells, which are rare, have been called **megakaryoblasts.** The cell undergoes a series of divisions in which the nucleus is replicated but the cytoplasm does not divide (**endomitosis**). At metaphase, the chromosomes become aligned in several planes on an increasingly complex multipolar spindle. With subsequent reconstitution, groups of chromosomes are incorporated into a huge lobulated nucleus. Thus a series of **polyploid** cells arise that in humans and rabbits may reach 64n in some megakaryocytes. In other animals a lesser degree of ploidy is shown, and even in humans and rabbits 16n nuclei are the more common. In general, cell and nuclear size are proportional to the degree of ploidy. The intriguing suggestion has been made that segmentation of the cytoplasm by demarcation membranes represents a delayed and modified cytokinesis. Cells of 4n and 8n ploidy, measuring 30 to 40 µm in diameter, frequently are called **promegakaryocytes.** The fully formed but not yet functional megakaryocyte consistently shows a clear marginal zone, whereas in platelet-forming megakaryocytes this zone disappears.

The nucleated thrombocytes are derived from a mononuclear stem cell, not from megakaryocytes. Maturation of thrombocytes is attended by clumping of the nuclear chromatin, appearance of cytoplasmic granules, elongation of the cell, and a decrease in cytoplasmic basophilia. The thrombocyte retains its nucleus and remains as a distinct complete cell, in contrast to the mammalian platelet, which is a cytoplasmic fragment.

Development of Monocytes

KEY WORDS: promonocyte, azurophil granule, macrophage

Monocytes originate from a pool of precursors in the bone marrow, most likely the same restricted stem cells that give rise to granular leukocytes. In cultures, cells from granulocytic spleen colonies yield monocytes as well as granulocytes.

Immature monocytes of the bone marrow (**promonocytes**) are rare and difficult to distinguish. They range from 8 to 15 µm in diameter and possess large round to oval nuclei with evenly dispersed chromatin and several nucleoli. The cytoplasm is fairly abundant and contains numerous free ribosomes but only scant endoplasmic reticulum. The prominent Golgi complex is associated with numerous small granules that represent the formative stages of azurophil granules.

The mature monocytes of the bone marrow closely resemble those of the blood, are somewhat smaller than promonocytes (9 to 11 μm in diameter), and contain fewer ribosomes and larger and more abundant **azurophil granules.** Azurophil granules contain a variety of hydrolytic enzymes and are primary lysosomes. Following release into the blood, the monocyte continues its maturation in the circulation and additional azurophil granules are formed.

Monocytes migrate into various tissues where they complete their maturation by transforming into **macrophages,** such as those of the peritoneum, alveoli of the lungs, or Kupffer's cells of the liver.

Marrow Lymphocytes

Lymphocytes arise from pluripotent stem cells in the marrow, then emigrate to populate the lymphatic organs and tissues. Restricted stem cells that reach the thymus proliferate there and are released as T-lymphocytes (T-cells). After being released from the thymus, the T-cells migrate to the spleen, where they complete their maturation and are released as long-lived lymphocytes. B-lymphocytes (B-cells) also originate in the marrow. In birds they migrate to the bursa of Fabricius, where they differentiate into B-cells. The mammalian equivalent of the bursa has not been identified, but the bone marrow itself may be the organ for differentiation of B-cells. These cells also appear to complete their development in the spleen. B- and T-cells circulate and recirculate through the blood and lymphatic organs. In humans, B-cells have a life span of at least several months.

Control of Blood Formation

KEY WORDS: hypoxia, erythropoietin

Erythropoiesis is under humoral control and is regulated mainly by a specific erythropoiesis-stimulating factor called erythropoietin. However, the fundamental stimulus for red cell pro-duction is **hypoxia,** since the rate of production of erythropoietin is inversely related to the oxygen supply of the tissues. **Erythropoietin** is a glycoprotein hormone mainly produced by the kidney, though this is not the sole source of erythropoietin since it can be produced in animals whose kidneys have been removed. The sites of extrarenal production of erythropoietin are not known, but small amounts of an erythropoietic-active substance have been detected in liver perfusates.

Erythropoietin increases synthesis of several species of ribonucleic acid (RNA) and protein, followed by the initiation of hemoglobin synthesis and differentiation of the restricted stem cell. Erythropoietin also appears to accelerate hemoglobin synthesis in those more differentiated cells that still are capable of synthesizing RNA and promotes release of reticulocytes from the marrow. Hormones other than erythropoietin have been implicated in blood formation. Testosterone stimulates red cell development and appears to be important for normal maintenance of red cell formation; estrogen has the opposite effect.

Whether there are individual hemopoietic hormones for each of the cell lines in bone marrow is unknown. There is evidence for circulating poietins that control the differentiation of granulocytes and megakaryocytes. These factors, granulopoietin and thrombopoietin, have not been characterized nor is their tissue of origin known. Agents (CFUs) capable of controlling the proliferation and maturation of specific CFUs have been demonstrated in T-lymphocytes.

Lymphatic Tissues

Scattered throughout the body are various lymphatic elements that form part of the body's defense system. Generally distributed so that noxious agents entering the body soon encounter them, lymphatic tissues are prominent in the connective tissue coats of the gastrointestinal, respiratory, and urogenital tracts. Lymphatic structures also are inserted into the lymph drainage and blood circulation, where they serve to filter lymph and blood. Eventually, all the body fluids are filtered through some form of lymphatic structure.

Lymphatic elements may be spread throughout connective tissue and form the lymphatic tissues, or they may be organized into discrete structures, the lymphatic organs.

Classification

KEY WORDS: reticular tissue, hemopoietic tissue, diffuse lymphatic tissue, nodular lymphatic tissue

Lymphatic tissue represents a specialization within the connective tissue compartment and, as for all connective tissues, can be classified according to the type of fiber that is present. On this basis, lymphatic tissue can be defined as a **reticular tissue.** It also contributes cells (lymphocytes) to the blood so it is a **hemopoietic tissue.** In common with bone marrow, the cellular content exceeds the intercellular material. Subdivision of lymphatic tissue into **diffuse** and **nodular** depends on the arrangement and concentration of the cells, not on differences in fiber types.

Cells of Lymphatic Tissues

KEY WORDS: fixed cell; reticular cell; free cell; small, medium, large lymphocyte; plasma cell, macrophage

The cells of lymphatic tissue are present as fixed and free cells. **Fixed cells** are the **reticular cells** responsible for the formation and maintenance of reticular fibers. The fixed cells of lymphatic tissue and reticular fibers, the two elements of the reticular network, are intimately related, and the fibers often reside in deep grooves in the cytoplasm of the reticular cells. By light microscopy, reticular cells appear as elongated or stellate elements with round or oval, palely stained nuclei and scant, lightly basophilic cytoplasm. The cytoplasm is more voluminous than is apparent under the light microscope, since the bulk of it is spread thinly along the reticular fibers. Electron microscopy reveals a variable amount of endoplasmic reticulum and a moderately well-developed Golgi element; other organelles are relatively inconspicuous. As in bone marrow, lymphatic reticular cells are incapable of giving rise to other cell types and show no special capacity for phagocytosis.

The remaining cells of lymphatic tissue are contained within the spaces of the reticular network and constitute the **free cells.** The bulk of these are lymphocytes, but macrophages and plasma cells also are present in variable numbers. The term *lymphocyte* encompasses a spectrum of cells that possess some general common features. As a class they show a rounded, centrally placed nucleus; their cytoplasm shows variable degrees of basophilia and lacks specific granules. The lymphocyte population customarily is divided into small, medium, and large lymphocytes on the basis of their size, nuclear morphology, and intensity of cytoplasmic staining. Although useful for purposes of description, such a subdivision is somewhat artificial since between the small and large types there is a continuum of cell sizes and morphologies.

Small lymphocytes are the most numerous. As seen in lymphatic tissues, these cells are 4 to 8 μm in diameter and contain a deeply stained nucleus surrounded by a thin rim of cytoplasm that may be expanded slightly at one side of the cell. Although rounded in shape in the blood or lymph, in tissues the cells are crowded together and assume various polyhedral shapes due to compression. The rounded or slightly indented nucleus contains a nucleolus that is barely discernible unless thin sections are examined. The chromatin is present as scattered masses of heterochromatin with some small patches of euchromatin. Electron microscopy shows a small Golgi complex, a few mitochondria and centrioles located in the region of the nuclear indentation, a moderate number of ribosomes, and a few lysosomes scattered throughout the cytoplasm. Granular endoplasmic reticulum is sparse.

Medium lymphocytes (prolymphocytes) range from 8 to 12 μm in diameter. Their nuclei are somewhat larger and more palely stained because of greater dispersion of the chromatin, and the nucleoli are larger and better defined. The cytoplasm is more voluminous and shows a greater basophilia because of an increased number of ribosomes.

Large lymphocytes (lymphoblasts) range in size from 15 to 20 μm. Occasionally even larger forms (25 to 30 μm) may be found, and some authors reserve the term *lymphoblast* for these cells. The nucleus is rounded, palely stained, and contains one or two prominent nucleoli, and the fine chromatin is more uniformly dispersed. The basophilic cytoplasm is abundant and contains free ribosomes and polysomes. The centrosomal region and Golgi body are more highly developed and mitochondria are abundant, but granular endoplasmic reticulum remains scanty.

In the development of lymphocytes, it generally is accepted that the direction of maturation is from large (lymphoblast) to small. However, this progression is complicated by the ability of small lymphocytes to respond to antigenic agents, reassume a blastlike appearance and character, and reproduce additional small lymphocytes and plasma cells.

Plasma cells (plasmocytes) vary in size from 6 to 20 μm in diameter. By light microscopy the cell presents a rounded, somewhat elongated or polyhedral form, depending on its location. The nucleus is round to oval and usually is eccentrically placed. This is most obvious in elongated cells, but in rounded cells the nucleus may be only slightly eccentric in its placement. The chromatin is dispersed in coarse heterochromatic blocks along the inside of the nuclear envelope, giving the nucleus a clock face or spoke wheel appearance. Binucleate cells may be seen. The cytoplasm is deeply basophilic except for a prominent pale area adjacent to the nucleus. This area represents a negative image of the Golgi body.

Occasionally, plasma cells contain globular or crystalline inclusions in their cytoplasm, the best known of which are Russell's bodies. These are round or ovoid acidophilic inclusions of variable size that represent incomplete antibody.

In electron micrographs the characteristic feature of plasma cells is the extensive development of the granular endoplasmic reticulum, which almost completely fills the cytoplasm. The cisternae may be flat and parallel or distended with flocculent material. Free ribosomes are numerous, and a well-developed Golgi apparatus and centrioles are present in the paranuclear area. Russell's bodies, when present, are contained within distended cisternae of the granular endoplasmic reticulum. Plasma cells are sessile and ultimately degenerate. Despite the massive amounts of endoplasmic reticulum, most antibody production is carried out by forms that are intermediate between lymphocytes and plasma cells. The precursors of plasma cells are B-lymphocytes.

The **macrophages** of lymphatic tissue are part of a system of mononuclear phagocytes widely spread throughout tissues and organs. The cells vary from 10 to 20 μm in diameter and have oval-, kidney-, or horseshoe-shaped nuclei in which one or more nucleoli are present. The cytoplasm is abundant and lightly basophilic and may be vacuolated or contain ingested material. Unless the cytoplasm does contain phagocytosed matter, the macrophage is difficult to distinguish from other large mononuclear cells including active fibroblasts. In electron micrographs, the cytoplasm shows numerous folds, processes, and invaginations of the surface and contains the usual assembly of organelles. The Golgi apparatus is conspicuous, lysosomes are numerous, and residual bodies may be prominent. As are macrophages elsewhere, those in lymphatic tissue are derived from blood monocytes.

Diffuse Lymphatic Tissue

KEY WORDS: reticular fiber, reticular cell, lymphocyte

Diffuse lymphatic tissue is a constituent of lymphatic organs and also is widely dispersed along mucous membranes. It appears as a rather loose aggregate of cells and shows no distinct demarcation from surrounding tissue with which it gradually merges. Basically, diffuse lymphatic tissue consists of a three-dimensional array of **reticular fibers** and their associated **reticular cells.** The two form a spongelike framework pervaded by large numbers of cells, chief of which are **lymphocytes** (see atlas figure 6-22).

Diffuse lymphatic tissue is particularly prominent in the connective tissue that underlies the epithelium of the intestine. Here the lymphatic tissue, in association with the lining epithelium, produces antibody that bathes the luminal surface. Any antigen that does penetrate the epithelial lining induces an immune response in the lymphatic tissue, the cellularity of which is related to the bacterial content of the intestines.

Nodular Lymphatic Tissue

KEY WORDS: solitary nodule, primary nodule, germinal center, secondary nodule, light pole, dark pole, cap, follicular dendritic cell, confluent lymphatic nodule, Peyer's patch

Nodular lymphatic tissue contains the same structural elements as diffuse lymphatic tissue, differing only in that the components are organized into compact, somewhat circumscribed structures. It may occur anywhere in connective tissue but is prominent along the digestive and respiratory tracts. Lymphatic nodules (also called follicles) may be present as **solitary nodules** or in masses forming confluent nodules as occur in the appendix and the Peyer's patches of the ileum (see atlas figure 6-23). Lymphatic nodules are prominent in organs such as the tonsils, lymph nodes, and spleen but are absent from the thymus.

In ordinary histologic sections, some lymphatic nodules appear as rounded collections of densely packed small lymphocytes; this type of nodule is called a **primary nodule.** Other lymphatic nodules contain a lightly staining central area surrounded by a deeply stained cuff or cap of closely packed small lymphocytes. The pale region has been called a **germinal center** and the whole structure a **secondary nodule** (see atlas figure 6-23).

There are few reticular fibers within the germinal center, and the free cells are supported by a cellular framework consisting of stellate reticular cells. The numerous processes of the reticular cells are joined by desmosomes. Reticular fibers are present in the cuff of cells at the periphery of the center, where they form concentric layers around the structure.

Germinal centers have dark and light poles. The **light pole** is sparsely populated by scattered small lymphocytes and reticular cells, while the **dark pole** is densely packed with large and medium lymphocytes, cells in transition to plasma cells, macrophages, mitotic cells, and the pyknotic nuclei of degenerating lymphocytes. Surrounding the center is a zone of small lymphocytes that usually is thicker at the light pole where it forms the **cap.** A thinner layer of lymphocytes covers the dark pole. The structure shows definite polarity: The light pole always is directed toward a surface — the capsule in lymph nodes, red pulp in the spleen, and the epithelium of a tonsil.

Germinal centers appear to be sites where lymphocytes are formed, but many of the newly formed cells die there. They also are the sites of antibody formation, and each germinal center appears to represent a clone of cells derived from an antigen-stimulated lymphocyte and active in the production of one specific antibody. Germinal centers produce B-cells that can migrate through the cap to leave the center and eventually pass to other lymphatic tissues. Areas where germinal centers develop contain **follicular dendritic cells,** which show numerous complex cytoplasmic processes that interdigitate with follicular lymphocytes. The cytoplasm contains many mitochondria, but ribosomes, lysosomes, and secretory granules are scarce. The nucleus is irregular and shows peripherally placed bars of heterochromatin and a distinct nucleolus. These cells are considered to be antigen-presenting cells that retain antigen on their surface for the stimulation of T-cells.

Germinal centers develop only after birth and in response to antigenic stimuli. They are absent in animals born and raised in a germ-free environment. Following a first exposure to antigen, germinal centers form de novo, then regress in the absence of antigen and eventually disappear. Upon a second stimulation by the same antigen, there is a rapid and marked production of germinal centers, which precedes a rise in circulating antibody. However, germinal centers are not essential for antibody formation, and it has been suggested that germinal centers arise only after repeated contact with antigen and may be involved in long-term (memory) antibody responses.

Aggregate or **confluent lymphatic nodules** occur in the appendix and are exemplified by Peyer's patches found in the lower half of the small intestine. **Peyer's patches** consist of many solitary nodules massed together to form grossly visible structures that underlie the intestinal epithelium. The light poles of their germinal centers are directed toward the epithelium. Individual nodules may be quite discrete and well defined, but usually they coalesce and can be distinguished only at their apices and by their germinal centers. Peyer's patches are prominent in children but undergo gradual regression with aging.

Interrelationships of Hemopoietic Cells

The current understanding of the interrelationships of the various blood cells is illustrated in Fig. 6-3. A pluripotent stem cell, present in the marrow and capable of unlimited self renewal, gives rise to several types of unipotent (restricted) stem cells. The latter have limited capacity for self renewal and each is committed to one line of development. Thus, there is a committed stem cell for each of the cell types seen in blood, and these give rise to the morphologic stages that can be recognized in any of the developmental lines. Several orders of restricted stem cells have been recognized, representing increasing stages of maturity. The morphologic identity of the restricted and pluripotent stem cells is undetermined.

Functional Summary

The obvious function of hemopoietic tissues is to provide blood with continuous replacement of cells. Separation of the replicating cells from their end products in the blood and sequestering them in specific hemopoietic tissues allows the establishment of environments best suited to each tissue. It ensures that replicating cells are not unduly influenced by the activities of other organs and tissues, as would occur if replication occurred within the bloodstream. It also provides the blood with small cells that can more easily circulate through fine capillary beds. Since there is no need to set aside, within the circulation, a population of cells concerned with replication, all the blood cells are functional and can serve the body's needs. Subdivision of hemopoietic tissue into lymphatic and bone marrow components allows separate conditioning of cells (such as T-lymphocytes) without, at the same time, exposing the remainder of the hemopoietic cells to the same conditioning factors.

Within bone marrow, yellow marrow fills in spaces unoccupied by active marrow, but, being very labile, this fatty marrow can quickly be replaced by hemopoietic marrow when demands for blood become insistent. The sinusoids of the marrow provide sites where newly formed blood cells can gain access to the circulation. Additional maturation of cells occurs within the sinusoids, and the cells held here serve as a reserve that can be mobilized as needed.

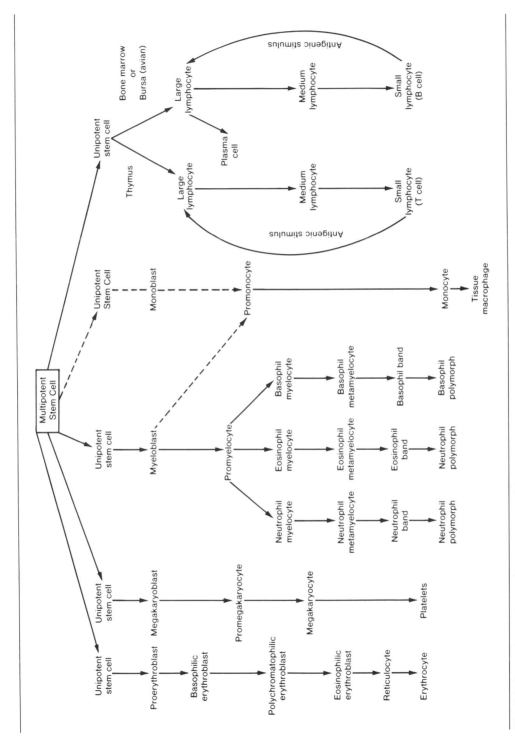

Fig. 6-3. Interrelationships of hemopoietic cell lines.

Clinical Correlations

Leukemia is believed to result from impaired differentiation of progenitor cells, leading to overproduction of hemopoietic cells that fail to mature. Immature cells build up and interfere with production of normal cells, leading to anemia, thrombocytopenia, and neutropenia, and are released into the blood to infiltrate other organs and tissues. Leukemias can be classified according to the cell line affected and subdivided into acute or chronic depending on the immaturity of the cell and the clinical course. Thus, acute or chronic granulocytic, lymphatic, and monocytic forms can be identified. Granulocytic leukemias most often involve neutrophil granulocytes, but eosinophilic and basophilic types have been reported. Lymphatic leukemias can be subdivided immunologically into B-cell, T-cell, and null cell varieties. A mixed myelomonocytic variety also occurs, illustrating the origin of granulocytes and monocytes from a common precursor.

In the acute leukemias the striking feature is the accumulation of blast cells in the marrow, which, in some cases, may be solidly packed with such cells. More commonly, some degree of differentiation persists and more mature forms (progranulocytes, granulocytes, large and small lymphocytes, monocytes) are present to indicate the cell line affected. Red cell formation may be markedly suppressed and represented only by a few polychromatophilic and eosinophilic normoblasts.

In chronic forms of leukemia, the marrow is densely packed with hemopoietic cells; neutrophil myelocytes are the characteristic cells, but there also may be an increase in promyelocytes and megakaryocytes. Myeloblasts rarely form more than 5 percent of the cells. Eosinophils are more numerous and basophils characteristically increased. Erythropoietic elements, while decreased, are not so severely depleted as in the acute forms. In chronic lymphocytic leukemia the marrow is replaced by small lymphocytes and may appear as a monotonous succession of these cells. Bleeding and anemia are more common than in granulocytic leukemia since red cell and platelet precursors are replaced.

Chapter 6

Atlas and Table of Key Features

Key Features of Bone Marrow Hemopoietic Cells

Cell	Diameter (μm)	Cytoplasm	Nucleus	Nucleolus
Myeloblast	10–13	Light blue, transparent; no granules	Round or oval with pale staining; fine vesicular chromatin	Yes
Promyelocyte	15–22	Light blue, transparent; scattered azurophil granules	Round or oval, may have slight indent, fine, lightly stained, dispersed	Yes
Myelocyte	12–18	Light blue, obscured by granules; specific granules are present (neutrophils, azurophil, eosinophils, basophils)	Round or oval, often with slight indent; chromatin more deeply stained and condensed	No
Metamyelocyte	12–16	Light blue, completely obscured by specific granules; a few azurophil granules present	Horseshoe- or kidney-shaped; coarse masses of deeply stained chromatin	No
Band	10–14	Filled with specific granules; a few azurophil granules present	Ribbon-like, twisted or coiled, no filaments; coarse, deeply stained chromatin	No
Megakaryocyte	50–80	Light blue, transparent; scattered azurophil granules	Large, convoluted, irregular; stains deeply; coarsely patterned	No
Proerythroblast	15–20	Deep blue, opaque; no granules	Round, occupies about three-fourths of cell; texture deeply stained, uniformly "granular"	Yes
Basophil erythroblast	12–16	Deep blue, opaque; may have blotchy appearance; no granules	Round, occupies about half of cell; coarsely clumped, deeply stained	No
Polychromatophilic erythroblast	10–12	Variable — slate gray to blue gray	Round, dense, compact, deeply stained	No
Acidophilic erythroblast (normoblast)	8–10	Pink or pink with slight blue-gray	Round, dense, pyknotic, often eccentric	No

185

Fetal Hemopoietic Tissue

Island of
developing
erythroid
cells

Hepatic
cells

Island of
developing
erythroid
cells

Fig. 6-4. Fetal hemopoietic tissue from developing liver. Note the islands of developing erythroid cells. (LM, ×1,000.)

Developing
granulocytes

Developing
granulocytes

Hepatic
cells

Fig. 6-5. Fetal liver containing regions of developing granulocytes. (LM, ×1,000.)

Young megakaryocyte

Hepatic cells

Developing granulocytes

Developing erythroid cells

Hepatic cell

Fig. 6-6. Fetal liver containing groups of developing granulocytes as well as erythroid cells. An immature megakaryocyte also is present. (LM, ×1,000.)

Bone Marrow

Megakaryocytes

Developing erythroid cells

Developing granular leukocytes

Fig. 6-7. A section of bone marrow demonstrating hemopoietic tissue. (LM, ×250.)

Sinusoid

Central
nutrient
artery

Sinusoid

Osteoblasts

Osteocyte

Compact
bone

Fig. 6-8. A section of bone marrow illustrating its relationship to bone and the central nutrient artery. (LM, ×250.)

Cytoplasm of
endothelial
cell

Migrating
erythroid
cell

Nucleus of
endothelial
cell

Sinusoid

Osteoblasts

Sinusoid

Compact
bone

Fig. 6-9. A section of bone marrow clearly demonstrating the relationship of sinusoids to the surrounding hemopoietic tissue. (LM, ×400.)

Hemopoietic Tissue

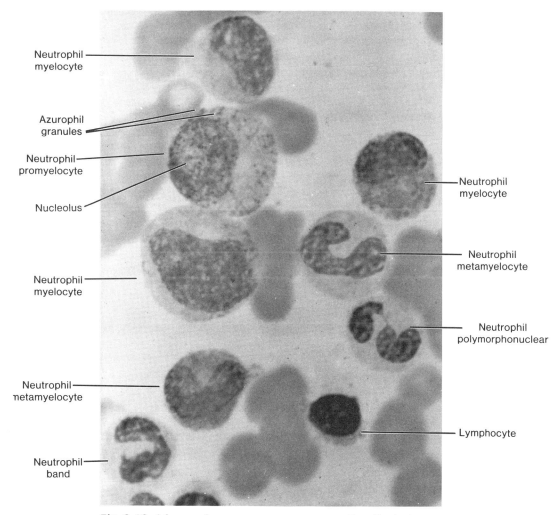

Fig. 6-10. A human bone marrow smear preparation illustrates several cell types typical of hemopoietic tissue. (LM, ×1,200.)

Fig. 6-11. Cells of hemopoietic tissue from a smear of human bone marrow. (LM, ×1,100.)

Fig. 6-12. Hemopoietic cells from a human bone marrow smear. (LM, ×1,000.)

Polychromatophilic
erythroblasts

Neutrophil
metamyelocyte

Eosinophil
metamyelocyte

Fig. 6-13. Hemopoietic cells from a human bone marrow smear.
(LM, ×1,000.)

Promyelocyte

Nucleolus

Basophilic
myelocyte

Fig. 6-14. Hemopoietic cells from a human bone marrow smear.
(LM, ×1,000.)

Fig. 6-15. Hemopoietic cells from a human bone marrow smear. (LM, ×1,000.)

Fig. 6-16. Hemopoietic cells from a human bone marrow smear. (LM, ×1,000.)

Neutrophil
myelocyte

Nucleus of
megakaryocyte

Fig. 6-17. Hemopoietic cells from a human bone marrow smear. (LM, ×1,000.)

Developing
platelets

Nucleus

Fig. 6-18. Several developing platelet fields in the cytoplasm of a megakaryocyte. (TEM, ×5,000.)

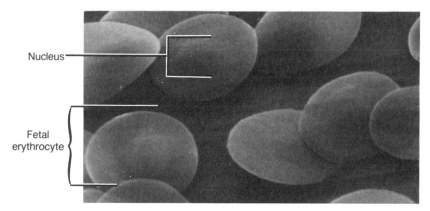

Nucleus

Fetal
erythrocyte

Fig. 6-19. Fetal erythrocytes from a sample of peripheral blood.
Each erythrocyte contains a central nucleus. (SEM, ×600.)

Neutrophilic
myelocyte

Eosinophilic
metamyelocyte

Eosinophil
polymorphonuclear
leukocyte

Normoblast
(eosinophilic
erythroblast)

Polychromatophilic
erythroblast

Fig. 6-20. Developing granulocytes and erythroid cells from hemopoietic tissue of fetal liver. (TEM, ×2,000.)

Polychromatophilic erythroblasts

Normoblast (eosinophilic erythroblast)

Fig. 6-21. Developing erythroid cells from fetal liver. (TEM, ×2,000.)

Lymphatic Tissue

Lymphocytes

Collagenous connective tissue

Fibroblast

Fig. 6-22. Diffuse lymphatic tissue in the loose connective tissue from a human eyelid. (LM, ×250.)

Lymphatic
nodule with
germinal
center

Fig. 6-23. A lymphatic nodule in the gastric mucosa. (LM, ×40.)

Review Questions and Answers

Questions

29. Describe the formation of blood in the embryo and fetus. What are the main cells formed at each stage?
30. What is the difference between reticular cells and reticulocytes?
31. What are the main cytologic changes that occur during erythropoiesis and granulocytopoiesis? (Do not describe specific stages.)
32. Describe the structure of the bone marrow sinusoids.
33. From what cells are platelets formed? How are platelets produced from these cells? What peculiar feature do these platelet-producing cells show?
34. What are colony-forming units?
35. Give a classification of lymphatic tissues.
36. Describe the germinal center. What is its function?
37. What type of granules are present in neutrophil granulocytes?

Answers

29. Blood formation in the embryo occurs first in the blood islands of the yolk sac and commences shortly after the formation of the germ layers. The main product of this activity is nucleated red cells. The second organ involved in hemopoiesis is the liver, which mainly produces non-nucleated erythrocytes; lesser numbers of granulocytes and megakaryocytes also are produced. During the splenic phase, the spleen produces erythrocytes, platelets, granulocytes, and lymphocytes. The bone marrow becomes the major blood-forming organ during the last three months of gestation and produces all types of blood cells.
30. The reticular cells are fixed cells that constitute part of the framework of both bone marrow and lymphatic tissues. They are large connective tissue cells responsible for the formation of the reticular fibers, which form the fibrous component of the hemopoietic tissues. Reticulocytes are erythrocytes in the last stages of development. They contain small amounts of residual ribonucleoprotein that, with special stains, can be precipitated and appears as a network within the cell.
31. During the development of red cells (erythropoiesis), the cell as a whole becomes progressively smaller; the cytoplasm first becomes more basophilic and then increasingly acidophilic as hemoglobin increases, and the content of ribosomes diminishes. The nucleus decreases in size, becomes more condensed, and ultimately is lost. During the process of granulocytopoiesis, the cells accumulate cytoplasmic granules of specific types. The nucleus becomes flattened and indented and finally assumes a lobulated form. The overall size of the cell decreases and nucleoli are lost.
32. The sinusoids of the bone marrow are thin-walled vessels of wide bore. The wall consists of three coats: (1) an endothelial lining of attenuated squamous cells united by junctions of the zonula adherens type; (2) a second coat consisting of a thin, discontinuous basal lamina on which the endothelial cells rest; and (3) reticular cells loosely applied to the exterior of the vessel to form an external coat of variable thickness.
33. Platelets are formed from megakaryocytes by segmentation of their cytoplasm. Small cytoplasmic vesicles appear between clusters of granules, coalesce, and elongate to form the demarcation membranes. The membranes surround each future platelet, which separate along the narrow clefts between them and are shed. The megakary-

ocytes are peculiar in that they arise from precursor cells by a series of nuclear divisions that occur without intervening periods of cytokinesis. This results in polyploid cells that may reach 64n.

34. Colony-forming units (CFUs) are the cells of bone marrow that give rise to spleen colonies when bone marrow is transfused into irradiated mice. The CFUs represent pluripotent and unipotent stem cells and are capable of repopulating all hemopoietic tissues. The CFU has the attributes of a stem cell — self renewal and the capacity for differentiation.

35. Lymphatic tissue may be classified as a reticular connective tissue on the basis of its content of reticular fibers or as a hemopoietic tissue because it contributes cells to the blood. It may be subdivided into diffuse and nodular types on the basis of its cellular organization.

36. Germinal centers are highly organized components of secondary lymphatic nodules. They show two distinct structural regions called the dark pole and the light pole. The dark pole contains a dense concentation of large and medium lymphocytes, macrophages, and plasma cells. The light pole is less densely populated and contains small lymphocytes and reticular cells. The dark pole is an area of active proliferation of lymphatic cells, but many of the newly formed cells appear to die there. Reticular fibers are scarce within both poles of the germinal center, and the cells are supported by a cellular framework formed by reticular cells. The germinal center contains B-lymphocytes, is closely associated with humoral immunologic responses, and may represent a clone of cells committed to responding to a single antigen.

37. The neutrophil granulocyte contains two types of granules: the specific granules and the azurophil granules. The azurophil granules are produced only at the promyelocyte stage and are formed at the concave face of the Golgi complex. Specific granules are produced during the myelocyte stage, are formed at the convex face of the Golgi, and become the dominant type of granule. The azurophil granules are lysosomes and contain the usual acid hydrolases associated with lysosomes. The specific granules contain different enzymes and possess proteins with antibacterial properties.

7 Muscle

Muscle is the basic tissue in which the property of contractility is preeminent. The purposeful movements of the body and the maintenance of posture are the result of contractions of muscles attached to the skeleton. Muscular contraction also is responsible for beating of the heart, breathing, constriction of blood vessels, movements of the intestines, emptying of the bladder, and other vital processes. The unit of structure of muscle is the muscle cell, which, because of its elongated shape, also is called a fiber. Functionally, the shape of the cell is important since a greater unidimensional contraction can be achieved by an elongated cell than by a globular cell of the same volume. Within a muscle mass, the fibers are oriented in the direction of movement.

Classification

KEY WORDS: **striated muscle, skeletal muscle, cardiac muscle, smooth muscle, visceral muscle, voluntary muscle, involuntary muscle**

Three kinds of muscle can be distinguished in vertebrates based on their morphology and function. Some muscles show a regular pattern of alternating light and dark bands that extend across the width of the fiber and have been called **striated muscles.** This is the kind of muscle associated with the skeleton and heart and thus forms **skeletal** and **cardiac muscle. Smooth muscle** lacks cross striations, occurs in the walls of viscera, and often is referred to as **visceral**

muscle. Functionally, muscle is either **voluntary** (under control of the will) or **involuntary** (not controlled by the will). Striated skeletal muscle is voluntary; smooth muscle is involuntary; and cardiac muscle is involuntary striated muscle.

Skeletal Muscle

Skeletal muscle is the most abundant tissue in the vertebrate body and forms those structures generally referred to as "the muscles." It permits a wide range of voluntary activities from the intricate and fine movements involved in writing to the rapid, powerful forces associated with jumping or throwing a ball. The power that can be generated by skeletal muscle is illustrated by the speed attained by a thrown ball which, at the moment it leaves the fingertips, may reach speeds of over 90 mph.

Organization

KEY WORDS: **fiber, multinucleated cell, fascicle, muscle, epimysium, perimysium, endomysium**

The smallest independent unit of striated muscle visible with the light microscope is the **fiber,** which is a long **multinucleated cell** (see atlas figures 7-9 and 7-10). Groups of parallel fibers form **fascicles** that can be seen with the naked eye. In turn, groups of fascicles make up an entire **muscle.** Fascicles vary in size with different muscles and in general are small in muscles associ-

199

ated with fine movements and large in muscles that perform actions demanding greater power.

At all levels of organization, muscle is associated with connective tissue (Fig. 7-1). The entire muscle is surrounded by a connective tissue sheath called the **epimysium.** Septa pass from the deep surface of the epimysium to invest each fascicle as the **perimysium;** delicate extensions of the perimysium wrap each fiber as the **endomysium.** Although given different names according to its association with different structural units of muscle, the connective tissue is continuous from one part to another. It consists of collagenous, reticular, and elastic fibers and contains several cell types including fibroblasts, macrophages, and fat cells. The endomysium is especially delicate and consists mainly of reticular fibers and thin collagen fibers; it carries blood capillaries and small nerve branches (see atlas figure 7-11). The larger blood vessels and nerves lie within the perimysium. The connective tissue not only binds the muscle units together but also acts as a harness and aids in integrating and transmitting the force of their contractions. The amount of connective tissue varies from muscle to muscle, being relatively greater in muscles capable of finely graded movements. Elastic tissue is most abundant in muscles that attach to soft parts such as the muscles of the tongue and face.

The Skeletal Muscle Fiber (Cell)

KEY WORDS: **banding, cross striation, A band, I band, Z line, H band, M line, sarcomere**

Generally, skeletal muscle fibers do not branch, but the muscles of the face and tongue may do so where the fibers insert into mucous membrane or skin. The fibers of skeletal muscle are elongated tubes that vary in shape and length. Some are cylindrical with rounded ends and appear to extend throughout the length of a muscle; others

Fig. 7-1. Portion of a muscle in transverse section to show the structural organization and the relationships of the connective tissue.

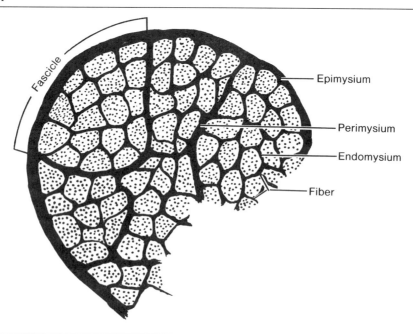

are spindle-shaped with narrowly tapering ends and apparently do not run the length of the muscle. One end of the fiber may attach to a tendon while the other unites with connective tissue in the belly of the muscle, or both ends may lie within the muscle mass. In transverse sections of fresh muscle the fibers are round or ovoid, but in fixed material they appear as irregular polyhedrons.

The fibers range between 10 and 100 μm in diameter. The size varies with the class of animal, decreasing through fish, amphibians, reptiles, mammals, and birds, and also varies from muscle to muscle and even within the same muscle. Longer fibers have the greater diameters and are associated with more powerful muscles. Some spacial arrangement of the fibers within a muscle has been noted, fibers of large diameter tending to be located more centrally. The size of the fibers changes with use, and fibers may hypertrophy (increase in size) in response to continued use or atrophy (decrease in size) with disuse.

The most outstanding histologic feature of skeletal muscle fibers is the presence of alternating light and dark segments that result in the **banding** or **cross striations** (Fig. 7-2) that are seen when the fiber is viewed in longitudinal section (see atlas figure 7-10). Under polarized light, the dark bands are anisotropic and are called **A bands,** whereas the light bands are isotropic and thus are called **I bands.** Running transversely through the center of the I band is a narrow dense

line, the **Z line** or Z disc. In good preparations, a pale narrow region, the **H band,** can be seen transecting the A band, with a dark **M line** within it. The relative length of each band depends on the state of contraction of the fiber. The length of the A band remains constant, whereas the I band is prominent in a stretched muscle and short in a contracted muscle (see Fig 7-5).

The contractile unit of the fiber is a **sarcomere,** defined as the distance between two successive Z lines. Within the sarcomere, as the I band becomes shorter, the Z lines approach the ends of the A bands.

Structure of Skeletal Muscle Fibers

KEY WORDS: sarcolemma, multinucleated cell, peripheral nuclei, sarcoplasm, satellite cell, myofibril, sarcoplasmic reticulum, sarcotubules, terminal cisternae, T-tubule, triad, T-system, junctional feet

Each skeletal muscle fiber is an elongated cell invested by a delicate membrane that, by electron microscopy, can be resolved into the plasmalemma and an adherent outer coat of glycoprotein. The plasmalemma of muscle is referred to as the **sarcolemma** but is no different from the limiting membrane of any cell. The outer glycoprotein layer corresponds to a basal lamina and is called the external lamina. It is associated with delicate reticular fibers that mingle with the reticular fibers of the endomysium.

Fig. 7-2. Banding pattern of striated skeletal muscle.

The striated muscle fiber is a **multinucleated cell.** The nuclei are elongated in the direction of the long axis of the fiber and, in adult mammalian muscle, are **peripheral,** located immediately below the sarcolemma (see atlas figures 7-9 and 7-10). The chromatin tends to be distributed along the inner surface of the nuclear envelope, and one or two nucleoli usually are present. The nuclei are fairly evenly spaced along the fiber but become more numerous and irregularly distributed in the area of attachment of the muscle to a tendon. Although the cytoplasm of the muscle cell is called the **sarcoplasm,** it corresponds to that of any cell. Many small Golgi bodies are present near one pole of the nucleus; lysosomes also usually take up a juxtanuclear position.

Closely associated with the muscle fiber are **satellite cells** that lie flattened against the fiber covered by the same basal lamina that invest the muscle cell. Although difficult to distinguish from muscle cells by light microscopy, satellite cells are more fusiform, their nuclei are more condensed, the chromatin is less dispersed, and nucleoli are lacking. The cytoplasm is scanty but may form a clear boundary between the nucleus of the satellite cell and the muscle fiber. In electron micrographs satellite cells show centrioles (not seen in muscle cells), scant endoplasmic reticulum, a small Golgi complex, and a few mitochondria near the ends of the nuclei. Satellite cells may represent survivors of the primitive myoblasts; they account for less than 4 percent of the muscle-associated nuclei.

Myofibrils are elongated, threadlike structures in the sarcoplasm and run the length of the muscle fiber. At 1 to 2 μm in diameter, myofibrils are the smallest units of contractile material that can be identified with the light microscope. In cross sections, myofibrils appear as small dots, while in longitudinal sections they give a longitudinal striation to the fiber. Each myofibril shows a banding pattern identical to that of the whole fiber (see atlas figure 7-12). Indeed, the banding of the fiber results from the bands on consecutive myofibrils being in register. Cross striations are restricted to the myofibrils and do not extend across the sarcoplasm between fibrils. The stria-

tions on adjacent fibrils are kept in alignment by a system of intermediate filaments composed of the protein desmin. Desmin also links the myofibrils to the cell membrane.

Associated with each myofibril is the **sarcoplasmic reticulum,** a modification of the smooth endoplasmic reticulum seen in other cells. The organelle consists of an extensive and continuous system of membrane-bound tubules called **sarcotubules** that form a mesh around each myofibril. At each junction of A and I bands, a pair of dilated sarcotubules, the **terminal cisternae,** pass around each myofibril and are continuous with the terminal cisternae of adjacent myofibrils. One of the pair of terminal cisternae serves an A band and the other serves an I band. From each of the cisternae, narrow, longitudinal sarcotubules extend over the A and I bands, respectively. Over the A band, the tubules form an irregular network in the region of the H band, while in the I band a similar confluence occurs at the region of the Z line (Fig. 7-3). Thus, each A and I band is covered by a "unit" or segment of sarcoplasmic reticulum. These units consist of the terminal cisternae at the A-I junctions, joined by longitudinal sarcotubules that anastomose in the region of the H and Z lines of their respective

Fig. 7-3. Diagrammatic representation of the sarcoplasmic reticulum and system of T-tubules in skeletal muscle.

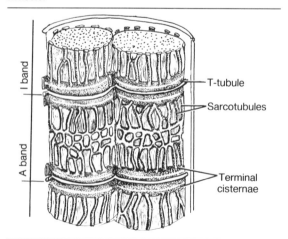

I band

A band

T-tubule

Sarcotubules

Terminal cisternae

A and I bands. The sarcoplasmic reticulum shows the same structure regardless of fiber type.

The pairs of cisternae at the A-I junctions are separated by a slender **T-tubule,** and the three structures — the T-tubule and two terminal cisternae — form the **triad** of skeletal muscle. In amphibians, the triad occurs at the Z line of each band rather than at the A-I junction as in mammals. T-tubules are inward extensions of the sarcolemma and penetrate into the muscle fiber to surround each myofibril. The T-tubules of one myofibril communicate with those of adjacent myofibrils to form a complete network across the fiber. The lumen of the T-tubule does not open into the cisternae but does communicate with the extracellular space at the surface of the sarcolemma. T-tubules are quite distinct from the sarcoplasmic reticulum and collectively make up the T-system.

The **T-system** rapidly transmits impulses from the exterior of the fiber to all the myofibrils throughout the cell, thereby producing a coordinated response. Passage of electrical impulses to the sarcoplasmic reticulum results in release of free calcium ions from the reticulum into the neighoring contractile elements, bringing about their contraction.

T-tubules and terminal cisternae are closely apposed. **Junctional feet** span the narrow gap between T-tubules and terminal cisternae, forming areas of low resistance through which impulses pass to the sarcoplasmic reticulum. In electron micrographs, the junctional feet appear as regularly spaced densities extending from the T-tubules to the terminal cisternae. These are matched by evenly spaced dimples on the cisternal membranes, corresponding to sites where the feet are located.

Structure of Myofibrils

KEY WORDS: myofilament, thick filament, myosin, thin filament, actin, tropomyosin, troponin

Under the electron microscope, the myofibril is seen to consist of longitudinal, fine **myofilaments,** of which two types have been identified,

differing in size and chemical composition. The thick filaments are 10 nm in diameter; thin filaments have a diameter of only 5 nm.

The **thick filaments** consist largely of **myosin** and are 1.5 μm long with a slightly thickened mid-portion and tapering ends. The mid-portion is smooth, whereas the ends are studded with many short projections. Myosin filaments can be dissociated into their constituent molecules, of which there are about 180 per filament, each consisting of a head and a tail. The tails of the molecules lie parallel and are so arranged that the smooth mid-portion of the filament consists of the tails only. The heads project laterally from the filament along its tapered ends and form a helical pattern along the filament. Most of the tail consists of light meromyosin, whereas the heads, with parts of the tails, consist of heavy meromyosin. **Thin filaments** are about 1 μm in length and are composed of globular subunits of **actin** attached end-to-end to form two longitudinal strands wound about one another in a loose helix. A second protein, **tropomyosin,** lies within the groove between the two actin strands. Still another protein, **troponin,** is bound to tropomyosin at intervals of 40 nm.

The arrangement of the thick and thin filaments is responsible for the banding pattern on the myofibrils (Fig. 7-4). The I band consists only of thin filaments, which extend in both directions from the Z line. The filaments on one side are offset from those of the other, and connecting elements appear to run obliquely across the Z line to create a zig-zag pattern. The structure and chemical composition of the Z line and the attachments of the thin filaments to it are not well understood. As the actin filament nears the Z line, it becomes continuous with four slender threads, each of which appears to loop within the Z line and join a thread from an adjacent actin filament. Several accessory proteins (α-actinin, Z protein, filamin, and amorphin) have been identified in the Z line. α-Actinin holds the actin filaments in register at the Z line.

The A band consists chiefly of thick filaments with slender cross-connections at their midpoints, which give rise to the M line (see atlas

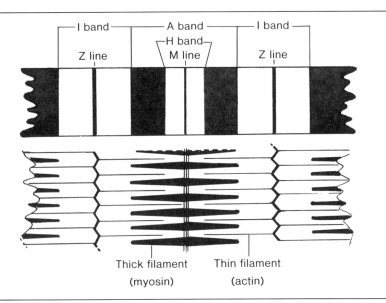

Fig. 7-4. Relationship of cross-banding to the arrangement of thin and thick filaments.

figures 7-12 and 7-13). A protein, myomesin, in the region of the M line holds the myosin filaments in register. Actin filaments extend into the A bands between the thick filaments; the extent to which they penetrate determines the width of the H band (which consists only of thick filaments) and depends on the degree of contraction of the muscle. At the ends of the A bands, where the thick and thin filaments interdigitate, the narrow space between filaments is traversed by cross-bridges formed by the heads of the myosin molecules.

The arrangement of the filaments also establishes the ultrastructural basis of the contractile mechanism (Fig. 7-5). During contraction, the A band remains constant in length, the length of the I and H bands decreases, and the Z lines approach the ends of the A bands. The changes result from alterations in the relative positions of the thick and thin filaments. No change in the lengths of the filaments is involved; the actin filaments slide past the myosin filaments to penetrate more deeply into the A band. As a result, the I and H bands become shorter. The Z lines are drawn closer to the ends of the A bands, thereby decreasing the length of each sarcomere

(the distance between successive Z lines) to produce an overall shortening of the myofilaments.

The sliding action of the filaments results from repeated "make and break" attachments between the heads of the myosin molecules and the neighboring actin filaments. The attachments are made at sites progressively further along the actin filaments, causing the filaments to slide past one another. The force resulting in movement of the filaments appears to be generated as the heads of the myosin change their angle of attachment to the actin filaments.

To translate the contraction of the sarcomere to contraction of an entire fiber, each sarcomere in the fiber must contract simultaneously and not in sequence. This simultaneous contraction — not only in a single fiber but throughout an entire muscle — is brought about by the T-system.

Fiber Types in Skeletal Muscle

KEY WORDS: type I, red fiber, slow twitch, type IIA, aerobic and anaerobic, type IIB, white, anaerobic, fast twitch, type IIC

Some skeletal muscles appear redder than others, reflecting the type of fibers present. Muscle fibers

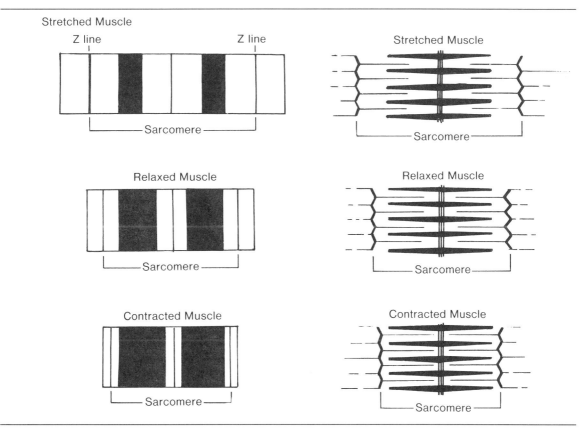

Fig. 7-5. Banding pattern and arrangement of thick and thin filaments in stretched, relaxed, and contracted muscle.

have been classed as red, white, and intermediate from their gross appearance, or as type I, IIA, IIB, and IIC on the basis of their histochemical reactions.

Type I fibers are **red fibers** (see atlas figure 7-16). These contain abundant myoglobin (a pigment similar to hemoglobin) and fat and are surrounded by many capillaries. They have numerous small mitochondria, are rich in oxidative enzymes, are low in myophosphorylase and glycogen, and metabolically are aerobic. The mitochondria are aggregated beneath the sarcolemma and form rows between myofibrils; they possess many closely packed cristae. The Z line is wide. The fibers do not stain when reacted for adenosinetriphosphatase (ATPase) at pH 9.4 but show

"reversal" and stain well (dark) when reacted at pH 4.6 or 4.3. Physiologically, type I fibers represent **slow twitch** fibers adapted to slow, repetitive contractions and are capable of long, continued activity. Type I fibers tend to be located deep in a muscle, closer to the bone.

Type IIA fibers also are red due to abundant myoglobin but contain less fat than type I fibers. They contain much glycogen and show both **aerobic and anaerobic** metabolism. Oxidative enzymes are present but their activity is slightly lower than in type I fibers. Myophosphatase activity is high, mitochondria are large but few in number, and Z lines are wide. ATPase activity is high (the fibers stain darkly) at pH 9.4 but is poor at pH 4.6 or 4.3.

Type IIB fibers are **white** in color and contain moderate amounts of glycogen but little myoglobin or fat. They are distinguished by their large diameters, poorer blood supply, decreased number of large mitochondria, and narrow Z lines. The fibers are rich in myophosphorylase but poor in oxidative enzymes. Metabolically they are **anaerobic.** After preincubation at pH 9.4, type IIB fibers show high ATPase activity but fail to stain at pH 4.3 and show only moderate reactivity at pH 4.6. Type IIB fibers represent **fast twitch** fibers adapted for rapid, short-lived activity. In comparison to types I and IIA fibers, type IIB fibers tire quickly.

Type IIC fibers also have been described. They appear to be similar to type IIB fibers except that their ATPase activity is inhibited only at a pH lower than 4.0. They have narrow Z lines and correspond to the intermediate fiber type. Type IIC fibers represent a fast twitch muscle fiber that is more resistant to fatigue than the type IIB fiber.

Type IID fibers also have been characterized.

Motor Nerve Endings

KEY WORDS: **motor unit, motor end plate, myoneural junction, synaptic trough, primary synaptic cleft, secondary synaptic cleft, junctional fold, synaptic vesicle**

Each skeletal muscle is supplied by one or more nerves that contain both motor and sensory fibers. A motor neuron and the muscle fibers supplied by it make up a **motor unit.** The size of the motor unit is determined by the number of muscle fibers served by a single nerve fiber and varies between muscles. Small motor units occur where precise control of muscle activity is required; large units are found in muscles used for coarser activities. In the intrinsic muscles of the eye, every muscle fiber is supplied by a nerve (forming small motor units), whereas in the major muscles of the limb, a single nerve fiber may supply 1,500 to 2,000 muscle fibers — a large motor unit. All the muscle fibers contained in one motor unit appear to be of the same histochemical type; thus there are type I and type II motor units.

Branches of a motor nerve end on the muscle fiber at a specialized region called the **motor end plate** or **myoneural junction** (Fig. 7-6). The junction appears as a slightly elevated plaque on the muscle fiber associated with an accumulation of nuclei. As the nerve approaches the end plate it loses its myelin sheath and ends in a number of bulbous expansions, the outer surfaces of which are covered by a continuation of the Schwann's cells. The nerve endings lie in shallow recesses, the **synaptic troughs (primary synaptic clefts),** on the surface of the muscle fiber. The sarcolemma that lines these clefts invaginates to form numerous **secondary synpatic clefts** or **junctional folds.** Acetylcholinesterase receptor is present on the outer edges of the secondary clefts, while acetylcholinesterase is located along the inner surface of the secondary cleft and in the sarcolemma in this area. Although the nerve and muscle fibers are intimately related at the junctions, their cell membranes remain separated by a glycoprotein layer derived from fusion of the basal laminae of the muscle fiber, nerve fiber, and Schwann's cells. This layer extends along the primary synaptic cleft and dips into each secondary cleft. Numerous large, vesicular nuclei and abundant mitochondria, ribosomes, and granular endoplasmic reticulum are present in the sarcoplasm that underlies the nerve terminal. The nerve terminals contain many mitochondria and a large number of **synaptic vesicles** that appear to be sites of acetylcholine, a neurotransmitter agent.

Sensory Nerve Endings

KEY WORDS: **muscle spindle, intrafusal fiber, extrafusal fiber, nuclear bag fiber, nuclear chain fiber, annulospiral ending, flower spray ending, motor end plate, trail ending**

Skeletal muscle contains many sensory endings, some of which are simple spiral terminations of nonmyelinated nerves that wrap about the muscle fibers and others that are highly organized structures called **muscle spindles** or neuromuscular spindles (Fig. 7-7). Each muscle spindle consists of an elongated, ovoid connective tissue capsule that encloses a few thin, modified skeletal

Fig. 7-6. Motor end plate.

muscle fibers associated with sensory and motor nerves. The modified muscle fibers traverse the capsule from end to end and form the **intrafusal fibers** to distinguish them from the ordinary muscle fibers (**extrafusal fibers**) outside the capsule (see atlas figures 7-16 and 7-17).

Two distinct types of intrafusal fibers are present. Both are striated over most of their lengths, but midway along the fibers the striations are replaced by aggregates of nuclei. One type of intrafusal fiber is larger, and its nonstriated region is occupied by a cluster of nuclei that produces a slight expansion of the fibers in this region; these form the **nuclear bag fibers.** The second type of fiber is thinner, and the nuclei in the central region form a single row, hence their name, **nuclear chain fiber.** Nuclear bag fibers extend beyond the capsule to attach to the endomysium of nearby extrafusal fibers. Nuclear chain fibers are the more numerous and shorter. They attach to the capsule at the poles of the spindle or to the sheaths of nuclear bag fibers. Since the central areas of the intrafusal fibers lack myofibrils, these regions are noncontractile.

Each spindle receives a single, thick sensory nerve fiber that gives off several nonmyelinated branches that end in a complex system of rings and spirals at the central regions of the intrafusal fibers. These **annulospiral endings** run beneath the basal lamina in grooves in the sarcolemma. **Flower spray endings** are cluster- or spray-like terminations of smaller sensory nerves that occur mainly on nuclear chain fibers. Intrafusal fibers also receive small motor nerve fibers that end either as **motor end plates** or as long, diffuse **trail endings** that ramify over the intrafusal fibers, making several contacts with them.

Muscle spindles serve as stretch receptors and are found mainly in slow-contracting extensor muscles involved in maintaining posture. They are present also in muscles used for fine movements. Stimulation by motor nerves maintains tension on the intrafusal fibers, resulting in a stretching of their nonstriated segments. The degree of stretch is sufficient to maintain the sensory nerve endings in this region in a state of excitation that is close to their thresholds. When a whole muscle is stretched, it causes increased tension on the intrafusal fibers and stretching of their nonstriated regions, resulting in the discharge of impulses by the sensory nerve. When the muscle contracts, tension on the spindle is reduced and sensory nerve endings cease firing. The frequency of the discharges by the nerve endings is proportional to the tension on the intrafusal fibers; together with the number of active spindles, a degree of muscle contraction appropriate to the stimulus is assured.

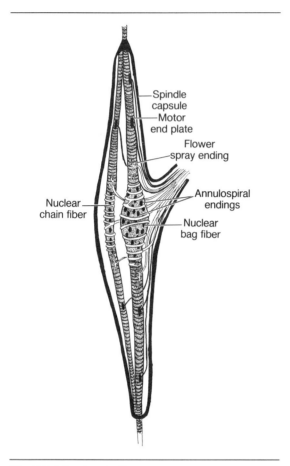

Spindle
capsule
Motor
end plate

Flower
spray ending

Nuclear
chain fiber

Annulospiral
endings

Nuclear
bag fiber

Fig. 7-7. Muscle spindle.

Tendon and Tendon-Muscle Junctions

KEY WORDS: collagen bundle, endotendineum, fascicle, peritendineum, epitendineum, fibroblast, tendon organ

Tendons consist of thick, closely packed **collagen bundles.** Surrounding each bundle is a small amount of loose, fibroelastic connective tissue, the **endotendineum.** Variable numbers of collagen bundles are collected into poorly defined **fascicles** wrapped in a somewhat coarser connective

tissue called the **peritendineum.** Groups of fascicles form the tendon itself, which is wrapped in a thick layer of dense irregular connective tissue, the **epitendineum.** The only cells present in the tendon are **fibroblasts** arranged in columns between the collagen fibers. Tendons are examples of dense regular connective tissue.

Where muscle and tendon join, the connective tissue of the endomysium, perimysium, and epimysium becomes strongly fibrous and blends with the connective tissue of the tendon. On the muscle side of the junction, the connective tissue fibers extend into indentations of the sarcolemma and are firmly attached to the basal lamina, to which the sarcolemma also attaches (see atlas figures 7-14 and 7-15). Within the muscle fiber, the actin filaments of the last sarcomere are anchored to the sarcolemma at the end of the fiber. Thus, contraction of the muscle fiber is passed to the sarcolemma, the basal lamina, and, by way of the connective tissue sheaths, to the tendon.

Tendon organs are encapsulated sensory receptors found at tendon-muscle junctions. The organ consists of a capsule of dense irregular connective tissue traversed by specialized collagen bundles that are continuous with collagen fibers outside the capsule. A single large sensory nerve pierces the capsule and gives rise to several nonmyelinated branches whose terminations entwine among the collagen bundles. The tendon organ senses stresses produced by muscle contractions, preventing them from becoming excessive.

Cardiac Muscle

Cardiac muscle occurs only in the heart, where it forms the muscle wall (myocardium). It resembles both smooth and skeletal muscle; both skeletal and cardiac muscle are striated, but like smooth muscle, cardiac muscle is involuntary. However, cardiac muscle is unlike either in many of its structural details and is unique in that its contractions are automatic and spontaneous, requiring no external stimulus.

Organization

KEY WORDS: **branching fiber, endomysium, perimysium**

As in skeletal muscle, the histologic unit of structure of cardiac muscle is the cell (fiber), but in cardiac muscle the cells are associated end-to-end to form long tracts, each about 80 μm long by 50 μm wide. The cells may divide at their ends before joining to adjacent fibers and thus form a network of **branching fibers.** A web of collagenous and reticular fibers is present between the muscle fibers and corresponds to an **endomysium,** but because of the branching fibers, it is more irregular than in skeletal muscle. Large bundles of fibers are wrapped in a coarser connective tissue of collagen and reticular fibers, forming a **perimysium,** as in skeletal muscle.

Fibers

KEY WORDS: **sarcolemma; central nuclei; A, I, M, H, and Z bands; actin and myosin filaments; sarcoplasmic reticulum; T-tubule; diad; Z line; peripheral coupling; subsarcolemmal cisternae**

Each cell (fiber) is enclosed in a **sarcolemma** external to which is an external lamina associated with fine reticular fibers. Each fiber contains one or two **central nuclei.** The same banding pattern seen in skeletal muscle is present on cardiac fibers, and **A, I, M, H,** and **Z bands** can be distinguished but are not as conspicuous as in skeletal muscle (see atlas figures 7-19 and 7-20). The banding pattern is due to the arrangement of **actin** and **myosin filaments,** but the aggregation of filaments into myofibrils is not well defined, and bundles of myofibrils often become confluent with those of adjacent bundles or are separated only by rows of mitochondria. The bundles of myofibrils diverge around the nuclei to leave a fusiform area of sarcoplasm at each pole. These areas are occupied by small Golgi elements and numerous large mitochondria that have closely packed cristae. Glycogen is a prominent feature of cardiac muscle.

The **sarcoplasmic reticulum** (Fig. 7-8) is neither as extensive nor as well developed as that of skeletal muscle (see atlas figure 7-22). The sarcotubules are continuous over the length of the sarcomere and anastomose freely to give a plexiform pattern with no special anastomosis at the H band. There are no terminal cisternae, and the reticulum makes contact with the **T-tubules** via irregular expansions of the sarcotubules. Since most T-tubules are apposed to only one cisterna at any point, the couplings of T-tubule to sarcoplasmic reticulum have been called **diads.** The T-tubules of cardiac muscle are located at **Z lines** rather than at A-I junctions, and their lumina are much wider than in the T-tubules of skeletal muscle (see atlas figure 7-22). The luminal surfaces of the cardiac T-tubules are coated by a continuation of the basal lamina of the sarcolemma. Sarcotubules at the periphery of the cell may be closely applied to the sarcolemma, and these couplings have been called **peripheral couplings** or **subsarcolemmal cisternae.** As in skeletal muscle, the functional unit of cardiac muscle is the sarcomere, demarcated by two successive Z lines.

Fig. 7-8. Diagrammatic representation of the sarcoplasmic reticulum and system of T-tubules in cardiac muscle.

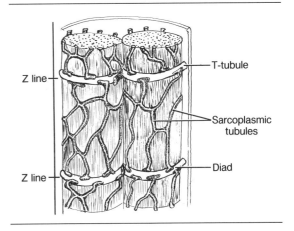

Intercalated Discs

KEY WORDS: Z line, desmosome, fascia adherens, nexus (gap) junction

At their end-to-end associations, cardiac muscle cells are united by special junctions that are visible under the light microscope as dark lines (see atlas figure 7-19). These are the intercalated discs that cross the fibers in stepwise fashion at the level of **Z lines** and thus have transverse and horizontal parts (see atlas figures 7-20 and 7-23). Along the transverse parts, the opposing cells are extensively interdigitated and at points are united by **desmosomes.** For the most part, the junction between cells is more extensive than that of a desmosome and thus is called a **fascia adherens.** The sarcoplasm immediately below the cell membrane contains a mat of filaments into which the actin filaments insert, thus binding the ends of the myofilaments to the sarcolemma. At irregular sites along the junctions, the membranes of opposing cells are united by **nexus (gap) junctions** (see atlas figures 7-21 and 7-23).

The longitudinal part of the intercalated disc is continuous with the transverse portion and also shows gap junctions that, however, are much more extensive. The gap junctions represent areas of low electrical resistance and allow rapid spread of excitation impulses from cell to cell.

Smooth Muscle

Smooth muscle is widely distributed throughout the body and plays an essential role in the functions of organs. It forms the contractile portion of the walls of blood vessels and of hollow viscera such as the digestive, respiratory, and reproductive tracts. Smooth muscle also is present in the skin, where it forms small muscles attached to hair follicles, and in the iris and ciliary body of the eye, the erectile tissue of the penis and clitoris, and the stroma of the ovary and prostate.

Smooth Muscle Fibers

KEY WORDS: cell, single central nucleus, myofibril, filaments, dense body, basal (external) lamina, gap junction (nexus), attachment plaque

Each smooth muscle fiber is an elongated **cell** with an expanded central region and tapering ends. The fibers vary in length in different organs, from 20 μm in small blood vessels to 500 to 600 μm in the pregnant uterus. A **single central nucleus** occupies the wide portion of the fiber about midway along its length, elongated in the long axis of the fiber (see atlas figure 7-24). In a contracted fiber the nucleus has a wrinkled or pleated outline. The fibers lack cross striations and in the usual histologic preparations appear homogeneous. However, longitudinal striations can be seen after maceration of the fibers in acid; these striations represent the **myofibrils.**

In electron micrographs, the sarcoplasm in the region of the nucleus shows long, slender mitochondria, a few tubules of granular endoplasmic reticulum, clusters of free ribosomes, and a small Golgi body at one pole of the nucleus. Unlike cardiac and skeletal muscle, only a rudimentary sarcoplasmic reticulum is present and a system of T-tubules is absent. The bulk of the cytoplasm contains closely packed, fine **filaments** arranged in bundles that run in the long axis of the fiber. Mitochondria and glycogen granules are interspersed between the myofilaments. Scattered throughout the sarcoplasm are a number of oval **dense bodies** into which the myofilaments (actin) appear to insert (see atlas figure 7-27). Desmin, the most abundant intermediate filament, and vimentin also insert into these anchoring points.

The sarcolemma is covered externally by a thick **basal** or **external lamina** consisting of proteoglycan associated with numerous fine collagenous and reticular fibers that blend with the surrounding connective tissue (see atlas figure 7-25). In some regions the basal lamina is lacking, and the membranes of adjacent smooth muscle cells are closely related in **gap junctions (nexuses)** through which excitation impulses spread from one fiber to another (see atlas figure 7-26). Areas of increased density, similar to the dense bodies, occur at intervals along the inner aspect of the sarcolemma, becoming more numerous along the ends of the fibers. These dense regions appear to be sites of attachment of myofilaments and intermediate filaments to the cell membrane and have been called **attachment plaques.** Between these areas the sarcolemma shows numerous caveolae, indicative of active micropinocytosis.

Myofilaments

KEY WORDS: thick filament, thin filament, actin, myosin

Thick and **thin filaments** have been demonstrated in smooth muscle by electron microscopy, and **actin** and **myosin** have been identified biochemically. However, myosin filaments have been difficult to identify in standard electron microscopic preparations, and it has been suggested that in smooth muscle, myosin is labile, aggregating into filaments only on initiation of contraction. Filamentous myosin has been shown in unfixed, rapidly frozen smooth muscle where regular arrays of thick myosin filaments have been seen surrounded by rosettes of actin. As in striated muscle, release of calcium ion in smooth muscle initiates contraction. In smooth muscle calcium ion is complexed to calmodulin (a calcium-binding protein), and this complex activates myosin light-chain kinase, an enzyme necessary for the phosphorylation of myosin, and permits it to bind to actin. Contraction then occurs. Myosin and actin of smooth muscle interact as in striated muscle, and a sliding filament mechanism appears to account for contraction of smooth muscle also.

Contraction of smooth muscle cells is associated with formation of blebs of the plasmalemma; the blebs are lost as the cells relax. The evaginations increase in size and number as the cell continues to shorten, and when the cell has reached 55 percent of its initial length, it is completely covered by blebs. In electron micrographs, the blebs are free of myofilaments, but filaments are prominent in the nonevaginated areas between attachment plaques.

In the contracted cell, the thick and thin filaments and the cytoplasmic dense bodies are ori-

ented obliquely to the long axis, criss-crossing the cell, whereas in the relaxed cell these components generally are parallel to the cell axis. The contractile elements unite with the attachment plaques and the dense bodies. During contraction, the contractile elements become obliquely oriented. As the cell shortens, its width must increase to accommodate the displaced volume, but this is opposed by the contraction pulling inward at the site of the attachment plaques. Those areas not directly subjected to the inward force bulge outward as blebs. The filaments between the dense bodies represent a contractile unit, several being strung together and anchored at either end in an attachment plaque.

Organization

Smooth muscle cells may be present as isolated units or small bundles in ordinary connective tissue, as in intestinal villi, the tunica dartos of the scrotum, and the capsule and trabeculae of the spleen. They also form prominent sheets in the walls of the intestines and arteries. In any one sheet of muscle, the fibers tend to be oriented in the same direction but are offset so that the thick portions of the fibers lie adjacent to the tapering ends of neighboring fibers. Thus, in transverse sections, the outlines of the fibers vary in diameter according to where along their lengths the fibers were cut. Nuclei are few and present only in the largest profiles, which represent sections through the expanded areas of the cells.

A thin connective tissue with few fibroblasts and consisting of fine collagenous, reticular, and elastic fibers extends between the smooth muscle cells and becomes continuous with a more dense connective tissue that binds the muscle cells into bundles or sheets. The latter connective tissue contains more abundant fibroblasts, collagenous and elastic fibers, and a network of blood vessels and nerves. The traction produced by contracting fibers is transmitted to the reticulo-elastic sheath about the cells and then to the denser connective tissue, permitting a uniform contraction throughout the muscle sheet. The reticular and elastic fibers of the reticulo-elastic sheath are products of the muscle fibers.

Development of Muscle

Skeletal muscle arises from mesenchyme in various parts of the embryo. Muscles of the limbs and trunk develop from myotomal mesenchyme; those of the head and neck arise in the mesenchyme of the branchial arches.

Initially the precursor muscle cells are rounded, noncontractile cells with single centrally placed nuclei. As the cells develop, they elongate and begin to synthesize myofilaments, creatinine kinase, and acetylcholine receptors, thus becoming identifiable as myoblasts. The spindle-shaped myoblasts contain numerous ribosomes, prominent Golgi regions, and rather short mitochondria, as well as a few myofilaments. The cells are actively mitotic.

By seven weeks' gestation the myoblasts begin to fuse with one another, end-to-end, to form primary myotubules. Primary myotubules are long cells, 8 to 15 μm wide, with multiple large, central nuclei, each with a prominent nucleolus (see atlas figure 7-18). The myoblasts that undergo fusion have ceased to synthesize deoxyribonucleic acid (DNA) and are postmitotic cells. Bulk synthesis of contractile proteins occurs in the myotubule, and organization of sarcomeres with clearly recognizable A and I bands and Z lines takes place. Actin filaments appear, closely associated with myosin filaments. Clusters of filaments appear, aggregate, increase in length and thicken, and soon show banding. Shortly after the appearance of myofilaments, transverse tubules appear at intervals of 1 to 5 μm. Fusion of Z bodies to which actin filaments are joined results in the appearance of Z lines, aligned with the T-system and units of the sarcoplasmic reticulum.

New generations of myoblasts continue to develop and either form new myotubules or fuse to the ends of older myotubules to form fibers that contain 50 to 100 nuclei. It is likely that new myotubules continue to form until their number equals that of the fibers of a given mature muscle. By the thirteenth week, the nuclei begin to move from the center of the tube to the periphery, and the cell becomes a myofiber. However, development of the fiber is not synchronous along its length, and the same structure may show features of a myotubule and a myofiber. The most mature regions are those in the middle of the cell, where fusion of myoblasts first occurred. The least mature areas are those at the ends. Thus, for a time the middle of the fiber might show peripheral nuclei, while at the ends, central nuclei are present as fusion of myoblasts continues. As the myotubule develops, the number of mitochondria increases and the cristae increase in number and are more tightly packed.

From the sixteenth week of gestation until birth, muscle fibers enlarge in length and width. The muscle mass continues to increase after birth until puberty. There is no evidence that the number of fibers increases postnatally, but the fibers do increase in length by the addition of new sarcomeres at the ends. Increase in girth is due to an increase in the number of myofibrils and the amount of sarcoplasm.

Histochemical fiber types can be recognized after the eighteenth or nineteenth week of gestation, and prior to this, all the myotubules react uniformly as type IIC. A few large type I fibers appear at about the twentieth week, but it is not until after the thirtieth week that type IIB, then IIA fibers differentiate from the type IIC. At birth, about 10 percent of the type IIC fibers persist. In adults, less than 3 percent are type IIC.

Cardiac muscle develops from mesenchyme (the myoepithelial mantle) that envelops the endocardial tube of the embryonic heart. The cells are stellate at first and joined by desmosomes. Unlike skeletal muscle cells, primitive cardiac muscle cells divide repeatedly. With the synthesis of myofilaments, the cells elongate and become myoblasts, which soon begin rhythmic contractions. Cell division continues into postnatal life but subsequently gives way to hypertrophy as the means of further growth. The sites of desmosomal unions between cells transform into the intercalated discs.

Formation of T-tubules characterizes the final stage of development of mammalian cardiac muscle. The tubules arise from invaginations of the sarcolemma late in the prenatal period in guinea pigs, sheep, and cattle but develop postnatally in the rat, mouse, and opossum. However, when considered relative to development of the external form rather than chronological age, the time at which cardiac T-tubules develop is the same for all mammals.

Smooth muscle arises from the mesenchyme at various sites in the embryo where smooth muscle ordinarily will occur in the adult. The undifferentiated cells in these areas continue to divide until they become confluent, after which individual cells, the myoblasts, differentiate. The myoblasts elongate and take on the fusiform shape characteristic of adult smooth muscle cells; early in development the myoblasts resemble fibroblasts. The cytoplasm contains abundant free ribosomes, granular endoplasmic reticulum, and mitochondria, and Golgi bodies are prominent.

Few filaments are present initially, but as the smooth muscle cell develops, bundles of thin filaments appear in association with dark bodies. Myosin can be detected in the bundles of filaments. Concomitant with the appearance of filaments, cytoplasmic organelles decrease in number. Dense areas along the cell membrane, plasmalemmal vesicles, and a basal lamina appear at the same time as or a little later than the thick filaments. In the newborn, myofilaments are small and usually restricted to the cytoplasm at the edge of the cell. Granular endoplasmic reticulum and Golgi elements are prominent and extend throughout the cell.

There is evidence that even in the adult (e.g., in the uterus), new smooth muscle cells arise by mitotic division. Generally, however, adult growth of smooth muscle is the result of hypertrophy.

The smooth muscle of the iris is commonly thought to be derived from cells near the margin of the optic cup and therefore is of ectodermal origin.

Functional Summary

Nerve impulses reaching the myoneural junctions of skeletal muscles cause release of acetylcholine contained within the synaptic vesicles. This neurotransmitter diffuses across the synaptic trough, the surface area of which is greatly increased by the junctional folds. Acetylcholine causes depolarization of the sarcolemma at the end plate, from which an excitation wave sweeps over the surface of the muscle fiber and, by means of the T-system, is delivered to all the myofibrils throughout the fiber. At the triads, the impulse is passed to the endoplasmic reticulum, causing release of calcium ions from the sarcotubules. Free calcium ions activate the myosin-actin interaction, apparently through the intervention of tropomyosin and troponin. Troponin is the calcium receptor that, in the presence of increased calcium ion, is thought to undergo structural changes, bringing about the interaction of myosin and actin. The energy for the cross-bridging between myosin and actin is obtained from the breakdown of adenosine triphosphate (ATP) by ATPase contained in the myosin fibrils. As the actin filaments slide past the myosin filaments to penetrate more deeply between them, the length of each sarcomere is reduced, resulting in an overall shortening of each myofibril and thus of each fiber. The tension generated is transmitted in succession to the sarcolemma, the external lamina, the connective tissue sheath, and then a tendon or other muscle attachment. Muscle spindles serve as stretch receptors and coordinate the degree of muscle contraction with the strength of the stimulus. Tendon organs sense the stresses produced by the muscle contractions and prevent them from becoming excessive.

The duration of the excitation wave at the myoneural junction is limited by the rapid breakdown of acetylcholine by the enzyme acetylcholinesterase, which is associated with the basal lamina of the junctional folds. With the end of the excitation wave, calcium is rebound in the sarcoplasmic reticulum, and ATPase activity and actin-myosin interactions cease, resulting in relaxation of the muscle.

Skeletal muscle fibers have limited capacity to regenerate but can repair minor injuries. It is thought that repair occurs through activation of satellite cells. These cells, which separate from the parent muscle fiber, divide and fuse with other satellite cells to form myotubules and new fibers that bridge small defects in the parent fiber. Adult muscle increases in mass by increase in the size of existing fibers, not by increase in the number of fibers. A shift occurs from the small- and medium-sized fibers of normal muscle to the large fiber groups, but few of the hypertrophied muscle fibers become larger than the largest normal fibers. Physiologic hypertrophy at first consists of an increase in the amount of sarcoplasm followed by an increase in the number of myofibrils.

Contraction of cardiac muscle occurs spontaneously, with no need for an external stimulus. However, the mechanism of contraction is identical to that of skeletal muscle and involves interaction of actin and myosin filaments. Cardiac muscle depends more on calcium and shows a relatively slower contraction time than does skeletal muscle; these characteristics may relate to the relatively poorer development of the sarcoplasmic reticululm. The high content of mitochondria and glycogen is related to the constant rhythmic expenditure of energy typical of cardiac muscle. Because of the numerous gap junctions between cardiac muscle cells, the fibers of cardiac muscle have an inherent capacity to conduct impulses, and electrically, the cells act as though there were no membranes between them. Rapid distribution of impulses throughout the cardiac muscle is aided by the many branchings that provide unions between adjacent fibers.

Thick and thin myofilaments have been identified in smooth muscle cells, but a sarcomere organization has not been demonstrated clearly. Contraction of smooth muscle is slower than in striated muscle, but the energy cost of an equivalent force is much less. Contraction of smooth muscle is somewhat unique in that forceful contractions can be sustained for long periods without fatigue of the muscle. An example of such contractions is those of the uterine muscle during parturition. This type of contraction differs from that of skeletal muscles, which are unable to sustain contraction without becoming fatigued, and cardiac muscle, which shows inherent intermittent contractions. Absence of an organized sarcoplasmic reticulum is related to the slow contractions exhibited by smooth muscle.

Nexus junctions permit free passage of impulses, and, as in cardiac muscle, smooth muscle frequently acts electrically as though there were no cell boundaries. Thus, a few motor neurons can control large numbers of smooth muscles. The connective tissue between and around smooth muscle bundles transmits the forces generated by individual cells as a coordinated force throughout the entire tissue. Smooth muscle cells of different organs may show differences with regard to size, organization (individual cells, bundles, or sheets of cells), and response to different stimuli.

Clinical Correlations

Myasthenia gravis is characterized by intermittent muscle weakness and represents a disease of the neuromuscular junction. It is associated with the attachment of Immunologlobulin G-type antibodies to the acetylcholine receptor sites on the postsynaptic membrane of the neuromuscular junction.

The muscular dystrophies are a group of genetically determined myopathies that follow a clinical course of progressive weakness. Many such myopathies with disordered morphology and physiology of muscle have been described. Central core disease is a disorder of the myofibrils in which clear zones appear in the fibers. The fibers retain their cross striations, but in the clear areas, the myofibrils appear compact and amorphous. The central cores of the myofibrils lack oxidative enzymes and phosphorylase activity. Type I fibers are predominantly involved in some patients; in others both type I and II fibers are affected. Electron micrographs show an absence of mitochondria in the cores, and the mitochondria appear as though squeezed to the periphery of the fiber because of the dense packing of the myofibrils in the cores.

Duchenne type muscular dystrophy is a common inherited muscle disease of male children due to a defect in the gene coding for a protein known as dystrophin. Its absence results in muscle cells slowly being replaced by connective tissue.

Ring fibers are characterized by a central zone of longitudinal myofilaments and a peripheral zone of radially arranged contractile protein. Ring fibers can be found in normal muscle, especially in the extraocular muscles, but are most frequently seen in myotonic muscular dystrophy. This genetic disorder causes diffuse muscle weakness most prominent in the distal limb muscles, neck, and face.

In fiber type disproportion, the muscles show a predominance of relatively small type I fibers and normal or large type II fibers, especially type IIB. Type I fibers may be disposed in groups and occasionally fill an entire fascicle. It has been suggested that the persistence of small type I fibers may represent a maturational arrest during development.

Pathologic hypertrophy of myocardial fibers occurs in response to the increased workload imposed by systemic hypertension. It is unlikely that the number of capillaries available in the heart is changed with the altered workload so that at some point the hypertrophied muscle outstrips the blood supply and chest pain results.

Atlas and Table of Key Features

Key Features of Muscle Types

Type	Cell Shape	Nuclei	Diameter	Striations	Other
Smooth	Small spindles	Central, single	Small with marked variation	Absent	Packed tightly, little connective tissue between fibers
Cardiac	Short branching, anastomosing cylinders	Central, usually single, may be double	Large, moderate variation	Present	Intercalated discs
Skeletal	Long cylinders	Peripheral, multiple	Large, uniform	Present	

Skeletal Muscle

Connective tissue

Longitudinal section of skeletal muscle cells

Cross section of skeletal muscle cells

Skeletal muscle nuclei

Skeletal muscle nuclei

Fig. 7-9. A section through the musculature of the human tongue demonstrates cross-sectional and longitudinal profiles of skeletal muscle cells. (LM, ×300.)

I band

Connective tissue

Width of muscle cell

A band

I band

Peripheral nucleus of muscle cell

Fig. 7-10. A longitudinal section of human skeletal muscle cells. (LM, ×1,000.)

Capillaries

Capillaries

Fig. 7-11. A longitudinal section of skeletal muscle. The specimen had its vasculature injected previously with colored gelatin. Note that each skeletal muscle fiber is enveloped by capillaries. Striations remain visible on individual skeletal muscle cells. (LM, ×250.)

A band

I band

M line

H band

Actin
filaments

Z line

Myosin
filaments

Myofibril

Fig. 7-12. Details of the banding on each myofibril shown in a
skeletal muscle cell. (TEM, ×26,000.)

Actin filaments

Myosin filaments

Z line

A band

M line

H band

Z line

Fig. 7-13. Details of a sarcomere from skeletal muscle. (TEM, ×49,000.)

Fig. 7-14. The tapering end of a skeletal muscle fiber at the muscle-tendon junction. The junctional surface is characterized by extensive microvillus-like foldings. The latter greatly increases the surface area for union with connective tissue elements. (SEM, ×400.)

Fig. 7-15. A region of the muscle-tendon junction similar to that shown in 7-14. Note the infolding of the cell membrane and the associated external lamina. (TEM, ×20,000.)

Fig. 7-16. A cross section of skeletal muscle stained with adenosinetriphosphatase at PH 10.4 demonstrates type I and type II skeletal muscle cells (fibers). Note the muscle spindle. (LM, ×250.)

Fig. 7-17. A cross section of a muscle spindle. Compare the diameters of extrafusal and intrafusal fibers. (LM, ×400.)

Development

Fig. 7-18. Developing skeletal muscle from an embryo illustrates myotubules. Note the concentration of nuclei centrally in myotubules and the banded individual myofibrils that can also be seen. (LM, ×400.)

Cardiac Muscle

Intercalated discs

Nucleus

Muscle fiber {

Fig. 7-19. A longitudinal section of cardiac muscle illustrates the banded appearance of these fibers and the presence of intercalated discs. (LM, ×400.)

Fig. 7-20. Two adjacent cardiac muscle cells illustrating individual banded myofibrils and portions of intercalated discs. Note the abundance of mitochondria between myofibrils. (TEM, ×6,000.)

Actin filaments

Myosin filaments

Nexus (gap) Junction

Mitochondrion

Fig. 7-21. A portion of an intercalated disc between two cardiac muscle cells showing a gap (nexus) junction. (TEM, × 100,000.)

T tubule

Mitochondria

T tubule

Glycogen

Z line

Smooth endoplasmic
reticulum
(sarcoplasmic
reticulum)

T tubule

Fig. 7-22. A portion of a cardiac muscle cell demonstrating T-
tubules and elements of the sarcoplasmic reticulum. (TEM,
×26,950.)

Fig. 7-23. An intercalated disc uniting ends of two cardiac muscle cells. (TEM, ×52,800.)

Smooth Muscle

Smooth muscle
in cross section

Smooth muscle
in longitudinal
section

Fig. 7-24. Smooth muscle cells from the wall of the oviduct as
viewed in longitudinal and cross section. (LM, ×400.)

Nucleus

Smooth
muscle
cell

Basal
lamina

Fig. 7-25. A longitudinal section through a smooth muscle cell
from the lamina propria of a human stomach. (TEM, ×3,000.)

Nucleus

Smooth
muscle
cell

Nexus
junctions

Nexus
junctions

Nucleus

Fig. 7-26. Cross-sectional profiles of several smooth muscle cells taken from the muscularis mucosae of a human stomach. (TEM, ×7,000.)

Nerve
process

Attachment
plaque

Nerve
processes

Smooth
muscle
cell

Filaments

Dense
bodies

Nerve
process

Fig. 7-27. Increased magnification of the nuclear region of a smooth muscle from a human stomach (longitudinal profile). (TEM, ×15,000.)

Review Questions and Answers

Questions

38. Briefly outline the arrangement of the connective tissue components of a skeletal muscle and relate it to the gross organization of a muscle. What function does the connective tissue serve?

39. Describe the banding pattern of striated muscle on the basis of the actin and myosin filaments.

40. What is the contractile unit of skeletal muscle? Describe it in terms of the banding pattern on the fiber.

41. Beginning with a whole muscle, outline the various levels of organization of its structural components.

42. What is the function of the sarcoplasmic reticulum? How does that of cardiac muscle differ from that of skeletal muscle?

43. How is an excitation stimulus transmitted from the sarcolemma throughout the muscle cell?

44. What is an intercalated disc?

45. Discuss the type (not mechanism) of contraction of smooth muscle and compare it to that of skeletal and cardiac muscle.

Answers

38. A whole muscle is wrapped in a connective tissue sheath called the epimysium, from which septa pass into the muscle to surround fascicles that consist of groups of muscle fibers. The connective tissue that surrounds fascicles is called the perimysium and in turn provides slips of connective tissue that surround the individual muscle fibers as the endomysium. The connective tissue forms a continuous harness that binds the muscle units together and integrates the contractions of the individual cells of the muscle to provide continuous force on a tendon or other structures.

39. The light I bands of the muscle fiber consist only of the actin filaments, which extend in both directions from the Z line, offset from one another on each side. The H band is a pale central region of the A band and consists only of myosin fibers joined at their midpoints by slender cross-connections. These cross-connections form the M line, which transects the H band. On either side of the H band, the dark portions of the A band consist of myosin filaments between which actin filaments are interdigitated. The width of the H band and the I band is determined by the degree to which the actin filaments are inserted between the myosin filaments. The width of the A band remains constant.

40. The contractile unit of a skeletal muscle is the sarcomere, defined as the distance between two successive Z lines. The mid-portion of the sarcomere consists of an entire A band. At either end, it will consist of half of each I band immediately adjacent to the A band.

41. A whole skeletal muscle consists of a variable number of fascicles that in turn are formed by groups of fibers. Each fiber is a cell and contains within its sarcoplasm a number of threadlike structures called myofibrils. In turn, the myofibrils are composed of myofilaments, which are of two types: thick and thin. The thick myofilaments consist of the linearly arranged tails of myosin molecules from which extend the globular heads of the molecule. The thin filaments consist of actin and are composed of globular subunits that form two longitudinal strands.

42. The sarcoplasmic reticulum stores the calcium ions required for the activation of myosin-actin interactions. Upon stimulation, calcium ion is released by the sarcoplasmic reticulum and is recaptured

following the termination of the stimulus. In skeletal muscle the sarcoplasmic reticulum is a more extensive organelle, and the terminal cisternae and T-tubules are located at the A-I junctions. The longitudinal sarcotubules form anastomoses at the level of the H bands and Z lines. In cardiac muscle the T-tubules are located at the levels of the Z lines, and terminal cisternae of the sarcoplasmic reticulum are lacking. The T-tubules and sarcoplasmic reticulum make contact at irregular intervals only via small expansions of the sarcotubules. The sarcoplasmic reticulum is not as extensive as in skeletal muscle, and the sarcotubules unite at random over the sarcomere with no special anastomosis at the H bands.

43. Impulses are transmitted from the sarcolemma by the system of T-tubules, which are invaginations of the sarcolemma. The T-tubules surround each myofibril and communicate with those of adjacent myofibrils, forming a complete network across the fiber and establishing a communication with the sarcolemma that extends throughout the whole fiber. The T-tubules are distinct from, and not part of, the endoplasmic reticulum.

44. Intercalated discs are the light microscopic representations of the end-to-end unions of cardiac muscle cells. They contain desmosomes and nexus (or gap) junctions.

45. Smooth muscle is capable of powerful contractions sustained for a considerable period of time without fatigue. An example of this is the contractions of the uterine musculature during parturition. Skeletal muscle, though capable of forceful contractions, is unable to sustain them for any length of time and soon becomes fatigued. The contractions of cardiac muscle, unlike either smooth or skeletal, are inherent and rhythmic and occur in the absence of external stimuli. However, cardiac muscle does not show sustained contractions, and the intervals between contractions represent periods of rest.

8 Nervous Tissue

Nervous tissue, one of the four basic tissues, consists of nerve cells (neurons) and supporting cells (neuroglia). Nerve cells are highly specialized to react to stimuli and conduct the excitation from one region of the body to another. Thus, the nervous system shows both irritability and conductivity, properties that are essential to the functions of nervous tissue — to provide communication and to coordinate body activities.

The nervous tissue of the brain and spinal cord makes up the central nervous system; all other nervous tissue constitutes the peripheral nervous system. Nervous tissue specialized to perceive external stimuli is called a receptor, from which sensory stimuli are carried by the peripheral nervous system to the central nervous system, which acts as an integration and communications center. Other neurons, the effectors, conduct nerve impulses from the central nervous system to other tissues, where they elicit an effect.

The specialized contacts between neurons are called synapses; the impulses are transferred between nerve cells by electrical couplings or chemical transmitters. Some neurons of the brain secrete substances (hormones) directly into the bloodstream and therefore the brain may be considered a neuroendocrine organ. Neurons also can stimulate or inhibit other neurons they contact.

Neurons

KEY WORDS: **perikaryon, dendrite, axon, neurofibril, neurofilament, neurotubule, chromophilic (Nissl) substance, axon hillock, melanin pigment, lipofuscin granule**

The nerve cell, or neuron, is the structural and functional unit of nervous tissue. Usually large and complex in shape, it consists of a cell body, the **perikaryon,** and several cytoplasmic processes (see atlas figures 8-7 and 8-8). **Dendrites** are processes that conduct impulses *to* the perikaryon and usually are multiple. The single process that carries the impulse *from* the perikaryon is the **axon** or axis cylinder.

The perikarya of different types of neurons vary markedly in size (4 to 140 μm) and shape and usually contain a large, central, spherical nucleus with a prominent nucleolus. The cytoplasm is rich in organelles and may contain a variety of inclusions. Bundles of **neurofibrils** form an anastomosing network around the nucleus and extend into the dendrites and axon (see atlas figure 8-7). Neurofibrils must be stained selectively to be seen with the light microscope. Ultrastructurally, neurofibrils consist of aggregates of slender **neurofilaments,** 10 nm in diameter, and microtubules that, although called **neurotubules,** appear to be identical to microtubules found in other cells. The perikarya of most neurons contain the characteristic **chromophilic (Nissl) substance,** which, when stained with dyes such as cresyl violet or toluidine blue, appears as basophilic masses within the cytoplasm of the perikaryon and dendrites (see atlas figure 8-8). It is absent from the axon and **axon hillock,** the region of the perikaryon from which the axon originates (see atlas figure 8-8B). In electron micrographs, Nissl substance is seen to consist of several parallel cisternae of granular endoplasmic reticulum (see atlas figure 8-9).

Small slender or oval mitochondria are scattered throughout the cytoplasm of neurons and contain lamellar and tubular cristae. Well-developed Golgi complexes have a perinuclear position in the cell. Although centrioles are seen occasionally, neurons in the adult do not divide.

Inclusions also may be found in the perikarya. Dark brown granules of **melanin pigment** occur in neurons from specific regions of the brain, such as the substantia nigra, locus ceruleus, and dorsal motor nucleus of the vagus nerve, and in spinal and sympathetic ganglia. More common inclusions are **lipofuscin granules,** which increase with age and are thought to be the by-products of normal lysosomal activity. The lipid droplets seen in many neurons represent storage material or may occur as the result of pathologic metabolism.

Nerve Processes

KEY WORDS: dendrite, dendritic spine (gemmule), axon (axon cylinder), axon hillock, collaterals, telodendrion, axoplasm, action potential

Nerve processes are cytoplasmic extensions of the perikaryon and occur as dendrites and axons. Each neuron has several **dendrites** that extend from the perikaryon, dividing repeatedly to form branchlike extensions. Although tremendously diverse in the number, size, and shape of dendrites, each variety of neuron has a similar branching pattern. The dendritic cytoplasm contains elongate mitochondria, Nissl substance, scattered neurofilaments, and parallel-running microtubules. The cell membrane of most dendrites forms numerous minute projections called **dendritic spines** or **gemmules** that serve as areas

for synaptic contact between neurons; an important function of dendrites is to receive impulses from other neurons. Dendrites provide most of the surface area for receptive synaptic contact between neurons, although in some neurons the perikaryon and initial segment of the axon also may act as receptor areas. The number of synaptic points on the dendritic tree varies with the type of neuron but may be in the hundreds of thousands. Dendrites play an important role in integrating the many incoming impulses.

A neuron has only one **axon (axis cylinder),** which conducts impulses away from the parent neuron to other functionally related neurons or effector organs. The axon arises from the **axon hillock,** an elevation on the surface of the perikaryon that lacks Nissl substance (see atlas figure 8-8B). Occasionally, axons may arise from the base of a major dendrite. Axons usually are much longer and more slender than dendrites and may or may not give rise to side branches called **collaterals,** which, unlike dendritic branches, usually leave the parent axon at right angles. Axons also differ in that the diameter is constant throughout most of the length and the external surface generally is smooth. Axons end in several branches called **telodendria,** which vary in number and shape and may form a network or basketlike arrangement around postsynaptic neurons.

The cytoplasm of the axon, the **axoplasm,** contains numerous neurofilaments, neurotubules, elongate profiles of smooth endoplasmic reticulum, and long, slender mitochondria. Since axoplasm does not contain Nissl substance, protein synthesis does not occur in the axon. Protein metabolized by the axon during nerve transmission is replaced by that synthesized in cisternae of granular endoplasmic reticulum in the Nissl substance of the perikaryon. Neurotubules are believed to carry the new protein down the axon.

Antegrade transport involves movement of material from the perikaryon to axon terminals and may be slow or fast. Fast transport (410 mm/day) involves transfer of membranous organelles, neurosecretory vesicles, calcium, sugars, amino acids, and nucleotides: Slow transport (1–6 mm/

day) includes movement of proteins, metabolic enzymes, and elements of the cytoskeleton. Retrograde transport is the transfer of proteins and small molecules from the axonal endings to the perikaryon and provides a route by which some toxins (tetanus) and viruses (herpes, rabies) can invade the central nervous system. Dendritic transport also occurs but is less well understood.

Axons transmit responses as electrical impulses called **action potentials,** which begin in the region of the axon hillock and the initial segment of the axon. An impulse behaves in an "all or none" fashion. Only when the threshold of activity is reached is the action potential transmitted along the axon to its terminations, which synapse with adjacent neurons or end on effector cells. An axon always induces a positive activity — for example, causing muscle to contract or stimulating epithelial cells to secrete. Impulses directed to another neuron may be excitatory or inhibitory.

Distribution of Neurons

KEY WORDS: gray matter, white matter, nuclei, ganglia

The central nervous system is divided into gray matter and white matter, reflecting the concentration of perikarya. **Gray matter** contains the perikarya of neurons and their closely related processes, whereas **white matter** is composed chiefly of bundles or masses of axons and their surrounding sheaths. In the spinal cord, gray matter has a central location surrounded by white matter; in the cerebral and cerebellar cortices, gray matter is at the periphery and covers the white matter. Aggregates of perikarya occur in the gray matter of the central nervous system and act as distinct functional units called **nuclei.** Similar aggregates or individual neurons located outside the central nervous system are called **ganglia.**

Types of Neurons

KEY WORDS: Golgi type I neuron, Golgi type II neuron, unipolar neuron, bipolar neuron, pseudounipolar neuron, multipolar neuron

Neurons may be divided into types according to their location, number of dendrites, and length and position of axons. In vertebrates, most neurons lie in the gray matter of the central nervous system. Some neurons have numerous, well-developed dendrites and very long axons that leave the gray matter to enter the white matter of the central nervous system and ascend or descend in the major fiber tracts of the brain or spinal cord, or leave the central nervous system and contribute to the formation of peripheral nerves. Neurons of this type conduct impulses over long distances and are called **Golgi type I neurons.** Other neurons whose axons are short and do not leave the region of the perikaryon are called **Golgi type II neurons.** These are especially numerous in the cerebellar and cerebral cortices and retina of the eye. They vary greatly in size and shape and have several branching dendrites. Golgi type II neurons primarily serve as association neurons — that is, they collect nerve impulses and disseminate them to surrounding neurons.

Individual neurons also can be classified by their number of dendrites. **Unipolar neurons** lack dendrites and have only a single process, the axon. Although common in the developing nervous system, they are rare in adults. **Bipolar neurons** have a single dendrite and an axon, usually located at opposite poles of the perikaryon. They are found in the retina, olfactory epithelium, and cochlear and vestibular ganglia. Neurons of all craniospinal ganglia originate as bipoplar neurons in the embryo, but during development, the dendrite and axon migrate to a common site in the cell body where they unite to form a single process. In the adult, this type of neuron is said to be **pseudounipolar.** The combined process, often called a dendraxon, may run for a short distance and then divide into two processes, one of which serves as a dendrite and receives stimuli from peripheral regions of the body, and the other of which acts as an axon and enters the gray matter of the central nervous system to synapse with other neurons. Although the process directed toward the periphery acts as a dendrite, it is unusual since morphologically, it resembles an axon. This functional dendrite is smooth and unbranched and usually receives nervous input from a receptor organ. **Multipolar neurons** are the most common type. They vary considerably in size and shape and are characterized by multiple dendrites.

Ganglia

KEY WORDS: **cranial ganglion, spinal ganglion, satellite cell, sensory ganglion, pseudounipolar neuron, glomerulus, autonomic ganglion, visceral motor efferent, multipolar neuron**

Ganglia are classified as cranial, spinal, and autonomic. Macroscopically, **cranial** and **spinal ganglia** appear as globular swellings on the sensory roots of their respective nerves. Each ganglion is enveloped by a connective tissue capsule and may contain perikarya of only a few neurons or as many as 55,000 (see atlas figures 8-22 and 23). A delicate network of collagenous and reticular fibers, accompanied by small blood vessels, extends between individual neurons and together with bundles of nerve processes, often separates the perikarya into groups. The perikarya are surrounded by two distinct capsules. The inner capsule is made up of a single layer of low cuboidal supporting cells called **satellite cells** (see atlas figure 8-22). The outer capsule lies immediately outside the basal lamina of the satellite cells and consists of a vascular connective tissue.

Cranial and spinal ganglia are **sensory ganglia** and contain **pseudounipolar neurons.** The perikarya appear spherical or pear-shaped and are 15 to 100 μm in diameter. They often show a large, central nucleus and a distinct nucleolus (see atlas figure 8-22). The dendraxon of the pseudounipolar neuron may become convoluted to form a **glomerulus** (see atlas figure 8-23). This nerve process then divides: One branch, a functional dendrite, passes to a receptor organ; the other, a functional axon, passes into the central nervous system. The perikarya of these pseudounipolar neurons do not receive synapses from other neurons.

Autonomic ganglia consist of collections of perikarya of **visceral efferent motor neurons** and are located in swellings along the sympathetic

chain or in the walls of organs supplied by the autonomic nervous system. They generally have a connective tissue capsule. The neurons usually are **multipolar** and assume various sizes and shapes (see atlas figure 8-24). Perikarya range from 15 to 60 μm in diameter; the nucleus is large, round, and often eccentrically placed in the cell; and binucleate cells are not uncommon. Lipofuscin granules are more frequent in neurons of autonomic ganglia than in craniospinal ganglia. The ganglia of larger sympathetic chains are encapsulated by satellite cells, but a capsule may be absent around ganglia in the walls of the viscera (see atlas figure 8-25). Unlike craniospinal ganglia, neurons of autonomic ganglia receive numerous synapses and are influenced by other neurons.

Nerve Fibers

KEY WORDS: **myelin, Schwann cell, neurilemma (sheath of Schwann), node of Ranvier, internode, internodal segment, neurokeratin, major dense line, intraperiod line, mesaxon, action potential, saltatory conduction**

A nerve fiber consists of an axon (axis cylinder) and a surrounding connective tissue sheath. Large nerve fibers are enclosed by a lipoprotein material called **myelin;** smaller nerve fibers may or may not be surrounded by myelin (see atlas figures 8-10, 8-13, and 8-16). Thus, nerve fibers may be classed as myelinated or unmyelinated (Fig. 8-1).

Axons of peripheral nerves are enclosed by a sheath of flattened cells called **Schwann cells.** These cells are thin, attenuated cells with flattened, elongate nuclei located near the center of the cells. Their cytoplasm contains a small Golgi complex, a few scattered profiles of granular endoplasmic reticulum, scattered mitochondria, microtubules, microfilaments, and at times, numerous lysosomes. The outer cell membrane is covered by a layer of proteoglycan. Schwann cells invest nerve fibers from near their beginnings almost to their terminations. The resulting **neurilemma (sheath of Schwann)** is continuous with the capsule of satellite cells that surrounds the perikarya of neurons in craniospinal ganglia.

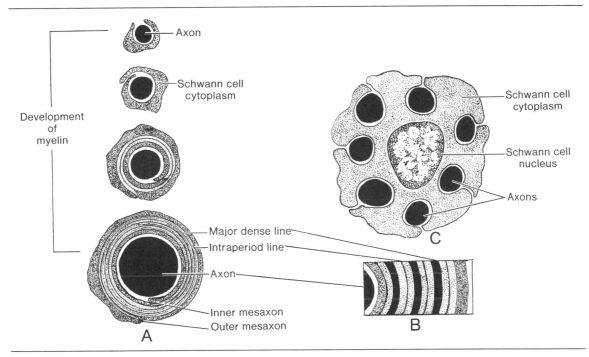

Fig. 8-1. Myelinated fiber (A, B) and nonmyelinated nerve (C).

Schwann cells produce and maintain the myelin on nerve fibers of the peripheral nervous system.

The neurilemmal and myelin sheaths are interrupted by small gaps at regular intervals along the extent of the nerve fiber. These interruptions represent regions of discontinuity between individual Schwann cells and are called **nodes of Ranvier** (see atlas figure 8-11). The neurilemmal and myelin sheaths are made up of a series of small individual segments, each of which consists of the region between two consecutive nodes of Ranvier and makes up one **internode** or **internodal segment.** An internode represents the area occupied by a single Schwann cell and its myelin. Myelin is not a secretory product of Schwann cells but a mass of lipoprotein that results from successive layering of the Schwann cell plasmalemma as it wraps around the axon. Myelin may appear homogeneous, but after some methods of preparation, it may be represented by a network of residual protein called **neurokeratin** (see atlas figure 8-12).

Ultrastructurally, myelin appears as a series of regular, repeating light and dark lines. The dark lines, called **major dense lines,** result from apposition of the inner surfaces of the Schwann cell plasmalemma (see atlas figure 8-14). The less dense **intraperiod lines** represent the fusion of the outer surfaces of the Schwann cell plasmalemma and lie between the repeating major dense lines. Oblique discontinuities often are observed in the myelin of peripheral nerves and form the Schmidt-Lantermann incisures or clefts. The clefts represent local separations of the myelin lamellae.

Unmyelinated fibers (axons) also are surrounded by Schwann cells. In electron micrographs, 15 or more unmyelinated axons are found in recesses in the plasmalemma of a single Schwann cell. The membrane of the Schwann cell closely surrounds each axon and is intimately associated with it (see atlas figures 8-13 and 8-16). As the cell membrane of the Schwann cell encircles the axon, it courses back to come in contact with itself. This point of contact is called the **mesaxon.** In myelinated nerves, the primary infoldings of the Schwann cell membrane at the axon-myelin junction is called the internal mesaxon. The junction between the superficial lamellae of the myelin sheath and the Schwann cell plasmalemma is the external mesaxon.

The speed with which an impulse is transmitted along a nerve fiber is proportional to the diameter of the fiber. The diameter of heavily myelinated nerve fibers is much greater than that of unmyelinated fibers, and therefore conduction is faster in myelinated fibers. Nerve fibers in peripheral nerves can be classed according to the diameter and speed of conduction. Type A nerve fibers are large, myelinated motor and sensory fibers, 3 to 20 μm in diameter, that conduct impulses at 15 to 120 m/second. More finely myelinated fibers with diameters up to 3 μm conduct impulses at 3 to 15 m/second and are type B fibers. They represent many of the visceral sensory fibers. Type C fibers are small, unmyelinated nerve fibers that conduct impulses at 0.5 to 2.0 m/second.

The first event in development of an **action potential** along a nerve fiber is a sudden increase in permeability to sodium ion, resulting in depolarization of the axon and development of a negative charge along the axon surface (Fig. 8-2A). The local current created between the depolarized and resting surface membranes causes an increased permeability of the membrane to sodium ion. A cycle of membrane activation is established that results in the transmission of the depolarization process (a nerve impulse) along the nerve fiber. Once depolarization occurs, it will pass along the entire cell membrane of the axon. The nerve impulse lasts for only a short time, and repolarization is brought about by a sodium pump mechanism in the cell membrane of the axon. The generation of a nerve impulse is an "all or nothing" phenomenon.

In the faster-conducting myelinated nerves, impulses travel from node to node; this method of impulse conduction is called **saltatory conduction** (Fig. 8-2B). Because depolarization occurs only at the nodes of Ranvier, nerve impulses jump from node to node across the intervening internodal segment. This explains, in part, the higher velocity of nerve transmission in myelinated nerve fibers.

Peripheral Nerves

KEY WORDS: mixed nerve, epineurium, fascicle, perineurium, endoneurium

Peripheral nerves consist of several nerve fibers united by surrounding connective tissue (see atlas figure 8-15). They are **mixed nerves** consisting of sensory (afferent) and motor (efferent) nerve fibers that may be myelinated or unmyelinated (see atlas figure 8-16). The sheath of connective tissue surrounding a peripheral nerve makes up the **epineurium** and unites several bundles of nerve fibers into a single unit, a peripheral nerve. The epineurium consists of fibroblasts, longitudinal collagen fibers, and scattered fat cells. Each bundle or **fascicle** of nerve fibers is enclosed by concentric layers of flattened, fibroblastlike cells and collagen fibers that form a dense connective tissue sheath called the **perineurium** (see atlas figure 8-16). Delicate collagenous fibers, reticular fibers, fibroblasts, and macrophages lie between individual nerve fibers within each fascicle and constitute the **endoneurium.** Small blood vessels are found primarily in the epineurium and perineurium, but in thicker regions of the endoneurium, they may occur as delicate capillary networks. The perineurium and epineurium of peripheral nerves become continuous with the meninges of the central nervous system.

Peripheral Nerve Endings

KEY WORDS: somatic efferent, motor endplate, motor unit, visceral efferent, receptor, free (naked) nerve ending, encapsulated nerve ending

Nerve endings increase the surface contact area between nervous and nonnervous structures and allow stimuli to be transmitted from nerve endings to muscles, causing them to contract, or to epithelial cells, causing them to secrete. When

Fig. 8-2. Schematic representation of action potential in (A) nonmyelinated and (B) myelinated fibers.

stimulated, dendrites at the periphery generate impulses that are transferred along the nerve fiber to sensory ganglia and ultimately to the central nervous system.

Peripheral efferent (motor) nerve fibers can be divided into somatic and visceral efferent groups. **Somatic efferent** fibers end in skeletal muscle as small, oval expansions called *motor end-plates* (see atlas figure 8-21). The skeletal muscle cells supplied by a single motor neuron constitute a **motor unit.** Muscles with a large number of motor units can make more precise movements than those with fewer units for the same number of muscle cells. **Visceral efferent** nerve fibers stimulate smooth muscle, cardiac muscle, and glandular epithelium. Visceral motor endings of smooth muscle terminate as two or more swellings that pass between individual muscle cells. In cardiac muscle, numerous thin nerve fibers end near the surface of individual muscle cells but form no specialized contacts with them. Endings in glands are from unmyelinated nerves and

form elaborate, delicate nets along the external surface of the basal lamina of the gland cells; fine branches penetrate the basal lamina and pass between individual epithelial cells.

Terminal peripheral nerve fibers that are excitable to stimuli are **receptors** and can transform chemical and physical stimuli into nerve impulses. Receptors vary in morphology, may be quite complex, and often are grouped into free (naked), diffuse, and encapsulated nerve endings.

Free (naked) nerve endings arise from myelinated and unmyelinated fibers of relatively small diameter. They are widely distributed and although most numerous in the skin, are present in the connective tissue of visceral organs, in deep fascia, in muscles, and in mucous membranes. As myelinated fibers near their terminations, they lose their myelin and form unmyelinated terminal arborizations. Unmyelinated nerve fibers end in numerous fibrils that terminate as small, knoblike thickenings. Many naked nerve endings act as pain receptors. A diffuse type of naked receptor encircles the base of hair follicles to form peritrichal nerve endings that are sensitive to hair movement. They are particularly well developed in the vibrissae of some mammals. In addition to the naked interepithelial nerve endings that terminate among epithelial cells, there are some endings that form concave neurofibrillar discs applied to a single modified epithelial cell of stratified squamous epithelium. These more specialized nerve endings are called the tactile discs of Merkel.

In **encapsulated nerve endings,** the terminals are enclosed in a capsule of connective tissue (Fig. 8-3; see atlas figures 8-19 and 8-20). They vary considerably in size, shape, location, and type of stimuli perceived. As the nerve fibers near their respective capsules, they generally lose their myelin and neurolemmal sheaths and enter the capsule as naked nerve endings. A number of encapsulated nerve endings, their locations, and proposal functions are summarized in Table 8-1.

Synapse

KEY WORDS: terminal bouton, calyx (basket ending), bouton en passage, synaptic vesicle, presynaptic membrane, synaptic cleft, postsynaptic membrane, subsynaptic web, threshold of excitation, gap junction

The site where impulses are transmitted from one neuron to another is called a synapse (Fig. 8-4) and may occur between axon and dendrite (axodendritic), axon and cell body (axosomatic), axon and axon (axoaxonic), dendrite and dendrite (dendrodendritic), dendrite and perikaryon (somatodendritic), or cell bodies of adjacent neurons (somatosomatic). The number of synapses associated with a single neuron varies according to the type of neuron. Small Golgi type II neurons (granule cells) of the cerebellum may have only a few synaptic points, whereas other neurons, such as Golgi type I (Purkinje cells of the cerebellum), may have several hundred thousand. Physiologically, excitatory and inhibitory synapses occur.

Synaptic endings of axons usually occur as small swellings at the tips of axon branches and are called **terminal boutons** (see atlas figure 8-17). The axon may end in thin branches that surround the perikaryon or dendrites of another neuron; these endings are called **calyces (basket endings).** Synaptic contacts also may occur at intervals along the terminal segment of an axon, forming **boutons en passage.**

Synaptic endings vary considerably in form from one type of neuron to another but generally show some common features. Each neuron is a distinct cellular unit, and there is no cytoplasmic continuity between cells. In some ways, synaptic points resemble desmosomes and may aid in maintaining contact between nerve cells. Ultrastructurally, the presynaptic area (terminal bouton) contains clusters of mitochondria and numerous membrane-bound, electron-lucent vesicles with diameters of 40 to 60 nm. These **synaptic vesicles** contain neurotransmitter substances such as dopamine, norepinephrine, acetylcholine, and serotonin; amino acids; and a number of peptides. The vesicles congregate near the **presynaptic membrane,** a slightly thickened area of the axon plasmalemma at the synaptic contact (see atlas figure 8-18). Pre- and postsynaptic membranes are separated by a narrow space, 20 to 30 nm wide, called the **synaptic cleft,** which may contain fine filaments and glycosaminoglycan. The **postsynaptic membrane** shows increased electron density and is slightly thickened, and its internal surface is associated with a network of dense filamentous material called the **subsynaptic web.** The cytoplasm of the postsynaptic region lacks synaptic vesicles and shows fewer mitochondria than are found in the presynaptic area.

As an action potential reaches the presynaptic area of an axon, the synaptic vesicles fuse at sites along the presynaptic membrane and release transmitter substance into the synaptic cleft. The transmitter substance reacts with special receptors in the postsynaptic membrane, causing an immediate increase in the permeability of the postneuronal membrane to sodium ion, thus changing the resting membrane potential. If the potential of the postsynaptic membrane rises above a certain level, the **threshold of excitation,**

Meissner's corpuscle

Corpuscle of Ruffini

Merkel's disc

End-bulb of Krause

Corpuscle of Vater-Pacini

Fig. 8-3. Diagram of types of sensory nerve endings.

Table 8-1. Encapsulated Sensory Nerve Endings

Name of receptor	Locations	Functions
Lamellated corpuscles of Vater-Pacini	Dermis of skin, periosteum, mesenteries, pleura, nipples, pancreas, tendons, joint capsules, ligaments, walls of viscera, penis, clitoris	Proprioception, pressure, vibration
Corpuscles of Meissner	Dermal papillae of digits, lips, genitalia, and nipples	Touch
End-bulbs of Krause	Dermis, conjunctiva, oral cavity	Cold, pressure
Genital corpuscles	Penis, clitoris, nipples	Touch, pressure
Corpuscles of Ruffini	Dermis, joint capsules	Heat
Neurotendinous endings (of Golgi)	Tendons	Proprioception
Neuromuscular spindles	Skeletal muscle	Proprioception

Fig. 8-4. Diagram of a synapse.

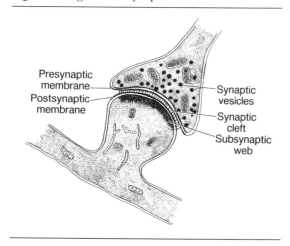

Presynaptic membrane
Postsynaptic membrane
Synaptic vesicles
Synaptic cleft
Subsynaptic web

an action potential is transmitted by the postsynaptic neuron. The first parts of the postsynaptic neuron to initiate an action potential are the axon hillock and initial segment of the axon. The initial segment of an axon is a few microns long and lacks a myelin sheath. In most neurons, the cell membrane of this region has a lower threshold of excitation than does that of the perikaryon or dendrites.

If transmitter substances decrease the permeability of the postsynaptic membrane, the threshold of excitation rises and the net effect is

inhibitory. Inhibition is thought to depend on the receptor sites in the postsynaptic membrane rather than specific neurotransmitter substances; transmitter substances that have an excitatory effect at one synapse may have an inhibitory influence at a synapse in a different site.

Acetylcholine is the transmitter substance most commonly found in the electron-lucent synaptic vesicles of the central nervous system and motor end-plates. Synaptic vesicles of most sympathetic postganglionic axons are characterized by electron-dense cores and contain catecholamines.

Electrical coupling is another means of transferring impulses in some types of synapses and occurs at **gap junctions.**

Neuroglia

KEY WORDS: astrocyte, protoplasmic astrocyte, fibrous astrocyte, end foot (foot process), oligodendrocyte, interfascicular oligodendrocyte, perineuronal satellite oligodendrocyte, microglia, ependyma, tela choroidea, choroid plexus, blood-brain barrier

Neurons form a relatively small proportion of the cells in the central nervous system. Most of the cells are nonneuronal supporting cells called neuroglia. Depending on the location in the central nervous system, neuroglia may outnumber neurons by as much as 50 : 1. Together, neuroglia account for over half the weight of the brain. Neuroglia generally are smaller than neurons and in light microscope preparations can be identified by their small, round nuclei, which are scattered among neurons and their processes. Neuroglia include ependymal cells, astrocytes, oligodendrocytes, and microglia. Astrocytes and oligodendrocytes often are collectively referred to as macroglia.

Morphologically, **astrocytes** are divided into protoplasmic and fibrous types. **Protoplasmic astrocytes** are found mainly in the gray matter and are characterized by numerous thick, branched processes. **Fibrous astrocytes** occur mainly in white matter and are distinguished by long, thin, generally unbranched processes (see atlas figure 8-30). The two forms of astrocyte may represent a single type that varies in morphology according to its location and metabolic state. In electron micrographs, astrocytes usually show an electron-lucent, largely organelle-free cytoplasm and euchromatic nuclei. The cytoplasm of the cell body and its processes contains bundles of intermediate filaments called glial filaments. Astrocytes may provide a framework to support the neurons and contribute to their nutrition and metabolic activity, but their precise function remains unknown.

The astrocyte processes vary considerably in appearance. Some are thick and long, others are thin and sheetlike. The processes often expand to form **end feet (foot processes)** that are aligned along the internal surface of the pia mater and around the walls of blood vessels. The largest concentration of end feet occurs beneath the pial surface, where they surround the brain and spinal cord to form a membranelike structure called the glia limitans.

Smaller neuroglial cells with fewer processes and more deeply stained nuclei are **oligodendrocytes,** of which there are two types. **Interfascicular oligodendrocytes** occur mainly in the fiber tracts that form the white matter of the brain and spinal cord. **Perineuronal satellite oligodendrocytes** are restricted to the gray matter and are closely associated with the cell bodies of neurons. The cytoplasm of both types of oligodendrocytes contains free ribosomes, short cis-

ternae of granular endoplasmic reticulum, an extensive Golgi complex, and numerous mitochondria. Large numbers of microtubules form parallel arrays that run throughout the cytoplasm of the cell body and into its processes.

Schwann cells are not present in the central nervous system; oligodendrocytes serve as the myelin-forming cells of this region. Myelinated nerve fibers of the central nervous system have nodes of Ranvier, but unlike peripheral myelinated fibers, they do not show incisures. The myelin sheath begins at the end of the initial segment of the axon, a few microns from the axon hillock, and ensheathes the rest of the axon to near its end. Each internodal segment of a nerve fiber in the central nervous system is formed by a single cytoplasmic process from a nearby oligodendrocyte, which wraps around the axon. Unlike Schwann cells of the peripheral nervous system, a single oligodendrocyte provides the internodal segments of the myelin sheath for several separate, but adjacent, axons (Fig. 8-5). In some regions, as in the optic nerve, a single oligodendrocyte may be responsible for the internodal segments on 40 to 50 axons. Because perineuronal satellite oligodendrocytes lie close to the perikarya of neurons, it has been proposed that oligodendrocytes influence the metabolism and nutrition of neurons, but this remains to be shown conclusively.

In the central nervous system, perineuronal satellite and interfascicular oligodendrocytes have the same relationship to perikarya and their

Fig. 8-5. Myelination in the central nervous system.

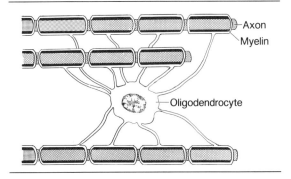

axons as that which exists between satellite cells and Schwann cells of peripheral nerve fibers. Schwann cells and satellite cells could be considered as neuroglial elements of the peripheral nervous system.

Small cells called **microglia** also are present in the central nervous system, and in areas of damage or disease, they are thought to proliferate and become phagocytic. As material is phagocytosed, the cells enlarge and then are called Gitterzellen or compound granular corpuscles. Monocytes appear to be the precursors of microglial cells, which thus are part of the mononuclear system of phagocytes with ultimate derivation from the bone marrow.

The **ependyma** lines the central canal of the spinal cord and ventricles of the brain. It consists of a simple epithelium in which the closely packed cells vary from cuboidal to columnar. The luminal surfaces of the cells show large numbers of microvilli and, depending on the location, may show cilia. Adjacent cells are united by desmosomes and zonula adherens; zonula occludens generally are not seen. Hence, cerebrospinal fluid in the central canal and ventricles can pass between ependymal cells to enter the parenchyma of the central nervous system. The bases of ependymal cells have long, threadlike processes that branch, enter the substance of the brain and spinal cord, and may extend to the external surface where they contribute end feet to the glia limitans.

The ependyma forms a secretory epithelium in the ventricles of the brain, where it is in direct contact with a highly vascular region of the pia mater, the **tela choroidea.** The modified ependyma and tela choroidea form the **choroid plexus,** which secretes cerebrospinal fluid. Ependymal cells of the choroid plexus are columnar and closely packed and bear numerous microvilli. Unlike those in other regions of the ependyma, cell apices here are joined by zonula occludens, which prevent passage of material between cells. Ependymal cells lie on a continuous basal lamina that separates them from a connective tissue that contains small bundles of collagenous fibers, pia-arachnoid cells, and numerous blood vessels.

Capillary endothelial cells in this region, unlike those elsewhere in the brain, have numerous fenestrations. Fluid readily moves through the capillary wall but is prevented from entering the ventricles by the zonula occludens. Ependymal cells secrete sodium ions into the ventricles, and chloride ions, water, and other substances follow passively. Protein and glucose concentrations are relatively low. Cerebrospinal fluid is formed continuously, moves slowly through the ventricles of the brain, and enters the subarachnoid space. It surrounds and protects the central nervous system from mechanical injury and is important in the metabolic activities of the central nervous system.

Certain substances in the blood are prevented from entering the central nervous system although they readily gain access to other tissues. Capillaries deep in the spinal cord and brain are sheathed by the end feet of astrocytes, and the nonfenestrated endothelial cells are united by occluding tight junctions. Additionally, the internal plasmalemma of the endothelial cells is thought to have special properties that prevent passage of these substances. Together, the tight junctions and internal plasmalemma of the endothelial cells form the **blood-brain barrier.**

Highly vascularized areas — the circumventricular organs — are present in specific regions along the midline of the walls of the ventricles. These organs include the organum vasculosum laminae terminalis, subfornical organ, subcommissural organ, and area postrema. Except for the subcommisural organ, the ependymal epithelium of these areas lacks cilia and contains stellate cells called tanycytes. Such regions are devoid of an internal (subependymal) layer and the external (subpial) layer of glial processes. The underlying capillaries are lined by a fenestrated endothelium. These regions lack the morphologic elements of a true blood-brain barrier and, except for the subcommissural organ, are able to accumulate vital dyes. Large molecules are thought to traverse these regions, which provide areas of exchange between the central nervous system and blood.

Spinal Cord

KEY WORDS: **gray matter, internuncial neuron, central canal, ependyma, white matter**

The spinal cord is subdivided into a central H-shaped region of gray matter and a surrounding layer of white matter. **Gray matter** consists mainly of perikarya of neurons, their dendrites, and surrounding neuroglial cells and is arranged into two dorsal and two ventral horns. The dorsal horns contain perikarya of multipolar neurons receiving sensory impulses that enter the spinal cord from the peripheral nervous system. Neurons of the dorsal horns transmit the impulses to other neurons in this and other areas of gray matter and are referred to as **internuncial neurons.** The multipolar neurons in the ventral horns are the largest in the spinal cord and transmit motor impulses from the spinal cord to the periphery (see atlas figure 8-26). In the thoracic and upper lumbar regions of the spinal cord, small multipolar neurons form an intermediolateral horn that provides preganglionic sympathetic fibers for the autonomic nervous system. The **central canal** of the spinal cord lies in the center of the crossbar of the H-shaped gray matter and is lined by **ependyma.**

The **white matter** consists mainly of myelinated axons and lacks the perikarya and dendrites of neurons. It is subdivided into anterior, lateral, and posterior funiculi by the dorsal and ventral horns of the gray matter. A funiculus consists of several tracts, each of which in turn contains several bundles of nerve fibers. Nerve fibers in each tract carry similar impulses, motor or sensory, that either ascend or descend along the long axis of the spinal cord.

Cerebellar and Cerebral Hemispheres

The cerebellar and cerebral hemispheres differ from the spinal cord in that the gray matter is located at the periphery and the white matter lies centrally. Both regions of the brain consist of an outer cortex of gray matter and a subcortical region of white matter.

Cerebral Cortex

KEY WORDS: **laminated appearance, pyramidal cell, apical dendrite, Betz cell, stellate (nonpyramidal) cell**

The cerebral cortex is 1.5 to 4.0 mm thick and contains about 14 billion neurons plus nerve processes and supporting glial cells. In all but a few regions it is characterized by a **laminated appearance.** Perikarya generally are organized into five layers. Starting at the periphery of the cerebral cortex, the general organization of neurons is molecular layer (I), external granular layer (II), external pyramidal layer (III), internal granular layer (IV), internal pyramidal layer (V), and multiform layer (VI).

The molecular layer (I) is a largely cell-free zone just below the surface of the cortex. Neurons of similar type tend to occupy the same layer in the cerebral cortex, although each cellular layer is composed of several different cell types. For convenience of description, these neurons often are placed in two major groups: pyramidal cells and stellate or nonpyramidal cells. The perikarya of **pyramidal cells** are pyramidal in shape and have large **apical dendrites** that usually are oriented toward the surface of the cerebral cortex and enter the overlying layers; the single axons enter the subcortical white matter (see atlas figure 8-27). They are found in layers II, III, V, and, to lesser extent, layer VI. Very large pyramidal-shaped neurons **(Betz cells)** are present in the internal pyramidal layer (V) of the frontal lobe. **Stellate (nonpyramidal) cells** lack the pyramid-shaped perikarya and the large apical dendrite. They occur in all layers of the cerebral cortex but are concentrated in the internal granular layer (IV). Impulses entering the cortex are relayed primarily to stellate cells and then transmitted to pyramidal cells in the various layers by the vertical axons of the stellate cells. Axons of pyramidal cells generally leave the cortex and extend to other regions of the brain and spinal cord.

The cerebral cortex functions in vision, hearing, speech, voluntary motor activities, and learning.

Cerebellar Cortex

KEY WORDS: molecular layer, stellate cell, basket cell, Purkinje cell layer, granule cell layer, mossy fiber, climbing fiber

The cerebellar cortex is characterized by three layers: an outer molecular layer, a middle Purkinje cell layer, and an inner granule cell layer.

The **molecular layer** is mainly a synaptic area with relatively few nerve cells. It consists primarily of unmyelinated axons from granule cells, the axons running parallel to the cortical surface. It also contains large dendrites of the underlying Purkinje cells and in its superficial portion contains small scattered neurons called **stellate cells.** Other small neurons located deep in this layer and adjacent to Purkinje cells are called **basket cells.**

The **Purkinje cell layer** is formed by the cell bodies of Purkinje cells — large, pear-shaped neurons aligned in a single row and characterized by large branching dendrites that lie in the molecular layer (see atlas figure 8-29). They represent Golgi type I neurons and number about 15 million. Three-dimensionally, the large dendritic trees occupy a narrow plane, reminiscent of fan coral, and are so arranged that each dendritic tree is parallel to its neighbor. A single small axon from the Purkinje cell passes through the granule cell layer and synapses with neurons in the central cerebellar area.

The **granule cell layer** consists of numerous closely packed, small neurons whose axons enter the molecular layer to synapse with dendrites of Purkinje cells. The granule cells represent Golgi type II neurons. They have small, round nuclei with coarse chromatin patterns and only scant cytoplasm; dendrites are short and clawlike (see atlas figure 8-28). The axons enter the molecular layer, bifurcate, and run parallel to the surface but perpendicular to the wide plane of the Purkinje dendritic tree. The axons of granule cells synapse with about 450 Purkinje cells in a relationship similar to that of wires coursing along telephone poles. Axons of granule cells also synapse with stellate and basket neurons in the molecular layer. Another type of small neuron, the Golgi cell, is found in the outer zone of the granule cell layer.

Two types of afferent nerve fibers enter the cerebellar cortex from outer regions of the central nervous system. These are the **mossy fibers,** which synapse with granule cells, and the **climbing fibers,** which enter the molecular layer and wind about the dendrites of Purkinje cells.

The cerebellum primarily modulates and coordinates the activities of skeletal muscle.

The gray matter of the spinal cord, cerebrum, and cerebellum consists of a complex, highly ordered meshwork of dendritic, axonal, and glial processes that envelop the perikarya of associated neurons. This network, called the neuropil, provides a vast area for synaptic contact and interaction between nerve processes and forms an organizing framework. It is important for coordinating activities in the central nervous system.

Meninges

KEY WORDS: dura mater, epidural space, subdural space, arachnoid, trabeculae, subarachnoid space, pia mater

In addition to the covering of bone supplied by the skull and vertebral column, the central nervous system is contained within three connective tissue membranes called meninges. The outermost, the **dura mater,** consists primarily of dense collagenous connective tissue. Around the brain it forms two layers and serves as a periosteum for the cranium and as the covering of the brain. The periosteal layer is rich in blood vessels, nerves, and cells. The inner layer is less vascular, and its interior surface is lined by a simple squamous epithelium. Where it covers the spinal cord, the dura is a single layer of dense irregular connective tissue that contains scattered elastic fibers. The outer surface is covered by a simple squamous epithelium, separated from the periosteum of the vertebrae by an **epidural space** filled by loose connective tissue that is rich in fat cells and veins.

The inner surface of the dura of the spinal cord is lined by a simple squamous epithelium. Between it and the next meninx, the arachnoid, is a narrow, fluid-filled **subdural space.**

The **arachnoid** is a thin, weblike, avascular membrane made up of fine collagenous fibers and scattered elastic fibers (Fig. 8-6). The outer region forms a smooth sheet while the inner surface gives rise to numerous strands **(trabeculae)** that extend into and blend with the underlying pia mater. The inner surface of the arachnoid, the trabeculae, and the external surface of the pia are covered by a simple squamous epithelium that also lines a large space, the **subarachnoid space,** which contains cerebrospinal fluid.

The **pia mater** is a thin, vascular membrane that closely invests the brain and spinal cord. Because the pia and arachnoid are closely related, they often are considered together as the pia arachnoid. The pia consists of delicate collagenous and elastic fibers, fibroblasts, macrophages, and scattered mesenchymal cells. Blood vessels entering and leaving the brain substance are invested by a sheath of pia mater. A perivascular space surrounds the vessels as they extend into the substance of the central nervous system and is continuous with the subarachnoid space.

Development of Nervous Tissue

Most of the nervous tissue arises from neuroectoderm on the dorsal surface of the embryonic disc, in the region called the neural plate. As a result of mitotic activity and cell growth, the lateral edges of the neural plate fold upward to form a neural groove (see atlas figures 8-31 and 8-32).

Fig. 8-6. Diagram of the pia arachnoid.

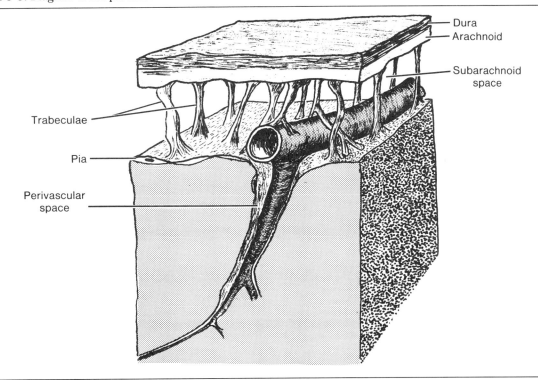

The edges of the fold converge, fuse, and create a hollow neural tube that separates from the overlying ectoderm. Differential proliferation of ectodermal cells along the internal aspect of the neural tube ultimately gives rise to the brain and spinal cord. Some of the proliferating cells differentiate into neurons; others become glial elements (as summarized below).

Cells of craniospinal and autonomic ganglia, pia and arachnoid, Schwann cells, satellite cells, chromaffin cells, and melanocytes

Three concentric zones become visible in the wall of the neural tube: an internal ependymal layer; a wide, intermediate mantle layer; and an outer marginal layer (see atlas figure 8-33). Cells of the ependymal layer divide, migrate to the mantle layer, and differentiate into neuroblasts or glioblasts. Neurons differentiate first, followed by astrocytes and later by oligodendrocytes.

In the spinal cord, the ependymal zone gives rise to the ependyma, the mantle zone becomes the gray matter, and the white matter develops from the marginal zone. Presumptive neurons in the mantle layer are apolar neuroblasts at first but become bipolar neurons as cytoplasmic processes develop at opposite ends of the cell body. As differentiation proceeds, one process (a primitive axon) elongates while the other is replaced by several small processes (primordial dendrites), and multipolar neurons develop. The axons enter into and form the marginal layer. Depending on the region, myelinization occurs after the differentiation of oligodendrocytes.

The regions of the neural tube that initially form the cerebral and cerebellar cortices show three zones similar to those in the spinal cord. Differentiating neurons in the mantle zone of the cerebral cortex migrate into the marginal zone to establish superficial cortical layers. The stratified appearance of the adult cerebral cortex results from successive waves of migration of neuroblasts into the marginal zone and the differentiation of different types of neurons in the cortex. Sensory areas of the cerebral cortex are typified by numerous granular cells (neurons), whereas motor areas are characterized by large numbers of pyramidal cells.

Initially, the developing cerebellar cortex also is arranged into ependymal, mantle, and marginal zones. As development progresses, some neuroblasts from the mantle zone migrate into the marginal zone of the cerebellar cortex to become Golgi and granular cells, while others remain in the mantle zone to form cerebellar nuclei. As this takes place, a second migration occurs and these Purkinje cells, together with cells from the first migration, establish the definitive cerebellar cortex.

As the neural tube closes, a second source of neurons, the neural crest, arises and gives origin to neurons and supportive (glial) elements. Along the crest of each neural fold, ectodermal cells lose their epithelial characteristics, detach, and migrate into the mesoderm that lies on either side of the neural tube; they then acquire the characteristics of mesenchymal cells. The neural crest is a major contributor to the peripheral nervous system and gives rise to neurons and supporting cells (glia and satellite cells) of spinal root ganglia; autonomic ganglia; Schwann cells; some neurons in the sensory ganglia of cranial nerves V, VII, IX, and X; and supporting cells, but not the neurons of the geniculate, acoustic, petrosal, and nodose ganglia. Other cells of the neural crest envelop the neural tube and contribute to formation of the meninges.

Functional Summary

An essential function of nervous tissue is communication. Nervous tissue is able to fulfill this role because of its ability to react to various stimuli and transmit the impulse from one region to another. Thus, the organism is able to react to the external environment and internal events to integrate and coordinate body functions. In cortical regions of the brain, complex relationships between different types of neurons provide intellect, memory, and conscious experience and serve for the interpretation of special impulses from the eye and ear into the sensations of sight and sound, respectively. All contribute to the personality and behavior of the individual.

Neurons are the structural and functional units of nervous tissue. They generally are complex in shape and usually have several cytoplasmic processes. Dendrites conduct nerve impulses to the perikaryon, and a single axon conducts impulses from the perikaryon to other neurons or effector organs. Receptor organs of nerve tissue convert mechanical, chemical, or other stimuli into nerve impulses that are transmitted along a physiologic dendrite to its cell body located in spinal or cranial ganglia. From ganglia the impulses are relayed to other neurons in the central nervous system. Nerve fibers of most somatic sensory neurons are large and myelinated, and impulses are relayed quickly to the central nervous system to elicit a response. Most effector and internuncial neurons are multipolar, and their numerous dendrites summate the excitatory and inhibitory impulses that influence a specific neuron. Dendrites of this type of neuron usually are unmyelinated. When the threshold of activity is attained, an action potential is generated in the region of the axon hillock and/or initial segment of the axon. These regions of the neuron have a lower threshold of excitation than the dendrites or perikaryon. The impulse is conducted by the axon to other neurons or an effector organ to elicit a response. The speed of conduction depends on fiber diameter and usually reflects the degree of myelinization, both in peripheral nerve fibers and those of the central nervous system. Myelin is formed by consecutive layerings of the plasmalemma of adjacent supporting cells. In the peripheral nervous system, myelin is formed by Schwann cells scattered at intervals along a single axon. Oligodendrocytes are responsible for myelinization in the central nervous system and form internodal segments on more than one axon. Myelin is thought to act as an insulating material to prevent the wave of depolarization (action potential) from traveling the length of the axolemma as occurs in unmyelinated nerve fibers. Depolarization occurs only at the nodes of Ranvier in myelinated nerves, and the impulses jump the internodal segment to adjacent nodes. This saltatory conduction partly explains the greater speed of nerve impulses transmitted by myelinated nerve fibers.

Communication between neurons and effector organs takes place at specific contact points called synapses, where nerve impulses are transferred directly to other cells by chemical transmitters or electrical coupling. The terminal axons of some neurons, such as those in the hypothalamic and paraventricular regions, may secrete peptides or other agents directly into the bloodstream. These neurons influence cells that are not in direct contact with them and thus act as endocrine cells.

Neurons are surrounded by supporting cells. In the peripheral nervous system, neurons are intimately associated with Schwann and satellite cells that, like astrocytes and oligodendrocytes of the central nervous system, provide structural and metabolic support to their associated neurons. The ependyma represents glial cells that form a simple epithelial lining for the ventricles of the brain and the central canal of the spinal cord. In some areas of the ventricles, ependyma comes in direct contact with vascularized regions of the pia mater to form the choroid plexus. The choroid plexus actively and continuously produces cerebrospinal fluid, which surrounds and cushions the brain and spinal cord and plays an important role in their metabolism. The meninges form protective coverings for the brain and spinal cord and contain numerous blood vessels that supply the structures of the central nervous system.

Clinical Correlations

Except for the bipolar neurons of olfactory epithelium, nerve cells are end cells and if lost for any reason, are not replaced. In the central nervous system, neuroglial cells (primarily astrocytes) fill any areas from which neurons are lost. Necrosis of neurons can result from a variety of noxious processes such as anoxia, viral infections, ischemia, and hypoglycemia. The affected neurons shrink and the triangular shape of their perikarya is accentuated. Nissl granules disappear, the cytoplasm becomes more acidophilic, and the nucleus becomes pyknotic before fragmenting. The necrotic cells may be removed by phagocytosis, but more frequently they undergo autolysis and disappear. Atrophy of neurons occurs in many slowly progressive degenerative diseases of nervous tissue. The neurons are smaller than normal, large amounts of lipofuscin accumulate in the cytoplasm, and finally, the neurons disappear. In advanced atrophy of the brain, the convolutions are more rounded, the sulci widened, and the pia arachnoid thickened. Loss of neurons is accompanied by disappearance of their axons and myelin sheaths so that the white matter of the brain is thinned.

When axons of peripheral nerves are dissociated from their perikarya by transection or severe crushing injuries, degenerative changes occur in the cell body and in the severed process. The axon and myelin sheath distal to the point of transection show changes known as Wallerian (secondary) degeneration. Within a few hours after injury, focal accumulations of mitochondria appear; neurofilaments and mitochondria become vesicular and begin to break up. By two days later the axon has a beaded appearance as it frag-

ments; simultaneously, myelin degenerates and is broken down into simpler lipids. The droplets of fat are taken up by phagocytes. The Schwann cells remain after the axon and myelin have been removed and form a neurilemmal tube surrounded by endoneurium and filled with debris. The Schwann cells proliferate, the wall of the tube thickens, and the original bore is reduced in size or obliterated; the tube forms a rounded cord. Wallerian degeneration also occurs in the central nervous system. The degenerated myelin and fragments of axons are removed by microglia.

Proximal to the point of injury, the perikaryon also shows degenerative changes, but these extend for only a short distance, perhaps one or two internodes in a clean incised wound. Within two or three days, the Nissl substance breaks down into dustlike particles, beginning near the nucleus and extending to the periphery of the cell. The nucleus becomes eccentrically placed and the whole cell may appear paler than normal. New axonal sprouts (neurites) may appear from the stump of the severed axon and grow along the neurilemmal tubes to restore the axon. If the neurites fail to associate with the tube, they shrink, an axon fails to develop, and the entire cell dies. Usually, only one neurite dominates. If appropriate contact with a receptor occurs, the neurite enlarges and remyelinization may take place, resulting in functional recovery.

Demyelination of axons between two nodes of Ranvier (segmental demyelination) can occur in diabetes mellitus and lead poisoning. Many segments may be involved, and nerve conduction is affected. The myelin may regenerate but will be thinner than normal. In multiple sclerosis myelin of the central nervous system is destroyed in part by the immune system. Its cause is unknown.

Most tumors of the central nervous system arise from glial cells and thus are called gliomas. Some gliomas consist of relatively well-differentiated cells that closely resemble astrocytes, oligodendrocytes, or ependymal cells; others contain cells that are pleomorphic or that are less well differentiated. The most common glioma, the astrocytoma, is derived from astrocytes. As in other tissues, the more primitive and undifferentiated the tumor, generally the more rapid is its growth. All these tumors infiltrate adjacent brain tissue, but neuroectodermal tumors do not metastasize to other organs. Tumors arising from neurons are less common but do occur. These tumors are expanding, space-occupying lesions, and their effects are mainly due to raised intracranial pressure, cerebral edema, and, where blockage of the flow of cerebrospinal fluid occurs, hydrocephalus.

Tumors of nerve roots and peripheral nerves may be solitary or multiple. Some of the tumors (neurofibromas) resemble fibromas and are believed to originate from the cells of the endoneurium or perineurium. In other tumors, the cells form distinctive palisading patterns across bundles of long spindle cells; these are believed to represent Schwann cells and are called schwannomas.

Atlas and Table of Key Features

Key Features of Primary Cell Types of Nervous Tissue

Location of Perikarya	Morphology	Other
Neurons of the peripheral nervous system		
Cranial and spinal ganglia	Large, round, pseudounipolar; distinct central nucleus with nucleolus	Each perikaryon surrounded by satellite cells
Sympathetic chain ganglia, parasympathetic ganglia, in walls of organs	Size variable, stellate; multipolar; nucleus often eccentric; lipofuscin granules common	Axons usually unmyelinated
Neurons of the central nervous system		
Gray matter of spinal cord	Multipolar, stellate; size variable; distinct nuclei and nucleoli	Perikarya occur in groups or columns
Gray matter of cerebral cortex	Multipolar; pyramidal with large apical dendrite; stellate cells with round nuclei; lack apical dendrite	Perikarya organized into 5 layers
Gray matter of cerebellar cortex	multipolar; Purkinje cell and small neurons of granule layer characteristic	Perikarya organized into 3 layers
Glia of the peripheral nervous system		
Schwann cells	Flattened, elongated; heterochromatic nucleus in center of cell	Envelop axon to form neurilemmal sheath; form myelin in peripheral nervous system
Satellite cells (amphicytes)	Single layer of low cuboidal cells; nuclei heterochromatic, cytoplasm clear and indistinct	Surround neuronal perikarya; continuous with neurilemma sheath
Glia of the central nervous system		
Fibrous astrocytes	Pale-staining ovoid or spherical nucleus, sparse chromatin; long thin, unbranched processes	Primarily in white matter

Key Features of Primary Cell Types of Nervous Tissue (continued)

Location of Perikarya	Morphology	Other
Protoplasmic astrocytes	Pale-staining ovoid or spherical nucleus, sparse chromatin; short, thick, branching processes	Primarily in gray matter
Interfascicular oligodendrocytes	Small cell (6–8 μm); ovoid or spherical, deeply staining nuclei; few processes	Envelop axons of white matter; form myelin in central nervous system
Perineuronal oligodendrocytes	Same as above	Gray matter; closely associated with perikarya of neurons
Ependyma	Simple cuboidal to columnar	Central canal of spinal cord; ventricles of brain

Neurons

Neurons

Nerve processes

Neurofilaments

Nucleus

Fig. 8-7. Multipolar neurons from the ventral horn of a human spinal cord. Note the abundance of surrounding nerve processes. (LM, ×400.)

Nucleolus

Chromophilic substance

Nucleus

Chromophilic substance

Axon hillock

Fig. 8-8. A. Ventral horn of human spinal cord stained with crystal violet to demonstrate chromophilic (Nissl) substance. (LM, ×400.) B. Similarly stained neurons in human spinal cord, one of which shows an axon hillock. (LM, ×400.)

Mitochondria

Chromophilic
(Nissl)
substance

Golgi
complexes

Fig. 8-9. A Nissl body in a neuron from the inferior olivary nucleus illustrates that Nissl consists in fact of parallel arrays of granular endoplasmic reticulum. (TEM, ×20,000.)

Peripheral Nerve

Myelin
sheaths

Myelin
sheaths

Fig. 8-10. A cross section of human peripheral nerve stained with osmium to demonstrate myelin sheaths. (LM, ×400.)

Fig. 8-11. A longitudinal section of human peripheral nerve stained with osmium illustrates several nodes of Ranvier. (LM, ×400.)

Fig. 8-12. A cross section of human sciatic nerve stained with Masson trichrome illustrates numerous axis cylinders and neurokeratin. (LM, ×400.)

Myelin

Axoplasm

Mitochondrion

Myelinated
nerve
fiber

Unmyelinated
nerve
fibers

Fig. 8-13. A cross section of a mixed peripheral nerve illustrating a myelinated and several unmyelinated nerve fibers. (TEM, ×8,000.)

Major
dense
line

Intraperiod
line

Fig. 8-14. A region of myelin showing major dense and intraperiod lines. (TEM, ×54,000.)

Perineurium

Collagen bundle

Schwann cell nuclei

Arteriole

Fig. 8-15. A small peripheral nerve within the connective tissue of a human tongue. (LM, ×250.)

Unmyelinated nerve fibers

Myelinated nerve fiber

Schwann cell nucleus

Fibroblast nucleus

Schwann cell nucleus

Unmyelinated nerve fiber

Fibroblast of perineurium

Fig. 8-16. A small mixed peripheral nerve demonstrating several myelinated and unmyelinated nerve fibers and the limiting perineurium. (TEM, ×2,000.)

Synapse

Fig. 8-17. A perikaryon of a human spinal neuron, the external surface of which is associated with numerous terminal boutons. (LM, ×1,000.)

Fig. 8-18. A region of dendritic spines illustrating both presynaptic and postsynaptic membranes. (TEM, ×39,000.)

Nerve Endings

Pancreatic tissue

Nerve fiber in core

Connective tissue lamellae

Fig. 8-19. A pacinian corpuscle found in a human pancreas. (LM, ×250.)

Meissner's corpuscle

Nerve fiber

Keratinized stratified squamous epithelium

Fig. 8-20. A Meissner's corpuscle within a connective papillae of human skin (palm). (LM, ×400.)

Nerve fibers

Motor end-plate

Skeletal muscle

Fig. 8-21. Motor end-plates of human skeletal muscle. (LM, ×400.)

Ganglia

Nuclei of satellite cells

Nuclei of satellite cells

Nucleolus
Nucleus
Cytoplasm
} Nerve cell body

Nuclei of fibroblasts of connective tissue capsule

Golgi complex

Fig. 8-22. A dorsal root ganglion associated with a human spinal cord (osmium stain). (LM, ×300.)

Perikaryon of neuron

Glomeruli

Nerve fibers

Fig. 8-23. Neurons within a human dorsal root ganglion. Note the dendraxons of these pseudounipolar neurons are convoluted and termed glomeruli. (LM, ×250.)

Nerve processes

Neurons

Nucleolus

Fig. 8-24. A human autonomic ganglion. Note that these neurons are multipolar. (LM, ×250.)

Nucleus

Unmyelinated
nerve
fibers

Cytoplasm

Fig. 8-25. An autonomic neuron from a submandibular gland. Note the associated unmyelinated nerve. (TEM, ×2,000.)

Central Nervous System

Nerve
processes

Neurons in
ventral
horn

Axis
cylinders

Gray
matter

White
matter

Fig. 8-26. Neurons in the ventral horn of a human spinal cord. (LM, ×400.)

Fig. 8-27. Pyramidal neurons from a human cerebral cortex. (LM, ×250.)

Fig. 8-28. The three layers of human cerebellar cortex. (LM, ×250.)

Dendritic tree

Purkinje cell

Fig. 8-29. A Purkinje cell from human cerebellum stained to show its dendritic tree. (LM, ×250.)

Glia

Fibrous astrocytes

Capillary

Foot process of fibrous astrocyte

Fig. 8-30. Fibrous astrocytes from white matter of a human spinal cord. (LM, ×300.)

Development

Neural folds

Developing brain

Fig. 8-31. The developing central nervous system of an opossum embryo. (SEM, ×40.)

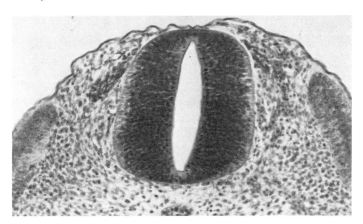

Fig. 8-32. Developing neural tube (spinal cord) from a pig embryo. (LM, ×250.)

Fig. 8-33. A section of developing spinal cord from a human embryo showing ependymal, mantle, and marginal layers. (LM, × 50.)

Review Questions and Answers

Questions

46. Define a nerve fiber as found in the peripheral nervous system.
47. Discuss the role of Nissl substance in a neuron.
48. Compare myelin in the peripheral and central nervous systems.
49. What role does myelin play in the transmission of a nerve impulse?
50. Briefly discuss the synapse and its role in nervous tissue.

Answers

46. A peripheral nerve fiber consists of an axon (axis cylinder) and a surrounding neurilemmal sheath (sheath of Schwann), derived from ectoderm. Nerve fibers may be classified as myelinated or unmyelinated depending on whether a myelin sheath is present.
47. Nissl substance is found throughout the cytoplasm of the perikaryon and dendrites of most neurons but is absent from the axon hillock and axon. It consists of cisternae of granular endoplasmic reticulum arranged in parallel. Nissl bodies represent the sites of protein synthesis in neurons. The protein is transported down the length of the axon for use in metabolism or repair in this region or in some instances is secreted. Protein synthesis does not occur in the axoplasm.
48. Myelin of the peripheral nervous system does not form a continuous sleeve but is in the form of internodal segments, each of which is produced and maintained by a single Schwann cell. It is not a secretory product but represents a mass of lipid-protein that results from the successive layering of the Schwann cell plasmalemma wrapped around the axon. Oblique discontinuities (clefts of Schmidt-Lantermann) are often observed in the myelin sheaths of peripheral nerves and represent local separations of myelin lamellae.

Myelin of the central nervous system also is arranged in numerous internodal segments around axons and, as in peripheral nerves, forms as the result of successive layering of a plasmalemma around an axon. Unlike myelin of the peripheral nerves, however, myelin in the central nervous system is formed and maintained by interfascicular oligodendrocytes. Whereas each internodal segment of myelin in the peripheral nervous system is formed by a single Schwann cell, in the central nervous system a single oligodendrocyte is responsible for the internodal segments on several separate but adjacent axons. Myelinated nerve fibers of the central nervous system lack the clefts of Schmidt-Lantermann.
49. The speed with which an impulse is transmitted along a nerve fiber is proportional to the diameter of the nerve fiber. The diameter of heavily myelinated nerve fibers is much larger than that of unmyelinated fibers and therefore the speed of impulse conduction is faster in myelinated nerves. In the unmyelinated nerve fibers, the action potential travels along the length of the axolemma, whereas in the faster-conducting myelinated nerves, the impulses are conducted from node to node, jumping the internodal segments (saltatory conduction). The myelin sheath is thought to act as an insulating material, and depolarization occurs only at the nodes of Ranvier. This explains, in part, the speed of nerve transmission by myelinated nerve fibers.
50. A synapse represents a specialized site of attachment between neurons or between nerve cells and effector cells where impulses are transferred from one cell to another. Im-

pulses may be transferred either by chemical transmitters or electrical coupling. Synapses may occur between axon and dendrite, axon and cell body, axon and axon, dendrite and dendrite, dendrite and perikaryon, or cell bodies of adjacent neurons. Both excitatory and inhibitory synapses occur. Although synapses vary in morphology in different types of neurons, they exhibit some common features. The presynaptic area generally contains numerous mitochondria and clusters of synaptic vesicles and is separated from the postsynaptic membrane by a narrow synaptic cleft that measures 20 to 30 nm in diameter. The postsynaptic cell membrane shows an increase in electron density and is slightly thickened, and its internal surface is associated with a subsynaptic web. The postsynaptic cytoplasm is further characterized by a lack of synaptic vesicles and contains only a few scattered mitochondria. In this type of synapse, as an action potential reaches the presynaptic area, the synaptic vesicles fuse at specific sites along the presynaptic membrane and release their contained transmitter substance into the synaptic cleft. If the transmitter substance acts to decrease the electrical polarization of the postsynaptic membrane, an action potential (impulse) in the postsynaptic neuron is likely to be generated. If, on the other hand, the effect of the transmitter substance on the postsynaptic membrane increases the electrical polarization, it acts to elevate the threshold of firing and is inhibitory. The excitatory or inhibitory nature of synapses depends on receptor sites in the postsynaptic membrane rather than on the neurotransmitter substances. Electrical coupling is another method by which impulses can be transferred between cells and usually occurs at gap junctions.

9 The Eye

Eyes are photoreceptors containing systems of convex surfaces that transmit and focus light on a surface sensitive to the intensity and wavelength (color) of light. Images formed there are transmitted to the brain, where they are interpreted, correlated, and translated into the sensation of sight. Eyes can regulate the amount of light admitted and change their focal lengths.

In the human, the eyes are almost spherical and are located in and protected by boney sockets provided with a padding of fat. Because the eyes are offset from each other, the images formed are correspondingly offset and provide for binocular vision. Integration of the binocular images results in a three-dimensional quality of sight through which depth and spacial orientation are recognized.

General Structure

The wall of the eyeball consists of an outer corneoscleral coat, a central coat called the uvea, and an inner coat called the retina.

The corneoscleral coat is divided into a smaller, transparent, anterior cornea that allows light to enter the eye and the sclera, a larger, white segment. The sclera is a tough fibrous layer that protects the delicate internal structures of the eye and helps maintain the shape of the eyeball.

The uveal coat consists of the choroid, ciliary body, and iris. The choroid is the vascular part of the uvea, immediately below the retina. It is continuous with the ciliary body, which forms a belllike structure around the interior of the eye-ball, just forward of the anterior margin of the retina. The ciliary body controls the diameter and shape of the lens, which focuses light on the retina. The iris, the last portion of the uvea, is continuous with the ciliary body and has a central opening, the pupil, whose diameter can be changed to regulate the amount of light passing into the eyeball.

The retina consists of pigment-containing photoreceptors that, on exposure to light, produce chemical energy that is converted into the electric energy of nerve impulses. A chain of conducting neurons in the retina transmits the impulses to the optic nerve. The optic disc is the point where nerve fibers from the retina gather to form the optic nerve and leave the eyeball.

The interior of the eyeball is subdivided into an anterior chamber, a posterior chamber, and a vitreal cavity. Each is filled with a transparent medium that helps maintain the shape and turgor of the eye. The anterior and posterior chambers are continuous through the pupil and contain a watery aqueous humor, which provides nutrients for the anterior structures of the eye. The large vitreal cavity is filled with a viscous, transparent gel called the vitreous humor or vitreous body. The general structure of the eye is shown in Fig. 9-1.

Corneoscleral Coat

The corneoscleral coat forms the outermost layer of the eyeball and consists of the cornea and sclera.

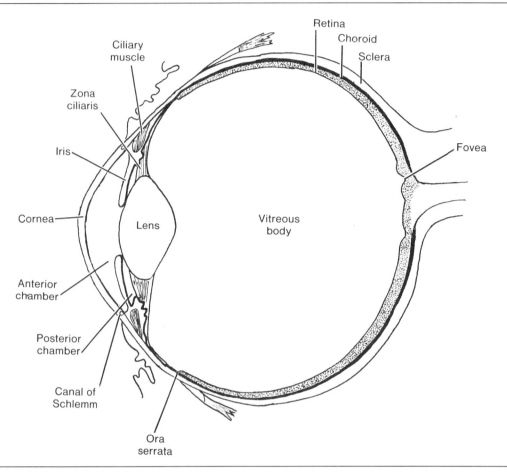

Fig. 9-1. General structure of the eye.

Sclera

KEY WORDS: fibrous outer tunic, lamina cribrosa

The sclera forms the tough, opaque, **fibrous outer tunic** of the posterior five-sixths of the eyeball. It varies in thickness in different regions but averages about 0.5 mm. It is composed of flat bundles of collagen that run in various directions parallel to the scleral surface. Delicate networks of elastic fibers and elongated, flattened fibroblasts extend between the collagen bundles. Melanocytes occur in the deeper layers. The sclera thins and forms a fenestrated membrane, the **lamina cribrosa,** at the point where fibers of the optic nerve penetrate the sclera to exit the eye. The sclera protects the interior of the eye, aids in maintaining its shape, and serves as the site of attachment for the extrinsic muscles of the eye.

Cornea

KEY WORDS: corneal epithelium, Bowman's membrane, substantia propria, keratocyte, Descemet's membrane, corneal endothelium

The transparent cornea is the most anterior part of the eye (see atlas figure 9-5). It is about 11 mm in diameter, approximately 0.8 mm thick near the center, and 1.00 mm at the periphery. Its curvature is considerably greater than that of the posterior sclera. The cornea is uniform in structure throughout and consists of corneal epithelium, Bowman's membrane, substantia propria, Descemet's membrane, and corneal endothelium.

The **corneal epithelium** is stratified squamous with a smooth outer surface and averages about 50 μm in depth (see atlas figure 9-6). It usually consists of five layers of large squamous cells that have few organelles but often contain glycogen. The superficial cells retain their nuclei, and their external surfaces form numerous fine ridges (microplicae) that help retain moisture on the corneal surface (see atlas figure 9-4). The epithelium lies on a distinct basal lamina. The lateral membranes of adjacent cells are extensively interdigitated and joined by numerous desmosomes. The corneal epithelium contains many free nerve endings and is very sensitive to a number of stimuli, especially pain.

The basal lamina of the corneal epithelium lies on the outer layer of the substantia propria and is called **Bowman's membrane;** it ends abruptly at the peripheral margin of the cornea. Bowman's membrane has a homogeneous appearance and consists of a feltwork of small collagen fibrils and lacks elastin. The membrane is well developed in humans but is absent in other primates and rabbits.

The **substantia propria,** or stroma, forms the bulk of the cornea (see atlas figure 9-6). It consists of numerous bundles of collagen fibers arranged in thin lamellae that run parallel to the corneal surface. The collagen bundles in each successive lamina run in different directions and cross at various angles. Adjacent lamellae are knit tightly together by interlacing collagenous fibers. The fibers, bundles, and lamellae of collagen are embedded in a matrix of sulfated proteoglycons rich in chondroitin sulfate and keratosulfate. These proteoglycans are not present in the sclera. Flattened fibroblast-like cells, the **keratocytes,**

are present between the bundles of collagen fibers. Blood vessels and lymphatics normally are absent in the substantia propria although occasional lymphoid wandering cells are seen.

Descemet's membrane is a homogeneous membrane, 6 to 8 μm thick, lying between the posterior surface of the substantia propria and the corneal endothelium. It may correspond to a thick basal lamina secreted by the corneal endothelium. It is resilient and elastic, although elastic fibers are not present, and appears to consist mainly of an atypical form of collagen.

The **corneal endothelium** lines the inner surface of the cornea and consists of a layer of large, hexagonal squamous cells (see atlas figure 9-6). The apices of the cells are joined by tight junctions, and the cytoplasm contains numerous mitochondria and vesicles. The cells appear active and may be involved in transporting material from the anterior chamber.

The transparency of the cornea is due to the uniform diameter and orderly arrangement of collagen fibers and to the properties of the ground substance. The cornea is avascular and depends on the aqueous humor and blood vessels of the surrounding limbus to supply its nutrients. Ion pumps of the corneal endothelial cells maintain a critical fluid level within the substantia propria. If excess fluid accumulates, the cornea becomes opaque. Corneal endothelial cells do not divide after birth and therefore are not replaced. Each person is born with a complete complement of corneal endothelial cells.

Limbus

KEY WORDS: **external scleral sulcus, internal scleral sulcus, scleral spur, trabecular meshwork, Schlemm's canal**

The limbus represents a zone of transition 1.5 to 2.0 mm wide between the transparent cornea and the opaque sclera. The outer surface bears a shallow groove, the **external scleral sulcus,** where the more convex cornea joins the sclera. A similar structure, the **internal scleral sulcus,** lies on the inner surface of the limbus. The **scleral spur** is a small ridge of tissue projecting from the posterior lip of the internal scleral sulcus and attached anteriorly to tissue that comprises the outflow system for fluid in the anterior chamber. The limbus is further characterized by the terminations of Bowman's and Descemet's membranes. The collagen fibers and bundles of the cornea become larger here and their arrangement more irregular as they blend with those of the sclera. Numerous small blood vessels form arcades in this region and nourish the peripheral portions of the avascular cornea.

Descemet's membrane is replaced by the spongy **trabecular meshwork** attached to the anterior part of the scleral spur. It contains numerous flattened, anastomosing trabeculae that consist of collagenous fibers and ground substance covered by an attenuated endothelium that is continuous with the corneal endothelium. The trabeculae form a labyrinth of spaces that communicate with the anterior chamber. Between the bulk of the limbal stroma and the trabecular meshwork, a flattened, endothelial-lined canal, **Schlemm's canal,** courses around the circumference of the cornea. Aqueous humor enters the trabecular spaces from the anterior chamber and crosses the endothelial lining of the trabeculae, the juxtacanalicular connective tissue, and, finally, the endothelium of the canal to enter its lumen. Several channels arise from the peripheral wall of the canal to join veins in the limbus and eventually drain to episcleral veins. Obstruction to the drainage of aqueous humor causes a rise in intraocular pressure, a characteristic of the condition called glaucoma.

Uveal Layer

The uvea, the middle vascular coat of the eye, is divided into choroid, ciliary body, and iris.

Choroid

KEY WORDS: suprachoroid lamina, perichoroidal space, vessel layer, choriocapillary layer, glassy (Bruch's) membrane

The choroid is a thin, brown, highly vascular membrane that lines the inner surface of the pos-

terior sclera. Its outer surface is connected to the sclera by thin avascular lamellae that form a delicate, pigmented layer called the **suprachoroid lamina.** The lamellae mainly consist of fine elastic fibers between which are numerous large, flat melanocytes and scattered macrophages. The lamellae cross a potential cleft, the **perichoroidal space,** between the sclera and choroid to enter the choroid proper.

The choroid proper consists of three regions. The outer **vessel layer** is made up of loose connective tissue with numerous melanocytes and contains the larger branches of the ciliary arteries and veins. The central **choriocapillary layer** consists of a net of capillaries lined by a fenestrated endothelium; these vessels provide for the nutritional needs of the outer layers of the retina. The choriocapillary layer ends near the ora serrata. The innermost layer of the choroid is the **glassy (Bruch's) membrane** that lies between the remainder of the choroid and the pigment epithelium of the retina. With the light microscope it appears as a homogeneous layer, 1 to 4 μm thick. Ultrastructurally it shows five separate strata made up of basal laminae of capillaries in the choriocapillary layer, the pigment epithelium of the retina, and between them, two thin layers of collagen separated by a delicate elastic network.

In some teleosts, a layer of cells rich in guanine crystals lies between the suprachoroid and the choroid. It extends to the iris and forms the argentum layer, which gives a silvery quality to the eyes of these species of fishes. A reflecting layer, the tapetum lucidum, lies between the choriocapillary and vessel layers of the choroid in several species; it is not present in humans, but is found in most other mammals. It may consist of several layers of fine fibers, as in herbivores, or of several layers of flattened cells characteristic of carnivores. This layer reflects light, causing the eyes to "glow" in the dark.

Ciliary Body

KEY WORDS: ciliary epithelium, inner nonpigmented cell, outer pigmented cell, blood-

aqueous barrier, aqueous humor, ciliary process, zonule fiber, ciliaris muscle

The ciliary body is located between the ora serrata of the neural retina and the outer edge of the iris, where it attaches to the posterior aspect of the scleral spur at the corneoscleral junction. It forms a thin triangle when seen with the light microscope and consists of an inner vascular tunic and a mass of smooth muscle immediately adjacent to the sclera. The internal surface is covered by **ciliary epithelium,** a continuation of the pigment epithelium of the retina that lacks photosensitive cells.

Ciliary epithelium consists of an **inner** layer of **nonpigmented cells** and an outer layer of pigmented cells, each resting on a separate basal lamina; it is unusual in that the cell apices of both layers are closely apposed (see atlas figures 9-8 and 9-9). The **outer pigmented cell** layer is separated from the stroma of the ciliary body by a thin basal lamina continuous with that underlying the pigment epithelium in the remainder of the retina. The basal lamina of the nonpigmented layer lies adjacent to the posterior chamber of the eye and is continuous with the inner limiting membrane of the retina. The basal plasmalemma of the nonpigmented cells shows numerous infoldings and is thought to be involved in ion transport. The cells contain numerous mitochondria and a well-developed, supranuclear Golgi complex. The adjacent pigmented cells of the outer layer also show prominent basal infoldings, and the cytoplasm is filled with melanin granules. The apices of cells of the inner, nonpigmented epithelium are united by well-formed tight junctions that form the anatomic portion of the **blood-aqueous barrier,** which selectively limits passage of materials between the blood and the interior of the eye.

The ciliary epithelium elaborates **aqueous humor,** which differs from blood plasma in its electrolyte composition and lower protein content. Aqueous humor fills the posterior chamber, provides nutrients for the lens, and, posteriorly, enters the vitreous humor. Anteriorly, it flows from the posterior chamber through the pupil into the anterior chamber and aids in nourishing the cornea. It leaves the anterior chamber via the trabecular meshwork and Schlemm's canal to the episcleral veins.

In its anterior part, the inner surface of the ciliary body is formed by 60 to 80 radially arranged, elongated ridges called **ciliary processes,** which are lined by ciliary epithelium and contain a highly vascularized stroma and scattered melanocytes (see atlas figure 9-7). **Zonule fibers,** which hold the lens in place, are produced mainly by the nonpigmented cell layer of the ciliary epithelium and are attached to its basal lamina. They extend from the ciliary processes to the equator of the lens (see atlas figures 9-7 and 9-9).

Most of the ciliary body consists of smooth muscle, the **ciliaris muscle,** which controls the shape and therefore the focal power of the lens. The muscle cells are organized into regions with circular, radial, and meridional orientations. Numerous elastic fibers and melanocytes form a sparse connective tissue between the muscle bundles (see atlas figures 9-7 and 9-8). The ciliaris is important in eye accommodation and when it contracts, it draws the ciliary processes forward, thus relaxing the suspensory ligament (zonule fibers) of the lens, allowing the lens to become more convex and to focus on objects near the retina.

Iris

KEY WORDS: pupil, anterior chamber, posterior chamber, myoepithelial cell, sphincter muscle

The iris is a thin disc suspended in the aqueous humor between the cornea and lens and has a central, circular aperture called the **pupil** (see atlas figure 9-5). The iris is continuous with the ciliary body at the periphery and divides the space between the cornea and lens into anterior and posterior chambers. The **anterior chamber** is bounded anteriorly by the cornea and posteriorly by the iris and central part of the lens. The **posterior chamber** is a narrow space between the peripheral part of the iris in front and the peripheral portion of the lens, ciliary zonule, and ciliary processes (see atlas figure 9-7). The two chambers communicate through the pupil. The anterior surface of the iris is irregular due to numerous fissures or crypts. The margin attached to the ciliary body forms the ciliary margin; that surrounding the pupil is the pupillary margin.

The stroma of the iris consists primarily of loose, vascular connective tissue with scattered collagenous fibers, melanocytes, and fibroblasts embedded in a homogeneous ground substance. The anterior surface lacks a definite endothelial or mesothelial covering but is lined in part by a discontinuous layer of melanocytes and fibroblasts. Tissue spaces of the stroma often appear to communicate with the anterior chamber. The posterior surface is covered by two rows of cuboidal, pigmented cells that are continuous with the ciliary epithelium (see atlas figures 9-7 and 9-15). Where it passes onto the posterior surface of the iris, the inner nonpigmented layer of the ciliary epithelium becomes heavily pigmented. Cells of the outer layer have less pigment and are modified into **myoepithelial cells** to form the dilator of the iris. The dilator of the pupil consists only of a single layer of radially arranged myoepithelial cells whose contraction increases the diameter of the pupil.

The **sphincter muscle** consists of a circularly arranged, compact bundle of smooth muscle cells near the pupillary margin. Contraction of the sphincter muscle reduces the diameter of the pupil. The iris acts as a diaphragm, modifying the amount of light that enters the eye, thus permitting a range of vision under a variety of lighting conditions.

The color of the iris is determined by the amount and distribution of pigment. In the various shades of blue eyes, melanin is restricted to the posterior surface of the iris, whereas in gray and brown eyes, melanin is found in increasing concentration within melanocytes present throughout the stroma of the iris. In albinos, melanin pigment is absent and the iris takes on a pink color due to the vasculature of the iridial stroma.

Retina

KEY WORDS: **pigment epithelium, neural retina (retina proper), ora serrata, macula lutea, fovea centralis, optic disc**

The retina, the innermost of the three tunics, is a delicate sheet of nervous tissue that forms the photoreceptor of the eye. The outer surface is in contact with the choroid; the inner surface is adjacent to the vitreous body. The posterior retina consists of an outer **pigment epithelium** and an inner **neural retina (retina proper)** (see atlas figures 9-16 and 9-17). The retina decreases in thickness anteriorly, and the nervous component ends at a ragged margin called the **ora serrata.** A thin prolongation of the retina covers the posterior aspect of the iris where it forms the iridia retinae. It also extends anteriorly to cover the ciliary processes as the ciliary epithelium. The forward extension of the retina consists only of the pigmented layer and an inner layer of columnar epithelial cells; the nervous component is lacking.

The neural retina is anchored only at the optic disc, where nerve fibers congregate before passing through the sclera to form the optic nerve, and at the ora serrata. Although cells of the pigment epithelium interdigitate with photoreceptor cells of the neural retina, there is no anatomic connection between the two components of the retina, and after trauma or disease, the neural retina may detach from the pigment epithelium.

The exact center of the posterior retina corresponds to the axis of the eye and at this point vision is most perfect. The region appears as a small, yellow, oval area called the **macula lutea.** In its center is a depression about 1.5 mm in diameter called the **fovea centralis** (see atlas figure 9-23), where the sensory elements are most numerous and most precisely organized. Nearer the periphery of the retina, neural elements are larger, fewer, and less evenly distributed. About 4.0 mm to the nasal side of the macula lutea is the **optic disc,** the site of formation and exit of the optic nerve (see atlas figure 9-24). Lacking photoreceptors, this area is insensitive to light and forms the "blind spot" of the retina.

Neural Retina

KEY WORDS: **three-neuron conducting chain, photoreceptor cell, bipolar neuron, ganglion cell, association neuron, glial cell**

Except for the extreme periphery and the fovea centralis, the neural retina is made up of the following layers, listed in order from the choroid, as seen with the light microscope: (1) layer of rods and cones; (2) external limiting membrane; (3) outer nuclear layer; (4) outer plexiform layer; (5) inner nuclear layer; (6) inner plexiform layer; (7) ganglion cell layer; (8) layer of nerve fibers; and (9) internal limiting membrane. The retina consists essentially of a **three-neuron conducting chain** that ultimately forms the nerve fibers in the optic nerve (Fig. 9-2). The neural elements of the conducting chain are **photoreceptors** (rod and cone cells), **bipolar neurons,** and **ganglion cells.**

When stimulated by light, photoreceptor cells transmit an action potential to the bipolar neu-

Fig. 9-2. Three-neuron chain system.

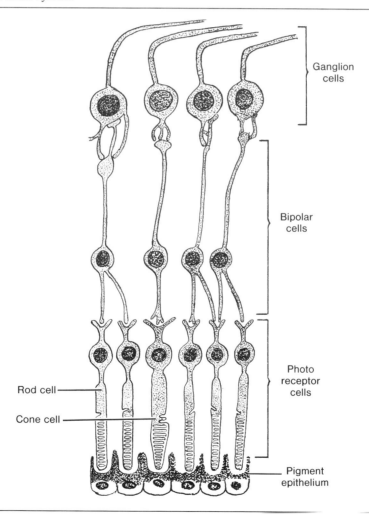

rons, which in turn synapse with ganglion cells. Unmyelinated axons from the ganglion cells enter the layer of retinal nerve fibers and unite at the optic disc to form the optic nerve, which transmits the impulse to the brain. Other intraretinal cells are either **association neurons** (horizontal cells, amacrine cells) or **glial cells.** These elements are organized into the various layers of the retina and can be summarized as shown in Table 9-1.

Glial Cells

KEY WORDS: Müller's cells, inner limiting membrane, outer limiting membrane

The largest and most prominent glial elements in the neural retina are **Müller's cells,** which extend between the outer and inner limiting membranes of the retina. Their cytoplasmic processes run between the cell bodies and processes of neurons in the retina and provide physical support for the neural elements. The basal lamina of Müller's cells lies adjacent to the vitreal body and forms the **inner limiting membrane** of the retina. The apices of Müller's cells are joined to adjacent photoreceptor cells by junctional complexes and form the **outer limiting membrane** (see atlas figures 9-17 and 9-18). The cytoplasm is rich in smooth endoplasmic reticulum and contains abundant glycogen. In addition to providing structural support, Müller's cells are thought to aid in the nutritional maintenance of other retinal elements and have been equated with astrocytes of the central nervous system.

A small number of spindle-shaped glial cells also are present around ganglion cells and between axons that form the nerve fiber layer of the retina.

Photoreceptor Cells

KEY WORDS: rod cell, rod proper, outer segment, rhodopsin, inner segment, ellipsoid, vitreal portion, myoid, outer fiber, cell body, inner fiber, spherule, synaptic ribbon, cone cell, iodopsin, cone pedicle

The two types of photoreceptors are rod cells and cone cells (Fig. 9-3). **Rod cells** are long, slender cells that lie perpendicular to the layers of the retina. They are 40 to 60 μm long and 1.5 to 3.0 μm wide, depending on their location in the retina, and number between 75 million and 170 million in each retina (see atlas figures 9-16 through 9-18). The scleral (outer) third of each rod, called the rod proper, lies between the pigment epithelium and the outer limiting membrane. The scleral end of the rods is surrounded by processes that extend from the underlying pigment epithe-

Table 9-1 Contents of Layers of Retina

Layers of Retina	Principal Contents
1. Layer of rods and cones	Inner and outer segments of rods and cones
2. External limiting membrane	Formed by junctional complexes between the scleral tips of Müller's cells and adjacent photoreceptor cells
3. Outer nuclear layer	Cell bodies and nuclei of rods and cones
4. Outer plexiform layer	Rod spherules, cone pedicles, dendrites of bipolar neurons, processes of horizontal cells
5. Inner nuclear layer	Nuclei of bipolar, horizontal, amacrine, and Müller's cells
6. Inner plexiform layer	Axons of bipolar neurons, dendrites of ganglion cells, processes of amacrine cells
7. Ganglion cell layer	Ganglion cells, scattered neuroglial cells
8. Nerve fiber layer	Nonmyelinated nerve fibers from ganglion cells, small neuroglial cells, processes of Müller's cells
9. Internal limiting membrane	Vitreal processes of Müller's cells and their basal lamina

Fig. 9-3. Diagram of rod and cone cells.

lial cells; the inner or vitreal end extends into the outer plexiform layer.

Each **rod proper** consists of outer and inner segments connected by a slender stalk containing nine peripheral doublets of microtubules. The doublets originate from a basal body in the vitreal end of the inner segment, but the connecting stalk differs from a typical cilium in that it lacks a central pair of microtubules (see atlas figure 9-11).

The **outer segment** contains hundreds of flattened membranous sacs or discs of uniform diameter. These sacs contain **rhodopsin,** the substance responsible for absorption of light. After exposure to light, rhodopsin changes its molecular configuration from *cis* to *trans* and breaks down, resulting in hyperpolarization of the plasmalemma of the rod cell, with formation of an electrical potential that is transferred to dendrites of associated bipolar cells. After stimulation, rhodopsin is rapidly reconstituted.

The **inner segment** consists of an outer scleral region called the **ellipsoid** (which contains numerous mitochondria) and a **vitreal portion** that houses the Golgi complex, free ribosomes, and myoid. Microtubules are numerous in both regions. The **myoid** region contains elements of granular and smooth endoplasmic reticulum and synthesizes and packages proteins that are transported down the connecting stalk to the scleral end of the outer rod segment to be used in the assembly of new membranous discs. Older sacs are shed from the tips of the rods during the morning hours and are replaced by new discs from below. The discarded discs are phagocytized and destroyed by cells of the pigment epithelium.

The remainder of the rod cell consists of an outer fiber, a cell body, and an inner fiber. The **outer fiber** is a thin process that extends from the inner segment of the rod proper to the **cell body,** which contains the nucleus. The **inner fiber** joins the cell body to the **spherule,** a pear-shaped synaptic ending that contains numerous synaptic vesicles and a **synaptic ribbon.** The latter consists of a dense proteinaceous plaque that lies perpendicular to the presynaptic surface, often bounded by numerous vesicles. The cell body and nucleus of the rods are located in the outer nuclear layer of the retina; the spherule lies within the outer plexiform layer.

Cone cells are 75 μm or more in length at the fovea, decreasing to 40 μm at the edge of the retina (see atlas figures 9-17 and 9-18). In the human, each retina contains between 6 million and 7 million cones. In general, cone cells resemble the rods but are flask-shaped with short, conical outer segments and relatively broad inner segments united by a modified stalk similar to that of rod cells. The membranous sacs of the

outer cone segments differ in that they may remain attached to the surrounding cell membrane and decrease in diameter as they approach the tip of the cone.

The inner segment, also called the ellipsoid portion, shows a region with numerous mitochondria and a myoid part that contains the Golgi complex and elements of smooth and granular endoplasmic reticulum. As in rods, the cones synthesize proteins that pass to the outer segments, where they are used in the formation of new membranous sacs (see atlas figure 9-22). Older sacs appear to be shed in the evening and are phagocytized in the pigment epithelial cells. Unlike those in rod cells, the sacs decrease in size as they approach the tip of the cone. The visual pigment of cone cells, **iodopsin,** is associated with the outer segments. Absorption of light and generation of an electrical impulse are similar to that occurring in rods. Cones function in color perception and visual acuity, responding to light of relatively high intensity. Detection of color is believed to depend on the presence of several pigments in the cones, whereas rods are thought to contain only one form of pigment.

Except for those in the outer fovea, cones lack an outer fiber, and the inner cone segment blends with the cell body. The nuclei of cone cells are larger and paler than those of the rods and form a single row in the outer nuclear layer, adjacent to the outer limiting membrane. Each cone has a thick inner fiber that runs to the outer plexiform layer where it forms a club-shaped synaptic ending, the **cone pedicle,** which synapses with processes from bipolar and horizontal neurons.

Bipolar cells

KEY WORDS: rod bipolar cell, flat cone bipolar cell, invaginating midget bipolar cell, flat midget bipolar cell

Like photoreceptor cells, bipolar cells lie perpendicular to the retinal layers with their cell bodies and nuclei in the inner nuclear layer of the retina. They give rise to one or more dendrites that extend into the outer plexiform layer, where they synapse with terminals of photoreceptor cells. A single axon extends into the inner plexiform layer and synapses with processes from ganglion cells. Several types of bipolar neurons have been described: **Rod bipolar cells** make contact with several rod cells; **flat cone bipolar cells** form synapses with several cone pedicles; **invaginating midget** and **flat midget bipolar cells** synapse with a single cone pedicle. Bipolar cells relay impulses from the rod and cone cells to the ganglion cells of the next layer.

Ganglion Cells

KEY WORDS: diffuse ganglion cell, midget ganglion cell

Dendrites of ganglion cells synapse with axons of bipolar neurons and represent the third and terminal link in the neuron chain. Axons of the various ganglion cells pass along the vitreal surface in the nerve fiber layer of the retina and join other axons at the optic disc to form the optic nerve. Although several morphologic varieties of ganglion cells have been described, two forms have been identified by their synaptic relations with bipolar neurons. **Diffuse ganglion cells** synapse with several types of bipolar cells, and **midget ganglion cells,** a monosynaptic type, synapse with a single midget bipolar cell.

Association Neurons

KEY WORDS: horizontal cell, amacrine cell

The cell bodies and nuclei of **horizontal cells** lie in the inner nuclear layer. Their dendrites enter the outer plexiform layer and synapse with a single cone pedicle. The axons also enter the outer plexiform layer and run parallel to the adjacent retinal layers to end on terminal twigs that synapse with several rod spherules. Although the functional significance of horizontal cells is not clear, because they synapse with cones of one area, with rods of another area, and with bipolar cells, it has been suggested that they may raise or lower the functional threshold of these cells.

Amacrine cells are pear-shaped neurons that lack axons but have several dendrites. The cell bodies lie in the inner nuclear layer, and their dendrites extend into the inner plexiform layer. Their function is unknown.

Fovea Centralis

The fovea centralis is a funnel-like depression on the posterior surface of the retina, in direct line with the visual axis (see atlas figure 9-23). At this point, those vitreal layers of the retina that are beyond the outer nuclear layer are displaced laterally, giving light an almost free pathway to the photoreceptors. The central region of the fovea, about 1.5 mm in diameter, consists only of cones that are longer and thinner than cones elsewhere in the retina. They are closely packed and number about 25,000 to 35,000. Vision is most acute in this part of the retina.

Pigment Epithelium

KEY WORDS: cylindrical sheath, elongated microvillus, lipofuscin granule, melanin granule, residual body, vitamin A

The pigment epithelium of the retina consists of a simple layer of hexagonal cells that tend to increase in diameter near the ora serrata (see atlas figure 9-19). Their basal cell membranes show numerous infoldings with associated mitochondria and are thought to be active in transport (see atlas figure 9-20). The basal lamina contributes to the glassy (Bruch's) membrane of the choroid as seen by the light microscope. The lateral cell membranes of adjacent cells show some interdigitations and, near the apex, are united by tight junctions. Two types of cytoplasmic processes arise from the apices of the cells: **Cylindrical sheaths** invest the tips of the rod and cone outer segments, and **elongated microvilli** extend toward photoreceptor cells. The cytoplasm is characterized by abundant mitochondria near the base of the cell and by many **lipofuscin** and **melanin granules** (see atlas figure 9-20). Pigment epithelial cells may show numerous **residual bodies** that contain remnants of phagocytized membrane material shed by rod outer segments.

Pigment epithelium absorbs light after it has

passed through the neural retina, thereby preventing reflection within the eye, and the apical tight junctions prevent undesirable substances from entering the intercellular spaces of the neural retina. The pigment epithelium also stores **vitamin A,** a precursor of rhodopsin, needed by the outer rod membranes.

Vascular Supply of the Retina

The outer nuclear and plexiform layers and the layer of rod and cone inner segments lack blood vessels. These parts of the retina are nourished by capillaries of the choriocapillary layer of the choroid. Nutrients cross the pigmented epithelium to enter the intercellular spaces of the outer neural retina. The inner layers of the retina are supplied by retinal vessels arising from the central retinal artery, which enters the eye in the optic nerve. Capillary networks from this source lie in the nerve fiber layer and in the inner plexiform layer.

Lens

KEY WORDS: capsule, anterior lens cell, lens fiber, lens substance, cortex, nucleus, zonule fiber

The lens is a transparent, biconvex epithelial body placed immediately behind the pupil between the iris and vitreous body (see atlas figure 9-5). It is about 10 mm in diameter and 3.7 to 4.5 mm thick. The posterior surface is more convex than the anterior surface. The lens consists of a capsule, anterior lens cells, and lens substance.

On its anterior and posterior surfaces, the lens is covered by a homogeneous, proteoglycon-rich **capsule** 10 to 18 μm thick (see atlas figures 9-10 and 9-11). A single layer of cuboidal cells, the **anterior lens cells,** lies immediately beneath the capsule and forms the epithelium of the lens, which is restricted to the anterior surface (see atlas figures 9-10 through 9-12); the posterior surface has no epithelium. The apices of the anterior lens cells face inward, toward the lens; the basal surfaces rest on a basal lamina. Anterior

lens cells are believed to contain ion pumps that maintain the proper fluidity of the lens. Near the equator of the lens, the cells increase in height and gradually differentiate into **lens fibers** that make up the bulk of the lens, referred to as the **lens substance** (see atlas figures 9-12 and 9-13). The lens grows throughout life by addition of new fibers to the periphery of the lens substance. The outer layers of the lens substance form the **cortex.** Nearer the center, the lens substance consists of condensed, concentrically arranged fibers that give it a more homogeneous appearance; this area is called the **nucleus** of the lens.

At the equator of the lens, the anterior lens cells elongate and push into the lens to lie beneath the epithelium anteriorly and the capsule posteriorly. As the cells increase in length, they lose their nuclei and their basal attachment to the capsule and become lens fibers that show a homogeneous, finely granular cytoplasm with few organelles (see atlas figure 9-13). They appear hexagonal in cross section and measure 7 to 10 μm in length (see atlas figure 9-14). The lateral membranes of the lens fibers (cells) in the cortex show large protrusions that interdigitate with concavities in adjacent fibers, in a ball and socket manner (see atlas figure 9-14). Nexus junctions are common at these points. The ball and socket joints maintain the relative positions of the fibers as the lens changes shape during focusing. The lens is avascular and derives nourishment totally from diffusion of material from the aqueous humor and vitreous body.

The lens is held in place by a system of fibers called **zonule fibers** that make up the suspensory ligament of the lens. Zonule fibers arise from the ciliary epithelium that covers the ciliary processes (see atlas figure 9-9) and attach to the lens capsule just anterior and posterior to the equator of the lens (see atlas figure 9-7). Zonule fibers consist of small bundles of fine filaments, approximately 12 nm in diameter, which may correspond to the microfibril component of elastic fibers (see atlas figures 9-11 and 9-13).

The thickness and convexity of the lens are controlled by the ciliary muscle. If the ciliary muscle contracts, the ciliary body and choroid are pulled forward and centrally, releasing tension on the zonule fibers, and the lens "sags" to become thicker and more convex. This permits focusing on near objects. When the ciliary muscle relaxes, the zonule fibers are placed under tension and the lens becomes thinner and less convex to focus on far objects.

Vitreous Body

KEY WORDS: hyaluronic acid, hyalocyte, hyaloid canal

The vitreous body is a colorless, transparent gelatinous mass that fills the vitreal cavity. It is 99 percent water and contains **hyaluronic acid** and other hydrophilic polysaccharides, as well as thin fibrils of collagen arranged randomly in a network. The fibrils are most prominent near the periphery. A few cells, the **hyalocytes,** and occasional macrophages are present in the outermost parts of the vitreous body. Hyalocytes may be responsible for the formation and maintenance of the vitreous body. A thin, cylindrical network of fibrils, the **hyaloid canal,** extends from the optic disc to the posterior surface of the lens. It represents the site of the embryonic hyaloid artery. The vitreous body provides nutrients to the lens and adjacent structures and maintains the correct consistency and shape of the eye.

Accessory Structures

Eyelids

KEY WORDS: conjunctiva, tarsal plate, tarsal (meibomian) gland, eyelash, zeisian gland, Moll's glands

The eyelids protect the anterior aspects of the eyes. They consist of a connective tissue core covered externally by thin skin. The interior surface of each lid and the anterior surface of each eye (except for the cornea) are covered by a mucous membrane called the **conjunctiva.** The palpebral conjunctiva lines the interior of the lid; the bulbar conjunctiva covers the anterior surface of the eye.

Both consist of a stratified columnar epithelium interspersed with goblet cells, resting on a dense connective tissue that is rich in elastic fibers and may contain numerous lymphocytes. The goblet cells provide mucus, which lubricates and prevents abrasion of the corneal epithelium. At the margin of the lid, the palpebral conjunctiva is continuous with the keratinized stratified epithelium of the skin. In some lower animals, a nictitating membrane is formed by the bulbar conjunctiva. It usually contains a core of connective tissue and smooth muscle, covered by conjunctival epithelium.

The external surface of the eyelid consists of skin — an external layer of keratinized stratified squamous epithelium and an inner layer of loose connective tissue with many elastic fibers. Fine hairs are present, associated with many small sebaceous and sweat glands. Skeletal muscle from the orbicularis oculi and superior levator palpebrae muscles is present in the substance of the lid. The curved **tarsal plate,** composed of dense fibrous connective tissue, is a major structure in the lid. It conforms to the shape of the eyeball and maintains the shape of the lid. Large sebaceous glands, the **tarsal (meibomian) glands,** are embedded in the tarsal plate, arranged in a single row with their ducts opening at the margin of the lid. Each gland consists of a long central duct surrounded by numerous secretory alveoli. They elaborate a lipid secretion that lubricates the lid margins.

The **eyelashes** are thick, short, curved hairs arranged in two or three irregular rows along the margin of the lid. Their follicles extend into the tarsal plate. Sebaceous glands associated with eyelashes are called the **zeisian glands;** the sweat glands located between the follicles are called **Moll's glands.**

Lacrimal Glands

KEY WORDS: compound tubuloalveolar, serous, myoepithelial cell, lacrimal duct, lacrimal sac, nasolacrimal duct

Lacrimal glands are well-developed, **compound tubuloalveolar** glands of the **serous** type (see atlas figure 9-25), located in the superior temporal region of the orbit. Each gland consists of several separate glandular units that empty into the conjunctival sac via six to twelve ducts. The secretory units consist of tall columnar cells with large, pale secretory granules. Numerous **myoepithelial cells** lie between the bases of the secretory cells and their basal lamina. The ducts are lined at first by simple cuboidal epithelium, which becomes stratified columnar in the larger ducts. Small accessory lacrimal glands can occur in the inner surface of the eyelid.

Secretions of the lacrimal gland moisten, lubricate, and flush the anterior surface of the eye and the interior of the eyelids. Excess tears collect at a medial expansion of the conjunctival sac, which is drained by the **lacrimal duct** to a lacrimal sac at the medial corner of each eye. The lacrimal duct is lined by stratified squamous epithelium. The **lacrimal sac** and the **nasolacrimal duct,** which drains the sac into the inferior meatus of the nasal cavity, are lined by pseudostratified columnar epithelium. The remainder of their walls consists of dense connective tissue.

Development of the Eye

Eyeball

The eyeball arises from neuroectoderm of the embryonic forebrain, surface ectoderm of the head, and mesenchyme that lies between or around these components (Table 9-2).

Eye development begins with the formation of shallow optic grooves on each side of the developing forebrain. As the neural tube closes, the optic grooves expand to form optic vesicles that remain attached to the brain by a hollow optic stalk. Thickenings of the surface ectoderm over the optic vesicles give rise to the lens placodes, which expand along their lateral walls to form the lens pits from which lens vesicles eventually form (see atlas figure 9-26). The walls of the lens vesicles consist of surface ectodermal cells. With loss of the superficial (epitrichial) cells of the surface ectoderm and of the connecting stalk to the surface, the underlying cuboidal cells of the lens vesicles come to form the definitive cells of the lens.

Simultaneously, the distal wall of the optic vesicle collapses into itself to form a double-walled optic cup in which the apices of the cuboidal cells in the two layers face each other. As the optic cup forms, the lens vesicle descends into the cavity of the cup, where it continues to develop. The optic cup remains attached to the brain by the optic stalk: The cup forms the retina, the stalk becomes the optic nerve.

Meanwhile, ingrowth of mesenchyme from the paraxial area helps separate the lens vesicle from the surface ectoderm. Part of the mesenchymal ingrowth differentiates into the corneal endothelium; the rest contributes to the anterior chamber. A second ingrowth of mesenchyme extends between the surface ectoderm and the corneal endothelium to form the substantia propria of the cornea (see atlas figures 9-29 and 9-30). The

Table 9-2 Contributions to the Eye

Embryonic Layer	Adult Structures
Neuroectoderm	Neural retina, pigment epithelium, epithelium over the iris, dilator and sphincter pupillary muscles, nervous and neuroglial elements of optic nerve
Surface ectoderm	Epithelium of cornea, lens
Mesenchyme	Substantia propria, endothelium of cornea, sclera, choroid, stroma and vessels of iris, ciliary body, ciliary process, ciliary muscle, sheaths of optic nerve; anterior, posterior, and vitreous chambers

surface ectoderm, previously a simple epithelium, is now two cells thick and forms the corneal epithelium (see atlas figure 9-31). A third ingrowth of mesenchyme extends into the optic cup from the lateral side near the lens and forms a loose, acellular matrix between the lens and corneal epithelium. The matrix behind the central cornea liquefies and an early anterior chamber is formed that, as it widens, separates the corneoscleral region from the developing iris. Bowman's and Descemet's membranes appear during the fourth month in humans, and collagen fibrils in the substantia propria reach their full thickness. As the corneal epithelium and a substantia propria develop, the cornea thickens to reach its full dimensions at the end of the first postnatal year.

The outer layer of the double-walled optic cup becomes highly pigmented to form the pigment epithelium of the retina (see atlas figure 9-28); endothelial cells in the adjacent, undifferentiated mesenchyme form the choriocapillaris. In humans, the collagenous portion of the glassy (Bruch's) membrane develops first, followed about six weeks later by the elastic part. Melanocytes have migrated from the neural crest into the outer layers of the choroid by the fifth month and later appear in its inner layer. The sclera arises as a condensation of mesenchyme around the optic cup, just external to the developing choroid. The condensation begins at the equator of the sclera and by the fifth month forms a complete layer.

The posterior four-fifths of the inner layer of the optic cup thickens due to cell proliferation and migration and forms the neural retina. The inner layer of the optic cup differentiates into inner and outer neuroblastic layers (see atlas figures 9-27 and 9-28). Cells of the inner layer develop into the neurons and glial elements of the adult retina; rods and cones arise from ciliated cells in the other neuroblastic layer. A marginal layer in the forming retina receives axons that extend posteriorly toward the optic stalk. Differentiation of retinal cells begins in the posterior region of the optic cup and gradually extends forward to the area of the (adult) ora serrata. Neuroblastic layers of the macular region develop first

so that the more peripheral, later developing axons must course around this region to reach the optic disc. Some retinal differentiation, especially of the macular region, continues after birth, and the density of the retinal pigment also increases postnatally.

Cells in the anterior one-fifth of the inner layer of the optic cup, beyond the region of the ora serrata of the adult eye, remain in a single layer. The cells lie apex-to-apex with cells of the pigment layer that extend to the margin of the optic cup and cover the developing ciliary region and iris.

The ciliary body arises from neuroectoderm of the anterior optic cup and its associated mesoderm. Neuroectoderm forms the outer pigmented and inner nonpigmented epithelia that cover the ciliary body and ciliary processes; mesenchyme forms the ciliary muscle, stroma, and blood vessels. As the ciliary muscle differentiates, folds appear in the outer layer of neuroectoderm, external to the margin of the optic cup. Each fold gives rise to a ciliary process, complete with a core of mesenchyme and blood vessels and covered by two epithelial layers in which the cells are arranged apex-to-apex. Zonule fibers develop within the vitreous and extend from the inner surface of the ciliary process to the lens capsule. In humans, they appear during the third month and form the suspensory ligament of the lens.

The iris also originates from neuroectoderm and mesenchyme. The double layer of epithelium covering the iris develops from the double cell layer of the optic cup. The smooth muscle of the sphincter and dilator muscles of the iris is unusual in that it develops from neuroectoderm. An ingrowth of mesenchyme at the edge of the optic cup provides the stroma and vasculature of the iris.

The optic nerve develops from axons of retinal ganglion cells, neuroectodermal cells, and mesoderm associated with the optic stalk. The mesoderm gives rise to the vascular components and connective tissue of the nerve, including the meninges. At first, the optic stalk contains an open ventral groove, the choroid fissure, through which mesenchyme enters the optic cup. Hyaloid vessels that supply the lens and inner surface of the retina during their development and axons from the brain to the retina also pass within the groove. As the choroid fissure closes, the optic stalk is transformed into the optic nerve with the central retinal (the previous hyaloid) artery at its center. That part of the hyaloid artery that supplied the lens degenerates and is resorbed. The mesenchyme filling the posterior aspect of the optic cup becomes the gelatinous, transparent vitreous.

The lamina cribrosa develops from neuroectoderm as a condensation of glial cells. It is strengthened by the mesenchymal component that gives rise to fibroblasts and collagenous septae that pass among the neuroglial cells.

Accessory Structures

Folds of integument adjacent to the eyeball differentiate to form the eyelid. Ectoderm on the exterior of the developing eyelid becomes the outer layer of stratified squamous epithelium (epidermis); that covering the cornea and anterior part of the sclera forms the conjunctiva. As development proceeds, the folds meet and fuse temporarily (see atlas figure 9-29). The epidermal union breaks down prior to the opening of the eyes, which, in some species, is delayed until well after birth. Eyelashes and sebaceous, sweat, and tarsal glands develop along the edge of each eyelid while they still are fused. The follicles of the lashes and their associated glands arise as epidermal ingrowths that then develop as hairs do elsewhere in the body.

Lacrimal glands develop as a series of solid cords of cells from the conjunctival epithelium. The cords grow, branch, and acquire lumina, thus establishing the ductal system. Secretory alveoli are the last components to form. The lacrimal sac and nasolacrimal duct first appear as a solid outgrowth of epithelium from the nasolacrimal groove; a second growth from the epithelium of each eyelid joins it. The distal end of the cord grows toward the nasal cavity and fuses with the nasal epithelium prior to acquiring a lumen.

Functional Summary

The corneoscleral coat, together with the intraocular pressure of the fluid contents within the eye, maintains the proper shape and size of the eyeball. Light entering the eye must cross several transparent media (cornea, aqueous humor, lens, and vitreous body) before reaching receptors in the retina. There are no blood vessels in the transparent elements, which rely on diffusion of materials for their nutrition. Peripheral regions of the cornea receive nutrients from adjacent vessels in the limbus; the remainder of the cornea depends on diffusion of nutrients from the aqueous humor. The lens receives all its nutrition from the aqueous humor, and it is thought to be secreted continuously into the posterior chamber by the ciliary epithelium. The aqueous humor enters the anterior chamber through the pupil and diffuses posteriorly into the vitreous chamber of the eye. From the anterior chamber the aqueous humor passes through the trabecular network into Schlemm's canal and then into adjacent episcleral veins. The aqueous humor supplies nutrients to the transparent media of the eye and is responsible for maintaining the correct intraocular pressure.

Stationary refraction occurs through the transparent cornea, in contrast to variable refraction that occurs in the lens as it changes shape to focus near or far obejcts on the retina during eye accommodation. The other media have negligible refraction. The lens is held in place by zonule fibers that extend from surrounding ciliary processes and focuses an inverted, real image on the retina. The convexity and thickness of the lens are controlled by the ciliary muscle acting through the ciliary processes and zonule fibers. If the ciliary muscle contracts, the ciliary body and choroid are pulled centrally and forward, releasing tension on the zonule fibers; this allows the lens to become thicker and more convex, enabling the eye to focus on near objects. When the ciliary muscle relaxes, the ciliary body slides posteriorly and peripherally, increasing the tension on the zonule fibers and making the lens thinner and less convex to focus on far objects.

The iris is continuous with the ciliary body at the periphery and divides the space between the cornea and lens into anterior and posterior chambers. The chambers communicate via the pupil, an aperture in the iris through which light passes into the lens and vitreous chamber. The dilator of the pupil consists of a single layer of radially arranged myoepithelial cells along the posterior surface of the iris. Contraction of these cells increases the diameter of the pupil. The sphincter of the iris consists of smooth muscle arranged around the margin of the iris that acts as a diaphragm to modify the amount of light entering the eye and permits vision under a variety of light conditions.

The rods and cones of the retina are the photoreceptors that collect visual impressions (light patterns) and translate them into nerve impulses. The membranous sacs of the outer rod segments contain rhodopsin, which, on exposure to light, changes from *cis* to *trans* and breaks down, producing hyperpolarization of the rod cell plasmalemma and formation of an electrical potential that is transferred to dendrites of associated bipolar cells. Rods have a lower threshold to light intensity than cones and are important in dark and light discrimination and in night vision.

The visual pigment associated with cone outer segments is iodopsin. Light absorption and generation of an electrical impulse in cones follow a sequence similar to that in rods. Cones serve for color perception and visual acuity, responding to light of relatively high intensity. Detection of color depends on the presence of different pigments in the cones. The central region of the fovea centralis consists only of cones and is in direct line with the visual axis of the eye. Here the inner layers of the retina that are beyond the outer nuclear layer are displaced laterally, allowing light almost a free pathway to the photoreceptors; in this portion of the retina vision is most acute.

The pigment epithelium of the retina absorbs light after it has passed through the neural retina and prevents reflection within the eye; melanocytes in the choroid, iris, and other regions of the eye serve a similar purpose. The cells of the pigment epithelium phagocytize the membranous sacs as they are shed from the tips of the outer cone and rod segments. Some components of the digested membranes are carried back to the photoreceptor cells to be reused. The pigment epithelium is a storage site for vitamin A, a precursor of rhodopsin, which is recycled to the membranes of the outer rod segments. Apical tight junctions between cells of the pigment epithelium form a barrier to prevent unwanted materials from entering the neural chain. The neurons are nourished by diffusion from capillaries in the choriocapillary layer of the choroid.

Basically, the retina represents a three-neuron chain of receptors (rods and cones), bipolar neurons, and ganglion cells equivalent to three-neuron sensory chains of the peripheral nervous system. Rods and cones can be equated with any other sensory receptors, bipolar neurons with craniospinal ganglia, and retinal ganglion cells with internuncial neurons in the spinal cord and brainstem. Thus, the arrangement of nervous elements in the sensory chain of the retina is identical to that in other sensory pathways. The retina represents an extension of the brain, modified to form a special receptor. Other neurons, horizontal cells, and amacrine cells in the retina serve as association neurons.

The eyelids are mobile folds of skin that protect the anterior of the eye from injury, desiccation, and excessive light. Lacrimal glands secrete tears that moisten and lubricate the anterior surface of the eye. Tears prevent the cornea from drying and flush the exposed surface of the eye and inner surface of the eyelid, washing away potentially dangerous agents.

Clinical Correlations

Trauma to one eye in which the iris or ciliary body is damaged may evoke a uveitis accompanied by giant cell formation in the opposite eye. Such a sympathetic uveitis is believed to result from release of antigens from the injured eye that stimulates an auto-immune response to which the second eye becomes a target organ.

Cataracts are opacities of the lens and are associated with chemical changes within the lens thought to be caused by alterations of the anterior lens cells. Loss of elasticity of the lens is common after age 40, resulting in disability to focus on near objects, a condition called presbyopia.

Glaucoma results from increased intraocular pressure due to impaired drainage or increased production of aqueous humor. It may be slowly progressive in older persons, leading to destruction of nerve fibers in the optic disc. Electron microscopy has shown the presence of abnormal collagen in the trabeculae and narrowing of intratrabecular spaces in the outer part of the trabecular meshwork, thus impeding outflow of aqueous humor.

There are several types and degrees of color blindness, the most common forms being an inability to detect the colors green and red. In these conditions two, rather than three, retinal pigments are present, the missing pigment being responsible for the inability to detect that color. Color blindness is hereditary and involves sex-linked recessive genes carried on the X chromosome.

With aging, the vitreous can shrink and pull way from the retina, causing breaks in the neural retina. Because there are no junctional attachments between cells of the neural retina and the underlying pigment epithelium, fluid from the vitreous cavity may seep through these breaks and separate the two layers, resulting in a detached retina. If not reattached surgically, the retina may degenerate and be replaced by glial cells. Retinal detachment may follow blows to the head, inflammation, or circulatory disturbances such as occur in diabetes and hypertension.

Atlas and Table of Key Features

Key Features of the Eye

Region	Epithelium	Major Components	Other Features
Sclera	None	Fibrous tunic	Lamina cribrosa
Cornea	Nonkeratinized stratified squamous	Bowman's membrane Substantia propria Descemet's membrane	Corneal endothelium
Choroid	None	Suprachoroid layer Choriocapillary layer Glassy membrane	Vessel layer Melanocytes
Ciliary body	Inner nonpigmented cells Outer pigmented cells	Ciliaris muscle Ciliary processes	Zonule fibers
Iris	Two layers of pigmented cells on posterior surface	Iridial stroma Sphincter muscle	Melanocytes
Neural retina	Pigment epithelium	Rods, cones, bipolar, and ganglion cells	Association neurons, glial cells
Lens	Anterior lens cells	Lens fibers	Lens capsule, zonule fibers
Vitreous body	None	Hyaluronic acid Thin collagen fibers	Hyalocytes

Fine ridges and processes of cell surface

Fig. 9-4. Features of three adjacent superficial cells covering the external surface of the cornea. (SEM, ×5,000.)

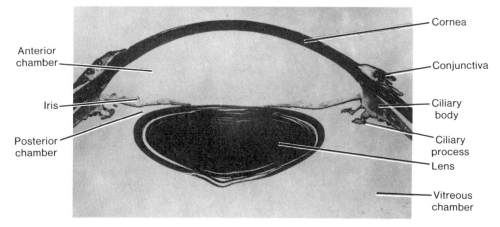

Cornea

Conjunctiva

Anterior chamber

Ciliary body

Iris

Ciliary process

Posterior chamber

Lens

Vitreous chamber

Fig. 9-5. A section through the anterior portion of a human eye illustrating the anterior chamber and lens. (LM, ×6.)

Corneal epithelium

Anterior limiting membrane

Substantia propria

Posterior limiting membrane

Corneal endothelium

Anterior chamber

Fig. 9-6. A photomicrograph of cornea showing its subcomponents. (LM, ×100.)

Anterior chamber

Iris

Posterior chamber

Zonule fibers

Lens

Sclera

Ciliary body

Ciliary processes

Zonule fibers

Fig. 9-7. A segment of human eye illustrating the relationship between iris, lens, and ciliary body. (LM, ×250.)

Smooth muscle of
ciliary body

Melanocytes

Ciliary
processes

Fig. 9-8. Increased magnification of the ciliary body shows the
abundance of smooth muscle as well as the epithelium covering
the ciliary processes (human eye). (LM, ×250.)

Zonule
fibers

Inner
columnar
epithelium

Outer
pigment
epithelium

Smooth
muscle of
ciliary body

Ciliary
epithelium

Erythrocytes
in vein

Fig. 9-9. Details of the ciliary epithelium from a human eye.
(LM, ×400.)

Fig. 9-10. A portion of a human lens showing lens capsule, lens epithelial cells, and lens fiber cells. (LM, ×250.)

Fig. 9-11. An electron micrograph of the lens capsule and epithelial cells. (TEM, ×4,500.)

Lens capsule

Lens epithelial cells

Nuclei of fiber cells

Fig. 9-12. A region of lens at its equator showing the transformation of anterior lens (epithelial) cells into fiber cells and their subsequent migration into the lens interior. (LM, ×125.)

Lens capsule

Zonule fibers

Fiber cell nuclei

Fig. 9-13. Ultrastructural features of fiber cells near the lens equator. The lens capsule and zonule fibers also are shown. (TEM, ×4,500.)

Ball and
socket
intercellular
process

Fiber
cells

Ball and
socket
intercellular
processes

Pyknotic
nucleus
of fiber
cell

Fig. 9-14. Ultrastructural features of more mature fiber cells taken from the lens cortex. Note the "ball and socket" intercellular processes. (TEM, ×6,000.)

Posterior chamber

Pigment epithelium

Sphincter smooth muscle

Stroma of iris

Fig. 9-15. A portion of iris illustrating the epithelium, sphincter, and stroma (human eye). (LM, ×250.)

Inner nuclear layer

Ganglion cell layer

Nerve fiber layer

Inner plexiform layer

Outer plexiform layer

Outer nuclear layer

Cones

Rods

Pigment epithelium

Outer limiting membrane

Fig. 9-16. A section through a human neural retina illustrating its subcomponents. (LM, ×250.)

Inner
nuclear
layer

Outer
plexiform
layer

Outer
nuclear
layer

Outer
limiting
membrane

Cones

Rods

Pigment
layer

Choriocapillary
layer

Fig. 9-17. A section of human retina showing the layer of rods
and cones and outer nuclear layer. (LM, ×250.)

Outer
limiting
membrane

Nucleus of rod

Nucleus
of cone

Cone

Rod

Pigment
epithelium

Fig. 9-18. Details of the cones, rods, and outer limiting membrane. Note the pigment epithelium of this human retina.
(LM, ×1,000.)

Rod and
cone
segments

Pigment
epithelium

Glassy
membrane

Choriocapillary
layer

Melanin
pigment
granules

Fig. 9-19. Pigment epithelium of a human retina. Note the underlying choriocapillary layer. (LM, ×1,000.)

Outer
rod
segment

Microvilli

Melanin
pigment
granules

Lipofuscin
granules

Mitochondria

Nucleus of
pigment
cell

Basal
lamina

Fig. 9-20. Melanin and lipofuscin granules within a human pigment epithelial cell. (TEM, ×6,000.)

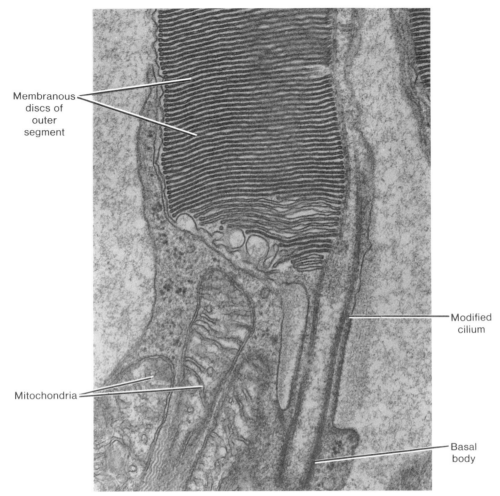

Membranous discs of outer segment

Modified cilium

Mitochondria

Basal body

Fig. 9-21. The junction between the outer and inner segment of a rod. (TEM, ×45,000.)

Fig. 9-22. Membranous discs of a cone outer segment. (TEM, ×56,000.)

Fig. 9-23. The fovea centralis of a neural retina. (LM, ×100.)

Sclera

Sclera

Lamina cribrosa

Fig. 9-24. A section through the optic disc of a human eye shows the exit of the forming optic nerve through the sclera at a region termed the lamina cribrosa. (LM, ×100.)

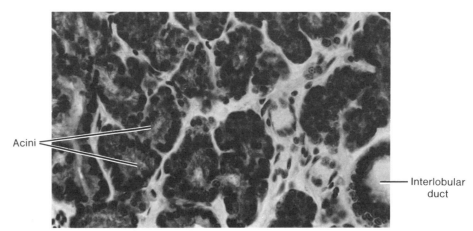

Acini

Interlobular duct

Fig. 9-25. A portion of human lacrimal gland showing numerous serous acini and an interlobular duct. (LM, ×250.)

Development

Ventricle

Wall of forebrain

Optic stalk

Lens placode

Intraretinal space

Invaginating optic vesicle

Fig. 9-26. Early eye development illustrating the invaginating optic vesicle as well as the lens placode. Note the intense mitotic activity in both. (LM, × 100.)

Surface ectoderm

Pigment epithelium

Developing neural retina

Mesenchyme

Lens

Fig. 9-27. Early eye development showing the lens, pigment epithelium, and developing neural retina. (LM, × 100.)

Lens

Pigment epithelium

Neural retina

Mesenchyme

Fig. 9-28. Increased magnification detailing the structure of the lens, neural retina, and pigment epithelium in developing eye. Note that the three-neuron chain has yet to form in the neural retina and that the lens appears immature. (LM, ×250.)

Fused eyelids

Lens

Cornea

Developing iris

Ventricles

Retina

Nasal cavity

Fig. 9-29. Later eye development showing the relationship between cornea, lens, and retina. Note that the eyelids are fused. (LM, ×50.)

Cornea

Proliferative zone of lens

Neural retina

Eyelids

Lens epithelium

Lens fibers

Vitreous

Sclera

Fig. 9-30. Eye development illustrating continued maturation of the lens and cornea. The retina remains immature in appearance. (LM, ×100.)

Surface ectoderm of embryo

Surface epithelium of cornea

Fig. 9-31. Features of the surface epithelium covering the cornea of a developing embryo. (SEM, ×250.)

Review Questions and Answers

Questions

51. Trace the flow of the aqueous humor and briefly discuss its function.
52. Briefly discuss the structure and function of the iris.
53. Describe the three-neuron conducting chain of the retina.
54. What is the function of the pigment epithelium of the retina?
55. Briefly describe the function of the accessory structures of the eye.

Answers

51. The ciliary epithelium is thought to elaborate the aqueous humor, which fills the posterior chamber of the eye and provides nutrients for the lens. Posteriorly, the aqueous humor enters, to a limited extent, the vitreous body, while anteriorly it flows through the pupil into the anterior chamber, where it aids in nourishing the cornea. The aqueous humor flows into the trabecular spaces from the anterior chamber, crosses the endothelium that lines the trabeculae, passes through the juxtacanalicular connective tissue, and finally traverses the endothelium of the Schlemm's canal to enter its lumen. Several channels arise from the peripheral wall of Schlemm's canal to join with veins in the limbus and eventually drain to episcleral veins. In addition to its nutritive role, the aqueous humor also is important for maintaining the proper intraocular pressure and shape of the cornea and eye, features that are essential for good vision.

52. The iris is a thin, circular disc suspended between the cornea and lens that divides the space between these structures into anterior and posterior chambers. It has a central, circular aperture, the pupil, through which the two chambers communicate, and at its margin the iris is attached to the ciliary body. The iris consists primarily of a loose, vascular connective tissue containing much ground substance and is covered on the posterior surface by two rows of pigmented cells. The outer cells of this pigmented layer constitute the dilator of the eye and are modified myoepithelial cells arranged radially in a single layer; contraction of the dilator increases the diameter of the pupil. A compact, circularly arranged bundle of smooth muscle cells is present near the pupillary margin and forms the sphincter muscle of the iris. Contraction of the sphincter muscle reduces the diameter of the pupil; thus the iris serves as a diaphragm to modify the amount of light entering the eye.

53. The conducting chain of neurons in the retina basically consists of three neuronal elements: photoreceptors (rods and cones), bipolar neurons, and ganglion cells. It is equivalent to other chains of sensory neurons found in the peripheral nervous system. The rods and cones, bipolar neurons, and ganglion cells are perpendicular to the retinal layers. Bipolar neurons make synaptic contact with rod and cone cells and relay impulses generated by these photoreceptors to the dendrites of the overlying ganglion cells, the third link in the neuron chain of the retina. Axons from the ganglion cells run along the vitreal surface in the nerve fiber layer of the retina before they join with other axons at the optic disc to form the optic nerve.

54. The pigment epithelium of the retina absorbs light after it has passed through the neural retina and prevents reflection within the eye. Its component cells actively phagocytize and break down the membranous sacs that are shed at the tips of the outer

rod and core segments. The pigment epithelium serves as a storage site for vitamin A (a precursor for rhodopsin), which, together with amino acids and proteins, is recycled back to the rods. Apical tight junctions between the cells of the pigment epithelium act as a barrier to prevent undesirable substances from entering the neural retina, which is nourished by diffusion from the capillaries of the choriocapillary layer of the choroid.

55. The primary accessory structures of the eye are the eyelids and the lacrimal glands, both of which protect the anterior surface of the eye. The eyelids are mobile folds of skin that provide protection from physical injury, excessive light, and desiccation, while the lacrimal glands secrete tears that moisten and lubricate the anterior surface of the eye. Together with the eyelids, tears prevent the cornea from drying out. Tears also flush the interior of the eyelid and the anterior surface of the eyeball, washing away potentially dangerous materials from this surface of the eye.

10 The Ear

The ear contains receptors specialized for hearing and for awareness of head position and movement. The ear is subdivided into the external ear, which receives and directs sound waves from the external environment; the middle ear, which transforms sound waves into mechanical vibrations; and the inner ear, where these mechanical vibrations are converted to nerve impulses and relayed to the brain to be interpreted as sound. The inner ear also contains the vestibular organs that function in balance. The general structure of the ear is shown in Fig. 10-1.

External Ear

KEY WORDS: **aurical (pinna), elastic cartilage, external auditory meatus, ceruminous gland, cerumen**

The **auricle (pinna)** of the external ear consists of an irregular plate of **elastic cartilage** surrounded by a thick perichondrium rich in elastic fibers. In humans the covering skin contains a few small hairs, their associated sebaceous glands, and an occasional sweat gland. The skin adheres tightly to the perichondrium except on the posterior surface, where a subcutaneous layer is present. In most mammals, the auricle is associated with sheets of skeletal muscle and in many species is mobile to aid in collecting sound waves and directing them into the external auditory meatus.

The **external auditory meatus** is about 2.5 cm long and follows an open S-shaped course. It consists of an outer part whose cartilaginous walls are continuous with the auricular cartilage and an inner portion whose walls are formed by the temporal bone. The external auditory meatus is lined by keratinized, stratified squamous epithelium that is continuous with the epidermis of the auricle. The epithelium is firmly anchored to the surrounding perichondrium or periosteum by dense collagenous connective tissue. Numerous small hairs are present in the epithelium of the outer part of the meatus and are associated with large sebaceous glands in the underlying connective tissue. A special form of coiled apocrine sweat gland, the **ceruminous gland,** occurs in the skin that lines the meatus. Depending on the state of activity, the secretory cells may vary in shape from cuboidal to columnar. Each secretory tubule is surrounded by a network of myoepithelial cells that lies between the basal lamina and the bases of the epithelial cells. The ducts may open directly on the surface or, together with adjacent sebaceous glands, into hair follicles. Their secretory product is **cerumen,** a waxy material that prevents drying of the skin that lines the external auditory meatus. Hairs and glands occur only along the roof of the inner (boney) part of the external auditory meatus.

Middle Ear

KEY WORDS: **tympanic cavity, auditory ossicle, tensor tympani, stapedius, auditory tube, tympanic membrane**

The **tympanic cavity** is an irregularly shaped space in the petrous portion of the temporal bone.

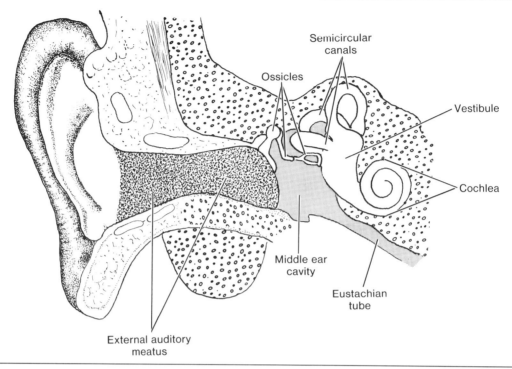

Fig. 10-1. Structure of the ear.

It is continuous anteriorly with the auditory (eustachian) tube and posteriorly with the mastoid air cells (cavities) of the temporal bone. The lateral wall consists chiefly of the tympanic membrane (eardrum), which forms a partition separating the tympanic cavity from the external auditory meatus. The inner, boney wall of the middle ear makes contact with the inner ear via two small, membrane-covered openings called the oval and round windows. The membrane of the oval window contains the base of an auditory ossicle, the stapes. The membrane that covers the round window often is referred to as the secondary tympanic membrane.

The tympanic cavity contains the **auditory ossicles,** a chain of three bones (malleus, incus, stapes) that unite the tympanic membrane of the middle ear with the oval window of the inner ear. The ossicles consist of compact bone and are united by small synovial joints. The bones are suspended in the air-filled tympanic cavity by thin strands of connective tissue called ligaments. Small skeletal muscles, the **tensor tympani** and **stapedius,** are associated with two of the ossicles; the tendon of the tensor tympani attaches to the malleus, and the tendon from the stapedius attaches to the stapes. The bulk of the muscles themselves is contained within small canals in the temporal bone.

The auditory ossicles, their suspending ligaments, and the inner walls of the tympanic cavity are covered by a thin mucous membrane that consists of a simple squamous epithelium lying on a thin layer of connective tissue. The mucous membrane is firmly attached to the periosteum of the temporal bone, lines the interior of the mastoid air cells, and covers the inner surface of the tympanic membrane. Where the tympanic cavity joins the auditory tube, the lining epithelium becomes ciliated columnar, interspersed with secretory cells.

The **auditory tube** (eustachian tube) is about 4 cm long and connects the anterior part of the tympanic cavity with the nasopharynx. The auditory tube acts as a passageway to ventilate the tympanic cavity and allows equalization of pressure between the middle ear and pharynx. Near the tympanic cavity the supporting wall consists of compact bone, whereas in its medial two-thirds, the auditory tube is supported by a J-shaped elastic cartilage. The boney portion is lined by a simple columnar epithelium that becomes ciliated pseudostratified columnar epithelium in the cartilaginous part. Cilia beat toward the pharynx. Goblet cells are present near the pharyngeal opening, and mixed, compound, tubuloalveolar glands often are found in the underlying connective tissue. A mass of lymphoid tissue, the tubal tonsil, fills the connective tissue and infiltrates the epithelium.

The **tympanic membrane** forms most of the lateral wall of the tympanic cavity and is made up of three layers. The outer layer consists of stratified squamous epithelium, which reflects onto the tympanic membrane from the external auditory meatus. Two layers of collagenous fibers and fibroblasts form the middle layer. In the external layer, the fibers are arranged radially, whereas those of the inner layer run a circular pattern. A simple squamous epithelium and its supporting connective tissue form the third layer and are continuous with the lining of the tympanic cavity. The fibrous layers of the tympanic membrane enter an encircling ring of fibrocartilage that unites the eardrum to the surrounding bone. The inner surface of the tympanic membrane attaches to the malleus (see atlas figure 10-7).

Sound waves received by the tympanic membrane cause it to vibrate slightly. The vibrations then are transmitted to the fluid-filled chambers of the inner ear via the ossicles. The tympanic membrane is about 18 times as large as the oval window of the inner ear, which contains the foot plate of the stapes. Because of this arrangement, the eardrum and auditory ossicles act as a piston that exerts pressure on the confined fluid of the inner ear. Thus, the tympanic membrane and auditory ossicles not only transmit vibrations but also are able to amplify weak forces of sound waves without expending energy.

The tensor tympani and stapedius muscles protect delicate structures in the inner ear by dampening ossicle movement resulting from loud or sudden noises. They also are thought to regulate the degree of tension in the tympanic membrane so that sounds of moderate intensity can be picked up in a noisy environment.

Inner Ear

KEY WORDS: **boney labyrinth, perilymph, membranous labyrinth, endolymph**

The inner ear consists of a system of canals and cavities within the petrous portion of the temporal bone. The compact bone surrounding the canals and cavities forms the **boney labyrinth** and is filled with a fluid called **perilymph.** A series of fluid-filled membranous structures, collectively called the **membranous labyrinth,** lie suspended in the perilymph. The membranous labyrinth is filled with **endolymph,** a fluid with an ionic composition similar to that of intracellular fluid, being rich in potassium ions and low in sodium ions. Perilymph resembles extracellular fluid, having a high content of sodium ions and a low concentration of potassium ions. Endolymph is produced by an area of the cochlear duct called the stria vascularis; the exact site of perilymph formation is unknown.

The boney and membranous labyrinths consist of two major components: the vestibular labyrinth, which contains sensory elements for equilibrium, and the cochlea, which contains sensory structures for hearing.

Vestibular Labyrinth

KEY WORDS: **semicircular canal, utricle, saccule, crista ampullaris, macula utriculi, macula sacculi, type I hair cell, kinocilium, type II hair cell, supporting cell, planum semilunatum, cu-**

pula cristae ampullaris, otolithic membrane,
otoliths (otoconia)

The vestibular labyrinth consists of three **semi-circular canals** that are continuous with an elliptical structure called the **utricle.** The utricle in turn unites with an anteromedial, spherical part of the vestibular system called the **saccule** by a thin duct that joins with a similar duct from the saccule. The two ducts unite to form the slender endolymphatic duct, which terminates as a small expansion called the endolymphatic sac.

Most of the membranous labyrinth that forms the vestibular portion of the inner ear is lined by a simple squamous epithelium. The remainder of this wall consists of fine connective tissue fibers and stellate fibroblasts. Thin trabeculae of connective tissue extend from the wall of the membranous labyrinth and cross the perilymphatic space to blend with the periosteum of the surrounding bone (see atlas figure 10-14). The trabeculae suspend the membranous component of the semicircular canals, utricle, and saccule in the perilymph contained within the osseous labyrinth. The perilymphatic connective tissue is rich in blood capillaries that supply the various segments of the membranous labyrinth.

In specific regions of each subdivision of the membranous labyrinth, the epithelium assumes a stratified appearance and serves in sensory reception (Fig. 10-2). The sensory epithelium of each semicircular canal is restricted to the dilated ampullary portion and together with an underlying core of connective tissue, forms a transverse ridge that projects into the lumen of the ampulla. The connective tissue contains many nerve fibers. These sensory neuroepithelial regions of the semicircular canals form the **cristae ampullaris** (see atlas figures 10-14 and 10-15). Similar raised regions of neuroepithelium are found in the utricle and saccule and form the **macula utriculi** and the **macula sacculi,** respectively (see atlas figures 10-14 and 16). The macula utriculi covers an area approximately 2 mm square along the superior-anterior wall. It lies on a plane perpendicular to the macula sacculi, which occupies an area measuring 2 × 3 mm on the anterior wall of the sac-

cule. The sensory epithelium of the cristae and maculae consists of type I and type II sensory hair cells (Fig. 10-3) and supporting (sustentacular) cells.

The **type I hair cell** is flask-shaped with a narrow apical region and a rounded base that contains the nucleus (Fig. 10-3). A large part of the cell is enveloped by a cuplike afferent nerve ending (calyx). Nearby efferent nerve endings may synapse with the nerve calyx but do not directly contact the type I hair cell; a narrow intercellular cleft, 30 nm wide, separates the hair cell from the nerve ending. The space narrows to approximately 5 nm at gap junctions that are scattered between the two compartments. Synaptic ribbons often are found in the cytoplasm of type I hair cells, immediately adjacent to the plasmalemma. Mitochondria are concentrated around the nucleus and at the cell apex, and numerous microtubules are present, especially in the apical region. The cytoplasm of the nerve calyx shows scattered mitochondria and many vesicles that range from 50 to 200 nm in diameter.

The apical membrane of the type I hair cell bears 50 to 100 large, specialized microvilli called "hairs" (see Fig. 10-3 and atlas figure 10-18). These nonmotile elements are limited by a plasmalemma, have cytoplasmic cores that contain numerous fine filaments, and are constricted at their base just before they join the rest of the cell. The longitudinal filaments leave the microvilli and enter into a thick mat of filaments that forms a terminal web in the apical cytoplasm of the cell. The microvilli progressively increase in height from about 1 μm on one side to about 100 μm on the opposite side of the cell. A single, eccentrically placed cilium is present on the apical surface and is peculiar in that the two central microtubules end shortly after originating from the basal body. The cilium is believed to be nonmotile and often is called a **kinocilium.**

Type II hair cells are simple columnar cells surrounded by numerous separate afferent and efferent nerve endings, rather than by a single afferent nerve ending as seen surrounding type I hair cells. The type II hair cell also bears a single, eccentrically placed, nonmotile cilium and 50 to

Ampullae of superior and
lateral semicircular canals

Macula utriculi

Macula sacculi

Endolymphatic
duct

Cochlear duct

Ampulla of posterior
semicircular canal

Fig. 10-2. Location of sensory regions in the membranous labyrinth (stippled areas).

100 large microvilli that are arranged identically to those of type I cells (see atlas figure 10-18). The cytoplasm contains scattered profiles of granular endoplasmic reticulum, abundant mitochondria, smooth-surfaced tubules, and numerous vesicles 20 nm in diameter. A well-developed Golgi complex occupies a supranuclear position. Synaptic ribbons are present in the cytoplasm of type II hair cells, immediately opposite the surrounding nerve terminals.

Adjacent columnar-shaped **supporting cells** (sustentacular cells) extend from the basal lamina to the free surface of the sensory epithelium (see atlas figure 10-16). They follow a very irregular course throughout the epithelium and in electron micrographs show a well-developed terminal web at the cell apex, a prominent Golgi complex, numerous secretory granules, and bundles of microtubules that extend from the basal cytoplasm to the terminal web. The microtubules form an integral part of the cytoskeleton and provide rigidity to the supporting cells. Although the func-

tion of the supporting cells is uncertain, it has been suggested that they are concerned with the metabolism of endolymph or that they contribute to the nutrition of hair cells. The supporting cells at the periphery of the sensory epithelium form a simple columnar layer, the **planum semilunatum,** which lacks hair cells.

The microvilli of the hair cells in the cristae are embedded in a gelatinous structure called the **cupula cristae ampullaris,** which is composed of viscous proteoglycans that project from the surface of the crista into the ampullary lumen of each semicircular canal (see atlas figures 10-14 and 10-15). Supporting cells in the sensory epithelium also may contribute to the cupula. The sulfated proteoglycans may be secreted by the planum semilunatum.

Microvilli of hair cells from the maculae of the utricle and saccule also are embedded in a viscous proteoglycan that forms the **otolithic membrane** (see atlas figure 10-16). Additionally, numerous crystalline bodies called **otoliths (otoconia)** are sus-

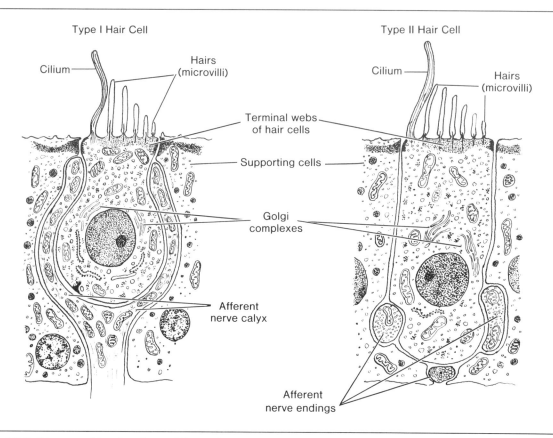

Fig. 10-3. Diagram of type I and type II hair cells.

pended in this layer (see atlas figure 10-17). These bodies consist of protein and calcium carbonate.

The gelatinous cupula of the cristae projects across the lumen of the ampullary region of the semicircular canal like a swinging door. During angular movement of the head, the cupula is displaced by the motion of endolymph contained within this part of the membranous labyrinth. Displacement of the cupula excites the sensory hair cells, which, in turn, generate an action potential that is received by surrounding nerve terminals. Similarly, gravitational forces on the otolithic membrane and the otoconia embedded in it cause a shearing action on the microvilli of the underlying hair cells in the macula. Linear acceleration also results in stimulation of hair cells in the macula.

Although the exact mechanism is unknown, the sensory epithelium in the vestibular organs transforms the mechanical energy of endolymph movement into the electrical energy of a nerve impulse. The bending or displacement of microvilli is thought to result in depolarization of hair cells, the impulse being transferred to surrounding nerve endings to result in the generation of a nerve impulse. Efferent nerve endings probably have inhibitory functions to control the threshold of activity of hair cells.

Cochlea

KEY WORDS: modiolus, spiral ganglion, spiral lamina, basilar membrane, spiral ligament, vestibular membrane, scala vestibuli, cochlear

duct, scala tympani, ductus reuniens, cecum cupulare, helicotrema

Like the vestibular portion of the inner ear, the cochlea consists of an outer portion of compact bone and a central membranous part contained in perilymph. The osseous part of the cochlea spirals for two and three-fourths turns around a cone-shaped axis of spongy bone called the **modiolus** (see atlas figure 10-8). Blood vessels, nerve fibers, and the perikarya of afferent bipolar neurons, called the **spiral ganglion,** lie within the boney substance of the modiolus. A projection of bone, the **spiral lamina,** extends from the modiolus into the lumen of the cochlear canal along its entire course. A fibrous structure, the **basilar membrane,** extends from the spiral lamina to the **spiral ligament,** a thickening of periosteum on the outer boney wall of the cochlear canal. The thin **vestibular membrane** extends obliquely across the cochlear canal from the spiral lamina to the outer wall of the cochlea.

The basilar and vestibular membranes divide the cochlear canal into an upper **scala vestibuli,** an intermediate **cochlear duct,** and a lower **scala tympani** (see atlas figure 10-9). A cross section of the cochlea is shown in Fig. 10-4.

The cochlear duct is part of the endolymphatic system and is connected to the saccule of the membranous labyrinth by the small **ductus reuniens.** The opposite end of the cochlear duct ends at the apex of the cochlea as the blindly ending **cecum cupulare.** The scala vestibuli and the scala tympani contain perilymph and communicate at the apex of the cochlea through a small opening called the **helicotrema.** At the base of the cochlea, the scala tympani is closed by the secondary tympanic membrane, which fills the round window. This membrane separates the perilymph in the scala tympani from the middle ear. The scala vestibuli extends through the perilymphatic channels of the vestibule to end at the oval window, which is closed by the foot of the stapes. Movement of the stapes in the oval window exerts pressure on the perilymph in the scala vestibuli. Because fluid cannot be compressed, waves of pressure either pass through the coch-

lear duct, displacing it to enter the scala tympani, or enter the scala tympani directly through the helicotrema. The pressure is released from the confined perilymphatic spaces of the cochlea by the elasticity of the secondary tympanic membrane, which bulges into the tympanic cavity of the middle ear (Fig. 10-5).

Cochlear Duct

KEY WORDS: basilar membrane, spiral crest, vestibular membrane, stria vascularis, marginal cell, basal cell, intraepithelial capillary, spiral prominence

The cochlear duct is a triangular space that follows the spiral course of the cochlea (see atlas figure 10-9). Its floor is formed by the basilar membrane and its roof by the vestibular membrane. The **basilar membrane** consists of a layer of collagen-like fibers embedded in an amorphous matrix and extends from the osseous spiral lamina of the modiolus to the **spiral crest,** a well-vascularized periosteal region along the outer wall of the cochlea. The **vestibular membrane** consists of two layers of simple squamous cells separated mainly by their basal laminae.

The outer wall of the cochlear duct is formed by a vascular area called the **stria vascularis** (see atlas figures 10-9 and 10-11). It occurs along the entire length of the cochlear duct and consists of a pseudostratified columnar epithelium that rests on a vascular connective tissue and contains basal and marginal cells. The epithelium is continuous with the simple squamous epithelium that lines the interior of the vestibular membrane.

Marginal cells show deep infoldings of the basal and lateral cell membranes and are associated with numerous mitochondria, suggesting that these cells are involved in fluid transport. They may participate in the elaboration of endolymph. **Basal cells** show few mitochondria or basal infoldings. The epithelium of the stria vascularis differs from that found elsewhere in the body in that it contains **intraepithelial capillaries.**

The epithelium of the stria vascularis is continuous below with a simple layer of attenuated

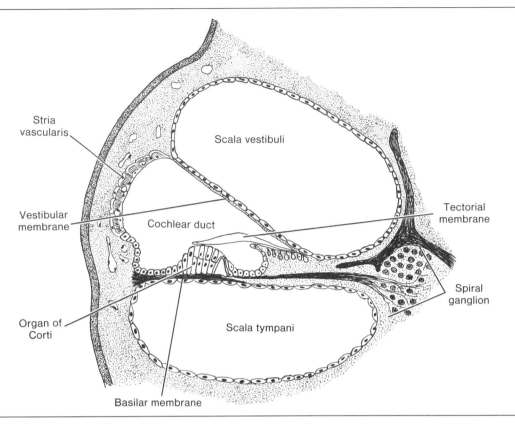

Fig. 10-4. Cross section of the cochlea.

cells that overlies the **spiral prominence,** a highly vascularized thickening of the periosteum. The spiral prominence lies beneath the stria vascularis and extends the length of the cochlear duct. The cells become cuboidal where the epithelium reflects onto the basilar membrane from the outer wall of the cochlear duct.

Organ of Corti

KEY WORDS: **supporting cell, inner pillar cell, outer pillar cell, inner phalangeal cell, outer phalangeal cell, border cell, inner spiral tunnel, spiral limbus, interdental cell, tectorial membrane, cells of Hensen, cells of Claudius, inner hair cell, outer hair cell**

The cochlear duct contains a region of specialized cells, the organ of Corti (Fig. 10-6), that trans-

forms vibrations of the basilar membrane into nerve impulses. The avascular organ of Corti extends along the length of the cochlear duct and lies on the basilar membrane. It consists mainly of supporting and hair cells. **Supporting cells** are tall and columnar and consist of inner and outer pillar cells, inner and outer phalangeal cells, border cells, cells of Hensen, and cells of Claudius.

Inner and **outer pillar cells** form the boundaries of the inner tunnel, a space that lies within and extends the length of the organ of Corti. In both types of pillar cells, the nucleus is located in the broad base. The elongated cell bodies contain numerous microtubules that form a cytoskeleton. Inner pillar cells are slightly expanded at the apex and extend over the outer pillar cells. The apices of the outer pillar cells also expand

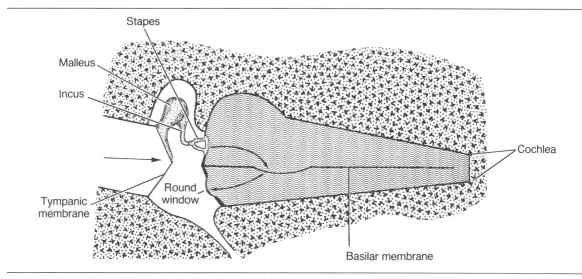

Fig. 10-5. Mechanics of hearing.

slightly to fit into the concave apical undersurface of the inner pillar cells. In addition to forming the boundaries of the inner tunnel, the pillar cells provide structural support for adjacent cells.

The phalangeal cells serve as supporting elements for the sensory hair cells (see atlas figure 10-10). The **inner phalangeal cells** form a single row immediately adjacent to the inner pillar cells and surround the sensory inner hair cells except at their apical regions. In contrast, the columnar **outer phalangeal cells** form three or four rows and support outer hair cells, which also are arranged in rows. The apex of each outer phalangeal cell forms a cuplike structure that surrounds the basal one-third of an outer hair cell. Afferent and efferent nerves are located at the base.

Each outer phalangeal cell gives rise to a slender cytoplasmic process filled with microtubules. The process extends to the surface, where it expands into a flat plate that attaches to the apical edges of the outer hair cell and is supported laterally by outer phalangeal cells and the outer hair cells in the adjacent row. The apical plates of the outer phalangeal cells provide additional support for the outer hair cells, the upper two-thirds of which are not supported by adjacent cells and are

surrounded by large, fluid-filled intercellular spaces. The fluid contained in these spaces is believed to be similar to that within the inner tunnel.

Border cells are supporting cells associated with the inner edge of the organ of Corti. These slender cells undergo a transition to the squamous cells that line the **inner spiral tunnel.** This space is formed by the **spiral limbus,** which consists of periosteal connective tissue that extends from the osseous spiral lamina and bulges into the cochlear duct. Vertically arranged collagenous fibers, often called auditory teeth, are contained within the substance of the limbus. **Interdental cells** are specialized cells along the upper surface of the spiral limbus. The cells extend between collagen fibers to reach the lumen of the cochlear duct. On the upper surface of the limbus, they form a continuous sheet and are united by tight junctions.

The interdental cells secrete a sheet of material that forms the **tectorial membrane,** which consists of a protein thought to be similar to epidermal keratin. The tectorial membrane extends over the interdental cells and beyond the substance of the spiral limbus to overlie the hair cells

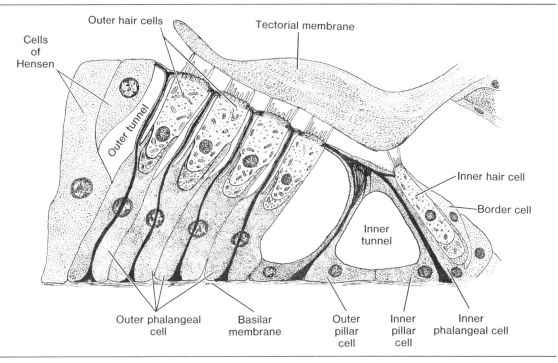

Fig. 10-6. Diagram of the organ of Corti.

of the organ of Corti (see atlas figures 10-10 and 10-13). The tips of microvilli extending from sensory hair cells are firmly embedded in the undersurface of the tectorial membrane.

Near the outer edge of the organ of Corti, immediately adjacent to the outer phalangeal cells, is another group of columnar supporting cells called **cells of Hensen** (see atlas figures 10-10 and 10-13). They decrease in height and transform into the adjacent **cells of Claudius,** which form the outer edge of the organ of Corti.

The sensory hair cells are divided into inner and outer hair cells. **Inner hair cells** form a single row along the inner aspect of the organ of Corti and extend the length of the cochlea (see atlas figures 10-10 and 10-12). Like type I hair cells of the vestibular labyrinth, the inner hair cells of the cochlea are short, flask-shaped cells with narrow necks. Well-developed microvilli extend from

the apical surface of the inner hair cells, but unlike type I hair cells, they lack a kinocilium. The microvilli are arranged in a U at the apical surface and contain numerous filaments that extend into a dense terminal web in the apical cytoplasm. Mitochondria aggregate just beneath the terminal web and also are scattered throughout the remainder of the cytoplasm, which contains scattered ribosomes and profiles of smooth endoplasmic reticulum. Numerous nerve endings synapse with the bases of the inner hair cells on a plane below the level of the nucleus.

The columnar **outer hair cells** usually form three or four rows and are supported by the apices of the outer phalangeal cells (see atlas figures 10-10 and 10-12). Microvilli are arranged in the shape of a W. There is no cilium. Mitochondria aggregate at the base of the outer hair cell, which makes contact with afferent and efferent nerve fibers. In all other respects, the outer hair cells are similar to the inner hair cells, and both are receptors of sound in the organ of Corti.

Development of the Ear

External Ear

Mesenchymal proliferation around the edges of the first and second pharyngeal arches, together with the surface ectoderm, gives rise to the auricle. The proliferations occur around the openings of the developing external auditory meati and gradually fuse to form the definite auricles.

The external auditory meatus develops from the first pharyngeal groove and the bounding arches. As the pharyngeal groove grows centrally, it forms a funnel-shaped pit lined by ectoderm and surrounded by cartilage. A thick epithelial plate forms in the ectoderm, growing from the base of the pit toward the developing tympanic cavity. Connective tissue between the two layers of epithelium develops from mesenchyme. Initially the eardrum lies horizontally, almost parallel to the floor of the meatus, but as the meatus continues to grow, the eardrum gradually becomes more erect.

Middle Ear

The tympanic cavity is derived from the first pharyngeal pouch and is lined by epithelium of endodermal origin. The distal part of the pouch, the tubotympanic recess, widens to form a provisional tympanic cavity. The narrow proximal connection to the region of the developing nasopharynx becomes the auditory tube. Mesenchyme from the first and second pharyngeal arches that lie above the provisional cavity becomes cartilaginous and forms the first models of the ossicles. These remain embedded in a spongy mesenchyme until the tympanic cavity widens and the mesenchyme degenerates. As this occurs, the epithelium expands to line the newly formed cavity and inner surface of the eardrum and to cover the ossicles in a mesentery-like fash-

ion. The ossicles thus are suspended in the tympanic cavity but actually lie outside the epithelium of the cavity. Each cartilaginous ossicle undergoes endochondral ossification.

The tensor tympani and stapedius muscles arise from mesenchyme of the first and second pharyngeal arches, respectively, and lie beyond the lining of the tympanic cavity. Ligaments supporting the ossicles develop from the mesenchyme that lies between the mesentery-like folds of the covering epithelium. The lining of the tympanic cavity continues to expand and eventually lines the mastoid air cells of the temporal bone.

Inner Ear

The epithelium of the inner ear is ectodermal in origin. Thickenings of the ectoderm, the auditory placodes, occur midway along both sides of the midbrain and invaginate to form cup-shaped auditory pits. These expand, lose their connections with the surface ectoderm, and become detached ovoid sacs called auditory vesicles or otocysts. A narrow, tubular recess, the endolymphatic duct, develops from the region last in contact with ectoderm, eventually expanding into a blind endolymphatic sac. The otocyst elongates and a tubular outgrowth at the ventral pole grows spirally for two and three-fourths turns into the surrounding mesenchyme. This is the cochlear duct, which remains connected to the saccule by a narrow ductus reuniens. The dorsal part of the otocysts expands and develops into the semicircular canals; the intermediate region forms the utricle and saccule.

The epithelial lining of the various segments of the membranous labyrinth is, at first, simple low columnar. As nerve fibers grow among the cells of the cristae ampullaris, maculae of the utricle and saccule, and organ of Corti, the epithelium thickens and differentiates into the special sensory and supporting cells. The supporting cells are thought to secrete and maintain the cupula cristae ampullaris and otolithic membranes in the maculae. Differentation of the organ of Corti progresses slowly, beginning as a thickening of the epithelium at the basal of the cochlea and progressing to the apex. Large inner and small outer ridges of epithelium form, both associated with a covering tectorial membrane. The small ridge gives rise to the supporting cells and inner and outer hair cells of the organ of Corti. The inner ridge involutes to form the lining of the spiral sulcus.

At first, the structures of the developing membranous labyrinth are embedded in mesenchyme that later undergoes chondrification and in turn is replaced by bone to form the boney labyrinth. Cartilage adjacent to the membranous labyrinth degenerates to form a syncytial reticulum that becomes the perilymphatic spaces filled with perilymph. In the region of the developing cochlear duct, the cartilage is resorbed so that the two perilymphatic spaces, the scala vestibuli and scala tympani, are formed on either side of the cochlear duct (see atlas figures 10-19 through 10-21). The modiolus of the cochlea develops directly from the mesenchyme as membranous bone.

Functional Summary

The pinna of the external ear collects sound and directs it into the external auditory meatus. Sound waves cause the tympanic membrane to vibrate slightly at the same frequency as the sound waves. Auditory ossicles suspended in the tympanic cavity of the middle ear conduct the vibrations to the perilymph channels of the inner ear. The force of the vibrations created by the sound waves is amplified with no expenditure of energy, because the tympanic membrane is much larger than the foot plate of the stapes. Together, the intervening ossicles act as a piston. With each movement, the foot plate of the stapes exerts pressure on the perilymph, which is confined to the scala vestibuli and scala tympani of the inner ear. The pressure waves pass through the perilymph from the scala vestibuli to the scala tympani and are released from the perilymphatic space by bulging of the secondary tympanic membrane into the air-filled tympanic cavity. As the pressure waves move from scala vestibuli to scala tympani, they must first pass through the intervening cochlear duct or travel to the helicotrema at the apex of the cochlea. When a pressure wave passes through the cochlear duct, the vestibular and basilar membranes are displaced slightly, creating strong shearing forces between microvilli at the apex of inner and outer hair cells and in the overlying tectorial membrane. The shearing action is thought to stimulate the hair cells, which in turn elicit a nerve impulse in the surrounding afferent nerve endings. Supporting cells, especially the pillar and phalangeal cells, provide strong structural support to the cell bodies of their hair cells so that the latter are not displaced by the shearing action on the microvilli.

Large areas of the basilar membrane vibrate at several frequencies, but sound waves of a given frequency produce a maximum displacement along specific regions of the basilar membrane. At low frequencies, maximum displacement occurs farther from the oval window. Because both efferent and afferent endings terminate on hair cells in the organ of Corti, both sensory reception and inhibition are said to occur. The inhibitory mechanism stems from the central nervous system and may aid in discrimination of loudness and pitch.

The two skeletal muscles of the middle ear, the tensor tympani and stapedius, dampen the movement of the ossicles and protect the delicate structures of the inner ear from loud and sudden noises. Contraction of these muscles may play a role in regulating the degree of tension placed on the tympanic membrane so that sounds of moderate intensity can be transmitted in a noisy environment.

Nerve impulses from the organ of Corti are transmitted via the bipolar neurons of the spiral ganglion to the cochlear division of the eighth cranial nerve. From here, impulses are relayed to appropriate regions of the brain to be interpreted as sounds.

The vestibular portion of the inner ear is important for coordinating and regulating locomotion and equilibrium. Types I and II hair cells of the cristae in the ampullary region of each semicircular canal are stimulated during angular movement of the head. Sensory stimulation of the receptors results from movement of endolymph and displacement of the cupula that overlies the cristae. Displacement of the cupula, in which microvilli of underying hair cells are embedded, causes a shearing force at the apices of the hair cells. Similarly, forces created during linear acceleration act on the otolithic membrane and its contained otoconia, again resulting in shearing forces being applied to the apices of hair cells. Hence, linear acceleration results in the stimulation of hair cells in the macula, while angular motion results in stimulation of hair cells in the cristae.

Hair cells of the vestibular organs, as well as those of the cochlea, transform mechanical movements of the endolymph (whether produced by displacement of the cupula, otolithic membrane, or basilar membrane) into the electrical energy of a nerve impulse. Bending or displacement of microvilli on the various types of hair cells is thought to result in depolarization of the hair cell, with the stimulus then being transferred to surrounding afferent nerve endings to generate a nerve impulse. Associated efferent nerve endings are thought to have an inhibitory action and may elevate the threshold of activity of hair cells.

Clinical Correlations

One of the most common diseases of childhood is otitis media, an inflammation of the middle ear cavity usually caused by a bacterial or viral infection, though allergies also have been implicated. A contributing factor to infection in children may be their short, straight auditory tube, which allows migration of infection from the nasopharynx to the middle ear cavity. In severe cases, inflammations may extend into the mucosal lining of the mastoid air cells, causing mastoiditis, or the large volume of exudate produced may rupture the eardrum. If the condition becomes chronic or if repeated infections occur, the mucous membrane may become thickened and fibrosed, there may be adhesion and thickening of ossicles, and rupture and scarring of the eardrum may occur, resulting in some loss of hearing.

Otosclerosis is a condition of unknown cause that results in changes in the temporal bone and fibrosis in the region of the oval window, resulting in fusion of the foot plate of the stapes that may cause severe hearing loss or even deafness.

Deafness may result from loss or lack of sensory elements in the inner ear. Developmental failure during formation of structures that make up the cochlea may occur as a result of viral infections during early pregnancy. German measles in the third month of pregnancy can be associated with nerve damage in the ear.

Destruction of cochlear elements can occur as the result of trauma, diabetes mellitus, or infections. A major cause of trauma is continued exposure to loud noise, especially music played through earphones, which results in excessive shearing forces on the delicate cochlear hair cells and tectorial membranes and their eventual destruction. Because these cells are not self-replacing, their loss results in accelerated and progressive hearing loss. Ossicles of the middle ear also are affected by the same type of continuous and excessive noise, which can cause a near arthritic condition or even eburnation of these delicate bones.

Atlas and Table of Key Features

Key Features of the Vestibular Labyrinth

Subdivision	Receptor Region	Neuroepithelium	Other Features
Semicircular canals	Cristae ampullaris	Type I and II hair cells	Cupula cristae ampullaris
Utricle (1)	Macula (of the utricle)	Type I and II hair cells	Otolithic membrane
Saccule (1)	Macula (of the saccule)	Type I and II hair cells	Otolithic membrane
Cochlear duct (1)	Organ of Corti	Inner hair cells Outer hair cells	Tectorial membrane Basilar membrane

Ear

Fig. 10-7. The eardrum as seen on its internal surface. (SEM, ×20.)

Fig. 10-8. Cochlea. (SEM, ×100.)

Scala
vestibuli

Vestibular
membrane

Cochlear
duct

Stria
vascularis

Tectorial
membrane

Osseous
spiral
lamina

Inner
tunnel

Scala
tympani

Fig. 10-9. A section through the cochlear duct illustrates its relationship to the scala vestibuli and scala tympani. (LM, ×100.)

Cochlear
duct

Cells of
Hensen

Outer
hair cells
Outer
phalangeal cells
Basilar
membrane

Outer
pillar cell
Scala
tympani

Tectorial
membrane

Inner
spiral sulcus

Inner
hair cell

Inner
phalangeal cell

Inner
pillar cell

Fig. 10-10. Cells and other components of the organ of Corti. (LM, ×250.)

Cochlear duct

Vestibular membrane

Intraepithelial capillaries

Connective tissue

Fig. 10-11. The stria vascularis. Note the intraepithelial capillaries. (LM, ×250.)

Fig. 10-12. The surface of the organ of Corti showing the arrangement of microvilli on inner and outer hair cells. They are separated by inner pillar cells. (SEM, ×1,350.)

Fig. 10-13. The external border of the tectorial membrane is attached to cells of Hensen. Note the exposed outer hair cells where the membrane is lifted up. (SEM, ×380.)

Ligaments of perilymphatic space

Macula utriculi

Perilymphatic space

Ampulla of semicircular canal

Cupula

Crista of semicircular canal

Fig. 10-14. A section through the vestibular portion of the inner ear illustrates both a macula utriculi and a crista within the ampulla of a semicircular canal. (LM, ×40.)

Sustentacular cells

Hair cells

Nerve fibers

Cupula

Connective tissue

Fig. 10-15. A region of a crista ampullaris showing both hair and sustentacular cells as well as the cupula. (LM, ×250.)

Otoconia

Hair cells

Connective tissue

Otolithic membrane

Sustentacular cells

Nerve fibers

Fig. 10-16. Hair cells and sustentacular cells of a macula utriculus. Note the underlying nerve fibers and the position of the otolithic membrane. (LM, ×250.)

Fig. 10-17. Otoconia on an otolithic membrane (compare with 10-16). (SEM, ×4,000.)

Microvilli on surface of supporting cells

Cilium

Microvilli (hairs)

Surface of hair cell

Fig. 10-18. The apices of vestibular hair cells. Note the single cilium and adjacent microvilli. (SEM, ×6,000.)

Development

Cochlear duct

Cartilaginous shell of cochlea

Cochlear duct

Fig. 10-19. A sagittal section through the cochlea of an embryo. Note the surrounding cartilage, which will be replaced by bone later in development. (LM, ×50.)

Fig. 10-20. Increased magnification of 10-19 illustrates the immature nature of the cochlear duct. (LM, ×100.)

Fig. 10-21. The cochlear duct later in development shows the differentiation of a tectorial membrane and the formation of a scala vestibuli and scala tympani. The organ of Corti has yet to differentiate fully. Compare with 10-9 and 10-10 of the adult. (LM, ×100.)

——————— *Review Questions and Answers* ———————

Questions

56. Briefly discuss the primary function of structures comprising the middle ear.
57. Describe the fluid dynamics of the cochlear division of the inner ear.
58. Compare the mechanisms of stimulation for sensory regions in the vestibular and cochlear regions of the membranous labyrinth.

Answers

56. The middle ear consists of an air-filled space called the tympanic cavity that is continuous anteriorly with the eustachian tube and posteriorly with mastoid air cells. The lateral wall of the tympanic cavity is formed by the tympanic membrane, and its inner boney wall makes contact with the inner ear via two small, membrane-covered apertures called the oval and round windows. The tympanic cavity contains a chain of auditory ossicles (malleus, incus, and stapes) and two small skeletal muscles, the tensor tympani and stapedius.

    The auditory tube connects the anterior portion of the tympanic cavity with the nasopharynx and serves as a passage to ventilate the tympanic cavity and allow pressure equilibration between the middle ear and throat.

    The tympanic membrane receives sound waves and transmits the resulting vibrations to the fluid-filled chambers of the inner ear via the auditory ossicles. The tympanic membrane is about 18 times as large as the oval window, which contains the foot plate of the stapes, and because of this relationship, the tympanic membrane and the auditory ossicles function as a hydraulic piston that exerts pressure on the confined fluid (perilymph) in the chambers

of the inner ear. These structures not only transmit the vibrations created by the sound waves to the inner ear but also amplify the weak forces of the sound waves without an expenditure of energy.

The tensor tympani and stapedius muscles protect delicate structures in the inner ear by dampening ossicle movement that results from loud or sudden noise. They also may regulate the degree of tension in the tympanic membrane, so that sound waves of moderate intensity can be transmitted in a noisy environment.

57. Movement of the foot plate of the stapes in the oval window (fenestra ovalis) exerts pressure on the perilymph in the scala vestibule. Because fluid in a confined space cannot be compressed, the waves of pressure either pass through the cochlear duct and displace it to enter the scala tympani, or enter the scala tympani directly by passing through the helicotrema. Pressure is released from the scala tympani of the cochlea by the elasticity of the secondary tympanic membrane, which bulges into the air-filled tympanic cavity of the middle ear. Pressure waves passing through the cochlear duct produce a slight displacement of the basilar membrane and the organ of Corti, creating a strong shearing force between the microvilli of the inner and outer hair cells and the overlying tectorial membrane. This shearing action is thought to depolarize the hair cells, which in turn generate nerve impulses in the surrounding afferent nerve endings.

58. Type I and type II hair cells of the cristae in the ampullary region of the semicircular canals are stimulated during angular movement of the head. Sensory stimulation of these receptors results from the movement of endolymph that displaces the gelatinous cupula cristae ampullaris, causing a shear-

ing force between the microvilli at the apices of the hair cells, which underly the cupula. Forces created during linear acceleration act on the otolithic membrane and the contained otoconia and result in a shearing force on the apices of the type I and type II hair cells in the maculae. In the cochlear region, a similar shearing force occurs between the microvilli on the inner and outer hair cells and the overlying tectorial membrane in which their tips are embedded. The shearing forces are generated by displacement of the basilar membrane and organ of Corti.

11 Cardiovascular and Lymph Vascular Systems

Unicellular animals acquire their oxygen and nutrients directly from the external environment by simple diffusion and other activities of their cell membranes. However, in multicellular animals most of the cells lie deep in the body, with no access to the external environment, and materials are carried to them through a closed system of branching tubes. Together with a muscular pump, the tubular system makes up the cardiovascular (blood vascular) system. The entire structure consists of a heart that acts as a pump, arteries that carry blood to organs and tissues, capillaries through which exchange of materials occurs, and veins that return the blood to the heart.

A second system of vessels, the lymph vascular system, drains interstitial fluid from organs and tissues and returns it to the blood. It lacks a pumping unit and is unidirectional, carrying lymph toward the heart only. There is no lymphatic equivalent of blood arteries.

Heart

The heart is a modified blood vessel that serves as a double pump and consists of four chambers. On the right side, the atrium receives blood from the body and the ventricle propels it to the lungs. The left atrium receives blood from the lungs and passes it to the left ventricle, from which it is distributed throughout the body. The wall of the heart consists of an inner lining layer, a middle muscular layer, and an external layer of connective tissue.

Endocardium

KEY WORDS: squamous (endothelial) cell, tight (occluding) junction, gap junction, subendothelial layer, subendocardial layer

The endocardium forms the inner lining of the atria and ventricles and is continuous with and comparable to the inner lining of blood vessels. It consists of a single layer of polygonal **squamous (endothelial) cells** with oval or rounded nuclei. **Tight (occluding) junctions** unite the closely apposed cells, and **gap junctions** permit the cells to communicate with one another. Electron micrographs show a few short microvilli (see atlas figure 11-1), a thin proteoglycan layer over the luminal surface, and the usual organelles in the cytoplasm. The endothelial cells rest on a continuous layer of fine collagen fibers, separated from it by a basement membrane. The fibrous layer is called the **subendothelial layer.** Deep to it is a thick layer of denser connective tissue that forms the bulk of the endocardium and contains elastic fibers and some smooth muscle. Loose connective tissue constituting the **subendocardial layer** binds the endocardium to the underlying heart muscle and contains collagen fibers, elastic fibers, and blood vessels. In the ventricles it also contains the specialized cardiac muscle fibers of the conducting system.

Myocardium

KEY WORDS: cardiac muscle, pectinate muscle, trabeculae carnea

The myocardium is the middle layer of the heart and consists mainly of **cardiac muscle** (see atlas figure 11-2). It is the thinnest in the atria and thickest in the left ventricle. The myocardium is arranged in layers that form complex spirals about the atria and ventricles. In the atria, bundles of cardiac muscle form a latticework and locally are prominent as the **pectinate muscles,** while in the ventricles, isolated bundles of cardiac muscle form the **trabeculae carnea.** In the atria, the muscle cells are smaller and contain a number of dense granules not seen elsewhere in the heart. These cells have properties associated with endocrine cells. They are most numerous in the right atrium and release the granules when stretched. The granules contain atrial natriuretic factor (ANF), which increases the glomerular filtration rate and excretion of sodium ions and water by acting on the medullary collecting tubules of the kidney.

Elastic fibers are scarce in the ventricular myocardium but are plentiful in the atria, where they form an interlacing network between muscle fibers. The elastic fibers of the myocardium become continuous with those of the endocardium and outer layer of the heart (epicardium).

Epicardium

KEY WORDS: visceral layer of pericardium, mesothelial cell, subepicardial layer

The epicardium is the **visceral layer of the pericardium,** the fibrous sac that encloses the heart. The free surface of the epicardium is covered by a single layer of flat to cuboidal **mesothelial cells,** beneath which is a layer of connective tissue that contains numerous elastic fibers. Where it lies on the cardiac muscle, the epicardium contains blood vessels, nerves, and a variable amount of fat. This portion is called the **subepicardial layer.**

The parietal layer of the epicardium consists of connective tissue lined by mesothelial cells that face those covering the epicardium. The two layers are separated only by a thin film of fluid, produced by the mesothelial cells, that allows the layers to slide over each other during contraction and relaxation of the heart.

Cardiac Skeleton

KEY WORDS: annuli fibrosi, dense connective tissue, trigona fibrosi, septum membranaceum

The so-called cardiac skeleton consists of several connective tissue structures to which the cardiac muscle is attached. The main part of the cardiac skeleton is formed by the **annuli fibrosi,** rings of **dense connective tissue** that surround the openings to the aorta and pulmonary artery. Also contributing to the skeleton are masses of fibrous tissue, the **trigona fibrosi,** that occur between the atrioventricular and atrial openings, and the **septum membranaceum,** which is the upper, fibrous part of the interventricular septum. The fibrous rings contain elastic fibers and some fat cells and, with aging, may calcify. In dogs the rings contain hyaline cartilage, and bone normally occurs in the annuli fibrosi in cattle.

Valves

KEY WORDS: chordae tendineae, papillary muscles

Valves are present between the atria and ventricles and at the openings to the aorta and pulmonary vessels. Regardless of their location, the valves are similar in structure. The atrioventricular valves are attached to the annuli fibrosi, the connective tissue of which extends into each valve to form its core. The valves are covered on both sides by endocardium that is thicker on the ventricular side. Scattered smooth muscle cells are present on the atrial side of the valves, while on the ventricular side, elastic fibers are prominent. Thin tendinous cords called **chordae tendineae** attach the ventricular sides of the valves to projections of cardiac muscle called **papillary muscles.** Valves of the pulmonary arteries and aorta are thinner but show the same general structure as the atrioventricular valves.

Conducting System

KEY WORDS: **specialized cardiac muscle, sinoatrial node, atrioventricular node, atrioventricular bundle, Purkinje fiber (cell), nodal cell**

The conducting system of the heart consists of **specialized cardiac muscle** fibers and is responsible for initiating and maintaining cardiac rhythm and for ensuring coordination of the atrial and ventricular contractions. The system consists of the sinoatrial node and the atrioventricular bundle.

The **sinoatrial node** is located in the epicardium at the junction of the superior vena cava and right atrium. Impulses initiated in the node spread throughout the ordinary cardiac muscle of the atria to reach the **atrioventricular node** located on the right side of the intra-atrial septum. From here, impulses travel rapidly along the **atrioventricular bundle** in the membranous part of the interventricular septum. The bundle divides into two trunks that pass into the ventricles, where they break up into numerous twigs that connect with the ordinary cardiac muscle fibers. Thus, the impulse is carried to all parts of the ventricular myocardium.

The specialized fibers of the atrioventricular bundle and its branches are called **Purkinje fibers (cells)** and differ from ordinary cardiac muscle in several respects (see atlas figure 11-2). Purkinje fibers are larger and contain more sarcoplasm, but myofibrils are less numerous and usually have a peripheral location. The fibers are rich in glycogen and mitochondria and often have two (or more) nuclei. Intercalated discs are uncommon, but numerous desmosomes are scattered along the cell boundaries. **Nodal cells** are smaller than ordinary cardiac muscle cells and contain fewer and more poorly organized myofilaments. Intercalated discs are lacking between cells of the sinoatrial nodes.

Blood Vessels

The blood vessels are variously sized tubes arranged in a circuit, through which blood is delivered from the heart to the tissues and back to the heart from all parts of the body. By this circulatory system, oxygen from the lungs, nutrients from the intestines and liver, and regulatory substances such as hormones are distributed to all the organs and tissues. Waste products also are emptied into the circulation and carried to organs such as the lungs and kidneys for elimination.

Structural Organization

KEY WORDS: **tunica intima, tunica media, tunica adventitia**

Although blood vessels differ in size, distribution, and function, structurally they share many common features. As in the heart, the walls of blood vessels consist of three major coats or tunics. Differences in the appearance and functions of the various parts of the circulatory system are reflected by structural changes in these tunics, or by reduction and even omission of some of the layers. From the lumen outward, the wall of a blood vessel consists of a tunica intima, tunica media, and tunica adventitia.

The **tunica intima** corresponds to and is continuous with the endocardium of the heart. It consists of an endothelium of flattened squamous cells resting on a basal lamina and is supported by a subendothelial connective tissue.

The **tunica media** is the equivalent of the myocardium of the heart and is the layer most variable both in size and structure. Depending on the function of the vessel, this layer contains variable amounts of smooth muscle and elastic tissue.

The **tunica adventitia** also varies in thickness in different parts of the vascular circuit. It consists mainly of collagenous connective tissue and corresponds to the epicardium of the heart, but it lacks mesothelial cells.

Arteries

As the arteries course away from the heart they undergo successive divisions to provide numerous branches whose calibers progressively decrease. The changes in size and the corresponding changes in structure of the vessel wall are continuous, but three classes of arteries can be distinguished: large elastic or conducting arteries; medium-sized muscular or distributing arteries; and small arteries and arterioles.

Elastic or Conducting Arteries

KEY WORDS: tunica intima, endothelial coat, caveolae, subendothelial layer, tunica media, elastic lamina, tunica adventitia, vasa vasorum

The aorta is the main conducting artery, but others in this class are the common iliacs and pulmonary, brachiocephalic, subclavian, and common carotid arteries. A major feature of this type of artery is the width of the lumen, which, by comparison, makes the wall of the vessel appear thin.

The **tunica intima** is relatively thick and is lined by a single layer of flattened, polygonal cells that rest on a complete basal lamina (see atlas figure 11-3). Adjacent endothelial cells may be interdigitated or overlap and are extensively linked by occluding and communicating junctions. The cells contain the usual organelles, but these are few in number. Peculiar membrane-bound, rod-shaped granules, consisting of several tubules embedded in an amorphous matrix, are present and have been shown to contain a factor (VIII) associated with blood coagulation that is synthesized by the cells and released into the blood. A proteoglycan layer, the **endothelial coat,** covers the luminal surface of the cell membrane. On the basal surface, the endothelial cells are separated from the basal lamina by an amorphous matrix. Numerous invaginations or **caveolae** are present at the luminal and basal surfaces of the plasmalemma, and the cytoplasm contains many small vesicles 50 to 70 nm in diameter. These are thought to form at one surface, detach, and cross to the opposite side, where they fuse with the plasmalemma to discharge their contents. In humans, about one-fourth of the total thickness of the intima is formed by the **subendothelial layer,** a layer of loose connective tissue that contains elastic fibers and a few smooth muscle cells.

The **tunica media** is the thickest layer and consists largely of elastic tissue that forms 50 to 70 concentric, fenestrated sheets or **elastic laminae,** each about 2 or 3 μm thick and spaced 5 to 20 μm apart (see atlas figure 11-4). Successive laminae are connected by elastic fibers. In the spaces between the laminae are thin layers of connective tissue that contain collagen fibers and smooth muscle cells arranged circumferentially. The smooth muscle cells are flattened, irregular, and branched and are bound to adjacent elastic laminae by elastic microfibrils and collagen fibers. An appreciable amount of amorphous ground substance also is present. Smooth muscle cells are the only cells present in the media of elastic arteries and synthesize and maintain the elastic fibers.

Elastic arteries are those nearest the heart, and because of the great content of elastic tissue, are expandable. As blood is pumped from the heart during its contraction, the walls of elastic arteries expand; when the heart relaxes the elastic recoil of these vessels serves as an auxiliary pumping mechanism to force blood onward between beats.

The **tunica adventitia** is relatively thin and contains bundles of collagen fibers and a few elastic fibers, both of which have a loose, helical arrangement (see atlas figure 11-4). Fibroblasts, mast cells, and rare longitudinally oriented smooth muscle cells also are present. Tunica adventitia gradually blends into surrounding loose connective tissue.

The walls of large arteries are too thick to be nourished only by diffusion from the lumen. Consequently, these vessels have their own small arteries, the **vasa vasorum,** that may arise as branches of the main vessel itself or derive from neighboring vessels. They form a plexus in the tunica adventitia and generally do not penetrate deeply into the media (see atlas figure 11-14).

Muscular or Distributing Arteries

KEY WORDS: tunica intima, endothelium, subendothelial layer, internal elastic lamina, tunica media, smooth muscle, external elastic lamina, tunica adventitia

The muscular or distributing arteries are the largest class, and except for the elastic arteries, the named arteries of gross anatomy fall into this category. All the small branches that originate from elastic trunks are muscular arteries, and the transition is relatively abrupt, occurring at the openings of the branching arteries. Compared to the luminal diameter, the walls of these arteries are thick and make up over one-fourth of the cross-sectional diameter. The thickness of the wall is due mainly to the large amount of smooth muscle in the media, which, by contraction and relaxation, helps to regulate the blood supply to organs and tissues. The general organization of these vessels is similar to that of elastic arteries, but the proportion of cells and fibers differs.

The **tunica intima** consists of an endothelium, a subendothelial layer, and an internal elastic lamina. The **endothelium** and **subendothelial layers** are similar to those of elastic arteries, but as the size of the vessel decreases the subendothelial layer becomes thinner. It contains fine collagen fibers, a few elastic fibers, and scattered smooth muscle cells that are longitudinal. The **internal elastic lamina** is a fenestrated band of closely interwoven elastic fibers that form a prominent, scalloped boundary between the tunica media and the tunica intima (see atlas figure 11-5). The basal surfaces of the endothelial cells send slender processes through discontinuities in the elastic lamina to make contact with cells in the tunica media.

The **tunica media** is the thickest coat and consists mainly of **smooth muscle** cells arranged in concentric, helical layers. The number of layers varies from three to four in smaller arteries to 10 to 40 in the large muscular arteries. The muscle cells are surrounded by basal laminae and communicate with each other by gap junctions. Reticular fibers and small bundles of collagen fibers interspersed with elastic fibers are present between the layers of smooth muscle. The number and distribution of elastic fibers correlate with the caliber of the artery. In the smaller vessels elastic fibers are scattered between the muscle cells, whereas in larger arteries the elastic tissue forms circular, loose networks. At the junction of the tunica media and the tunica adventitia, the elastic tissue forms a second prominent fenes-

trated membrane called the **external elastic lamina** (see atlas figure 11-5).

The **tunica adventitia** is prominent in muscular arteries and in some vessels may be as thick as the media. It consists of collagen and elastic fibers that are longitudinal in orientation. This coat continues into surrounding loose connective tissue with no clear line of demarcation.

Small Arteries and Arterioles

Small arteries and arterioles differ from large muscular arteries only in size and the thickness of their walls. The distinction between small arteries and arterioles is mainly one of definition: Arterioles are those small arteries with a diameter less than 250 to 300 μm and in which the media contains only one or two layers of smooth muscle cells (see atlas figures 11-6 through 11-8).

In the progression from distributing artery to arteriole, the subendothelial connective tissue progressively decreases until in arterioles, a subendothelial layer is lacking and the tunica intima consists only of endothelium and a fenestrated internal elastic lamina. The endothelial cells are joined by occluding junctions. Basal processes make contact with smooth muscle cells through the fenestrations in the elastic lamina. The thin basal lamina becomes indistinct in the smallest arterioles. The layers of smooth muscle of the media progressively decrease in number, and, at a diameter of about 30 μm, the muscle coat of arterioles consists of a single layer of circumferentially oriented cells. The internal elastic membrane is thin and disappears in terminal arterioles; there is no definite external elastic lamina. Tunica adventitia also decreases in thickness, becoming extremely thin in the smallest arterioles.

Compared to the luminal size, the walls of arterioles are thick. Because of the smooth muscle in the media, arterioles control the blood to capillary beds they feed and are the main regulators of blood pressure. Precapillary sphincters are simply the terminal arteries that give rise to capillaries.

Capillaries

Capillaries are the smallest functional units of the blood vascular system and are inserted between arterial and venous limbs of the circulation. They branch extensively to form elaborate networks, the extent of which reflects the activity of an organ or tissue. Highly branched, closely packed networks of capillaries are present in the lungs, liver, kidneys, glands, and mucous membranes. Based on the appearance of the endothelium and basal lamina in electron micrographs, capillaries are classed as continuous or fenestrated. Regardless of the type, the basic structure of capillaries is the same and represents an extreme simplification of the vessel wall. The tunica intima consists of endothelium and a basal lamina; the tunica media is absent and the tunica adventitia is greatly reduced.

Continuous Capillaries

KEY WORDS: **continuous endothelium, continuous basal lamina, tunica adventitia, pericytes**

Continuous capillaries are the common type of capillary found throughout the connective tissues, muscle, and central nervous system. Their lumina range from 5 to 10 μm in diameter and in the smaller vessels may be encompassed by a single endothelial cell. In larger capillaries three or four cells may enclose the lumen. The wall consists of a **continuous endothelium** and a thin tunica adventitia. The endothelial cells rest on a **continuous basal lamina** and show the same features as endothelial cells elsewhere in the vascular tree (see atlas figure 11-9). They contain the usual organelles, caveolae and vesicles, a proteoglycan layer, a few short microvilli on the luminal surfaces, and a variable number of membrane-bound granules. Multivesicular bodies also can be found. Adjacent cells may abut each other or overlap obliquely or in sinuous interdigitations. At intervals, adjacent cell membranes unite in occluding junctions, but it is not certain that these form complete belts as in other epithelia.

The **tunica adventitia** is thin and contains some collagen and elastic fibers embedded in a small amount of ground substance. Fibroblasts, macrophages, and mast cells are present also.

Pericytes are irregular, branched, isolated cells that occur at intervals along capillaries, enclosed by the basal lamina of the endothelium. The cells resemble fibroblasts and characteristically contain a few dense bodies and numerous cytoplasmic filaments. Actin and myosin have been demonstrated in the cytoplasm by immunohistochemistry, indicating a contractile function. However, their exact function is unknown.

Fenestrated Capillaries

KEY WORDS: **fenestra, diaphragm, continuous basal lamina**

Fenestrated capillaries have the same structure as the continuous type but differ in that the endothelial cells contain numerous **fenestrae** (pores) that appear as circular openings, 70 to 100 nm in diameter (see atlas figures 11-10 and 11-11). Fenestrae may be distributed at random or in groups and usually are closed by thin **diaphragms** that show central, knoblike thickenings. Each diaphragm is a single-layered structure — thinner than a single unit membrane — so it would appear unlikely that it is formed by apposition of two cell membranes. The **basal lamina** is **continuous** across the fenestrae on the basal side of the endothelium (see atlas figure 11-11). The fenestrated capillaries of the renal glomerulus differ in that the pores lack diaphragms and the basal lamina is much thicker than in other capillaries.

Diffusion

Exchange of nutrients and wastes between tissues and blood occurs across the thin endothelium of capillaries. It has been estimated that no active cell lies more than 30 or 40 μm away from a capillary. The most important way materials cross the endothelium is by diffusion, and the total capillary surface available for exchange has been calculated to be over 100 square meters. Lipid-soluble materials diffuse directly through the endothelial cells; water and water-soluble materials are transmitted through water-filled, physiologic "pores" that may be the equivalent of the cytologic pores of the fenestrated capillaries. In the continuous capillaries, caveolae and cytoplasmic vesicles have been implicated in transepithelial transport of water-soluble materials; pinocytosis also may contribute to transfer of substances of high molecular weight. Fluid exchange also occurs through intercellular clefts between endothelial cells.

Metarterioles

Metarterioles are intermediate between capillaries and arterioles and control the flow of blood through capillary beds. They also are called capillary sphincter areas or precapillary arterioles. Although poorly defined morphologically, their lumina generally are wider than those of the capillaries they serve, and circularly arranged smooth muscle cells are scattered in their walls.

Sinusoids

KEY WORDS: gaps, discontinuous basal lamina, phagocyte

Sinusoids are thin-walled vessels that are much wider and have lumina that are more irregular in outline than those of capillaries. Sinusoids are found in the liver, spleen, bone marrow, and some endocrine glands. Their endothelia are attenuated and may be continuous as in the marrow, or the cells may be separated by **gaps** and rest on a **discontinuous basal lamina.** Sinusoids often are associated with **phagocytes** either as a component of the lining, as in the liver, or closely applied to the exterior of the wall, as in the spleen. The endothelial cells themselves show no greater capacity for phagocytosis than do endothelial cells in other vessels. They do show more active endocytosis and more numerous lysosomes than are found in endothelia elsewhere.

Veins

The venous side of the circulatory system carries blood from the capillary beds to the heart, and in their progress, the veins gradually increase in size and their walls thicken. Their structure bas-

ically is the same as that of arteries, and the three coats — tunica intima, media, and adventitia — can be distinguished but are not as clearly defined. In general, veins are more numerous and larger than the arteries they accompany, but their walls are thinner because of a reduction of muscular and elastic elements. Since their walls are less sturdy, veins tend to collapse when empty and in sections may appear flattened, with irregular, slitlike lumina.

Structurally veins vary much more than arteries. The thickness of the wall does not always relate to the size of the vein, and the same vein may differ structurally in different areas. Histologic classification of veins is less satisfactory than for arteries, but several subdivisions usually are made — namely, venules and small, medium, and large veins.

Venules

KEY WORDS: continuous endothelium, pericyte, thin adventitia, incomplete tunica media

Venules arise from the union of several capillaries to form vessels 10 to 50 µm in diameter. The junctions between venules and capillaries are important sites of fluid exchange between tissues and blood.

The tunica intima consists of a thin, **continuous endothelium,** the cells of which are loosely joined by poorly developed intercellular junctions (see atlas figure 11-7). The thin basal lamina is pierced by **pericytes** that appear to make contact with the endothelial cells.

The tunica media is missing in the smallest venules, and the relatively **thin adventitia** contains a few collagen fibers, scattered fibroblasts, mast cells, macrophages, and plasma cells. As the vessels increase in size to reach diameters of 50 µm, circularly oriented, scattered smooth muscle cells begin to appear and form a somewhat discontinuous and **incomplete tunica media.** The adventitia increases in thickness and consists of longitudinally arranged collagen fibers that form an open spiral around the vessel. Fibroblasts often are irregular in shape and bear thin processes.

Small Veins

KEY WORDS: continuous endothelium, tunica media, tunica adventitia

Small veins vary from about 0.2 to 1.0 mm in diameter. The tunica intima consists only of a **continuous endothelium** that rests on a thin basal lamina. Circular smooth muscle fibers make up a **tunica media** which contains one to four layers of cells. Between the smooth muscle cells is a thin network of elastic and collagen fibers. The **tunica adventitia** forms a relatively thick coat and contains longitudinally oriented collagen fibers and some thin elastic fibers.

Medium Veins

KEY WORDS: thin tunica intima, narrow subendothelial layer, tunica media, thick tunica adventitia, vasa vasorum, valve

The medium class of veins includes most of the named veins of gross anatomy except for major trunks. They vary in size from 1 to 10 mm in diameter. The **thin tunica intima** consists of endothelial cells resting on a basal lamina, but a **narrow subendothelial layer** may be present and contains fine collagen fibers and scattered thin elastic fibers. The elastic fibers may form a network at the junction of tunica intima and media, but a poorly defined internal elastic lamina is formed only in the larger vessels. In most medium veins the **tunica media,** though well developed, is thinner than in corresponding arteries (see atlas figure 11-12). The **thick tunica adventitia** forms the bulk of the wall and is larger than the tunica media. It consists of collagen and elastic fibers and frequently contains longitudinal smooth muscle cells. **Vasa vasorum** are present in the larger vessels of this class.

Most medium veins are equipped with **valves,** pocketlike flaps of tunica intima that project into the lumen, their free edges oriented in the direction of flow (see atlas figure 11-13). They consist of a core of connective tissue covered on both sides by endothelium. A rich network of elastic fibers is present in the connective tissue beneath the endothelium on the downstream side of the valves. As blood flows toward the heart, the valves are forced against the vessel wall, but with backflow, the valves are forced outward against each other to occlude the vessel and prevent reversal of blood flow.

Large Veins

KEY WORDS: thick tunica adventitia, vasa vasorum, thin tunica media, tunica intima

In large venous trunks (venae cavae; renal, external iliac, splenic, portal, and mesenteric veins) the **thick tunica adventitia** forms the greater part of the wall (see atlas figure 11-14). It consists of a loosely knit connective tissue with thick, longitudinal bundles of collagen and elastic fibers. Smooth muscle layers, also longitudinal, are present and are especially well developed in the inferior vena cava. **Vasa vasorum** are present and may extend into the media. A **thin tunica media** is poorly developed and may even be absent; otherwise it has the same organization as that in medium veins. The **tunica intima** is supported by a subendothelial layer that may become prominent in larger trunks.

Veins with Special Features

Some veins lack a tunica media, such as the trabecular veins of the spleen; veins of the retina, bone, and maternal placenta; most meningeal and cerebral veins; and those of the nail bed. Veins in the pregnant uterus contain smooth muscle in all three coats; in the intima the fibers run longitudinally rather than circularly, as they do also in the tunica intima of the saphenous, popliteal, femoral, umbilical, and internal jugular veins. At their junctions with the heart, the adventitia of the pulmonary veins and venae cavae are provided with a coat of cardiac muscle; the fibers run longitudinally and circularly about the vessels for a short distance.

Arteriovenous Anastomoses

In addition to their capillary connections, arteries and veins may unite by shunts called arteriovenous anastomoses. Generally these arise from side branches of arterioles that pass directly to venules. They are thick-walled, muscular vessels of small caliber that usually are coiled and surrounded by a connective tissue sheath. They are plentiful in the plantar and palmar surfaces, fingertips, toes, lips, and nose and also occur in the thyroid. When open, the anastomoses shunt blood around the capillary bed and thus regulate the blood supply to many tissues.

Carotid and Aortic Bodies

KEY WORDS: epithelioid (glomus) cells, chemoreceptor

Carotid bodies are encapsulated structures that occur on each side of the neck at the bifurcations of the common carotid arteries. They consist of masses of large, polyhedral **epithelioid (glomus) cells** that are closely related to a rich network of sinusoidal vessels. The cells have large, pale nuclei and light, finely granular cytoplasm. In electron micrographs, the granules show dense cores and contain catecholamines and 5-hydroxytryptamine. A second cell type, the type II glomus cell, appears much the same as type I but lacks granules. Many nerves ramify throughout the structures. Carotid bodies act as **chemoreceptors** and monitor blood for changes in oxygen and carbon dioxide content, pH, and pressure.

Aortic bodies are similar structures that lie close to the aorta between the angle of the subclavian and carotid arteries on the right, and near the origin of the subclavian artery on the left. They are thought to have functions similar to those of carotid bodies. Both of these structures are derived from the neural crest.

Lymph Vascular System

The lymph vascular system consists of endothelial-lined tubes that recover intercellular fluid not picked up by the blood vascular system and return it to the blood. The fluid (lymph) carried by the lymphatics is a blood filtrate formed as fluid crosses the blood capillaries into the tissues. Unlike the blood vascular system, lymph flow is unidirectional — from tissues to the union of the

lymphatic and blood vascular systems at the base of the neck.

The lymphatic vascular system begins in the tissues as blindly ending capillaries that drain into larger collecting vessels and then into two main lymphatic trunks. Lymph nodes occur along the course of the vessels and filter the lymph. Lymphatics are present in most tissues but are absent from bone marrow, the central nervous system, coats of the eye, internal ear, and fetal placenta.

Lymph Capillaries

KEY WORDS: thin continuous endothelium, discontinuous basal lamina, anchoring filament

Lymph capillaries are thin-walled, blind tubes that branch and anastomose freely to form a rich network in organs and tissues. They are wider and more irregular than blood capillaries. The wall of a lymph capillary consists only of a **thin continuous endothelium** and a **discontinuous basal lamina** that is present only in patches or may even be absent. Adjacent endothelial cells may overlap, but junctional complexes are few and clefts occur between the cells. Externally, the endothelium is surrounded by a small amount of collagenous connective tissue. Fine filaments run perpendicularly from the collagen bundles and attach to the outer surfaces of the endothelium as **anchoring filaments** that maintain the patency of the vessel.

Collecting Lymph Vessels

KEY WORDS: tunica intima, tunica media, tunica adventitia, valve

Collecting lymph vessels differ from lymph capillaries in size and the thickness of their walls. Although three coats — intima, media, and adventitia — are described as in blood vessels, they are not clearly delineated.

The **tunica intima** consists of an endothelium supported by a thin network of longitudinal elastic fibers. The **tunica media** is composed of smooth muscle with a predominantly circular arrangement, though some fibers run longitudinally. Between the muscle fibers are a few fine elastic fibers. The **tunica adventitia** is the thickest coat and consists of bundles of collagen fibers, elastic fibers, and some smooth muscle cells, all of which have a longitudinal orientation.

Valves are numerous along the course of lymphatic vessels and occur at closer intervals than in veins. They arise in pairs as folds of the intima, as in veins.

Lymphatic Trunks

KEY WORDS: tunica intima, subendothelial layer, internal elastic lamina, tunica media, tunica adventitia

Collecting lymphatic ducts ultimately gather into two main trunks, the thoracic and right lymphatic ducts. The thoracic duct is the longer and has a greater field of drainage. It begins in the abdomen, passes along the vertebral column, and opens into the venous system at the junction of the left jugular and subclavian veins. It receives lymph from the lower limbs, abdomen, left upper limb, and left side of the thorax, head, and neck. The right lymphatic duct receives lymph only from the upper right part of the body and empties into the brachiocephalic vein.

The structure of the trunks is the same, generally resembling that of a large vein. The **tunica intima** consists of a continuous endothelium supported by a **subendothelial layer** of fibroelastic tissue with some smooth muscle. Near the junction with the tunica media, the elastic fibers condense into a thin **internal elastic lamina.** The thickest layer is the **tunica media** which contains more smooth muscle than does the media of large veins. The fibers have a predominantly circular arrangement and are separated by abundant collagenous tissue and some elastic fibers. The **tunica adventitia** is poorly defined and merges with the surrounding connective tissue. It contains bundles of longitudinal collagen fibers, elastic fibers, and occasional smooth muscle fibers. The wall of the thoracic duct contains nutrient blood vessels similar to the vasa vasorum of large blood vessels.

Development of the Cardiovascular System

Initially, the developing embryo is nourished by simple diffusion of nutrients, at first from the uterine fluids and later, after implantation, from maternal blood lakes. With growth, these sources are unable to meet the nutritional needs of the mass of cells in the embryo, so a vascular system arises early in development.

Heart

The earliest cardiac structure appears as an aggregation of splanchnic mesoderm to form two longitudinal strands. Each acquires a lumen and becomes a simple, endothelial-lined tube lying in a fold of mesoderm. The tubes fuse to form a single, saccular cardiac primordium, and the mesodermal folds merge into a single surrounding coat (see atlas figure 11-15). The endothelial tube gives rise to the endocardium; the myocardium and epicardium arise from the outer layer of mesoderm. Myofibrils first appear as loosely arranged groups of filaments within the cytoplasm of differentiating cardiac muscle cells of the myocardium (see atlas figure 11-16). Later in development the myofibrils acquire distinct Z bands prior to the appearance of A and I bands (see atlas figure 11-17). Following fusion of the two endocardial tubes, the single primitive heart tube grows more rapidly than the pericardial cavity. Because the two ends are anchored to surrounding tissues, elongation of the cardiac tube cannot occur and a cardiac loop is formed (see atlas figure 11-18). The cephalic end gives rise to the bulbus cordis, the caudal end to the presumptive ventricle.

At first the endothelial tube is separated from the myocardial layer by a jellylike fluid that is invaded by mesenchyme and transformed into the subendocardial layer. The cells at the external surface of the myocardium flatten into a mesothelium and together with a sublayer of connective tissue form the epicardium. The remainder of the myocardial coat forms an outer compact layer of cardiac muscle and an inner layer of loosely arranged trabeculae. In mammals the entire muscle wall becomes compact except for the trabeculae carneae of the ventricles, which persist as remnants of the spongy layer.

According to some investigators, the atrioventricular node is the first part of the conducting system to develop, arising from cardiac muscle cells around the atrioventricular canal. From this the atrioventricular bundle arises. An alternative view suggests that the bundle arises first, from muscle on the dorsal wall of the atrioventricular canal, then spreads to form the atrioventricular node and the right and left limbs of the bundle. The sinoatrial node is the last to appear, from a narrow muscular band in the lateral surface of the superior vena cava. Later in fetal life, the node is incorporated into the wall of the atrium.

Vessels

The earliest blood vessels arise from extraembryonic mesenchyme, appearing first as blood islands in the yolk sac and body stalk. Initially the islands form solid cords, but the outermost cells flatten to become the first endothelial cells, while the innermost become free and form the first primitive blood cells. This process of canalization occurs in several places, and by growth and union, the isolated vascular spaces unite to form a network of vessels that, at this stage, consists of simple endothelial tubes. The first vessels of the embryo form in a similar fashion. After circulation is established, further extension of blood vessels occurs by endothelial budding and growth of preexisting vessels. Formation of capillary-like vessels precedes development of definite arteries and veins. Smooth muscle and connective tissue coats are acquired by differentiation of surrounding mesenchyme.

Lymphatic vessels arise quite separately as isolated spaces in the mesenchyme. Cells bordering the spaces flatten to become endothelial cells. By progressive unions, the spaces link up to form continuous, branching channels that ultimately lead to a complete set of lymphatic vessels. In the larger lymphatics, the outer tunics are derived from the surrounding mesenchyme.

Functional Summary

The myocardium of the heart provides the propelling force that moves blood through the systemic and pulmonary circulations. Cardiac muscle is characterized by its ability to contract spontaneously without external stimulus. The heart has a system of specialized fibers that regulate the contractions into rhythmic beats coordinated throughout the chambers of the heart. The contraction impulse is initiated in the sinoatrial (SA) node, the pacemaker of the heart. The cells of the SA node are unique in that they spontaneously reach the threshold at which an action potential is automatically triggered. The impulse passes through ordinary cardiac muscle fibers of the atria to reach the atrioventricular node where it is delayed, allowing the atria to complete their contractions before the impulse is passed to the ventricles. The impulse then is conducted rapidly along the atrioventricular bundle and by its branches is spread throughout the ventricular myocardium. The granular cells of the atria secrete the peptide hormone ANF, which plays a role in regulating blood pressure and volume and in controlling the excretion of water and sodium. Thus the heart functions, to a limited extent, as an endocrine organ.

Flow of blood from the heart is intermittent, and the arteries immediately joining the heart are subjected to pulses of high pressure. Because of the large amounts of elastic tissue in their walls, the large conducting vessels can expand and absorb the forces without damage.

During the intervals between contractions, the elastic recoil of the vessel wall serves as an additional propelling mechanism, helps smooth out the blood flow, and protects delicate capillaries and venules from severe changes in pressure.

Distribution of blood to organs is controlled largely by muscular arteries. The caliber of these vessels is regulated by the degree of contraction of the tunica media in response to changes in blood pressure and the demands of organs. Pressure in a capillary bed is controlled by arterioles: The amount of blood flow is controlled by the opening and closing of shunts formed by arteriovenous anastomoses.

Exchange of material between blood and tissues occurs at the level of capillaries and venules. Passage of fluid across capillary walls depends partly on blood pressure and partly on colloidal osmotic pressure in the capillaries. Blood pressure promotes passage of fluid into tissues; osmotic pressure promotes resorption. At the arterial end of capillary beds, blood pressure is greater than osmotic pressure and fluid is driven out of the vessel; at the venous end osmotic pressure is the greater and fluid is driven into the vessel. Venules, with their thin walls and loosely joined endothelial cells, also are important sites of fluid exchange. Lipid-soluble materials readily diffuse through endothelial cells, whereas water-soluble materials pass through pores and intercellular clefts. The so-called physiologic pores may correspond to the fenestrae of fenestrated endothelium or to caveolae and cytoplasmic vesicles of continuous capillaries. Bulky material, including whole cells, readily crosses the walls of sinusoids.

Blood is returned to the heart via the veins, which are able to constrict or enlarge and store large quantities of blood. From 70 to 75 percent of the circulating blood is contained in the veins, and much of it can be made available to organs as needed. Blood is moved along the veins by the massaging action of muscles and fascial tissues and by special arrangements of vessels in the soles of the feet that act as pumps when pressure is exerted on them. Blood flows away from the area of compression but is prevented from flowing backward by the valves.

Although most of the fluid filtered from the blood capillaries is resorbed by them, about 10 percent is not recovered by the blood vascular system, and it is this fluid that is recovered by the lymphatics. Substances of high molecular weight such as proteins pass into the blood capillaries with difficulty but are recovered by lymphatic capillaries almost unhindered. Lymphatic channels are one of the main routes by which nutrients, especially fats, are absorbed from the gastrointestinal tract.

Blood vascular endothelium serves as a permeability barrier — a moderator of selective transport — and has important functions in maintaining the fluidity of blood. The endothelium provides a physical surface to which platelets do not normally stick, so it prevents their aggregation; it also synthesizes prostacyclin, an agent that inhibits platelet adhesion. However, endothelium also contains thromboplastic substances and antihemophilic factor VIII of the blood coagulation system. Thus, the endothelium is also equipped to initiate clotting and repair minor defects to prevent leakage of blood. The luminal surface bears a negative charge, as do red cells, thus preventing their aggregation on the wall of the blood vessel and resulting eddying and turbulent flow.

Clinical Correlations

Atheroma can occur in arteries of all sizes, including arterioles. Coronary atherosclerosis is a progressive disease marked by patchy thickening of the tunica intima with consequent narrowing of the lumen. The initial event appears to be chronic injury to the endothelium with exposure of subendothelial connective tissues, to which platelets adhere. Among other substances, platelets release an agent that is mitogenic for smooth muscle cells, which then migrate into the subendothelial layer and proliferate. Smooth muscle cells are the major constituent and primary cellular component of atheromatous plaques. Lipid accumulates in and between the cells, especially those close to the internal elastic lamina. Thin plates of collagen, produced by the muscle cells, appear in the superficial parts of the plaque, and lipid accumulates here also. Infiltration by granulocytes is common and "foam cells" — lipid-laden macrophages — may appear around the lipid deposits. Cholesterol crystals may also be present.

As the plaque develops, the deeper parts are converted to a structureless mass of lipid and tissue debris, and the necrosis gradually extends into the overlying fibrous tissue. Deep to the plaque, the internal elastic lamina becomes fragmented, and lipid deposits, necrosis, and fibrosis extend into the media. Calcification of the plaque may occur. Eventually the affected area of the media deep to the plaque becomes thinned and atrophic; the intima becomes thickened and, as can occur in the aorta, may become thicker in places than the media.

Coronary atherosclerosis is one of the more common diseases of the vascular system and is the main factor in most cases of angina pectoris, myocardial infarction, cardiac failure, and sudden death. Coronary atheroma shows the features of similar lesions in other arteries. Any of the main branches of the coronary arteries may be involved, but the most severe lesions tend to develop in the first 3 to 3½ cm of the left coronary artery or its anterior interventricular branch. Branches that have penetrated the myocardium are rarely involved. Occlusion of a coronary vessel can result in infarction (death) of the segment of the heart served by that vessel. The muscle fibers undergo coagulation necrosis, and the area becomes firm and dull. Microscopically, the dead cells become homogeneous, and the cross striations and details of cellular architecture are lost. The infarct is invaded by granular leukocytes and macrophages and over the next weeks or months, if the patient lives, the necrotic muscle is replaced by fibrous scar tissue.

Atlas and Table of Key Features

Key features of arteries and veins

Arteries	Tunica intima	Tunica media	Tunica adventitia	Other
Large	Thick subendothelial layer with elastic fibers and smooth muscle; internal elastic lamina prominent	Major coat; 40–60 elastic laminae; smooth muscle, fibrous connective tissue between laminae	Thin; no external elastic lamina	Compared to lumen, wall is thin; vasa vasorum extend through adventitia and about one-third of the way through media
Small and medium	Thin subendothelial layer present; prominent internal elastic lamina	Major coat; up to 40 layers of smooth muscle, some elastic tissue	May equal thickness of media; external elastic lamina present	Muscular (distributing) arteries, including most of named arteries
Arteriole	Thin, no recognizable subendothelial layer; internal elastic lamina	Forms the main coat; 1–5 layers of smooth muscle	Thin; no external elastic lamina; fibroelastic	Wall (relative to lumen) is thicker than in any other vessel
Capillaries				
Continuous	Endothelium plus basement membranes; pericytes, tight junctions, desmosomes	Absent	Scant reticular fibers	5–10 μm in diameter
Fenestrated	Endothelial cells bear openings in cytoplasm, usually closed by diaphragm	Absent	Scant reticular fibers	In glomeruli, fenestrae not closed by diaphragm
Veins				
Venule	Endothelium only; no internal elastic lamina	Very thin; 1–3 layers of smooth muscle cells	Thick compared to total wall; wholly collagenous	
Small and medium	Thin; subendothelial layer lacking in smaller veins	Thin; layer of smooth muscle, elastic fibers, and collagen fibers	Well developed; thick fibroelastic layer; no elastic lamina	
Large	Thicker than in small veins; a delicate internal elastic lamina may be present	Thin or even lacking	Thickest coat; fibromuscular; no elastic lamina	

Heart

Endothelial surface

Clump of microvilli

Microvilli

Leukocyte

Fig. 11-1. Surface features of endothelial cells from the endocardium of the heart. (SEM, ×1,000.)

Cardiac muscle cell

Myocardium

Purkinje cells

Endocardium

Fig. 11-2. A region of endocardium that contains Purkinje cells. Compare the size and staining intensity of these cells with cardiac muscle cells forming the myocardium. (LM, ×250.)

Arteries

Endothelial cells

Microvilli

Fig. 11-3. Surface features of endothelial cells lining the aorta. (SEM, ×1,000.)

Elastic laminae

Lumen

Vasa vasorum

Tunica adventitia

Fat cells

Fig. 11-4. A section through the wall of the aorta stained with orcein to selectively demonstrate elastic laminae. (LM, ×40.)

Internal elastic lamina

Tunica intima

Tunica media

Tunica adventitia

External elastic lamina

Fig. 11-5. A section through the wall of a muscular artery stained with orcein to selectively demonstrate elastic laminae. (LM, ×200.)

Smooth muscle cell

Endothelial cell

Tunica media

Collagen fiber

Fibroblast nucleus

Fig. 11-6. A section through the wall of a small artery. (LM, ×250.)

Arteriole

Smooth
muscle
cells

Venule

Collagen
fibers

Erythrocyte

Fibroblast
nuclei

Endothelial
cell

Fig. 11-7. A region of loose connective tissue containing an arteriole and venule. (LM, ×250.)

Internal
elastic
lamina

Lumen

Endothelial
cell

Smooth
muscle
cell

Smooth
muscle
cell

Basal
lamina

Collagen
fiber

Fig. 11-8. A portion of a wall from an arteriole. (TEM, ×6,000.)

Fig. 11-9. A capillary from the lamina propria of a human stomach. Note the erythrocyte within its lumen. (TEM, ×5,000.)

Fig. 11-10. A capillary lined by fenestrated endothelium from a pancreatic islet. (TEM, ×6,000.)

Fenestrations

Fenestrations

Basal lamina

Fig. 11-11. Fenestrated endothelium from a capillary within a parathyroid gland. (TEM, ×15,000.)

Veins

Internal elastic lamina

Tunica media

Lumen

Tunica adventitia

External elastic lamina

Fig. 11-12. A segment of wall from a human medium-sized vein stained with orcein to selectively demonstrate elastic laminae. (LM, ×100.)

Endothelial cell

Boundaries of endothelial cell

Valve

Fig. 11-13. A whole mount preparation of a vein illustrating a valve. The intercellular cement between endothelial cells has been impregnated with silver and stains black. (LM, ×250.)

Tunica intima

Tunica media

Vasa vasorum

Tunica adventitia

Fig. 11-14. A portion of the wall of human inferior vena cava stained with orcein selectively demonstrates scattered elastic laminae. (LM, ×40.)

Development

A

B

Fig. 11-15. Ventral views of the forming cardiac tube showing
the presumptive bulbus and cordis and ventricle. Note the region
of fusion in A. (SEM, ×200.)

C

Fig. 11-15. (continued.)

Fig. 11-16. Myofibrilogenesis in a differentiating cardiac muscle cell. The myofibril consists of a loose arrangement of filaments. (TEM, ×18,000.)

Fig. 11-17. A myofibril in a cardiac muscle cell later in development that shows distinct Z bands. A and I bands have yet to form. (TEM, ×18,000.)

A   B

Fig. 11-18. A. The initial bending of the cardiac tube during heart formation. (SEM, ×80.) B. Further bending and counterclockwise movement of the cardiac tube during heart formation. (SEM, ×80.)

Review Questions and Answers

Questions

59. List the layers that comprise the walls of the heart and name the corresponding structures in the blood vessels.

60. What is the most prominent coat in the large conducting arteries? What tissue component characterizes this coat? What functional advantage does this give to the arteries?

61. Of what does the conducting system of the heart consist? What is its function?

62. How do veins differ from arteries?

63. Name two types of capillaries and describe the structural changes that distinguish them. How do sinusoids differ from capillaries?

64. How is blood flow through a capillary bed controlled?

Answers

59. Layers comprising the wall of the heart are the endocardium, myocardium, and epicardium and correspond to the tunica intima, tunica media, and tunica adventitia of blood vessels.

60. Conducting arteries show a prominent tunica media, characterized by the abundance of elastic tissue that is arranged in sheets or laminae. Because of the large amount of elastic tissue, the conducting arteries are expansile and able to absorb the force of the blood as it is ejected from the heart. The recoil of the elastic wall serves as a propelling mechanism for blood during the periods between the heart beats, thus helping to smooth out the blood flow and protect the delicate capillaries and venules from violent changes in pressure.

61. The conducting system of the heart consists of the sinoatrial node, the atrioventricular node, and the atrioventricular bundle and its branches. Each of these components consists of modified cardiac muscle fibers. The conducting system is responsible for the coordination of the intrinsic contractions of the cardiac muscle, ensuring the maintenance of cardiac rhythm and coordination of the atrial and ventricular contractions.

62. Veins are more numerous and generally of greater size, and their walls are thinner than those of arteries mainly because of a reduction in the muscular and elastic elements. Veins also are much more variable in their structure — the thickness of their walls does not necessarily relate to the overall size of the vein, even in the same vein. Usually, but not invariably, the tunica adventitia forms the prominent layer in the wall of the veins.

63. Capillaries are classed as continuous or fenestrated based on the appearances of the endothelium and basal lamina. Continuous capillaries are characterized by an uninterrupted, continuous lining of endothelial cells resting on a complete basal lamina. Fenestrated capillaries are characterized by fenestrae or pores in the endothelial cells and a continuous basal lamina. The fenestrae usually are closed by a thin diaphragm. Sinusoids are more irregular in outline and have wider bores than other capillaries. These vessels show a loose arrangement of the endothelium, and gaps are present between adjacent endothelial cells. The basal lamina is discontinuous. Phagocytes usually are closely associated with the walls of sinusoids. In all types of capillaries, the walls consist of tunica intima and an attenu-

ated tunica adventitia; the media is lacking.

64. Blood flow through a capillary bed is controlled by the activity of the arterioles and by the operation of the arteriovenous anastomoses. The distribution of blood to the organs or tissues in which the capillary bed lies is controlled by the muscular distributing arteries.

12 Lymphatic Organs

Lymphatic organs are divided into primary (central) and secondary (peripheral) organs. Primary lymphatic organs are the first to develop and include the thymus in mammals and the thymus and bursa of Fabricius in birds. The mammalian equivalent of the bursa is unknown but probably is the bone marrow, although the spleen and the lymphatic tissue associated with the gastrointestinal tract (Peyer's patches, lamina propria of small intestine, appendix) have been considered also. The secondary lymphatic organs are the lymph nodes, spleen, tonsils, and lymphatic tissues associated with the gastrointestinal tract. Lymphatic organs consist of accumulations of diffuse and nodular lymphatic tissues that are organized into discrete structures. The lymphatic tissues that compose the organs are isolated from the surrounding tissues by a well-defined capsule.

Tonsils

Tonsils are aggregates of lymphatic nodules associated with the pharynx and oropharynx and are present in reptiles, birds, and mammals. In amphibians, tonsils are poorly developed and are present as lymphoid masses in the roof of the pharynx. Similar masses of tissue in reptiles and birds are better organized into the pharyngeal tonsils. A ring of lymphatic tissue, in varying degrees of completeness, is present at the entrance to the esophagus and respiratory tract in mammals, reaching its greatest development in hu-

mans. Depending on the species, the structures are spread through different areas — oropharynx, nasopharynx, and tongue — and form the palatine, pharyngeal, and lingual tonsils, respectively. Palatine tonsils are absent in the rat and mouse, pharyngeal tonsils are lacking in the rabbit, and the cat, dog, and sheep have no lingual tonsils. The general structure of a tonsil is shown in Fig. 12-1.

Tonsils do not filter lymph; they have no afferent vessels leading to them, nor do they have an internal system of sinuses for the filtering of lymph. However, at the inner surfaces of the tonsils, plexuses of blindly ending lymph capillaries form the beginnings of efferent lymphatic vessels. Tonsils contribute to the formation of lymphocytes, many of which migrate through the covering epithelium and appear in the sputum as salivary corpuscles. Bacteria that penetrate the lymphoid tissue of the tonsils act as antigens to stimulate the production of antibodies.

Palatine Tonsils

KEY WORDS: **stratified squamous epithelium, crypt, partial capsule**

The palatine tonsils are paired, oval lymphatic organs located laterally at the junction of the oral cavity and oropharynx. A **stratified squamous epithelium** continuous with that of the oral cavity and oropharynx covers the free surface of the tonsil and is very closely associated with the lymphatic tissue (see atlas figures 12-7 and 12-8).

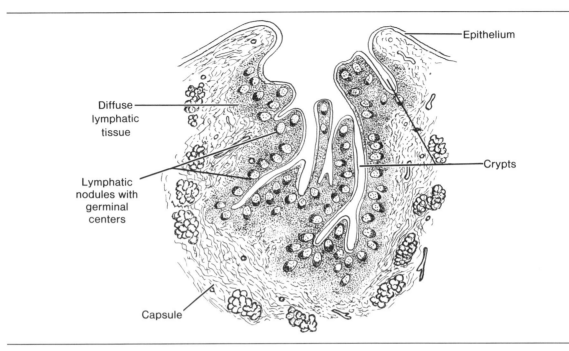

Fig. 12-1. General structure of a tonsil.

Deep invaginations of the epithelium form the tonsillar **crypts** that reach almost to the base of the tonsil (see atlas figure 12-7). Secondary crypts may branch from these deep pockets and also are lined by stratified squamous epithelium that tends to thin out in the deeper parts of the crypts. Lymphatic nodules, many with prominent germinal centers, usually are arranged in a single layer beneath the epithelium, embedded in a mass of diffuse lymphatic tissue. Large numbers of lymphocytes infiltrate the epithelium, especially that lining the lower ends of the crypts, often to such an extent that the demarcation between epithelium and lymphatic tissue is obscure.

A **partial capsule** beneath the basal surface of the tonsil separates it from surrounding structures to which the capsule adheres. Septae of loosely arranged collagen fibers extend from the capsule into the tonsillar tissue and partially divide the crypts and their associated lymphatic

tissue from one another. Fibers from the septae spread out and become continuous with the reticular fibers of the lymphatic tissue. The connective tissue is infiltrated by lymphocytes of various sizes, plasma cells, and mast cells. Neutrophil granulocytes may be present and are numerous during inflammation of the tonsils. Small mucous glands lie outside the capsule, and their ducts drain to the free surface of the tonsil or, rarely, empty into a tonsillar crypt.

Lingual Tonsils

KEY WORDS: root of the tongue, crypt, stratified squamous epithelium, mucous gland

The lingual tonsils form nodular bulges in the **root of the tongue,** and their general structure is similar to that of the palatine tonsil. **Crypts** are deep, may be branched, and are lined by **stratified squamous epithelium** that invaginates from the surface. The associated lymphatic tissue consists of diffuse and nodular types. **Mucous glands** embedded in the underlying muscle of the tongue drain by ducts, most of which open into the bases of the crypts.

Pharyngeal Tonsil

KEY WORDS: nasopharynx, pseudostratified ciliated columnar epithelium

The pharyngeal tonsil is located on the posterior wall of the **nasopharynx.** Its surface epithelium is a continuation of that lining the respiratory passages — namely, **pseudostratified ciliated columnar epithelium** that contains goblet cells (see atlas figures 12-9 and 12-10). Patches of squamous epithelium may be present, however, and tend to become more common with aging and smoking. The crypts are not as deep as in the palatine tonsils, and the epithelium forms numerous shallow folds. A thin capsule separates the pharyngeal tonsil from underlying tissues and provides fine septae that extend into the substance of the tonsil. Small mucoserous glands lie beneath the capsule and empty onto the surface of the folds.

Lymph Nodes

Lymph nodes are small encapsulated lymphatic organs set in the course of lymphatic vessels. They are absent in fish, amphibians, and reptiles, although nodular collections of lymphatic tissue about blood vessels have been described in toads, and rudimentary structures like lymph nodes have been reported in crocodiles. In aves simple aggregates of lymphatic tissue occur beside the terminal part of the cervical duct and in the abdomen superior to the genital gland. Lymph nodes are most characteristic of mammals, in which they show their fullest development. They are prominent in the neck, axilla, groin, and mesenteries and along the course of large blood vessels in the thorax and abdomen. In some animals, the lymph nodes of the mesentery are aggregated into a single large organ called the pancreas of

Anselli. This appears to be a general feature of rodents and carnivores, but no similar organ is found in humans.

Structure

KEY WORDS: hilus, afferent lymphatic, efferent lymphatic, diffuse lymphatic tissue, nodular lymphatic tissue, capsule, trabeculae, reticular network, cortex, outer cortex, deep (inner) cortex, thymus-dependent area, follicular dendritic cell, medulla, medullary cord

Grossly, lymph nodes appear as flattened, ovoid or bean-shaped structures with a slight indentation at one side, the **hilus,** through which blood and lymphatic vessels enter or leave (Fig 12-2). Lymph nodes are the only lymphatic structures that are set into the lymphatic circulation and thus are the only lymphatic organs to have afferent and efferent lymphatics. **Afferent lymphatics** enter the node at multiple sites, anywhere over the convex surface; **efferent lymphatics** leave the node at the hilus. Both sets of vessels have valves that allow unidirectional flow of lymph through a node. The valves of afferent vessels open toward the node; those of efferent vessels open away from the node.

Essentially, lymph nodes consist of accumulations of **diffuse** and **nodular lymphatic tissue** enclosed in a capsule that is greatly thickened at the hilus. The **capsule** consists of closely packed collagen fibers, scattered elastic fibers, and a few smooth muscle cells that are concentrated about the entrance and exit of lymphatic vessels. From the inner surface of the capsule, branching **trabeculae** of dense irregular connective tissue extend into the node and provide a kind of skeleton for the lymph node (see atlas figure 12-11). The spaces enclosed by the capsule and trabeculae are filled by an intricate, three-dimensional **reticular network** of reticular fibers and their associated reticular cells. The meshes of the network are crowded with lymphatic cells, so disposed as to form an outer cortex and an inner medulla.

The **cortex** forms a layer beneath the capsule and extends for a variable distance toward the

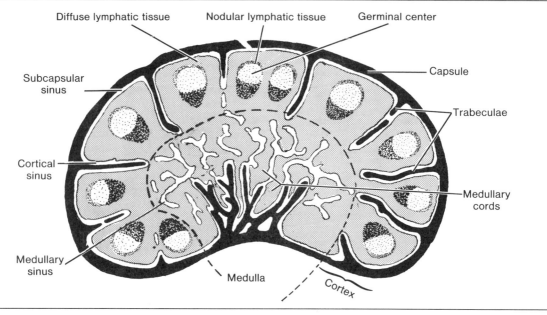

Fig. 12-2. General structure of a lymph node.

center of the node. It consists of lymphatic nodules, many with germinal centers, set in a bed of diffuse lymphatic tissue. Trabeculae are arranged fairly regularly and run perpendicular to the capsule, subdividing the cortex into several irregular "compartments." However, trabeculae do not form complete walls but rather represent bars or rods of connective tissue, and compartmentalization of the cortex is incomplete. All the cortical areas communicate with each other laterally and above and below the plane of section where trabeculae are deficient.

The cortex usually is divided into an **outer cortex** that lies immediately beneath the capsule and contains nodular and diffuse lymphatic tissue, and a **deep (inner) cortex** that consists of diffuse lymphatic tissue only. There is no sharp boundary between the two zones, and their proportions differ from node to node and with the functional status of the node. In general, B-lymphocytes are concentrated in the nodular lymphatic tissue, while T-cells are present in the diffuse lymphatic tissue. The deep cortex becomes depleted of cells after thymectomy and has been called the **thymus-dependent area.** This area also contains **follicular dendritic cells,** a rather bizarre cell type with a pale-staining nucleus, few cytoplasmic organelles, and numerous, long processes that interdigitate with similar projections from nearby lymphocytes. They represent a form of antigen-presenting cell. The deep cortex continues into the medulla without interruption or clear demarcation.

The **medulla** appears as a paler area of variable width, generally surrounding the hilus of the node. It consists of diffuse lymphatic tissue arranged as irregular **medullary cords** that branch and anastomose freely. Medullary cords contain abundant plasma cells, macrophages, and lymphocytes. The trabeculae of the medulla are more irregular arranged than those of the cortex.

Lymph Sinuses

KEY WORDS: subcapsular (marginal) sinus, cortical (trabecular, intermediate) sinus, medullary sinus

Within the lymph node is a system of channel-like spaces, the lymph sinuses, through which lymph percolates. Lymph enters the node through afferent lymphatic vessels that pierce the capsule anywhere along the concave border and empty into the **subcapsular (marginal) sinus,** which separates the cortex from the capsule (see atlas figure 12-12). The sinus does not form a tubular structure but is present as a wide space extending beneath the capsule, interrupted at intervals by the trabeculae. The subcapsular sinus is continuous with similar structures, the **cortical (trabecular, intermediate) sinuses,** which extend radially into the cortex, usually along the trabeculae (see atlas figure 12-12). These in turn become continuous with **medullary sinuses** that run between the medullary cords and trabeculae of the medulla (see atlas figures 12-11 and 12-16). At the hilus, the medullary and subcapsular sinuses unite, penetrate the capsule, and become continuous with the efferent lymphatics.

In sections, sinuses appear as regions in which the reticular net is coarser and more open. Stellate cells supported by reticular fibers crisscross the lumen and are joined to each other and to the cells bordering the lumen by slender processes. Numerous macrophages are present in the luminal network and also project from the boundaries of the sinus. The cells that form the margins of the sinuses and extend through the sinus space generally are regarded as flattened reticular cells. However, they also have been considered to be attenuated endothelial cells akin to those that line the lymphatic vessels with which they are continuous.

Sinuses in the cortex are less numerous than in the medulla and are relatively narrow. Those in the medulla are large and irregular and show repeated branchings and anastomoses. They run a tortuous course in the medullary parenchyma and account for the irregular cordlike arrangement of the lymphatic tissue in this area.

Blood Vessels

KEY WORDS: postcapillary venule, high endothelium

The major blood supply reaches the node through the hilus and only occasionally do smaller vessels enter from the convex surface. The arteries (arterioles) at first run within the trabeculae in the medulla but soon leave these and enter the medullary cords to pass to the cortex. Here they break up into a rich capillary plexus that distributes to the diffuse lymphatic tissue and also forms a network around the nodules.

The capillaries regroup to form venules that run from the cortex and enter the medullary cords as small veins. These in turn are tributaries of larger veins that pass out of the node at the hilus. In the deep cortex, the venules take on a special appearance and have been called **postcapillary venules.** These vessels are characterized by a **high endothelium** that varies from cuboidal to columnar and at times appears to occlude the lumen. The walls of these vessels often are infiltrated with small lymphocytes that generally are presumed to be passing into the lymph node. The cells pass between adjacent endothelial cells, indenting their lateral walls as they cross through the endothelium. The significance of the tall endothelium is not known, but it has been suggested that as the lymphocytes sink deeper between them, the adjacent endothelial cells resume their original relationship to each other above the lymphocytes and seal off the interendothelial cleft, thereby limiting the loss of plasma from the venule.

Spleen

The spleen embodies the basic structure of a lymph node and can be regarded as a modified, enlarged lymph node inserted into the blood flow. Unlike lymph nodes, the spleen has no afferent lymphatics and no lymphatic sinus system, and the lymphatic tissue of the spleen is not arranged into cortex and medulla. It does have a distinctive pattern of blood circulation and specialized vascular channels that facilitate the filtering of blood.

Structure

KEY WORDS: capsule, hilus, trabeculae, reticular network, splenic pulp, white pulp, red pulp, splenic sinusoid

The spleen (Fig. 12-3) is enclosed in a well-developed **capsule** of dense irregular connective tissue (see atlas figure 12-17). Elastic fibers are present between bundles of collagen fibers and are most abundant in the deeper layers of the capsule. Smooth muscle fibers also may be present in small groups of cords, but the amount varies with the species. They are prominent in horses, carnivores, and ruminants, but few smooth muscle fibers are found in the splenic capsule in humans and rodents. On the medial surface of the spleen, the capsule is indented to form a cleftlike **hilus** through which blood vessels, nerves, and lymphatics enter or leave the spleen.

Broad bands of connective tissue, the **trabeculae,** extend from the inner surface of the capsule and pass deeply into the substance of the spleen to form a rich branching and anastomosing framework. As in lymph nodes, the trabeculae subdivide the organ into communicating compartments. The spaces between trabeculae are filled by a **reticular network** of fibers and associated reticular cells. The meshes vary in size and tend to be smaller around blood vessels and aggregates of lymphatic tissue.

The substance of the spleen is called the **splenic pulp,** and sections from a fresh spleen show a clear separation of the tissue into rounded or elongated grayish areas set in a greater mass of dark red tissue. Collectively, the scattered gray areas form the **white pulp** and consist of diffuse and nodular lymphatic tissue. The dark red tissue is the **red pulp** and consists of diffuse lymphatic tissue that is suffused with blood. The large number of red cells present imparts the color to the red pulp. In many species, including humans, the red pulp contains large, branching,

thin-walled blood vessels called **splenic sinusoids** (sinuses); such spleens are said to be sinusal (see atlas figures 12-18 and 12-19). Animals such as the cat and opossum lack splenic sinusoids so their spleens are classed as asinusal.

White Pulp

KEY WORDS: periarterial lymphatic sheath, lymphatic nodule, splenic follicle, marginal zone, interdigitating cell

The white pulp generally is associated with the arterial supply of the spleen and forms the **periarterial lymphatic sheaths** that extend about the arteries, beginning as soon as the vessel leaves the trabeculae to enter the splenic pulp. The sheaths have the structure of diffuse lymphatic tissue and contain the usual cellular elements of lymphatic tissue. Small lymphocytes, mostly T-cells, make up the bulk of the cells. Here and there along the course of the sheath, the lymphatic tissue expands to incorporate **lymphatic nodules** that resemble the cortical nodules of lymph nodes. They represent sites of B-lymphocytes and many contain germinal centers. The lymphatic nodules of the spleen are called **splenic follicles** (see atlas figure 12-23). At the periphery of the lymphatic sheath, the reticular net is more closely meshed than elsewhere, and the reticular fibers and cells form concentric layers that tend to delimit the lymphatic tissue from the red pulp. This forms the **marginal zone** (see atlas figure 12-23). Cells similar to the follicular dendritic cells of lymph nodes are present in the white pulp of the spleen. These dendritic-like cells are called **interdigitating cells** and also represent antigen-presenting cells.

In the rat and rabbit the periarterial lymphatic sheaths are well developed and the lymphatic nodules are small and numerous. In the dog and cat, however, the sheaths are poorly developed but lymphatic nodules are large.

Red Pulp

KEY WORDS: splenic sinusoid, splenic cord

The red pulp is a diffuse lymphatic tissue associated with the venous system of the spleen. The

Fig. 12-3. General structure of the spleen.

reticular meshwork is continuous throughout the red pulp and is filled with large numbers of free cells, including all of those usually found in the blood. Thus, in addition to the cells of lymphatic tissue, the red pulp is suffused with red cells, granular leukocytes, and platelets. Occasionally macrophages can be seen that contain ingested red cells or granulocytes, or that are laden with a yellowish-brown pigment, hemosiderin, derived from the breakdown of hemoglobin (see atlas figure 12-22).

The red pulp is riddled with large, irregular blood vessels, the **splenic sinusoids,** between which the red pulp assumes a branching, cordlike arrangement to form the **splenic cords** (see atlas figure 12-19). The sinusoids have wide lumina (20 to 40 μm diameter), and their walls have a unique structure (Fig. 12-4). Almost the entire wall is made up of elongated, fusiform endothelial cells that lie parallel to the long axis of the vessel (see atlas figures 12-20 and 12-21). The cells lie side by side around the lumen but are not in contact and are separated by slitlike spaces. Outside the endothelium, the wall is supported by a basement membrane that is not continuous but forms widely spaced, thick bars that encircle the sinusoid. The bars of basement membrane are joined to each other by thinner strands of the same material and are continuous with the reticular network of the splenic cords (see atlas figures 12-18 and 12-19).

Blood Supply

KEY WORDS: **trabecular artery, central artery, penicillar artery, sheathed capillary, open circulation, closed circulation, pulp vein, trabecular vein**

The architecture of the spleen is best understood in relation to the blood circulation, which shows some special features (Fig. 12-5). Branches of the splenic artery enter the spleen at the hilus, divide, and pass within trabeculae into the interior of the organ. These branches have an overlapping, segmental arrangement, with each main branch serving a defined area of the spleen. The **trabecular arteries,** as they now are called, branch repeatedly, finally leaving the trabeculae as **central arteries** that immediately become surrounded by the lymphatic tissue of the periarterial lymphatic sheath. Where the sheath expands to form nodules, the central artery (more appropriately, the follicular arteriole) is displaced to one side and assumes an eccentric position in the nodule (see atlas figures 12-23 and 12-24). Only rarely does the vessel retain a central position in the nodular tissue. Throughout its course in the white pulp, the central artery provides numerous capillaries that supply the sheath, then pass into the marginal zone surrounding the white pulp. How these capillaries end is not certain. Many arterial branches appear to open directly into the marginal zone, often ending in a funnel-shaped terminal part. There is no direct venous return, and the white pulp is associated only with the arterial supply. Although the term *artery* commonly is used for the different levels of the splenic vasculature, once the vessel has reached lymphatic tissue, it is actually an arteriole.

The central artery continues to branch, and its

Fig. 12-4. Structure of a splenic sinusoid.

Bars of
basement
membrane

Endothelial
cells

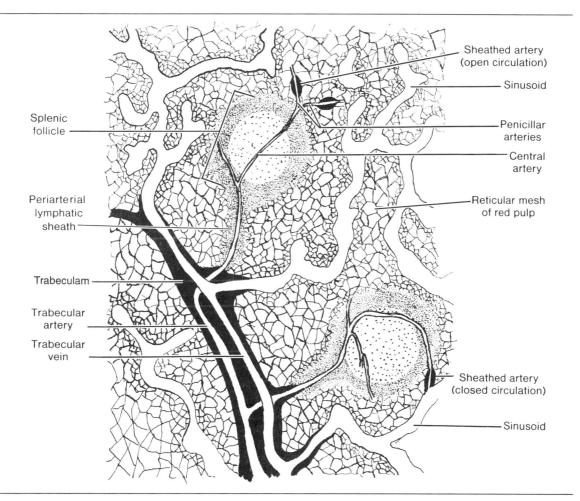

Fig. 12-5. Blood supply of the spleen.

attenuated stem passes into a splenic cord in the red pulp, where it divides into several short, straight **penicillar arteries,** some of which show a thickening of their wall and now form **sheathed capillaries.** The sheath consists of compact masses of concentrically arranged cells and fibers that become continuous with the reticular network of the red pulp. Close to the capillary, the cells of the sheath are rounded, while at the periphery of the sheath the cells become stellate. The cells of the sheath are avidly phagocytic.

Not all the capillaries are sheathed, and occa-

sionally a single sheath may enclose more than one capillary. Sheathed capillaries are prominent in dogs, pigs, reptiles, and birds, are less well developed in humans, and are lacking in rodents. Sheathed capillaries may continue as simple capillaries or they may divide to produce two to four nonsheathed, terminal capillaries. How these end still is a matter of some debate and has led to the "open" and "closed" theories of circulation. According to the **open circulation** theory, the capillaries empty into the meshwork of the red pulp in the splenic cords. The blood then slowly seeps through the red pulp and finds its way into the venous system through the walls of the splenic sinusoids. The **closed circulation** theory holds that the capillaries open directly into the lumina of the venous sinusoids; blood leaves the sinusoid at the capillary end and re-enters at the venous end because of a decreasing pressure gradient between the two ends of the sinusoid. A compromise between the two views suggests that a closed circulation in a contracted spleen becomes open when the spleen is distended.

Splenic sinusoids drain into **pulp veins,** which are supported by a thin muscle coat and, more externally, are surrounded by reticular and elastic fibers. A sphincter-like activity of the smooth muscle has been described at the junction of the pulp veins and sinusoids. Pulp veins enter trabeculae where, as **trabecular veins,** they pass in company with the artery. Trabecular veins unite and leave at the hilus as the splenic vein.

The spleen has no afferent lymphatics, but efferents arise deep in the white pulp and converge on the central arteries. The lymphatics enter trabeculae and form large vessels that leave at the hilus. Areas of the spleen supplied by sinusoids (i.e., the red pulp) lack lymphatics.

Thymus

Thymic tissue is present in all vertebrates except cyclostomes (lampreys and hagfish). In humans the thymus is a bilobed, encapsulated lymphatic organ situated in the superior mediastinum dorsal to the sternum and anterior to the great vessels that emerge from the heart. The thymus is the only primary lymphatic organ in mammals and is the first organ of the embryo to become lymphoid. Unlike the spleen and lymph nodes, it is well developed and relatively large at birth. The greatest weight (30 to 40 g) is achieved at puberty, after which the organ undergoes progressive involution and is partially replaced by fat and connective tissue.

The general structure of the thymus is shown in Fig. 12-6.

Structure

KEY WORDS: lobe, capsule, septum, lobule, cortex, medulla, reticular network, epithelial reticular cell, cytoreticulum

In humans the thymus consists of two **lobes** closely applied and joined by connective tissue. Each lobe arises from a separate primordium, and there is no continuity of thymic tissue from one lobe to the other. A thin **capsule** of loosely woven connective tissue surrounds each lobe and provides **septa** that extend into the thymus, subdividing each lobe into a number of irregular **lobules.** Each lobule consists of a **cortex** and **medulla** (see atlas figures 12-25 and 12-26). In the usual sections, the medulla may appear as isolated, pale areas completely surrounded by denser cortical tissue. However, serial sections show that the lobules are not isolated by the septa; the medullary areas are continuous with one another throughout each lobule.

The free cells of the thymus are contained within the meshes of a **reticular network,** which, however, differs from that of other lymphatic tissues. In the thymus the reticular cells take origin in endoderm rather than mesenchyme and are not associated with reticular fibers. These **epithelial reticular cells** are stellate in shape with greatly branched cytoplasm that contains few organelles. The large round or oval euchromatic nuclei show one or more small but prominent nucleoli. The cytoplasmic processes are in contact with the processes of other reticular cells and at their points of contact are united by desmosomes. Thus, the stroma of the thymus consists of a **cytoreticulum** composed of epithelial cells. Reticular fibers are found only in relation to blood vessels.

Cortex

KEY WORDS: lymphocyte, no lymphatic nodules, reticular cell, macrophage

The cortex consists of a thick, deeply stained layer extending beneath the capsule and along the septa. Most of the cells of the cortex are **lympho-**

Capsule

Septa

Cortex

Medulla

Hassall's corpuscle

Fig. 12-6. General structure of the thymus.

cytes that are closely packed with little intervening material between them (see atlas figure 12-26). Because of mutual compression, the cells appear polyhedral in shape. Large, medium, and small lymphocytes are present, the latter being the most abundant; they are indistinguishable from small lymphocytes found elsewhere. Large lymphocytes tend to concentrate in the outer cortex beneath the capsule and represent stem cells that have newly emigrated from the bone marrow. They form only a small part of the cell population. Small lymphocytes become increasingly more numerous toward the deeper cortex, where degenerating cells with pyknotic nuclei also are found. Unlike lymph nodes, there are **no lymphatic nodules** in the cortex of the thymus, nor is there an internal sinus system.

Reticular cells in the cortex are highly branched, but their processes are obscured by the mass of lymphocytes. They form a continuous layer at the periphery of the cortex, separating it from the capsule and septa. These epithelial reticular cells contain tonofilaments and membrane-bound structures that appear to be secretion granules. **Macrophages** are consistently present in small numbers, scattered throughout the cortex. They are difficult to distinguish from reticular cells by light microscopy unless phagocytosed material can be seen in their cytoplasm. In electron micrographs they are distinguished from epithelial reticular cells by the lack of desmosomes. Macrophages that have engulfed degenerating cells can be found scattered throughout the thymus and tend to increase in number toward the junction of the cortex and medulla.

Medulla

KEY WORDS: **pleomorphic reticular cell, dendritic interdigitating cell, small lymphocyte, thymic corpuscle**

The medulla occupies the central region of the thymus, where it forms a broad, pale band of tissue that is continuous throughout each lobule. Often, however, it appears to be isolated within a lobule, surrounded by a complete layer of cortex. Lymphocytes are less numerous than in the cortex, and the epithelial reticular cells are not as widely dispersed or as highly branched. The **reticular cells** tend to be **pleomorphic** and vary from stellate cells with long processes to rounded or flattened cells with many desmosomes and abundant tonofilaments. **Dendritic interdigitating cells** are found in the medulla and cortico medullary region. They act as antigen-presenting cells for more mature T-lymphocytes.

The free cells of the medulla are mainly **small lymphocytes,** but a small and variable number of macrophages are present. Plasma cells, mast cells, and eosinophil granulocytes can be found. Mitotic figures are rare. Collagen and reticular fibers extend for short distances from blood vessels and wind between the epithelial cells.

Rounded or ovoid epithelial structures, the **thymic corpuscles,** are a prominent feature of the medulla (see atlas figures 12-26 and 12-27). These bodies vary in size from 10 to 100 μm or more in diameter and consist of flattened epithelial reticular cells, wrapped about one another in concentric lamellations, that are joined by numerous desmosomes. Many contain granules of keratohyalin. The cells at the center of the structure undergo hyalinization or necrosis and may become lysed to leave a cystic structure. Some of the cells at the periphery of the corpuscle retain their connections with the surrounding cytoreticulum. The function of the thymic corpuscles is unknown; they have been regarded purely as degenerated structures, but there is some evidence that they may be secretory bodies. Although considered characteristic of the thymus, similar structures occur in the palatine tonsils of the dog and horse. Thymic corpuscles are poorly developed in mice but are prominent in the thymi of humans, guinea pigs, and rats.

Blood Supply

KEY WORDS: **corticomedullary junction, cortical capillary, blood-thymic barrier**

The arteries to the thymus penetrate the organ within the connective tissue of the septa. Arteriolar branches from these vessels run along the **corticomedullary junction** and provide arterioles and capillaries to the medulla and capillaries to the cortex; vessels larger than capillaries are not found in the cortex. Within the cortex, the capillaries run toward the capsule, where they form branching arcades before passing back through the cortex to drain into venules and thence into veins that accompany the arterioles in the corticomedullary region and medulla. The veins leave via the septa and ultimately unite to form a single thymic vein.

The **cortical capillaries** are enveloped by a collar of connective tissue that forms part of the **blood-thymic barrier.** This envelope in turn is surrounded by a continuous layer of epithelial reticular cells. The perivascular connective tissue space varies in width and is traversed by reticular fibers that accompany the vessel. Within the perivascular space are granular leukocytes, plasma cells, macrophages, and lymphocytes. The blood-thymic barrier in the cortex thus consists of the capillary endothelium and its basal lamina, the perivascular connective tissue sheath, and the layer of epithelial reticular cells and their associated basal lamina. There is little movement of macromolecules across this barrier, and cortical lymphocytes develop in relative isolation from antigens. Vessels of the medulla and corticomedullary junction are permeable to circulating macromolecules.

Involution

Growth of the thymus during fetal life is very rapid, and the organ attains its greatest relative size by the time of birth. It continues to grow, at a lesser rate, until puberty, after which it undergoes progressive involution. The organ decreases in weight, loses cortical lymphocytes, and shows an increase in the size and number of thymic corpuscles. The septa also increase in width. The cortical areas become infiltrated by fat cells, and the replacement may become extensive. By the time involution commences, T-cells have disseminated into the secondary lymphatic tissue throughout the body. The thymic parenchyma does not disappear completely even in old age, and the thymus maintains some activity in the adult.

Other Constituents

The thymi of birds, reptiles, and amphibians frequently show a number of peculiar structural elements, the significance of which is not known. Among these structures are cystlike spaces lined by cells with brush borders, cilia, or mucus-producing cells or by reticular cells that contain microvillus-lined vacuoles. Most peculiar are the "myoid" cells, which have an imperfect resemblance to striated muscle. These cells may resemble embryonal or adult muscle fibers complete with typical banding patterns: Z lines and A, I, and M lines have been described. It is not known whether these various inclusions have functional significance or represent aberrant differentiation of embryonal elements.

Dendritic (Antigen-Presenting) Cells

Dendritic (antigen-presenting) cells arise in the bone marrow, but unlike monocytes (macrophages) have low levels of lysosomal enzymes. In contrast, they have high levels of class II major histocompatibility complex (MHC) molecules essential for presenting new antigens to T-lymphocytes. Dendritic cells have the capacity to ingest foreign proteins, process (partially digest) the antigens, and insert selected portions of an antigen into their cell membrane, thereby retaining the product for long periods of time. Dendritic cells are found in lymph nodes, spleen, thymus, mesenteries, and skin (Langerhans' cells), and under mucosal surfaces. Despite the morphologic similarities of exhibiting fine ramifying cytoplasmic processes and containing relatively few lysosomes, each dendritic antigen-presenting cell appears to have developed specialized surface receptors for a given specific microenvironment at the site in which it is found. After a period of time, they leave the specific environment (skin, for example), make their way to lymphoid tissue, and gradually present the antigens collected in a specific environment to T-lymphocytes. Thus, the dendritic antigen-presenting cells play a very important role in the immune system by monitoring a number of different environments.

Development of Lymphatic Organs

The thymus arises as a pair of endodermal outgrowths from the third pharyngeal pouch, with some contribution from the fourth also. Each outgrowth extends caudally and medially and by the eighth week lies in the midline beneath the upper part of the sternum. Initially, each outgrowth has a slitlike lumen surrounded by several layers of tall cuboidal or columnar cells. As the cells proliferate, the lumina disappear. Centrally, the cells become stellate and loosely arranged but retain their cytoplasmic connections with one another. These form the epithelial reticular cells of the thymic cytoreticulum.

At about 8 weeks, the thymic rudiment is seeded by blood-borne stem cells that originate in the yolk sac and fetal liver; lymphoid stem cells capable of repopulating the thymus are present in the bone marrow also. The migration of stem cells appears to be guided by chemotactic agents liberated by the thymic reticular cells. The stem cells give rise to the thymic lymphocytes, which, by the fourteenth week of gestation, are arranged into cortex and medulla. It is not known whether the lymphoid progenitor cells are already differentiated as T-cell precursors at the time of seeding, or whether differentiation occurs in the thymus.

Mesenchyme surrounding the thymic primordium condenses to form the capsule and also invades the cellular mass to provide the septa.

Lymph nodes develop locally in vascular mesenchyme at sites normally occupied by lymph nodes, and their formation is related closely to development of the lymph vascular system. Aggregates of mesenchymal cells form around loops of lymphatic capillaries, in close association with lymphatic sacs. At the periphery of the aggregates, lymphatic vessels form isolated spaces that are separated by slender bridges of connective tissue. As the lymph spaces gradually fuse to form the marginal (subcapsular) sinus, the connective tissue outside the sinus and in the bridges condenses to form the capsule and trabeculae. As they fuse, the sinuses follow the courses of the developing trabeculae, subdivide, and develop into the trabecular and medullary sinuses. The mesenchymal aggregates give rise to the reticular cells and fibrous network of the cortex and medulla. The entire mass is seeded by lymphocytes from the bone marrow and thymus, and the cells take up their characteristic locations in the nodes.

The spleen first appears as several thickenings in the cranial end of the greater omentum. With growth, the primordia fuse to form a lobulated spleen that extends into the body cavity. As the organ expands, it loses its lobulated appearance. Mesenchymal cells in the body of the cellular mass differentiate into reticular cells that provide the splenic reticular stroma. The outermost connective tissue gradually condenses to form the capsule from which mesenchymal projections condense to form the trabeculae. At this stage (eighth to ninth week) the spleen consists of a meshwork of reticular cells surrounded by a thin capsule. This spleen rudiment is seeded by lymphocytes from the bone marrow and thymus. Enlargement of the white pulp to form nodules occurs late, and during much of development, lymphatic tissue mainly forms periarterial lymphatic sheaths. Germinal centers appear only after birth. The fetal spleen is hemopoietic, producing erythrocytes and granular leukocytes, but in humans this function ceases just before birth.

Functional Summary

The assembly of lymphatic tissue — lymphatic organs spread throughout the connective tissue — constitutes the immune system that protects the body against invading foreign macromolecules and constantly monitors the circulating fluids (blood and lymph) for abnormal components. Antigenic material evokes a specific defense reaction, the immune response, that gives rise either to B-cells that produce specific antibodies or to a variety of T-cells that attack foreign cells directly, release nonspecific toxic agents, assist B-cells in the production of antibody, or direct macrophage response and maturation. Antibodies may act by binding to the antigen to neutralize it, inhibit the entrance of the antigen into a cell, enhance its phagocytosis, or initiate its lysis. Germinal centers are associated with production of humoral antibody, especially during a secondary response, and may represent a clone of B-cells geared to the production of a single antibody. Stimulation by antigen results in proliferation and differentiation of lymphocytes, some of which go on to react against the antigen, while others remain as committed memory cells. On a second exposure to the same antigen, memory cells react swiftly and with great efficiency.

Tonsils are the major bulwark against oral and pharyngeal routes of infection. They contribute to the formation of lymphocytes, are able to mount immunologic responses, and take part in the immunologic defenses of the body. Tonsils appear to be especially valuable sources of interferon, an antiviral factor, and may be of greater importance in fighting infection than has been recognized previously.

Lymph nodes contribute to the production of lymphocytes as indicated by the mitotic activity, especially in germinal centers. The lymphocytopoietic activity of quiescent nodes does not seem to be great, and the bulk of the cells in an unstimulated node are recirculating lymphocytes. B- and T-cells enter the node through the postcapillary venules, but some also enter through afferent lymphatics. Once in the parenchyma, B-cells home in on the lymphatic nodules of the outer cortex; T-cells make their way to the deep cortex and the region of the thymus-dependent area. The cells remain in the lymph node for variable periods of time, then leave to recirculate in the blood and other lymphatic organs. Only small lymphocytes recirculate.

Lymph nodes form an extensive filtration system that removes foreign particles from the lymph, preventing their spread through the body. A single lymph node can remove 99 percent of the particulate matter presented to it, and lymph usually passes through several nodes before entering the bloodstream. Sinuses form a settling chamber through which lymph flows slowly, while baffles of crisscrossing reticular fibers form a mechanical filter and produce an eddying of the lymph. Most of the lymph that enters a node flows centrally through the sinuses, where it comes into contact with numerous phagocytes. Filtration by a lymph node may be impaired if the number of particles is excessive or if the organism is exceptionally virulent. Agents not destroyed in a lymph node may disseminate throughout the body, and the node itself may become a focus of chronic infection.

Lymph nodes are immunologic organs and participate in humoral and cellular immune responses. Antigen accumulates about and within primary nodules and at the junction of the deep and outer cortex. Some of the antigen appears to be held on the surfaces of macrophages and follicular dendritic cells and thus is available to react with T- and B-cells as these move into the node and sort out within the parenchyma.

Antigens that evoke antibodies react with uncommitted B-cells to elicit their activation and proliferation. The first antibody-producing cells appear in the cortex, then migrate into medullary cords where they accumulate as plasma cells. After this cortical response, intense antibody formation occurs in newly formed germinal centers. This is the primary response, elicited on first exposure to an antigen, and takes several days to develop. Relatively few cells respond and a low titer of antibody results. On a second exposure to the same antigen, a rapid and greatly enhanced production of antibody occurs. This is the secondary response, marked by an explosive development of germinal centers that expand rapidly because of the presence of conditioned memory cells produced during the primary response.

Cell-mediated responses (rejection of foreign grafts, reaction to molds, fungi, and some bacteria) involve the T-cells. The deep cortex of the draining nodes become very thick, and lymphoblasts in this area divide rapidly. After a short lag, small lymphocytes leave the nodes, infiltrate the affected region, and destroy the antigen. Committed T-cells also are disseminated throughout the body as memory cells and form part of the recirculating pool of small lymphocytes. Since an associated humoral response also develops, newly formed germinal centers appear in the cortex.

A splenic reservoir function is highly developed in those species in which the splenic capsule is muscular; in such animals, the spleen can store large numbers of red cells that can be given up to the circulation as needed. In the dog, the spleen can accommodate up to one-third of the circulating mass of erythrocytes; in the horse it has been estimated that the spleen can deliver to the circulation a volume of blood equal to 40 percent of the resting circulating volume. Normal humans have no significant splenic reservoir of erythrocytes (only 30 to 40 ml), but there are indications that even this small volume can be mobilized. About one-third of the platelets in the body are sequestered in the spleen, where they form a reserve available on demand.

The spleen serves as a filter for blood, removing particulate matter that is taken up by macrophages in the marginal zone, splenic cords, and sheathed capillaries. The sinusoidal endothelium and the reticular cells of the reticular net have no special phagocytic powers and contribute little to the clearing of foreign materials from the blood.

The spleen also forms the graveyard for worn out red cells and platelets and possibly for granular leukocytes as well. As the blood filters through the splenic cords, it comes under constant scrutiny and monitoring by macrophages. Viable cells are allowed to pass through the spleen, but damaged or aged cells are retained and phagocytosed. Several factors are probably involved in the recognition of old cells. As the cell ages, changes in the surface may permit antigenic reaction with opsonizing antibodies that enhance phagocytosis. The sinusoidal wall is a barrier to the re-entrance of cells into the circulation, since the cells must insinuate themselves through the narrow slits between sinusoidal endothelial cells. Normal cells are pliant and able to squeeze through the interendothelial clefts, but cells such as spherocytes or sickled red cells are unable to pass through the sinusoidal barrier. As red cells age, their membranes become more permeable to water, and the relatively slow passage through the red pulp may allow the cells to imbibe fluid, swell, and become too rigid to pass into the sinusoids. Red cells that have been excluded are phagocytosed, and the cells appear to be taken up intact without prior lysis or break down. Components of the red cells that can be reused in production of new blood cells are recovered by the spleen; it is especially efficient in conserving iron freed from hemoglobin and returning it to accessible stores.

A "pitting function" has been described for the spleen. Red cells that contain rigid inclusions (malarial parasites or the iron-containing granules of siderocytes, for example) but that are otherwise normal are not destroyed, but the inclusions are removed at the wall of the sinusoid. The flexible part of the erythrocyte passes through the sinusoidal wall, but the rigid inclusion is held back by the narrow intercellular clefts and is stripped from the cell. The rigid portion remains in the splenic pulp and is phagocytosed; the rest of the cell enters the lumen of the sinusoid.

The spleen has great importance in the immune system, mounting a large scale production of antibody against blood-borne antigens. However, antigen introduced by other routes also evokes a response in the spleen, since an antigen soon finds its way into the bloodstream. The reactions in the spleen are the same as those occurring in lymph nodes and include primary and secondary responses. In the primary response, clusters of antibody-forming cells first appear in the periarterial lymphatic sheaths, then increase in number and concentrate at the edge of the sheath. Immature and mature plasma cells appear, and germinal centers develop in the splenic nodules. Ultimately, plasma cells become numerous in the marginal zone between white and red pulp and in the red pulp cords, either by direct emigration from the white pulp or indirectly via the circulation. During a secondary response, germinal center activity dominates, occurs almost immediately, and is of large scale.

The spleen has important hemopoietic functions in all vertebrates and in lower forms is the primary blood-forming organ, producing all types of blood cells. In most mammals, the spleen produces red cells, platelets, and granulocytes only during embryonic life, but production of lymphoid cells continues throughout life. In some conditions (leukemia and some anemias) the red pulp contains islets of hemopoietic tissue, even in the adult. This probably results from sequestration of circulating stem cells from the blood rather than from activation of an indigenous population of potential stem cells in the spleen. In some mammals, splenic production of red cells and granulocytes continues during adult life. In the bat, production of red cells and granulocytes by the spleen is conspicuous during hibernation, when there is very little activity in the bone marrow.

Removal of the spleen (splenectomy) emphasizes its primary functions. The peripheral blood shows an increase in the number of platelets and abnormal erythrocytes. Older erythrocytes often contain Howell-Jolly bodies that normally would have been removed by the splenic cord-sinus system. Following splenectomy, individuals are at risk of developing bacterial septicemia. Under normal circumstances, blood-borne vectors would stimulate the immune component of the spleen and prevent infection via the blood.

The thymus is essential for production of T-cells, lymphocytes that are involved in cell-mediated immune responses such as rejection of foreign grafts and immunologic responses to fungi, viruses, and certain bacteria. Although not directly involved in elaborating conventional antibodies, T-cells do cooperate with B-cells in producing antibodies against antigens such as foreign red cells. All these responses are impaired in animals that have been thymectomized at birth. There is a marked decrease in the number of circulating small lymphocytes, and the deep cortex of lymph nodes and the periarterial lymphatic sheaths of the spleen fail to develop. The hagfish has no thymus and appears to be nonimmunocompetent.

Most of the lymphocytes in the thymus seem to be inert and acquire immunologic capabilities after passage through the spleen. T-cells have a long life span and recirculate between lymphatic organs (except for the thymus), lymph, and blood. Thymic lymphocytes show a high rate of mitotic activity, but many die within the thymus or emigrate to other organs.

Thymic tissue contained in diffusion chambers and transplanted into thymectomized newborn animals partly prevents or reverses the effects of thymectomy. Permeable molecules but not whole cells diffuse from the chamber, indicating the presence of a thymic-produced humoral factor. Several peptides have been isolated from thymic extracts and appear to have some regulatory and stimulating effects on the thymus. The best characterized of these is thymosin, an agent that restores T-cell deficiencies in thymectomized mice; it is regarded as a hormone that induces T-cell differentiation. Other agents have been described: thymopoietin, which induces T-cell maturation; thymic humoral factor, which enhances T-cell mediated graft rejection; and serum thymic factor, which induces development of surface markers on T-cells. The agents appear to be produced locally in the thymus, possibly by the reticular epithelial cells, and to have local effects on the lymphocyte population in the thymus.

In addition to encapsulated lymphatic tissue, an equally large amount of nonencapsulated lymphoid tissue occurs in the walls of the respiratory, urogenital, and gastrointestinal tracts that provides immunologic protection along these mucosal surfaces. Here it is generally referred to as mucosa-associated lymphoid tissue (MALT); if specifically associated with the gastrointestinal tract it is termed gut-associated lymphoid tissue (GALT).

Clinical Correlations

Nonneoplastic enlargement of lymph nodes can occur from reaction to stimuli or from accumulation of phagocytosed material. Continued irritation, as with drainage of an area of chronic infection, can lead to aggregation of macrophages, which may fill the cortical and medullary sinuses (sinus hyperplasia). Features of an immune response are present, and the lymphatic nodules increase in size and number but remain discrete (follicular hyperplasia). Germinal centers are prominent, postcapillary venules are distinct and crowded with lymphocytes, and plasma cells are numerous in the medullary cords. Overall, the architecture of the node is preserved and even exaggerated.

Particulate matter carried to a node is engulfed by macrophages associated with the sinuses and medullary cords and may persist almost indefinitely. In anthracosis, carbon taken up by macrophages forms a black mass that replaces lymphatic tissue but causes little stromal thickening; silicosis causes a marked increase in fibrous tissue at the expense of lymphatic tissue and the enlarged nodes become hard.

Lymphomas are tumors of lymphoid tissue and may occur in any lymphoid mass. Hodgkin's disease is the most common malignant lymphoma and is marked by progressive enlargement of lymph nodes with gradual loss of normal architecture. The nodular lymphatic tissue is replaced by diffuse sheets of lymphocytes among which are large, rounded or oval Sternberg-Reed cells. These large cells (20–40 μm diameter) have binucleate nuclei or nuclei so deeply indented that they appear binucleate; the two nuclei or two half nuclei form a mirror image. This cell is considered diagnostic of Hodgkin's disease, in which

there are early depression of T-cell function and impaired cell-mediated immunity.

Atrophy of the spleen occurs with aging and involves the red and white pulp. Homogeneous thickening (hyalinization) of the walls of small arteries and arterioles is common and increases with age. The resulting ischemia causes atrophy of the pulp and an increase in the amount of reticular fibers. Blockage of sinusoids by sickle cells in sickle cell anemia results in infarcts, and ultimately the spleen may become a small fibrous remnant.

Splenomegaly accompanies increased functional activity and is a common secondary phenomenon in many diseases. Increase in the white pulp occurs as a result of antigenic stimulation. Splenomegaly may occur as a result of the resumption of a role in hemopoiesis, as in anemias arising from replacement of bone marrow by fibrous tissue or tumor. In chronic myeloid leukemia the spleen may be grossly enlarged and packed with the same type of cells that are present in the blood. The cells accumulate mainly due to sequestration of blood-borne cells. The white pulp is largely obscured and replaced by the expansion of the red pulp.

The spleen is commonly involved in amyloidosis, in which a homogeneous, waxy material is deposited in the splenic nodules, converting them to translucent globules — the "sago spleen." Amyloid is an extracellular, fibrillary material. Slow and progressive enlargement occurs in Gaucher's disease, a deficiency of the lysosomal enzyme beta-glucuronidase. As a result, glucocerebrosides from the normal breakdown of red cells accumulate in macrophages. The spleen shows huge numbers of large macrophages (Gaucher's cells), usually with one but sometimes two or three nuclei and abundant cytoplasm with irregular vacuolated appearance.

Atlas and Table of Key Features

Key Features of Lymphatic Organs

	Tonsil	Lymph node	Spleen	Thymus
Capsule	Partial, at base	Yes	Yes	Thin
Trabeculae	No	Yes	Yes	Forms thin septae
Lymphatic tissue arranged as cortex and medulla	No	Yes	No	Yes
Nodular lymphatic tissue	Yes	Yes	Yes	No
Special features	Crypts; closely associated with overlying epithelium Palatine and lingual: stratified squamous, nonkeratinized Pharyngeal: pseudostratified, ciliated columnar	Subscapsular, trabecular, and medullary sinuses; only lymphatic organ with afferent and efferent lymphatics	Lymphatic tissue arranged as red and white pulp; splenic follicles (nodules) associated with central arteries; sinusoids in red pulp	Thymic corpuscles in medulla; stroma is a cytoreticulum of endodermal origin

Lymphatic Organs — Tonsils

Surface epithelium

Crypt

Germinal center

Secondary nodule

Fig. 12-7. A section of human palatine tonsil showing a deep crypt and a covering of stratified squamous epithelium. (LM, ×20.)

Lymphocytes

Stratified squamous epithelium

Fig. 12-8. Increased magnification of the stratified squamous epithelium covering the surface of a human palatine tonsil. (LM, ×250.)

Fig. 12-9. Surface features of a human pharyngeal tonsil. Note the abundance of cilia. (SEM < ×2,000.)

Fig. 12-10. A section through the surface epithelium covering a human pharyngeal tonsil (compare with 12-9). (LM, ×400.)

Lymph Node

Capsule

Germinal
center

Medullary
cords

Medullary
sinus

Lymphatic
nodule

Trabeculae

Fig. 12-11. A segment of human lymph node demonstrating its
capsule and trabeculae as well as medullary cords. (LM, ×250.)

Capsule

Subcapsular
sinus

Diffuse
lymphatic
tissue

Cap of small
lymphocytes

Trabeculum

Cortical
sinus

Germinal
center

Fig. 12-12. A region of human lymph node near the capsule
showing a well-defined subcapsular sinus. (LM, ×250.)

Reticular
fibers

Germinal
center

Fig. 12-13. A portion of human lymph node stained with silver to demonstrate selectively the supporting framework of reticular fibers. (LM, ×400.)

Medium
sized
lymphocyte

Small
lymphocytes

Large
lymphocyte

Fig. 12-14. Lymph node showing different sizes of lymphocytes. (LM, ×400.)

Fig. 12-15. A region of lymph node showing small lymphocytes and a macrophage. (LM, ×400.)

Fig. 12-16. The medulla of a human lymph node demonstrating the trabecular and medullary sinuses. (LM, ×100.)

Spleen

Central artery

Lymphatic nodule

Peritoneum

Capsule

Red pulp

Venous sinusoids

Fig. 12-17. A segment of spleen near the capsule illustrates a region of red pulp as well as a lymphatic nodule (white pulp). (LM, ×100.)

Lumen of sinusoid

Bars of basement membrane

Bars of basement membrane

Fig. 12-18. A region of red pulp of spleen stained with periodic acid-Schiff (PAS) illustrates the bars of basement membrane supporting the endothelial cells of sinusoids. (LM, ×300.)

Sinusoids

Sinusoid

Billroth's
cord

Basement
membrane

Fig. 12-19. A region of splenic red pulp clearly demonstrating a
longitudinal profile of a sinusoid and an adjacent splenic (Billroth's) cord. (LM, ×250.)

Neutrophil

Erythrocytes

Processes of
macrophage

Macrophage

Endothelial
cells

Neutrophil

Erythrocyte

Macrophage

Fig. 12-20. Endothelial cells comprising a sinusoidal wall in the
red pulp of a spleen. (SEM, ×3,000.)

Sinusoid

Sinusoid

Sinusoids

Lumen of
sinusoid

Macrophages

Nuclear
regions of
endothelial
cells

Region of
Billroth's
cord

Erythrocytes

Billroth's
cord

Sheathed
artery

Fig. 12-21. Several profiles of sinusoids within the red pulp of a
spleen. (SEM, ×700.)

Heterophagic
vacuole
with remnants of
a red blood cell

Mitochondria

Nucleus of
macrophage

Fig. 12-22. A macrophage from the red pulp of a spleen. Note the phagocytosed red blood cell. (TEM, ×2,500.)

Lymphatic
nodule

Central
artery

Marginal
zone

Marginal
zone

Fig. 12-23. A region of splenic white pulp illustrating a lymphatic nodule and a central artery. (LM, ×250.)

Smooth muscle cell of central artery

Endothelial cells of central artery

Small lymphocytes

Fig. 12-24. Small lymphocytes within the white pulp of a spleen. Note the endothelial cells of the central artery. (TEM, ×1,500.)

Thymus

Fig. 12-25. A section of human thymus showing the central medulla and surrounding cortex. (LM, ×10.)

Cortex

Medulla

Medulla

Cortex

Thymic corpuscle

Fig. 12-26. Increased magnification details the cortex and medulla of a human thymus. (LM, ×50.)

Fig. 12-27. Thymic corpuscles from the medulla of a human thymus. (LM, ×250.)

—————— *Review Questions and Answers* ——————

Questions

65. Given a section of a lymphatic organ, how would you identify it as a lymph node, a tonsil, or the thymus?
66. What constitutes the thymus-blood barrier?
67. What is the orientation of germinal centers in tonsils, spleen, lymph nodes, and thymus?
68. Describe a splenic sinusoid. In what part of the spleen are these structures found?
69. What is the distribution of T-lymphocytes in the lymphatic organs? What is their function?

Answers

65. The presence of a complete capsule and compartmentalization of the tissue by septae or trabeculae would eliminate the possibility of the tissue being a tonsil. Although both the thymus and lymph node show a cortex and medulla, the cortex of the thymus lacks lymphatic nodules, which usually are prominent in a lymph node and often contain germinal centers. Also lacking in the thymus is an internal system of lymphatic sinuses, which are prominent in a lymph node and consist of marginal (subcapsular), cortical (trabecular), and medullary sinuses. The medulla of the thymus appears rather homogeneous and contains thymic (Hassall's) bodies. That of the lymph node is arranged in irregular cords separated by the medullary sinuses. In the absence of a complete capsule and trabeculae, the tonsil could be identified by the close association of lymphatic tissue to an overlying epithelium that is deeply invaginated to form crypts. The lymphatic tissue contains lymphatic nodules, many of which contain germinal centers and usually are arranged in a single row immediately beneath the epithelium.

66. The thymus-blood barrier exists in the cortex of the thymus, which is supplied only by capillaries. The barrier consists of the capillary endothelium and its basal lamina, the perivascular connective tissue sheath, and a complete investing layer of epithelial reticular cells and their associated basal laminae.

67. In the tonsil the germinal centers are oriented so that the light pole is directed toward the covering epithelium. In the lymph nodes, the light poles are directed toward the capsule and the subcapsular sinus. The light pole in the spleen is oriented toward the red pulp, and since the thymus lacks lymphatic nodules there are no germinal centers (see Chapter 6).

68. The splenic sinusoids are irregular, tortuous blood vessels whose walls consist only of fusiform, longitudinally oriented endothelial cells and a discontinuous basement membrane. The endothelial cells are not united by any type of junction and so have large gaps between them. The basal lamina forms widely spaced bars that encircle the endothelial cells. All other elements of a blood vessel wall are lacking. Sinusoids are found in the red pulp of the spleen.

69. T-lymphocytes are found in the deep or inner cortex of the lymph nodes (the thymic-dependent area), in the periarterial lymphatic sheaths of the spleen, and generally in the thymus. They function in the cell-mediated immune responses and cooperate with B-cells in the production of conventional antibodies.

13 Skin

The skin covers the exterior of the body and constitutes a large organ with several functions. It protects the body from mechanical injury and loss of fluid, acts as a barrier against noxious agents, aids in temperature regulation, excretes various waste products, and, through its receptors for sensations of heat, cold, touch, and pain, provides information about the external environment.

Structure

KEY WORDS: epidermis, dermis, appendage, integument, thick skin, thin skin, epidermal ridge, dermal papilla

The skin consists of a surface layer of epithelium called the **epidermis** and an underlying layer of connective tissue, the **dermis** (corium). A loose layer of connective tissue, the hypodermis, attaches the skin to underlying structures but is not considered a component of skin. The **appendages** of the skin — hair, nails, and sweat and sebaceous glands — are local specializations of the epidermis. Together, the skin and its appendages form the **integument.**

The thickness of the skin varies in different parts of the body, and the proportions of dermis and epidermis also differ. Between the scapula, the dermis is especially thick, whereas on the palms of the hands and soles of the feet, the epidermis is thickened. The terms **thick skin** and **thin skin** refer to the thickness of the epidermis and not to the thickness of the skin as a whole

(see atlas figures 13-4 and 13-5). In thick skin the epidermis is especially well developed, whereas in thin skin it forms a relatively narrow layer.

At its junction with the dermis, the epidermis forms numerous ridgelike extensions, the **epidermal ridges,** that project into the underlying dermis (see atlas figure 13-5). Complementary projections of the dermis fit between the epidermal ridges and form the **dermal papillae.** The surface patterns of the skin, such as the fingerprints, reflect the pattern of the dermal papillae.

Epidermis

KEY WORDS: stratified squamous epithelium, keratinocyte, keratinization, melanocyte, pigmentation, layers (strata)

The epidermis forms the surface layer of the skin and consists of **stratified squamous epithelium.** The cells, **keratinocytes,** undergo an orderly progression of maturation and **keratinization** to produce a superficial layer of dense, flattened, dead cells at the surface. A smaller population of cells, the **melanocytes,** is associated with **pigmentation** of the skin. A third cell type, the Langerhans' cell, makes up a small part of the cell population and is regarded as an antigen-presenting cell. The epidermis lacks blood vessels and is nourished by diffusion of material from vessels in the underlying dermis.

The epidermis can be divided into several **layers (strata)** that reflect the sequential differentiation of keratinocytes as they progress from the base of the epidermis to the surface where they arc cxfoliatcd. In thick skin, thc layers are stratum basale, stratum spinosum, stratum granulosum, stratum lucidum, and stratum corneum (Fig. 13-1). In thin skin the layers are narrower and less well defined and stratum lucidum is absent.

Stratum Basale

KEY WORDS: columnar epithelial cell, growing layer, stratum germinativum

Stratum basale abuts the underlying dermis, separated from it only by a basement membrane. It consists of a single row of **columnar epithelial cells** that follows the contours of the ridges and papillae. Stratum basale is the **growing layer** of the epidermis and most, but not all, of the mitotic activity occurs in this layer. For this reason, stratum basale often is called the **stratum germinativum** (see atlas figure 13-5).

Each cell of stratum basale is limited by a typical trilaminar membrane and is joined to adjacent cells by numerous desmosomes. At the basal surfaces, hemidesmosomes attach the cells to the underlying basement membrane, which, in turn, is anchored to the dermis by short filaments (see atlas figure 13-8). The cytoplasm of the basal ker-

Fig. 13-1. Structure of thick skin.

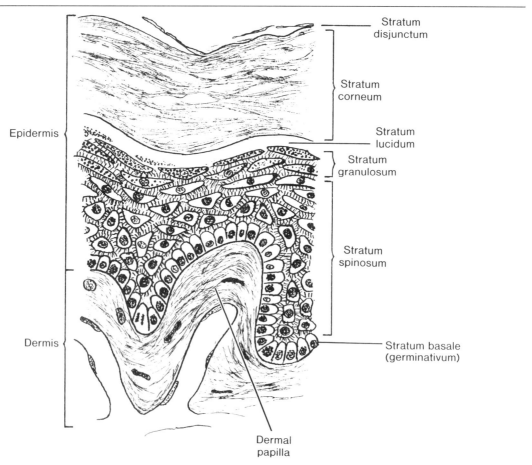

atinocytes is fairly dense and contains many scattered tonofilaments (keratin). Clusters of ribosomes are prominent and the cells contain a moderate number of mitochondria, some profiles of granular endoplasmic reticulum, and a few Golgi saccules.

Stratum Spinosum

KEY WORDS: prickle cell, membrane-coating granule, stratum malpighii

Stratum spinosum consists of several strata of irregular, polyhedral cells that become somewhat flattened in the outermost layers (see atlas figure 13-5). The cells are closely applied to each other and joined at all surfaces by desmosomes. During tissue preparation, the cells tend to shrink and pull apart except at the points of attachment. Thus, the cells appear to have numerous short, spiny projections that extend between adjacent cells and commonly are called **prickle cells** (see atlas figure 13-6). The projections are not areas of cytoplasmic continuity between cells but are sites of typical desmosomes.

In addition to the organelles seen in the basal cell, prickle cells in the upper layers of stratum spinosum contain ovoid granules, 0.1 to 0.5 μm in diameter, called **membrane-coating granules.** These consist of parallel laminae bounded by a double membrane and are rich in glycols and phospholipids that help maintain the barrier function of the skin. Tonofilaments (keratin) are numerous and may form dense bundles that extend into the spinous processes, ending in the dense plaques of desmosomes (see atlas figure 13-7). Stratum spinosum and stratum basale often are grouped together as **stratum malpighii.**

Stratum Granulosum

KEY WORDS: keratohyalin granules

Stratum granulosum contains three to five layers of flattened cells whose long axes are parallel to the surface of the skin (see atlas figure 13-5). The cells are distinguished by the presence of amorphous, densely packed particles, the **keratohyalin granules,** that vary in size and shape. The granules are not limited by membranes and are

associated closely with bundles of filaments (see atlas figure 13-7). Chemically, they contain large amounts of sulphur-containing amino acids. The granules increase in number and size in the outermost layers of stratum granulosum and the cells show evidence of degenerative changes. The nuclei stain more palely and the contacts between adjacent cells become less distinct. The cells of the granular layer are viable but undergo programmed death as they pass into the succeeding horny layer. Membrane-coating granules increase in number in the cells of stratum granulosum. These rod-shaped granules fuse with the plasmalemma and empty their contents into the intercellular space. The lipid-rich contents act as a barrier between cells of this layer and those toward the surface and contribute to the sealing effect of skin, preventing water loss and entrance by foreign substances between cells.

Stratum Lucidum

KEY WORDS: loss of nuclei, thickened plasmalemma, thick skin

Stratum lucidum forms a narrow, undulating, lightly stained zone at the surface of stratum granulosum (see atlas figure 13-5). It consists of several layers of cells so compacted together that outlines of individual cells cannot be made out. Traces of flattened nuclei may be seen, but generally this layer is characterized by the **loss of nuclei.** Only a few remnants of organelles are present, and the main constituent of the cytoplasm is aggregates of tonofilaments (keratin) that now have a more regular arrangement, generally parallel to the skin surface. The **plasmalemma is thickened** and more convoluted, and the amount of intercellular material is increased. Stratum lucidum is prominent in the **thick skin** of the palms and soles but is absent from the epidermis in other parts of the body.

Stratum Corneum

KEY WORDS: squame, keratin, soft keratin, desquamation, stratum disjunctum

Stratum corneum forms the outermost layer of the epidermis and is composed of scalelike cells, often called squares, that become increasingly flattened as they approach the surface. **Squames** are enclosed by a thickened, modified cell envelope and represent the remains of cells that have lost their nuclei, all their organelles, and their desmosomal attachments to adjacent cells. The cells are filled with **keratin,** which consists of tightly packed bundles of filaments embedded in an opaque, structureless material (see atlas figure 13-7). The keratin filaments of stratum corneum consist of "soft" keratin as distinct from the "hard" keratin of nails and hair. **Soft keratin** has a lower sulphur content and is somewhat more elastic than hard keratin. The outermost cells of stratum corneum are constantly shed or **desquamated**; this region often is referred to as **stratum disjunctum.**

The life span of keratinocytes in their passage from basal layer to desquamation is between 40 and 55 days. As the keratinocytes progress toward the surface, they become much broader and flatter so that ultimately, only four surface squames are needed to cover the same area as 100 columnar basal cells. Thus, a low rate of mitosis (less than seven per 1000 basal cells) can maintain the surface layer.

Pigmentation

KEY WORDS: melanin, melanocyte, epidermal-melanin unit, melanosome

Skin color is determined by the pigments carotene and melanin and by the blood in the capillaries of the dermis. Carotene is a yellowish pigment found in the stratum corneum and in fat cells of the dermis and hypodermis. Melanin, a brown pigment, is present mainly in the cells of stratum basale and the deeper layers of stratum spinosum.

Melanin is formed in specialized cells of the epidermis, the **melanocytes,** which originate from cells that emigrated from the neural crest during development. Melanocytes are scattered throughout the basal layer and send out numerous fingerlike cytoplasmic processes that extend between the cells of stratum spinosum. Each melanocyte maintains a functional relationship with

36 keratinocytes in stratum spinosum. The combination of melanocytes and keratinocytes forms an **epidermal-melanin unit.** In electron micrographs, epidermal melanocytes can be distinguished by the lack of tonofilaments and the content of melanin granules (**melanosomes**) in various stages of development. Melanocytes also contain the usual array of cytoplasmic organelles. While melanocytes lack desmosomal junctions with neighboring cells, they are affixed to the basement membrane by hemidesmosome-like junctions.

Mature melanosomes are transferred from melanocytes via their processes to the cells of the basal layer and stratum spinosum. In humans, melanosomes frequently aggregate above the nuclei of basal cells, but in the superficial layers of the epidermis the granules are more evenly dispersed and become progressively finer. Since epidermal cells constantly are shed from the surface, melanocytes must provide for continued renewal of melanin. Although melanocytes may die and be replaced by division of neighboring cells, this is a random event, and there does not appear to be a regular cycle of replacement of melanocytes.

The number of melanocytes and the size of the melanosomes is somewhat greater in negroid and mongolian skin than in caucasian, but not sufficiently to account for the differences in skin color. Caucasoid melanosomes are less completely melanized and are packaged in groups, the melanosome complexes, surrounded by a membrane. The larger negroid melanosomes are more widely dispersed within cells and do not form membrane-bound complexes. The distribution of pigment within the epidermis also differs, being concentrated in the lower zones of the malpighian layer in caucasian skin and distributed through all cells of this layer in negroid skin. The smaller melanosomes of caucasians are degraded by lysosomes before they reach the upper strata.

The degree of pigmentation varies in different parts of the body. The axilla, circumanal region, scrotum, penis, labia majora, nipples, and areola are areas of increased pigmentation. In contrast, the palms and soles contain little or no pigment. Freckles represent local areas of pigmentation but paradoxically, contain fewer melanocytes than adjacent paler skin. Pigmentation of freckles and the areola and nipples may be intensified with pregnancy. A general increase in melanization occurs from exposure to sunlight, at first by darkening of existing melanin and later by increased formation of new melanin. The activated melanocytes produce larger melanosomes.

A deficiency of melanin also may occur. The white spotted patterns of piebald animals and of piebaldism in humans result from abnormalities in the morphology of melanocytes in which the length and number of the cell processes is deficient. Complete albinism results from an inability of the melanocytes to synthesize melanin, not from an absence of melanocytes.

Other Cell Types

KEY WORDS: Langerhans' cells, Merkel's cells

Two other cell types present in the epidermis are Langerhans' and Merkel's cells. **Langerhans' cells** are present throughout the epidermis but are especially numerous in the upper layers of stratum malpighii. In routine sections the cells have darkly stained, large, convoluted nuclei surrounded by a clear cytoplasm. With special stains they are seen to be stellate cells that extend long cytoplasmic processes into stratum spinosum. In electron micrographs, the nucleus shows a highly irregular outline, and the abundant cytoplasm lacks tonofilaments, desmosomes, and melanosomes (see atlas figure 13-19) but is characterized by membrane-bound, rod-shaped granules with a regular, granular interior. Some of these granules appear to be continuous with the cell membrane. Langerhans' cells trap antigens that penetrate the skin and transport them to regional lymph nodes. These antigen-presenting cells originate in bone marrow, probably from a monocyte precursor.

Merkel's cells tend to lie close to sensory nerve endings in stratum basale. Morphologically, they resemble cells of stratum spinosum, but in electron micrographs, they are distinguished by indented nuclei, prominent Golgi complexes, and numerous dense-cored vesicles. The vesicles tend to concentrate basally at the site where nerve endings approach. The function of Merkel's cells is unknown. They may play a role in sensory processes and have been compared to polypeptide- and hormone-containing cells, but a definite relationship with these has not been established.

Dermis

KEY WORDS: reticular layer, papillary layer, dermal papilla, arrectores pilorum muscle

The dermis (corium) varies in thickness in different regions of the body. It is especially thin and delicate in the eyelids, scrotum, and prepuce; very thick in the palms and soles; thicker on the posterior than anterior aspects of the body; and thicker in men than in women. The dermis is tough, flexible, and highly elastic and consists of a feltwork of collagen fibers with abundant elastic fibers. The connective tissue is arranged into deep reticular and superficial papillary layers.

The **reticular layer** is the thicker, denser part of the dermis and consists of interwoven bundles of collagen fibers that mostly run parallel to the surface. Below, the reticular layer merges indistinctly into the subcutaneous tissue, which generally contains many fat cells. Collagen in the reticular layer is mostly type I with a small amount of type II. The **papillary layer** lies immediately below the epidermis and extends into it in the form of the dermal papillae. The papillary layer is not clearly demarcated from the reticular layer, but its fibers and bundles of collagen tend to be thinner and more loosely arranged. This layer also has a more cellular appearance. Most of the collagen is type III. Just below the epidermis, reticular fibers are present and have a vertical orientation. Elastic fibers are found deeper in the papillary layer.

Dermal papillae are small, conical projections with rounded or blunt apices that fit into corresponding pits on the undersurface of the epidermis. They are especially prominent on the palmar surface of the hands and fingers, where they are closely aggregated and arranged in parallel lines that correspond to the surface ridges of the epidermis. Capillary loops are present in the papillae and in some, especially those in the palms and fingers, nerve endings and tactile corpuscles are present (see atlas figures 13-10 and 13-11).

Smooth muscle is present in the deeper parts of the reticular layer in the penis, scrotum, perineum, and areola. On contraction, the muscle produces wrinkling of the skin in these areas. The **arrectores pilorum muscles** are small bundles of smooth muscle associated with hairs. Many mammals have an extensive subcutaneous layer of skeletal muscle, the panniculus carnosus, that permits voluntary movement of large areas of skin.

Dermatoglyphics

Skin ridges are normal features in the fingers, hands, feet, and toes in humans, apes, monkeys, and opossum. They act as antislip devices and also are thought to improve the sense of touch. The ridges form three main patterns: arches, loops, and whorls. Loops are the most common pattern on the fingers and arches the rarest. The ridge patterns on the toes are similar to those on the fingers, but arches are more numerous and whorls are fewer. The ridge pattern is established early in life and is permanent. In any individual the pattern varies from digit to digit, and it is unlikely that in a group of unrelated persons, the sequence of patterns would be identical.

Appendages of the Skin

The appendages of the skin are derived from the epidermis and in humans include hair, nails, and sweat and sebaceous glands. In other animals, the epidermis gives rise to claws, hooves, beaks, feathers, quills, scales, salt glands in certain marine reptiles and birds, and shells in turtles.

Nails

KEY WORDS: body (nail plate), root, proximal nail fold, lateral nail fold, eponychium, hyponychium, lunule, nail bed, nail matrix, hard keratin

The nails (Fig. 13-2) are hard, elastic, keratinized structures that cover the dorsal surfaces of the tips of the fingers and toes. Each nail consists of a visible **body (nail plate)** and a proximal part, the **root**, which is implanted into a groove in the skin. The root is overlapped by the **proximal nail fold,** a fold of skin that continues along the lateral borders of the nail, where it forms the **lateral nail fold.** Stratum corneum of the proximal nail fold extends over the upper surface of the nail root and for a short distance onto the surface of the body of the nail where it forms a thin cuticular fold called the **eponychium.** At the free border of the nail, the skin is attached to the underside of the nail, forming the **hyponychium**.

The nail is a modification of the cornified zone of the epidermis and consists of several layers of flattened cells with shrunken, degenerate nuclei. The cells are hard, tightly adherent, and, throughout most of the body of the nail, clear and translucent. The pink color of the nails is due to transmission of color from the underlying capillary bed. Near the root, the nail is more opaque and forms a crescentic area, the **lunule,** which is most visible on the thumb, becoming smaller and more hidden by the proximal nail fold toward the little finger. The lunule represents the region from which nail formation occurs.

Beneath the nail lies the **nail bed,** which corresponds to the stratum malpighii of the skin. It consists of prickle cells and a stratum basale resting on a basement membrane. The underlying dermis is thrown into numerous longitudinal ridges that are very vascular. Near the root, the ridges are smaller and less vascular. The nail bed beneath the root and lunule is thicker, actively proliferative, and concerned with growth of the nail; it is called the **nail matrix.** The nail bed beneath the rest of the nail is thinner and not involved with nail growth. Cells in the deepest layer of the matrix are cylindrical and show frequent mitoses, while above them are several layers of polyhedral cells and flattened squames that represent the differentiating cells of the nail. Nail keratin has a higher sulphur content than the keratin of the epidermis and is called **hard keratin**.

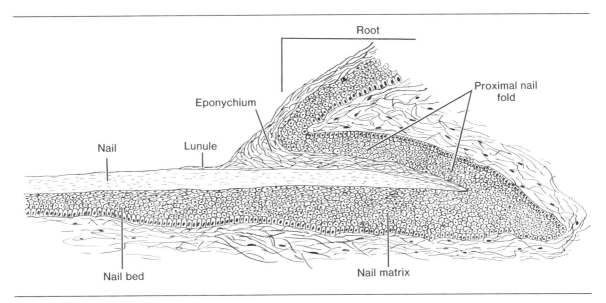

Fig. 13-2. Longitudinal section of a nail.

Hair

KEY WORDS: **lanugo, vellus hair, terminal hair**

Hairs are present on almost all surfaces of the skin except for the palmar surfaces of the hands, plantar surfaces of the feet, margin of the lip, prepuce, glans penis, clitoris, labia minora, and inner surfaces of the labia majora. They consist of elastic, keratinized threads that vary in length and thickness in different regions of the body and in different races. From the middle of fetal life, the skin of the human is covered by fine hair called **lanugo;** this mostly is shed by birth and is replaced by downy vellus hair. **Vellus hairs** are retained in most regions, where they appear as short, soft, colorless hair such as that on the forehead. In the scalp and eyebrows, vellus hairs are replaced by coarser **terminal hair** that also forms the axillary and pubic hair and, in the male, the hair of the beard and chest. Modified hairs form the spines and quills of porcupines, hedgehogs, and echidnas, and a closely packed mat of hair forms the "horn" of the rhinoceros.

Structure of Hair

KEY WORDS: **shaft, medulla, cortex, cuticle, root, hair bulb, papilla**

Each hair consists of a root embedded in the skin and a hair **shaft** projecting for a variable distance above the surface of the epidermis (see atlas figure 13-12). In cross section the shaft appears round or oval and is made up of three concentric layers. The **medulla** (core) is composed of flattened, cornified, polyhedral cells in which the nuclei are pyknotic or missing. There is no medulla in thin fine hair (lanugo), and a medulla may be absent in hairs of the scalp or extend only part of the way along the shaft. The bulk of the hair consists of the **cortex,** which is composed of several layers of intensely cornified, elongated cells tightly compacted together. Most of the pigment of colored hair is found in the cortex and is present in the cells and the intercellular spaces. Variable accumulations of air spaces are present between and within the cells of the cortex. Together with fading of pigment, increase in the number of airspaces is responsible for graying of the hair. The outermost layer is thin and forms the **cuticle.** It consists of a single layer of clear, flattened, squamous cells that overlap each other, shingle fashion, from below upwards (see atlas figure 13-13).

The **root** of the hair is embedded in the skin. At the lower end, the root expands to form the **hair bulb,** which is indented at its deep surface by a conical projection of the dermis and called a **papilla** (see atlas figure 13-14). Papillae contain blood vessels that provide nourishment for the growing and differentiating cells of the hair bulb.

The structure of the root differs somewhat from that of the shaft. In the lower part of the root, the cells of the medulla and cortex tend to be cuboidal in shape and contain nuclei of normal appearance. At higher levels in the root, nuclei become indistinct and finally are lost. The cells of the cortex become progressively flattened toward the surface of the skin.

Hair Follicle

KEY WORDS: inner epithelial root sheath, cuticle of root sheath, Huxley's layer, trichohyalin granules, Henle's layer, outer epithelial root sheath, glassy (vitreous) membrane

The root of each hair is enclosed within a tubular sheath called the hair follicle, which consists of an inner epithelial component and an outer connective tissue portion. The epithelial component is derived from the epidermis and consists of inner and outer root sheaths. The connective tissue sheath is derived from the dermis.

The **inner epithelial root sheath** corresponds to the superficial layers of the epidermis that have undergone specialization to produce three layers. The innermost layer is the **cuticle of the root sheath,** which abuts the cuticle of the hair shaft. The cells are thin and scalelike and are overlapped from above downward; the free edges of the cells interlock with the free edges of the cells of the hair cuticle. Immediately surrounding the cuticle of the root sheath are several layers of elongated cells that form **Huxley's layer.** The cells contain granules that are similar to keratohyalin granules but differ chemically; they are called **trichohyalin granules.** Huxley's layer is surrounded

by **Henle's layer,** a single row of clear, flattened cells that contain keratin filaments. The cells of these three layers are nucleated in the distal parts, but as the sheath approaches the surface, the nuclei are lost.

The **outer epithelial root sheath** is a direct continuation of stratum malpighii. The cells of the outermost layer are columnar and arranged in a single row and at the surface become continuous with stratum basale of the epidermis. The inner layers of cells are identical to and continuous with the prickle cells of stratum spinosum.

The connective tissue portion of the follicle consists of three layers. A narrow clear band, the **glassy (vitreous) membrane,** is closely applied to the columnar cells of the outer epithelial root sheath and equates with the basement membrane. The middle layer consists of fine, circularly arranged collagen fibers. The outermost layer is poorly defined and contains collagen fibers arranged in loose, longitudinal bundles, interspersed with some elastic fibers.

A bulbous expansion of the hair root surrounds the papilla. The cells of the hair bulb are not arranged in layers but form a matrix of growing cells. Matrix cells at the tip of the papilla differentiate into the medulla of a hair. Those on the slopes develop into the cortex and medulla. Laterally, cells of the bulb form the inner epithelial root sheath. Pigmentation occurs from the activity of melanocytes present in the matrix.

The structure of a hair and hair follicle are shown in Fig. 13-3.

Hair Cycle

No hair grows forever; each cycles through a proliferative phase (anagen), a period of decreasing growth (catagen), and a resting phase (telogen). The cyclic activity continues throughout life, but the phases of the cycle change with age. At about the fifth month of gestation, all the hairs are in anagen, a uniformity of growth not seen again. Between 8 and 10 weeks before birth, some hair sites have reached catagen and telogen phases. The frontal and parietal scalp areas show the first shedding events; in the occipital region hairs remain in anagen until after birth. From about 6

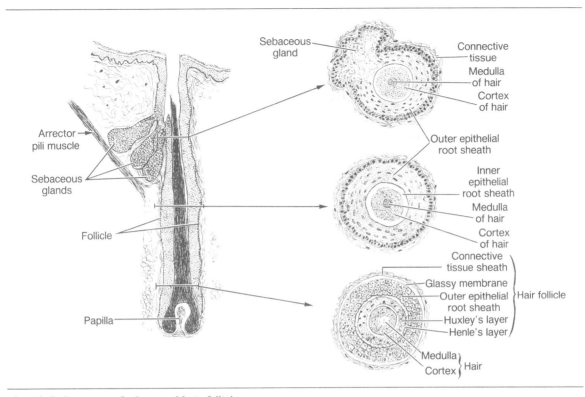

Fig. 13-3. Structure of a hair and hair follicle.

weeks before birth, telogen hairs again appear in the frontal and parietal scalp, indicating a second cycle of hair growth.

All hairs usually enter telogen immediately after birth, giving rise to a second period of shedding. After this, the phases are more irregular. About 18 weeks after birth, cycles are associated with individual hairs or groups of hairs. In adults hair cycles vary with body region. The total hair cycle in the scalp extends over 300 weeks with telogen occupying 18 to 19 weeks.

Sebaceous Glands

KEY WORDS: alveolus, holocrine, sebum

Sebaceous glands occur in most parts of the skin and are especially numerous in the scalp and face and around the anus, mouth, and nose. They are absent from the palms of the hands and soles of the feet. Generally, sebaceous glands are associated with hairs and drain into the upper part of the hair follicle, but on the lip, glans penis, inner surface of the prepuce, and labia minora, the glands open directly onto the surface of the skin, unrelated to hairs. The glands vary in size and consist of a cluster of two to five oval alveoli drained by a single duct.

The secretory **alveoli** lie within the dermis and are composed of epithelial cells enclosed in a well-defined basement membrane and supported by a thin connective tissue capsule. Cells abutting the basement membrane are small and cuboidal and contain round nuclei. The entire alveolus is filled with cells that, centrally, become larger and polyhedral and gradually accumulate fatty material in their cytoplasm. Nuclei become compressed and pyknotic and finally disappear (see atlas figure 13-15). Secretion is of the **holocrine** type, meaning the entire cell breaks down and cellular debris, along with the secretory product, is released as **sebum.** Myoepithelial cells are absent from sebaceous glands, but the glands are closely related to the arrectores pilorum muscle. In the nipple, smooth muscle bundles are present in the connective tissue between alveoli.

The short duct of a sebaceous gland is lined by stratified squamous epithelium that is a continuation of the outer epithelial root sheath of the hair follicle. Replacement of secretory cells of the alveolus comes mostly from division of cells close to the walls of the ducts, near their junctions with the alveoli. Some replacement comes from cells at the periphery of the alveoli.

Sweat Glands

KEY WORDS: eccrine sweat gland, simple tubular, coiled, dark cell, clear cell, myoepithelial cell, apocrine sweat gland

Two classes of sweat glands are distinguished: ordinary or eccrine sweat glands and apocrine glands, such as those of the axilla and circumanal region.

Eccrine sweat glands are distributed throughout the skin except in the lip margins, glans penis, inner surface of the prepuce, clitoris, and labia minora. Elsewhere the numbers vary, being plentiful in the palms and soles and least numerous in the neck and back. Each gland is a **simple tubular** structure. The deep part is tightly **coiled** and forms the secretory part located in the dermis (see atlas figure 13-16). The secretory part consists of a simple epithelium resting on a thick basement membrane.

Two types of cells, clear cells and dark cells, are present. The **dark cells** are narrow at their bases and broad at the luminal surface; in electron micrographs they show numerous ribosomes, secretory vacuoles, and few mitochondria. These cells secrete glycoproteins, which have been identified in secretory vacuoles. **Clear cells** are broad at their bases and narrow at the apices. Intercellular canaliculi extend between adjacent clear cells, which contain glycogen, considerable smooth endoplasmic reticulum, and numerous

mitochondria, but few ribosomes. The plasmalemma at the base of the cell shows extensive, complex infoldings. Clear cells appear to secrete sodium chloride, urea, uric acid, ammonia, and water.

Eccrine glands empty via ducts onto the surface of the skin, on the summit of the skin ridges. The ducts consist of a stratified cuboidal epithelium.

Myoepithelial cells are present in the secretory portion, located between the basal lamina and the bases of the secretory cells. These stellate cells are contractile and are believed to aid in the discharge of secretions. The gland empties into a narrowed duct that at first is coiled, then straightens as it passes through the dermis to reach the epidermis. The lining of the duct consists of two layers of cuboidal cells. At their luminal surfaces, the cells of the inner layer show aggregations of filaments organized into a terminal web. The epithelium lies on a basal lamina, but myoepithelial cells are lacking. In the epidermis, the duct consists of a spiral channel that is simply a cleft between the epidermal cells; those cells immediately adjacent to the duct are circularly arranged.

Apocrine sweat glands are enlarged, modified eccrine sweat glands. Their secretions are thicker than those of the ordinary sweat glands, and their histologic structure differs in several respects (see atlas figure 13-17). Apocrine glands also are coiled, tubular glands lined by cuboidal cells, but the tubes are wider. Their myoepithelial cells are larger and more numerous and there is only one type of secreting cell, which resembles the dark cells of the eccrine glands. The ducts are similar to those of ordinary sweat glands but empty into a hair follicle rather than onto the surface of the epidermis. Secretion by apocrine glands is of the merocrine type and involves no loss of cellular structure. Although retained, the term apocrine is misapplied to these glands.

The ceruminous (wax) glands of the external auditory canal are apocrine glands in which the secretory portion and the duct may branch. Glands in the margins of the eyelids (Moll's glands) also are apocrine but differ in that the terminal portions show less coiling and have wider lumina.

Development of Skin

Skin has a dual origin: the epidermis and its appendages arise from ectoderm, and the dermis is formed from mesoderm. Initially, the surface of the embryo is covered by a single layer of cuboidal cells resting on a basal lamina. Only a few desmosomes unite the loosely arranged cells. With proliferation, two layers are formed: an outer periderm and an inner basal layer.

The periderm is the outermost layer in the 2- to 6-month-old fetus and covers the "epidermis proper" prior to keratinization. It consists of a single layer of flattened, polygonal cells that in humans bear microvilli on their free surfaces (see atlas figure 13-18). The periderm protects the epidermis and may serve in some exchange capacity between the fetus and amniotic fluid. Bleblike projections form on the surfaces of the periderm cells, reaching maximum development at the beginning of the sixth week and thereafter decreasing in size. At the same time blebbing occurs, the cell envelope shows alterations similar to those that occur in the keratinization of adult epidermal cells. When keratinization of the epidermis is complete, the periderm sloughs and the cells become mixed with sebaceous secretions to form part of the vernix caseosa, a greasy coating found on the surface of the newborn's skin.

The basal layer is the only layer of epidermis proper in the 1- and 2-month-old fetus. It forms the germinative layer from which all the epidermal cells arise. During the first two months, peridermal and epidermal cells are filled with glycogen and have few organelles. In the second month, bundles of filaments develop in the epidermal cells, along with desmosomes and hemidesmosomes. More extensive filaments, presumed to be keratin, spread throughout the cytoplasm. Basal cells are the first to lose glycogen and attain adult morphology, and as they proliferate, additional layers are added between the periderm and the basal layer. The first intermediate cells appear at 9 to 10 weeks and the layer

is fully developed by 11 weeks. Second and third layers are added in the fourth month.

The cytoplasm of the intermediate cells is filled with glycogen, but desmosomes and filaments also are prominent. As the number of intracellular filaments increases, the amount of glycogen diminishes. The outermost intermediate cells accumulate laminar granules at their upper borders, then differentiate into cells with cornified envelopes, bundles of keratin filaments, and small amounts of glycogen in their cytoplasm. Once the granular layer has formed, true cornified cells appear and a thin stratum corneum becomes evident by the end of 6 months. Thus, at the end of the second trimester, all the layers of the epidermis are established.

Melanocytes migrate into the epidermis from the neural crest during the second month and synthesize melanin in the fourth month. Langerhans' cells arrive in the epidermis from the bone marrow during the third month, and Merkel's cells are first recognized in special regions (nail bed, fingertips) in the sixteenth week. The first surface ridges are formed on the palmar and plantar surfaces of the tips of the digits at about the thirteenth week. The ridges later extend over the entire volar surfaces of the hands and feet. The pattern that develops at this time remains for life.

Dermis arises as a condensation of adjacent mesenchyme. The cells differentiate and fibroblasts and collagen and elastic fibers appear. The dermis soon is well defined and organized into papillary and reticular layers. Initially, the dermoepidermal junction is smooth, but dermal ridges soon appear and can be identified by the third to fourth month of gestation.

All the epidermal appendages (e.g., nails, hair, feathers, quills, sweat glands, sebaceous glands) arise as outgrowths of the primitive epidermis. Hairs arise from solid cords of epidermis (hair buds) that grow into the dermis at an angle (see atlas figure 13-19). Each hair bud has an outer layer of columnar cells and an inner core of polygonal cells. The deepest part of the hair bud swells to form the hair bulb, which comes to sit, cuplike, over a small mound of mesenchyme that forms the papilla of the hair. The primitive dermal connective tissue along the length of the hair bud condenses to form the connective tissue sheath of the hair follicle. Cells at the periphery of the hair bud give rise to the epidermal portions of the root sheath; the inner cell mass forms the substance of the hair.

Sebaceous glands arise from thickenings of the outer root sheath (see atlas figure 13-19). Solid buds of cells grow into the surrounding mesenchyme, branching into several flask-shaped alveoli. The lining cells, derived from stratum germinativum, proliferate, pushing older cells toward the center where they elaborate fats, degenerate, and form sebum. A cellular bulge on the root sheath, below the origin of the sebaceous glands, provides for the attachment of the arrectores pilorum muscles, which arise independently from mesenchyme.

Sweat glands also begin as solid downgrowths of epidermis (see atlas figure 13-20). As these elongate, the deeper portions become coiled to form the secretory parts of the glands. A lumen develops in each cord, which now forms a tube that opens onto the surface. It is lined by a double layer of epithelium. Myoepithelial cells associated with the secretory portions of the glands arise locally from the same epidermal bud. Some sweat glands develop from superficial epidermal swellings on hair follicles; their ducts empty into the uppermost part of the follicle.

Functional Summary

The outer, horny layer of the epidermis is highly impermeable to water and rather inert chemically. It is this portion of the epidermis that acts as the main barrier to mechanical damage, desiccation, and invasion by bacteria. Contents of membrane-coating granules contribute to or constitute the primary intercellular barrier to water. Epidermis has a high capacity for self-renewal, the new cells being derived mainly from stratum basale. The main function of melanin is to protect the germinal cells from the effects of ultraviolet irradiation. It has been suggested that melanin may capture harmful free radicals generated in the epidermis by ultraviolet light. Accumulation of melanin above the nuclei of basal cells affords maximum protection of the genome from the effects of irradiation. Poorly melanized skin is more subject to sunburn, degenerative changes, and skin cancer after chronic exposure to sunlight than is darker skin.

The dermis provides mechanical strength, due to the high content of collagen fibers; elastic fibers provide elasticity. The vascular supply is contained within the dermis, and the epidermis is nourished by diffusion from this vascular bed. The area of contact between dermis and epidermis is increased by the dermal papillae, which facilitate exchange of nutrients from the capillaries in the papillary layer of the dermis. They also provide an interlocking surface to more tightly secure the epidermis to the dermis.

In furred animals, hairs serve as insulation and aid in temperature regulation by minimizing heat loss and gain. Erection of hairs by arrectores pilorum muscles contributes to thermal insulation by allowing incorporation of an air blanket in the fur. In humans, hair contributes little to this function, which is served mainly by the subcutaneous fat and the much thicker epidermis, a relatively poor conductor of heat. Hairs in humans mainly are concerned with cutaneous sensations of touch. Each hair follicle is elaborately innervated, and some of the nerve endings are associated with tactile discs of the Merkel type. In some mammals, tylotrich hairs ("feelers") are present in special patches of epithelium of the face.

The nerve endings associated with these hairs show especially rapid conduction of impulses.

Humans and equine and bovine species regulate body temperature by evaporation of sweat from eccrine sweat glands. In dogs, eccrine glands are confined to the pads of the paws, and temperature regulation is accomplished by panting. Lizards and birds also depend on panting for reduction of body heat. Sebum from sebaceous glands acts as a lubricant for the skin, protects it from drying, and aids in waterproofing. It also has some slight antibacterial activity, but the effect appears to be minimal. Nails not only have a protective function, they also serve as rigid bases for the support of the pads at the ends of the digits and thus may have a role in tactile mechanisms.

Clinical Correlations

Pathologic changes in the skin may involve the epidermis, dermis, or both. Acanthosis is a progressive hyperplasia of the epidermis, leading to an increased number of layers with a generalized thickening of stratum spinosum. Frequently, there is an associated elongation of the epidermal ridges. Stratum granulosum may be increased or decreased; stratum corneum usually is increased. Keratin turnover or maturation may be abnormal and appears as hyperkeratosis in which stratum corneum forms an abnormally thick layer. There usually is an associated hypertrophy of stratum granulosum. Parakeratosis is associated with rapid turnover of cells of stratum granulosum, resulting in a decrease in keratin in individual cells and failure of stratum corneum to form. The superficial squames retain their pyknotic nuclei, and instead of forming a compact stratum corneum, form a layer of loosely applied cells.

Atrophy of the epidermis often accompanies chronic or repeated insults. The individual cells become smaller, fewer layers of cells are formed, and there is slight keratinization. Epidermal ridges are poorly developed, and eventually the epidermis consists only of two to three layers of cells with a smooth epidermal-dermal junction.

The dermis shows atrophic changes in some diseases and with aging. Collagen is reduced in amount, stains poorly, and often is loosely arranged, and the dermal papillae are somewhat flattened. With pronounced atrophy, connective tissue support for vessels in the papillae is lost

and the blood vessels become dilated. Specific degeneration of the papillary layer may occur in which the collagen fibers become fragmented and indistinct, and there is an increase in the amount of elastic tissue. Eventually the zone is replaced by an amorphous, basophilic material — hence the name basophilic degeneration.

Exceptionally thick, dense collagen fibers and an overall increase in the depth of the dermis occurs in scleroderma. Elongation of the dermal papillae into the epidermis may occur in acanthosis.

Severe sunburn causes damage to the epidermis and dermis alike. Within 6 hours of exposure, nuclear, nucleolar, and cytoplasmic changes are evident in the basal cells, then extend throughout the epidermis by 72 hours. The cells show clumping of tonofilaments, reduction in the number of desmosomes, fragmentation of the nucleus, and formation of lipid droplets, cytoplasmic vacuolation, and edema; keratinosomes are absent or reduced in number. Langerhans' cells are markedly affected and at exposures lower than those that affect keratinocytes are almost eliminated. Those that remain are severely damaged. Necrosis of keratinocytes and sloughing of the epidermis usually occurs about 96 hours after overexposure to sunlight. With each episode of prolonged exposure and impairment, the epidermis becomes thinned. Premalignant changes also occur in the cells of the basal layer, and excessive exposure to sunlight is a frequent cause of skin cancers. Mild to moderate vasodilation and perivascular accumulation of monocytes and granular leukocytes occur early in the dermis. With each period of excessive exposure to sunlight, cumulative, progressive, irreversible changes occur in the dermis. Collagen fibers degenerate and fragment and are replaced by elastic fibers, and eventually the skin shows changes of premature aging and becomes dry and wrinkled.

Acne is an inflammatory disorder of sebaceous glands and their ducts, affecting mainly the skin of the face, chest, and upper back. The initial lesion consists of blockage of the opening of hair follicles and the duct of the sebaceous glands by a plug of sebum, cellular debris, and desquamated cells. The lesion is called a comedo (black-head), the blackened tip being due to deposition of melanin. Although the duct is blocked, secretion of sebum continues and the gland becomes increasingly distended. In rare cases, the pressure may cause atrophy of the gland. Commonly, the contents are associated with a bacterium, *Corynebacterium acne*, which produces a lipase that splits the neutral fats of sebum into free fatty acids. These form highly irritant substances that induce an intense inflammatory reaction in and about hair follicles. With infiltration by granular leukocytes, a pustule forms that, with healing, can form a scar.

Atlas and Table of Key Features

Key Features of Thick and Thin Skin

	Epidermis	Dermis	Other
Thick skin	Shows five layers: stratum corneum, stratum lucidum, stratum granulosum, stratum spinosum, and stratum germinativum	Papillary and reticular layers very thick	Only on palms of hand, soles of feet; contains eccrine sweat glands, the only glands present in thick skin
Thin skin	Lacks stratum lucidum; stratum corneum, stratum granulosum, and stratum spinosum are thinner	As for thick skin, depth varies with area; thick dermis in skin between scapulae; delicate dermis over eyelids, scrotum, penis; thinner on anterior surface of body than on posterior surface	Contains hair follicles, eccrine sweat and sebaceous glands; apocrine sweat glands in axilla and groin

Integument — Epidermis

Fig. 13-4. The epidermis of human thin skin (thigh). (LM, ×250.)

Keratinized stratified squamous epithelium (epidermis)

Stratum basale

Keratin layer

Stratum spinosum

Dermis

Fig. 13-5. The epidermis of human thick skin (palm). (LM, ×100.)

Duct of sweat gland

Stratum granulosum

Dermal papilla

Epidermal ridge

Stratum corneum

Stratum lucidum

Stratum spinosum

Stratum basale

Dermis

Fig. 13-6. Cells from the stratum spinosum of human palmar epidermis. (LM, ×1,000.)

Stratum granulosum

Stratum corneum

Keratohyalin granules

Stratum spinosum

Tonofilaments

Desmosomes

Desmosomes

Fig. 13-7. Cytoplasmic portions of cells comprising the epidermis of thin skin. Note the abundance of desmosomes. (TEM, ×8,000.)

Mitochondria

Hemidesmosomes

Collagen

Nucleus of
fibroblast

Nucleus of
cell in
stratum
basale

Hemidesmosomes

Basal
lamina

Fig. 13-8. The interface between epidermis and dermis of thin
skin. Note the position of the basal lamina and the abundance of
hemidesmosomes. (TEM, ×7,000.)

Granular
endoplasmic
reticulum

Desmosomes

Tonofilaments

Tonofilaments in
spinosal cell

Nucleus of
Langerhans
cell

Multivesicular
body

Plasmalemma

Fig. 13-9. An antigen-presenting cell (Langerhans' cell) from the
epidermis of thin skin. (TEM, ×10,000.)

Duct of sweat gland

Vasculature of dermal papillae

Duct of sweat gland

Blood vessels around duct of sweat gland

Duct of sweat gland

Epidermis

Dermis

Duct of sweat gland

Fig. 13-10. A segment of human thick (palmar) skin injected with colored gelatin to illustrate the associated vasculature. (LM, ×100.)

Stratum spinosum

Meissner's corpuscle

Nerve fibers

Stratum corneum

Fig. 13-11. A Meissner's corpuscle from a dermal papilla of human thick (palmar) skin. (LM, ×400.)

Hair

Hair
shaft

Erythrocyte

Edge of
sloughing
squame

Fig. 13-12. A hair shaft emerging from a follicle within the epidermis. (SEM, ×1,000.)

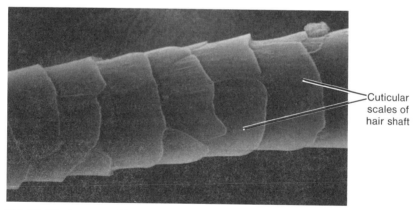

Cuticular
scales of
hair shaft

Fig. 13-13. A region of hair shaft showing the outer cuticular
scales. (SEM, ×2,000.)

Connective tissue papilla of hair follicle

Hair bulb

Matrix

Inner root sheath

Outer root sheath

Fig. 13-14. The bulb of a human hair follicle. (LM, × 100.)

Glands

Ducts

Degenerating cells

Sebaceous cells

Basal cells

Basal cells

Alveolus of sebaceous gland

Fig. 13-15. A human sebaceous gland from the eyelid. (LM, × 100.)

Secretory
tubule
of sweat
gland

Duct of
sweat
gland

Fig. 13-16. An eccrine sweat gland from human thin skin. (LM, ×250.)

Secretory
tubule

Dermis

Fat cells

Duct of
sweat gland

Fig. 13-17. A human apocrine sweat gland from the axilla. Note that the secretory tubule is larger and the lumen more dilated when compared to that of an eccrine sweat gland (see 13-16). (LM, ×100.)

Development

Cell

Nuclei

Fig. 13-18. The periderm covering fetal skin. (SEM, ×300.)

Epidermis

Developing
sebaceous
gland

Dermis

Developing
hair
follicle

Fig. 13-19. A developing hair follicle and sebaceous gland of
human fetal thin skin. (LM, ×250.)

Fig. 13-20. Developing sweat glands of human thin skin. (LM, ×250.)

———— *Review Questions and Answers* ————

Questions

70. Define the terms *thick skin* and *thin skin*. What are the main differences between them?
71. Briefly outline the structure of the hair follicle and relate its components to the epidermis and dermis.
72. What contributes to the color of the skin?
73. What functions are served by the integument?

Answers

70. The terms *thick skin* and *thin skin* refer to the thickness of the epidermis. In thick skin, the epidermis is well developed and its component layers are well defined. In thin skin the epidermis is thinner, its layers are more poorly established, and a stratum lucidum is lacking. Thin skin also contains hair follicles and associated sebaceous glands.

71. The hair follicle surrounds the hair and is composed of an outer component, derived from the dermis, that consists of a poorly defined outer layer of collagenous and elastic fibers; a middle layer of circularly arranged connective tissue fibers; and an inner, homogenous glassy membrane. The glassy membrane forms a boundary with the epithelial component of the hair follicle and is equivalent to the epithelial basement membrane. Immediately adjacent to the glassy membrane are layers that represent a direct extension of the stratum malpighii (stratum basale and stratum spinosum), which forms the outer epithelial root sheath. Interior to this is the inner epithelial root sheath, which represents modifi- cations of the stratum granulosum and stratum corneum.

72. The color of the skin depends mainly on the presence and distribution of melanin, which gives a brown coloration. Melanin is produced by the melanocytes found scattered in the stratum basale and is distributed via their cytoplasmic processes to the cells of the basal layer and stratum spinosum. In the white race melanin tends to be confined to the lower regions of the malpighian layer, whereas in the black race it is distributed through all layers of the epidermis. Carotene, a pigment in the stratum corneum and the fat cells of the dermis and hypodermis, also contributes to the color of the skin, as does the blood in the capillaries of the dermis.

73. The integument consists of the skin and its appendages (hair, nails, and sweat and sebaceous glands). The skin forms a protective, waterproof covering that is chemically inert and acts as a barrier against penetration by noxious agents. It also prevents water loss from the body. Hairs in lower animals serve as insulation against heat loss but have little function in this regard in humans, where they are largely concerned with cutaneous sensation. The skin, especially the epidermis, is a relatively poor conductor of heat and in humans the paucity of hair is compensated for by an increase in the thickness of the epidermis. Temperature is regulated mainly by the evaporation of sweat produced by the sweat glands. Sebum elaborated by the sebaceous glands acts as a lubricant for skin, prevents drying, and aids in waterproofing. Nails protect the ends of the digits and may have a role in tactile mechanisms by providing a firm base for the pads of the fingertips.

14 Respiratory System

The respiratory tract consists of respiratory and conducting portions. Respiratory tissue, located in the lungs, is that portion of the tract where exchange of gases between air and blood occurs and is characterized by a close relationship between capillary blood and air chambers. The conducting portion delivers air to the respiratory tissue and is characterized by rigid walls that keep the airways open. This part of the tract consists of nasal cavities, pharynx, larynx, trachea, and various subdivisions of the bronchial tree. Parts of the conducting system are within the lungs (intrapulmonary) and parts are outside the lungs (extrapulmonary).

Nose

KEY WORDS: pseudostratified ciliated columnar epithelium, goblet cell, olfactory epithelium, lamina propria, venous sinus, mucoperiosteum, mucoperichondrium

The skin that covers the external surface of the nose extends for a short distance into the vestibule of the nasal cavity, where stiff hairs and their associated sebaceous glands aid in filtering the inspired air. More posteriorly, the vestibule is lined by nonkeratinized stratified squamous epithelium (see atlas figure 14-2). Throughout most of the remainder of the nasal cavity, the respiratory passage is lined by **pseudostratified ciliated columnar epithelium** that contains **goblet cells,** but a specialized **olfactory epithelium** is present in the roof of the nasal cavities (see atlas figures 14-5 and 14-6).

A layer of connective tissue, the **lamina propria,** underlies the epithelium and is separated from it by a basement membrane. Contained within the lamina propria are mucous glands, serous glands, and thin-walled **venous sinuses** (see atlas figures 14-4 and 14-6). The venous sinuses warm incoming air and are especially prominent in the lamina propria that covers the middle and inferior conchae. Lymphatic tissue is present and becomes prominent near the nasopharynx. The deep layers of the lamina propria fuse with the periosteum or perichondrium of the nasal bones and cartilages, and at these sites, the nasal mucosa forms a **mucoperiosteum** or **mucoperichondrium,** respectively.

The surface of the epithelial lining is bathed by a film of mucus that constantly is moved toward the pharynx by the action of the ciliated epithelial cells (see atlas figures 14-3 and 14-4). The mucus is derived from surface goblet cells and secretions from mucoserous glands in the lamina propria. The layer of mucus helps to moisten the air and trap particulate matter. The same type of mucosa extends into the paranasal sinuses, but here the epithelium is thinner, there are fewer goblet cells, the lamina propria is thinner and contains fewer glands, and venous sinuses are absent.

Olfactory Epithelium

KEY WORDS: **pseudostratified columnar epithelium, supporting (sustentacular) cell, olfactory cell, bipolar nerve cell, olfactory vesicle (knob), olfactory hair, fila olfactoria, basal cell, olfactory gland**

Olfactory epithelium (Fig. 14-1) occurs in the roof of the nasal cavities, where it extends over the superior conchae and for a short distance on either side of the nasal septum. It also is a **pseudostratified columnar epithelium,** but it lacks goblet cells and is much thicker than the respiratory lining epithelium (see atlas figure 14-6).

Three primary cell types are present: supporting cells, basal cells, and sensory or olfactory cells. **Supporting (sustentacular) cells** are tall with narrow bases and broad apical surfaces that bear long, slender microvilli. An oval nucleus is located just above the center of the cell. Apically, well-developed junctional complexes join the supporting cells to adjacent olfactory cells. **Olfactory cells** are the sensory component and are **bipolar nerve cells** evenly distributed among the supporting cells (see atlas figure 14-5). They are spindle-shaped with rounded nuclei located centrally in an expanded area of cytoplasm. Apically, the cell tapers to a single slender process (a modified dendrite) that extends between the supporting cells to reach to the surface, where it expands into a

bulblike **olfactory vesicle (knob).** Six to eight long **olfactory hairs** extend from the olfactory vesicle and pass parallel to the surface of the epithelium, embedded in a film of fluid (see atlas figure 14-5). The processes are modified, nonmotile cilia and appear to be the excitable component of the sense organ. For a short distance from their origins, the processes have a typical ciliary structure but then narrow abruptly, and the microtubules decrease in number and change from doublets to singlets. Basally, the olfactory cells narrow to a thin process, an axon, that passes into the lamina propria, where, with similar fibers, it forms small nerve bundles (see atlas figure 14-6). These collect as the **fila olfactoria** that pass directly to the olfactory bulb.

Basal cells are short, pyramidal cells crowded between the bases of sustentacular and olfactory cells. They are undifferentiated cells that give rise to either of the other two types of cells.

The olfactory cells are unique among neurons in that they are in direct contact with the external environment and, unlike other neurons, constantly are replaced every 30 to 60 days. New olfactory cells arise from differentiation of the basal cells. Between the surface and the basal cells lie variable numbers of progressively more differentiated receptor neurons, accounting in part for the thickness of the olfactory epithelium.

Rich plexuses of blood vessels and branched, serous, tubuloalveolar glands are present in the lamina propria. The glands are the **olfactory glands** (of Bowman), whose watery secretions flush the surfaces of the olfactory epithelium to prevent continuous stimulation by a single odor and also serve as a solvent for odorous materials (see atlas figure 14-6).

Pharynx and Larynx

KEY WORDS: **nasopharynx, pseudostratified ciliated columnar epithelium, goblet cell**

The nasal cavities continue posteriorly into the pharynx, which has nasal, oral, and laryngeal parts. The most superior part, the **nasopharynx,** is directly continuous with the nasal cavities and is lined by the same respiratory passage epithelium — that is, **pseudostratified ciliated col-**

Fig. 14-1. Diagram of olfactory epithelium.

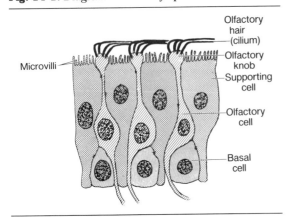

Microvilli

Olfactory hair (cilium)

Olfactory knob

Supporting cell

Olfactory cell

Basal cell

umnar epithelium with goblet cells. In areas subject to abrasion, a nonkeratinizing stratified squamous epithelium may occur, such as on the edge of the soft palate and posterior wall of the pharynx where these surfaces make contact during swallowing. The underlying connective tissue contains mucous, serous, and mixed mucoserous glands and abundant lymphatic tissue. The lymphatic tissue is irregularly scattered throughout the connective tissue and also forms tonsillar structures: the pharyngeal tonsils in the posterior wall of the nasopharynx, the tubal tonsils around the openings of the eustachian tubes into the nasopharynx, and the palatine and lingual tonsils at the junctions of the oral cavity and oropharynx.

The larynx connects the pharynx and trachea. Its framework consists of several cartilages, of which the thyroid, cricoid, and arytenoid are hyaline, while the epiglottis, corniculate, and tips of the arytenoid are elastic. This scaffold of cartilages is held together and to the hyoid bone by sheets of dense connective tissue that form the cricothyroid and thyroid membranes. The lining epithelium varies with location. The anterior surface and about half of the posterior surface of the epiglottis are covered by stratified squamous nonkeratinizing epithelium that may contain a few taste buds. The vocal cords also are covered by stratified squamous epithelium, but elsewhere, the larynx is lined by the respiratory passage type of epithelium. The lamina propria of the larynx is thick and contains mucous and some serous or mucoserous glands.

Trachea and Extrapulmonary Bronchi

KEY WORDS: rings of hyaline cartilage, smooth muscle, pseudostratified ciliated columnar cell, goblet cell, brush cell, small granule cell, short cell, adventitia

The walls of the trachea and its terminal branches (the primary bronchi) are characterized by the presence of C-shaped rings of hyaline cartilage that maintain patency of the airway. The spaces between successive rings are filled with fibroelastic connective tissue, and the gaps between the arms of the cartilages are filled with bundles of smooth muscle. The gaps are directed posteriorly, and in section, the trachea and extrapulmonary bronchi appear flattened. The lining consists of pseudostratified ciliated columnar epithelium with numerous goblet cells that rests on a thick basal lamina (see atlas figures 14-7 and 14-8). Cilia beat toward the pharynx.

In addition to the ciliated and goblet cells, several other cell types have been described in the tracheobronchial epithelium. Brush cells contain glycogen granules, show long straight microvilli on their apical surfaces, and, basally, make contact with nerve processes. They are rare in humans and their function is unknown, but they may be sensory cells, exhausted goblet cells, or intermediates between short cells and mature ciliated cells. Small granule cells are few and scattered. They appear to be part of a population of diffuse neuroendocrine cells able to take up and store amines and amine precursors. Short cells occur in the depths of the epithelium between the bases of the other cell types and are undifferentiated cells that give rise to goblet and ciliated cells. A network of dendritic cells lies along the base of the tracheal epithelium. They function as antigen-presenting cells capable of binding and presenting antigens to T-lymphocytes. The lamina propria contains many small seromucous glands and occasional accumulations of lymphatic tissue. External to the cartilage is a fibroconnective tissue coat, the adventitia, which contains elastic collagenous and reticular fibers, blood vessels, and nerves.

Intrapulmonary Air Passages

KEY WORDS: intrapulmonary bronchus, plates of hyaline cartilage, pseudostratified ciliated columnar, goblet cell, submucosa, simple ciliated columnar, bronchiole, ciliated cuboidal, terminal bronchiole, Clara cell, surfactant, neuroepithelial body

The primary bronchi divide to give rise to several orders of intrapulmonary bronchi in which the C-shaped cartilaginous rings of the primary bronchi are replaced by irregular plates of hyaline cartilage that completely surround the structure. Thus, the intrapulmonary bronchi are cylindrical and are not flattened on one side as are the main bronchi and trachea. Internally, the large intrapulmonary bronchi are lined by a mucous membrane that is continuous with and identical to that of the trachea and primary bronchi: **pseudostratified ciliated columnar** epithelium with **goblet cells.** The lamina propria contains some diffuse lymphatic tissue and is separated from the epithelium by a prominent basal lamina. Beneath the lamina propria, a sheet of irregularly arranged smooth muscle fibers runs around the bronchus in open left- or right-handed spirals. The muscle layer separates the lamina propria from the connective tissue of the **submucosa,** which lies immediately internal to the plates of cartilage. Mucous and mucoserous glands are present in the submucosa, their ducts penetrating the muscle layer to open onto the epithelial surface (see atlas figure 14-9).

With successive divisions, the intrapulmonary bronchi progressively decrease in size, and although they retain the basic structure outlined above, the layers of their walls become thinner. The smallest of the intrapulmonary bronchi show only isolated cartilage plates and no longer are surrounded by cartilages. The epithelium is reduced to **simple ciliated columnar** with goblet cells. Mucous and mucoserous bronchial glands are present as far down as cartilages extend.

When the diameter of the tube reaches about 1 mm, cartilage disappears from the wall and the structure becomes a **bronchiole.** Glands and lymphatic tissue also disappear, but smooth muscle is fairly prominent and becomes the major supporting element (see atlas figures 14-10 through 14-15). The lining epithelium varies from ciliated columnar with goblet cells in the large bronchioles to **ciliated cuboidal** with no goblet cells in the **terminal bronchioles.** Terminal bronchioles are the smallest branches of the purely conducting system (see atlas figure 14-14). Scattered among the ciliated cells are a few nonciliated cells whose apical surfaces bulge into the lumen and bear a few microvilli. These are the **Clara cells,** also called bronchiolar secretory cells, which secrete **surfactant,** a phospholipid that al-

ters the surface tension of the fluid layer covering the cell surface.

Neuroepithelial bodies are innervated, epithelial corpuscles scattered throughout the intrapulmonary airways and even extending into alveoli. They are not present in the trachea. The corpuscles appear as ovoid or triangular bodies, 20 to 40 μm wide, set into the respiratory epithelium, where they extend from lumen to basement membrane. Basally, the neuroepithelial body is closely related to a capillary. The whole structure is richly innervated, and many of the nerve endings make contact with cells of the corpuscle.

The neuroepithelial bodies contain 4 to 10 tall, nonciliated cells with a slightly acidophilic cytoplasm that gives a positive argyrophil (silver) reaction. The oval nuclei are basally located and oriented in the long axis of the cells, which contain numerous mitochondria, moderately well-developed granular endoplasmic reticulum, small Golgi complexes, and some glycogen and multivesicular bodies. Characteristic of these cells are numerous dense-cored vesicles. The neuroepithelial bodies are believed to be chemoreceptors that react to the composition of inhaled air. When the oxygen tension of the inspired air decreases, the neuroepithelial body releases dense-cored vesicles that contain serotonin, a potent vasoconstrictor. Thus, during local hypoxia, blood could be shunted from poor to better oxygenated and ventilated areas of the lungs.

Respiratory Tissue

KEY WORDS: **respiratory bronchiole, alveolar duct, alveolar sac, alveolus, interalveolar septum, alveolar pore, blood-air barrier, pulmonary epithelial cell (type I pneumonocyte), septal cell (type II pneumonocyte), alveolar macrophage**

Exchange of gases between air and blood occurs only when air and blood are in close relation. Such a condition occurs first in the **respiratory bronchioles,** which form a transition between the purely conducting and purely respiratory regions of the tract. The walls of respiratory bronchioles consist of collagenous connective tissue with interlacing bundles of smooth muscle and elastic fibers (see atlas figures 14-13 and 14-15). The larger respiratory bronchioles are lined by simple cuboidal epithelium with only a few ciliated cells; goblet cells are lacking. Many of the cuboidal cells are Clara cells. In the smaller bronchioles, the epithelium becomes low cuboidal without cilia. Alveoli bud from the walls of the respiratory bronchioles and represent the respiratory portions of these airways. The alveoli become more numerous distally. Respiratory bronchioles end by branching into alveolar ducts. **Alveolar ducts** are thin-walled tubes from which numerous alveoli or clusters of alveoli open around the circumference so that the wall becomes little more than a succession of alveolar openings (see atlas figure 14-15). Appearances of a tube persist only in a few places, where small groups of cuboidal cells intervene between successive alveoli and cover underlying bundles of fibroelastic tissue and smooth muscle. The alveolar ducts end in irregular spaces surrounded by clusters of alveoli called **alveolar sacs** (see atlas figure 14-15).

Alveoli are thin-walled, polyhedral structures that are open at one side to allow air into their cavities (see atlas figures 14-13 and 14-14). Adjacent alveoli are separated by a common **interalveolar septum,** whose most conspicuous feature is a rich network of capillaries that bulge the septal wall to expose most of the capillary surface to alveolar air. Reticular and elastic fibers form a tenuous framework for the septa. Small openings in the septal wall, **alveolar pores,** permit communication and equalization of air pressure between alveoli. On each side, the alveolar wall is covered by an attenuated epithelium beneath which is a basal lamina. In many areas the epithelial basal lamina is separated from the basal lamina of the capillary by a space of only 15 to 20 nm; in other regions the two laminae are fused. Thus, at its thinnest, the **blood-air barrier** consists of a thin film of fluid, the attenuated epithelium of the alveolar lining cell, the fused basal laminae, and the endothelium of the capillaries within the septal wall (see atlas figures 14-18 and 14-19).

Several types of cells are present in the septa. The attenuated squamous cells that form a continuous lining for the alveolar wall are called **pulmonary epithelial cells** or **type I pneumonocytes** (see atlas figures 14-16 through 14-20). In addition to these are septal cells, alveolar macrophages, and the endothelial cells that line blood capillaries. **Septal cells (type II pneumonocytes)** are rounded or cuboidal cells that may lie deep in the surface epithelium or bulge into the alveolar lumen between pulmonary epithelial cells. Their free surfaces have short microvilli, and laterally, the cells are united to pulmonary epithelial cells by junctional complexes (see atlas figures 14-16 and 14-17). The most distinctive feature of the septal cells is the presence of multilamellar bodies in their cytoplasm. These bodies consist of thin, concentric lamellae thought to be the storage sites of surfactant.

Alveolar macrophages are present within the interalveolar septa and alveolar lumina (see atlas figure 14-21). Many contain particles of inhaled material and have been called "dust" cells. As with all macrophages, the alveolar macrophages originate from blood monocytes. Most of these cells ultimately are eliminated via the air passages and appear in the sputum; a few may migrate into lymphatics and escape the lungs by this route.

Pleura

The pleura are thin membranes made up of collagenous and elastic fibers, covered by a single layer of mesothelial cells (see atlas figures 14-22 and 14-23). The layer lining the wall of the thoracic cavity is the parietal pleura, which reflects from the thoracic wall onto the surface of the lungs, where it becomes the visceral pleura. The pleura secrete a small amount of fluid between the two layers to permit friction-free movement.

Development of the Respiratory System

During the fourth week of gestation, the respiratory passages first appear as an endodermal bud arising from the caudal end of the laryngotracheal groove. As the lung bud grows, it becomes covered by mesenchyme that later differentiates into blood vessels and the cartilage, smooth muscle, and connective tissues that support the walls. The endoderm provides the lining epithelium for the entire respiratory tract. The lung bud grows caudally and undergoes successive divisions, the first branches representing the main bronchi. Subsequent divisions provide finer and finer branches of a complex respiratory tree, ultimately ending in small expansions called infundibula. These minute pouches eventually become the definitive alveoli.

During their development, the lungs undergo considerable change in appearance, and histologically, three phrases can be identified. The first or glandular phase extends from the fifth to the seventeenth week and consists mainly of development of the branching air passages (see atlas figures 14-24 and 14-25). The repeated divisions of the endodermal tubes within a bed of mesenchyme give the lung the appearance of a gland. The tubes are lined by undifferentiated columnar cells that have few organelles but are rich in glycogen and contain fat. Nuclei are variable in size and show one or two nucleoli. Mitoses are common. The cells are united at their apices by tight junctions and desmosomes. Even in the earliest stages, the epithelial cells are separated from the mesenchyme by a delicate basement membrane. The cells later become cuboidal, and by the thirteenth week, cilia and goblet cells appear, first in the trachea and then progressively at more distal levels. By 16 weeks Clara cells are differentiating and endocrine cells can be found.

The canalicular phase extends from the seventeenth to the twenty-sixth week and is marked by rapid growth of the tubular elements to provide the finer twigs of the respiratory tree, and by delineation of the respiratory parts (see atlas figure 14-26). The terminal buds (infundibula) becomes less spherical and are intimately related to capillary networks. Transformation of tubules to canaliculi is accompanied by flattening of the epithelium and considerable cytodifferentiation. Osmiophilic lamellar bodies associated with production of surfactant appear in some of the epithelial cells, which now have fairly well developed endoplasmic reticulum and plentiful ribosomes. These cells, identifiable as type II pneumonocytes, appear at the fifth to sixth month of gestation. During this phase, the cells reduce their height, and their intercellular junctions lie at the lower half of the cell rather than at the apex as in the glandular phase. These low cells are the precursors of type I pneumonocytes of saccules and alveoli.

The terminal sac (alveolar) phase extends from the twenty-sixth week until term. By this time respiratory bronchioles can be recognized as tubes lined on one side by flattened epithelium and on the other by a ciliated cuboidal epithelium. Branches that had been buds lined by cuboidal epithelium now are clusters of five to six generations of saccules lined by flattened epithelial cells closely associated with capillaries. The septa between capillaries are thick, but gradually thin.

At birth, alveoli are small and shallow, and only a few solitary alveoli are present in respiratory bronchioles. Inflation of alveoli occurs after birth with the onset of respiration, first in the hilar region, then in the central portion of the lungs. Only after several hours of breathing are distal alveoli inflated. New alveoli continue to be formed after birth, and it is not until about the eighth postnatal year that the adult number of alveoli is attained.

Functional Summary

The stiff hairs in the vestibule of the nose help prevent particulate matter in the inspired air from reaching the rest of the respiratory passages. Mucus secreted by goblet cells in the respiratory lining and by glands in the lamina propria of the conducting portion provides a sticky blanket that traps particles and, along with the serous secretions from these glands, prevents drying of the mucosal surface. The secretions also humidify the air. The beat of the cilia moves the fluid blanket toward the mouth, both in the nose and lower respiratory tract. The large venous plexuses in the nasal cavities warm the incoming air. In several species, including humans, periodic engorgement of the venous plexus occurs, alternating on either side of the nasal cavity. This results in temporary obstruction to flow on the one side, allowing the mucosa to recover from the drying effects of air. In humans the periods of occlusion occur approximately hourly.

The olfactory epithelium serves for the sense of smell, the sensory component being the olfactory cells. The olfactory hairs borne by these cells form the excitable element of the sense organ. Glands in this area secrete a watery fluid that serves as a solvent for materials and flushes the olfactory epithelium to prevent continuous stimulation by a single odor.

Patency of the conducting portion, from the trachea to the smallest intrapulmonary bronchus, is maintained by cartilage in the walls. In the trachea and main bronchi, the fibroelastic tissue between cartilages gives pliability and longitudinal extensibility to these structures. This is essential for the accommodations these structures make for the incursions of the lung during breathing.

Beginning with the small bronchi, the epithelium progressively simplifies and becomes thinner. Ciliated cells persist farther along the resiratory tree than do mucus-secreting cells, and this may ensure that the sites of gaseous exchange do not become coated with a viscid, mucoid material that would impede or prevent the passage of gases. Significantly, cells that produce surfactant begin to appear at about the level at which goblet cells disappear. Surfactant reduces the surface tension of the fluid layer. During late phases of expiration, bronchioles close, so that provision of a nonsticky fluid of decreased surface tension may be important for the reopening of bronchioles.

The small granule cells are part of a widespread diffuse endocrine system, with the cells apparently secreting various agents (perhaps hormones) that may have a role in regulating the secretion of mucus or surfactant.

The neuroepithelial bodies appear to be specifically adapted to respond to oxygen tension and adjust capillary flow to areas of high oxygen content.

The mucous secretions and cilia of the respiratory tree serve the same protective functions as in the nasal passages. Additionally, the mucosubstances have antiviral and antibacterial properties. The lymphoid tissue associated with the larger respiratory passages gives immunologic protection by producing immunoglobulin A (IgA) antibodies. Secretory IgA is assembled by mucosal cells of bronchial glands and mucosa; the secretory protein is produced by the serous cells of the submucosal glands.

Exchange of gases occurs where air and blood are closely approximated — in the alveoli. The barrier between air in the alveoli and blood in the capillaries of the alveolar septa consists only of a thin film of fluid, an extremely attenuated cytoplasm of the alveolar lining cell, the conjoined basal laminae plus the endothelium of the capillary. Surfactant-secreting cells also are present in the alveolar lining. Without surfactant the alveolus tends to collapse because of the surface tension of the fluid that bathes the alveolar epithelium. Particulate matter that reaches the alveoli is removed by alveolar macrophages that, through their role as phagocytes, provide the main defense against microorganisms. During phagocytosis the cells release hydrogen peroxide and other peroxide radicals to destroy foreign organisms. Cigarette smoking triggers an inappropriate release of peroxide by alveolar macrophages, resulting in damage to normal respiratory and connective tissues. Phagocytosis by macrophages is greatly depressed in smokers, and the cells show twice the normal volume with a marked reduction in surface-to-volume ratios. The density of lysosomes also decreases.

Each lung is enclosed in a sac formed by the pleural membranes. The outer (parietal) layer lines the inner surface of the thoracic wall; the inner (visceral) layer covers the surface of the lungs. The space between the two layers is under negative pressure, and the two layers are separated only by a thin film of fluid. As the thoracic wall moves out to increase the size of the thoracic cage, the parietal pleura is taken along, passively. The combined effects of surface tension and negative pressure result in the visceral pleura being drawn outward also. Since the visceral pleura is firmly attached to the lungs, they are expanded, the air pressure within the lungs decreases, and air flows into the lungs. Expiration of air occurs as the result of elastic recoil of the lungs when the thoracic wall relaxes.

Clinical Correlations

Acute rhinitis is the common inflammatory lesion of the nasal cavities, exemplified by the common cold. The nasal mucosa is thickened by edema, the blood vessels of the lamina propria are dilated, the goblet cells are hyperactive, and the glands of the lamina propria are enlarged and show excessive secretion. Granulocytes are sparse until secondary bacterial infection occurs, when the exudate becomes mucopurulent and thickened. There is variable loss of the superficial ciliated epithelium.

Chronic inflammation of the larynx and trachea often is associated with smoking. The mucous glands become swollen and squamous metaplasia is common. In heavy smokers, the entire larynx, including the epiglottis and upper trachea, can become lined by stratified squamous epithelium instead of the normal pseudostratified columnar. Development of cancer of the larynx frequently is associated with such squamous metaplasia.

Chronic bronchitis is primarily a reaction to chronic irritation of the bronchial epithelium, leading to hypertrophy and hyerplasia of the mucous glands within the bronchial wall. The number of goblet cells also increases, at the expense of ciliated cells, and goblet cells appear in terminal bronchioles where they normally do not occur. The increase in goblet cells leads to excessive production of mucus. With the loss of ciliated cells, mucus accumulates even down into alveolar spaces, where it tends to stagnate and become infected. One of the most common irritants is tobacco smoke, and in chronic smokers, ciliary action is impaired and the ciliary beats are uncoordinated. The cilia also are physically damaged, many showing clubbed and deformed ends.

Emphysema is a permanent enlargement of respiratory passages and air spaces beyond the terminal bronchioles. The disease may begin in respiratory bronchioles that become greatly enlarged and ballooned out, with no involvement of alveolar ducts and alveoli early in the disease. The condition may also arise as a permanent enlargement of alveoli and alveolar ducts initially, followed by enlargement of respiratory bronchioles. Emphysema is most pronounced at the apices of the lungs and along their margins, but in severe cases the entire lung substance may be involved. The airways supplying the emphysematous space often are the sites of carbon deposition and almost always show inflammatory changes with peribronchiolar infiltration by lymphocytes or granular leukocytes. Portions of septa often show chronic inflammation and the parent airway often is constricted. Emphysema is associated with pneumoconiosis in coal miners and workers exposed to inhalation of carbon dust generally. Tobacco smoking also is implicated in the etiology of emphysema; not only is the incidence increased among smokers, the disease also occurs at an earlier age and with increased severity.

Atlas and Table of Key Features

Key Features of the Respiratory System

Division	Part	Epithelium	Support	Other Features
Extrapulmonary conducting	Nose Main portion	Pseudostratified ciliated columnar with goblet cells (respiratory lining epithelium)	Hyaline cartilage and bone	Lamina propria forms a mucoperiosteum; contains seromucous glands and large venous sinuses
	Olfactory region	Pseudostratified columnar with 3 cell types: basal, supporting, olfactory	Bone of nasal concha	Lamina propria contains serous glands, venous sinuses, and nerves; forms a mucoperiosteum
	Pharynx Nasal	Respiratory lining epithelium	Skeletal muscle	Lamina propria contains mucous, serous, and mucoserous glands; abundant lymphatic tissue; pharyngeal tonsils
	Oral	Stratified squamous, nonkeratinized	Striated muscle	As above; palatine tonsils

Key Features of the Respiratory System (continued)

Division	Part	Epithelium	Support	Other Features
	Laryngeal	Stratified squamous to middle of posterior surface of epiglottis, and vocal cords; respiratory lining epithelium elsewhere	Cartilage; dense regular connective tissue	Epiglottis, corniculate cartilage, tips of arytenoid are elastic cartilage, rest are hyaline; epithelium over epiglottis may contain taste buds
	Trachea and main bronchi	Respiratory lining epithelium	C-shaped hyaline cartilages; fibroelastic connective tissue	Supporting connective tissue divided into lamina propria and submucosa by elastic tissue; seromucous glands in submucosa; scattered lymphatic tissue
Intrapulmonary conducting	Intrapulmonary bronchi	Respiratory lining epithelium in largest; ciliated columnar with goblet cells in smallest	Irregular, discontinuous plates of hyaline cartilage decreasing in smaller bronchi	Smooth muscle increasingly prominent as cartilage disappears; mucoserous glands and lymphatic tissue in submucosa
	Bronchioles	Ciliated columnar with goblet cells in largest to ciliated columnar with no goblet cells in smallest; Clara cells appear	Smooth muscle	Connective tissue decreased in amount; no glands or lymphatic tissue present
Transitional from conducting to respiratory	Respiratory bronchioles	Simple cuboidal, some ciliated, no goblet cells; Clara cells	Thin layer of fibroelastic connective tissue; few smooth muscle cells	Alveoli bud out from wall
	Alveolar ducts	Cuboidal, nonciliated between successive alveoli	Thin, delicate connective tissue	

Key Features of the Respiratory System (continued)

Division	Part	Epithelium	Support	Other Features
Respiratory	Alveolar sacs	Thin squamous epithelium; type II pneumonocytes, phagocytes	Elastic and reticular fibers	Formed by clusters of alveoli
	Alveoli	Attenuated squamous cells, type II pneumonocytes, macrophages	Reticular and elastic fibers	Closely approximated to capillaries; blood-air barrier consists of cytoplasm of type I pneumonocyte, common basement membrane, cytoplasm of endothelial cells

Nose

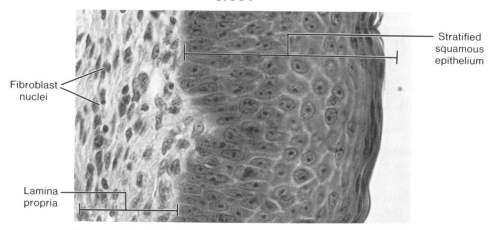

Fig. 14-2. Keratinized stratified squamous epithelium lining the vestibule of the human nose. (LM, ×300.)

Fig. 14-3. Surface features of the epithelium covering the human inferior concha. (SEM, ×400.)

Lamina propria

Serous (Bowman's) gland

Cilia

Ciliated pseudostratified columnar epithelium

Venous sinus

Compact bone

Fig. 14-4. Ciliated pseudostratified columnar epithelium lining a nasal concha. Note the supporting bone. Compare the epithelium shown in this figure with 14-3. (LM, ×250.)

Microvilli

Olfactory hairs
(nonmotile cilia)

Olfactory
vesicles

Fig. 14-5. Surface features of olfactory epithelium showing olfactory vesicles and cilia from underlying sensory bipolar neurons. (SEM, ×5,700.) Inset: Cell bodies of olfactory bipolar neurons stained by immunohistochemistry for olfactory marker protein. (LM, ×500.)

Bowman's glands

Nerves

Olfactory epithelium

Venous sinus

Fig. 14-6. A region of the superior concha showing olfactory epithelium and glands. Note the nerves and venous sinus in the lamina propria. (LM, ×250.)

Conducting Airways

Lamina propria

Venule

Diffuse lymphatic tissue

Cross section of elastic fibers

Ciliated pseudostratified columnar epithelium

Cilia

Goblet cells

Fig. 14-7. The mucosal lining of a human trachea. (LM, ×400.)

Apex of
nonciliated
cell

Cilia

Erythrocyte

Lymphocyte

Fig. 14-8. Apices of ciliated and nonciliated cells from the epithelial lining of the trachea. Note the erythrocyte and lymphocyte on the epithelial surface. (SEM, ×2,000.)

Smooth
muscle

Ciliated
pseudostratified
columnar
epithelium

Smooth
muscle

Bronchial
glands

Hyaline
cartilage

Fig. 14-9. A section through a human intrapulmonary bronchus. (LM, ×100.)

Lamina propria

Ciliated simple columnar epithelium

Cilia

Fig. 14-10. A longitudinal section of a bronchiole. (LM, ×400.)

Cilia

Apices of nonciliated cells

Apices of nonciliated cells

Cilia

Cilia

Fig. 14-11. Surface features of a bronchiole. Note the folded appearance as well as ciliated and nonciliated cells. Compare with 14-10 and 14-12. (SEM, ×1,000.)

Smooth muscle

Ciliated simple columnar epithelium

Pulmonary arteriole

Alveolus

Smooth muscle

Fig. 14-12. A cross section of a bronchiole in a human lung. (LM, ×100.)

Lung (Respiratory Portion)

Alveoli

Respiratory bronchioles

Pulmonary arteriole

Bronchiole

Terminal bronchiole

Alveoli

Fig. 14-13. A segment of human lung showing different types of bronchioles and numerous alveoli. (LM, ×40.)

Alveolus

Terminal
bronchiole

Pulmonary
arteriole

Fig. 14-14. Human lung showing a terminal bronchiole and several alveoli. (LM, ×40.)

Terminal
bronchiole

Respiratory
bronchiole

Alveolar
duct

Alveolar
sac

Alveolar
duct

Pleura

Fig. 14-15. A segment of human lung illustrating the progression of terminal bronchiole to respiratory bronchiole to alveolar duct. (LM, ×40.)

Type II pneumonocyte

Type I pneumonocyte

Cell junctions

Type I pneumonocyte

Cell junction

Type II pneumonocytes

Fig. 14-16. The interior of an alveolus demonstrating types I and II pneumonocytes. (SEM, ×2,000.)

Lipid droplets

Nucleus of Type II pneumonocyte

Cytosomes (multilamellar bodies)

Nucleus of endothelial cell

Capillary

Type I pneumonocyte

Tight junction

Lumen of alveolus

Fig. 14-17. A section through an alveolus shows type I and II pneumonocytes and an adjacent capillary. (TEM, ×4,000.)

Lumen of alveolus

Cytoplasm of Type I pneumonocyte

Fused basal laminae

Erythrocyte

Cytoplasm of fibroblast

Nucleus of Type I pneumonocyte

Cytoplasm of endothelial cell

Collagen

Fig. 14-18. A section of alveolar wall demonstrates the close association between the type I pneumonocyte and the endothelial cell. Note the fused basal laminae. (TEM, ×4,000.)

Lumen of alveolus

Type I pneumonocyte

Fused basal laminae

Nucleus of endothelial cell

Lumen of capillary

Junction between Type I pneumonocytes

Cytoplasm of endothelium

Fused basal laminae

Lumen of capillary

Fig. 14-19. The junction between type I pneumonocytes (compare with 14-20). (TEM, ×5,000.)

Type I pneumonocyte

Cell junctions

Cell junction

Type I pneumonocyte

Fig. 14-20. The interior surface of an alveolus showing the junction between type I pneumonocytes. (SEM, ×10,000.)

Lumen of capillary

Lipid droplets

Lysosomes

Lumen of alveolus

Lumen of capillary

Collagen

Nucleus of alveolar macrophage

Pseudopodia

Capillary lumen

Fig. 14-21. An alveolar macrophage within the lumen of an alveolus. (TEM, ×2,500.)

Pleura

Lumen of
alveolus

Lumen of
alveoli

Collagen
fibers
Elastic
membrane
Mesothelium

Visceral
pleura

Fig. 14-22. A section of visceral pleura stained with orcein to selectively demonstrate the elastic membrane. (LM, ×3,000.)

Fig. 14-23. A region of visceral pleura showing the mesothelium, elastic lamina, and collagen layer. (TEM, ×3,000.)

Development

Primary bronchus

Cartilage

Fig. 14-24. A portion of fetal lung showing the early glandular phase of development. (LM, ×250.)

Parietal pleura

Vertebral bodies

Intrapulmonary bronchi

Fig. 14-25. A region of fetal lung later in the glandular phase of development (compare with 14-24). (LM, ×100.)

Vertebral body

Distal bronchioles

Intrapulmonary bronchi

Fig. 14-26. Fetal lung showing the early canalicular phase of development. Note the appearance of bronchioles. (LM, ×100.)

——— *Review Questions and Answers* ———

Questions

74. What structures constitute the extrapulmonary conducting portion of the respiratory tract? What types of epithelium are present and where do they occur?
75. Describe the changes in the air that occur in the nose and relate the changes to structures in the nasal cavity.
76. Where does gas exchange occur? What features are necessary for gas exchange and how are these met?

Answers

74. The extrapulmonary air passages consist of the nasal cavities; nasal, oral, and laryngeal pharynx; larynx; trachea; and main bronchi. The main type of epithelium present is pseudostratified ciliated columnar epithelium with goblet cells. Other types include keratinizing and nonkeratinizing stratified squamous in the vestibule of the nose, olfactory epithelium in the roof of the nasal cavities, and stratified squamous nonkeratinizing in the oro- and laryngo-pharynx, anterior surface of the epiglottis, margins of soft palate, and posterior wall of nasopharynx where this wall contacts the soft palate. The remainder of the passage is lined by the pseudostratified columnar type.

75. As the air enters the nostrils it is strained by stiff hairs that, with their associated sebaceous glands, help remove particulate matter. As it passes along the nasal passages, the air is warmed, moistened, and further depleted of particles. Warming results from the numerous venous sinuses in the lamina propria. Moisture is added from the fluid bathing the mucosal surface, contributed to by goblet cells and glands in the lamina propria. The fluid film also traps particulate materials, which are carried toward the mouth by the cilia. In the roof of the nasal cavities, any odorous materials stimulate the olfactory epithelium, resulting in the sense of smell.

76. Gas exchange occurs in the alveoli. Requirements for gas exchange are a close approximation of blood and air and a large surface area. These conditions are met in the alveolus by the presence, in the alveolar septum, of a rich capillary network that is closely apposed to the septal wall. The barrier between air in the alveolus and blood in the capillary is exceedingly thin and is composed of a molecular layer of fluid, an extremely attenuated alveolar epithelium, the endothelium of the blood capillary, and their fused basal laminae.

15 Digestive System

The digestive or alimentary tract consists of the oral cavity, pharynx, esophagus, stomach, small and large intestines, rectum, and anal canal. In addition to the digestive tract proper, there are associated glands that lie outside the tract but that are connected to it by ducts.

General Structure

KEY WORDS: **mucous membrane, mucosa, lining epithelium, lamina propria, muscularis mucosae, submucosa, muscularis externa, adventitia, serosa**

Throughout its extent, the alimentary tract shows several features that represent basic components. The innermost tissue layer of the digestive tract is called a **mucous membrane** or **mucosa** and consists of a **lining epithelium** and an underlying layer of fine, interlacing connective tissue fibers that form the **lamina propria.** A muscular component of the mucosa, the **muscularis mucosae,** is found only in the tubular portion of the tract. Immediately beneath the mucosa is a layer of dense irregular connective tissue consisting of coarse, loosely woven collagen fibers and scattered elastic fibers. This layer is the **submucosae,** which houses larger vessels and nerves and provides the mucosa with considerable mobility. Where it is absent, the mucosa is immobile and firmly attached to underlying structures. In the tubular portion of the tract, a thick layer of smooth muscle, the **muscularis externa,** forms an outer supporting wall that in turn is surrounded either by connective tissue, an **adventitia,** or a layer of connective tissue covered by mesothelium called a **serosa.**

Oral Cavity

The irregularly shaped oral cavity consists of the lips, cheek, tongue, gingiva, teeth, and palate. The mucosa consists of a stratified squamous epithelium and a rather dense lamina propria. A submucosa may be present in some regions of the oral cavity.

Lip

KEY WORDS: **vermillion border, papilla, labial gland**

The external surface of the lip is covered by thin skin and contains sweat glands, hair follicles, and sebaceous glands. At the **vermillion border,** the lip is covered by a nonkeratinized, translucent, stratified squamous epithelium that lacks hair follicles and glands (see atlas figure 15-4). Its lamina propria projects into the overlying epithelium to form numerous tall connective tissue **papillae** that contain abundant capillaries. The combination of tall vascular papillae and translucent epithelium accounts for the red hue of this part of the lip. The red portion is continuous with the oral mucosa internally and with thin skin externally. Because glands are lacking, the red portion of the lips is kept moist by licking.

The inner surface is lined by nonkeratinized

(wet) stratified squamous epithelium that over-lies a compact lamina propria with numerous connective tissue papillae. Between the oral mu-cosa and the skin are the skeletal muscle fibers of the orbicularis oris muscle. Coarse fibers of connective tissue in the submucosa connect it to the underlying muscle. The ducts of numerous mixed mucoserous **labial glands** in the submu-cosa empty onto the internal surface of the lip and provide moisture and lubrication for this re-gion. They can be identified as small bumps when the tongue is pressed firmly against the interior of the lip.

Cheek, Palate, and Gingiva

A similar mucous membrane lines the interior of the cheek, soft palate, floor of the mouth, and underside of the tongue. The mucosa of the cheek and soft palate, like that in the lips, is attached to underlying skeletal muscle fibers by coarse connective tissue elements of the submucosa, al-lowing considerable mobility to the oral mucosa in these regions. Mucoserous glands, adipose tis-sue, larger blood vessels, and nerves are present in the submucosa. The cheek and soft palate con-tain a core of skeletal muscle, the buccinator and palatine muscles, respectively. Externally, the cheek is covered by thin skin. Where the non-cornified stratified squamous epithelium of the oral cavity reflects over the posterior aspect of the soft palate to enter the nasopharynx, it changes to a typical respiratory passage epithelium.

The hard palate, gingiva, and dorsum of the tongue, which are subjected to mechanical trauma during chewing, lack a submucosa and are covered by cornified, stratified squamous ep-ithelium (see atlas figure 15-10). In these areas, the lamina propria is immobilized by its attach-ment to underlying structures. Where the mu-cosa attaches directly to bone, it forms a mucoperiosteum. The mucosa of the gingiva (gums) is attached directly to the periosteum of alveolar bone, and a similar attachment occurs in the midline raphe of the hard palate and where the hard palate joins the gingiva. A submucosa is present under the rest of the hard palate and

contains abundant adipose tissue anteriorly and small mucous glands posteriorly.

Tongue

KEY WORDS: **papilla, lingual tonsil, filiform papilla, fungiform papilla, taste buds, circum-vallate papilla, serous glands (of von Ebner), fol-iate papilla**

The mucous membrane of the tongue is firmly bound to a core of striated muscle and there is no submucosa. The skeletal muscle forms inter-woven fascicles that run in all three planes, each perpendicular to the other. The undersurface of the tongue is smooth whereas the anterior two-thirds of the upper surface shows numerous small protuberances called **papillae.** The poste-rior one-third lacks papillae but shows mucosal ridges and moundlike elevations. The latter result from the underlying lymphatic tissue of the **lin-gual tonsils.**

Four types of papillae are associated with the anterior portion of the tongue. **Filiform papillae** are 2 to 3 mm long and contain a conical core of connective tissue that is continuous with the un-derlying lamina propria (see atlas figures 15-5 and 15-6). The covering stratified squamous ep-ithelium shows variable degrees of cornification. The mushroom-shaped **fungiform papillae** are scattered singly between the filiform type (see atlas figures 15-5 and 15-7). They are most nu-merous near the tip of the tongue, where they appear as small red dots. The color is due to the richness of capillaries in their connective tissue cores. **Taste buds** may be associated with this type of papilla. **Circumvallate papillae,** the larg-est of the papillae, are located along the V-shaped sulcus that divides the tongue into anterior and posterior parts. They number 10 to 14 in hu-mans. The circumvallate papillae appear to have sunk into the mucosa of the tongue and are sur-rounded by a wall of lingual tissue, from which they are separated by a deep furrow. Each con-tains a large core of connective tissue with nu-merous vessels and small nerves. Occasionally, small serous glands may be present. The epithe-lium over the lateral surfaces of these papillae contains numerous taste buds (see atlas figure 15-8). **Serous (von Ebner's) glands** open into the bottom of the furrow. Their thin serous secretions continuously flush the furrow and provide an environment suitable for sensory reception by the taste buds. **Foliate papillae** are rudimentary in humans but in species such as the rabbit are well developed and contain many taste buds. They form oval bulges on the posterior, dorsolateral aspect of the tongue and consist of parallel ridges and furrows. Taste buds lie in the epithelium on the lateral surfaces of the ridges, and serous glands drain into the bottoms of the adjacent furrows.

Taste Buds

KEY WORDS: **taste pore, supporting (sustentacular) cell, neuroepithelial cell, taste hair**

Taste buds are present in fungiform, circumvallate, and foliate papillae and may be scattered in the epithelium of the soft palate, glossopharyngeal arches, pharynx, and epiglottis. They appear as lightly stained, oval structures that extend from the basement membrane almost to the surface of the lining epithelium (see atlas figure 15-9). A small **taste pore** allows for communication with the external environment. Taste buds consist of **supporting (sustentacular) cells,** between which are **neuroepithelial cells;** the cells surround the taste pore somewhat like the segments of an orange. Both types of cells have large microvilli called **taste hairs** that project into the taste pore and are embedded in an amorphous, polysaccharide material. Neuroepithelial cells are stimulated by substances that enter the taste pore. The sensation is transmitted to club-shaped nerve endings that pass between both cell types of the taste bud but apparently make synaptic contact only with neuroepithelial cells. Peripheral and basal cells, also associated with taste buds, are thought to represent undifferentiated progenitors of the supporting and neuroepithelial cells.

Four taste sensations are perceived: bitter, sweet, salty, and sour (or acid). The sensations may be detected regionally in the tongue — sweet and salty at the tip of the tongue, sour at the sides of the tongue, and bitter in the area of the circumvallate papillae — but structural differences in taste buds in these areas have not been seen.

Salivary Glands

KEY WORDS: **major salivary glands, minor salivary glands, saliva, lysozyme, IgA, secretory piece**

Salivary glands of the oral cavity can be divided into major and minor glands; all are compound tubuloalveolar glands. The **major salivary glands** are the parotid, submandibular, and sublingual glands and lie outside the oral cavity. Numerous smaller, intrinsic salivary glands are present in the oral cavity and make up the **minor salivary glands** (Table 15-1), which secrete continuously to moisten the mucosa of the oral cavity, vestibule, and lips.

Saliva is a mixture of secretions from both groups of salivary glands and contains water, ions, mucins, immunoglobulins, desquamated epithelial cells, and degenerating granulocytes and lymphocytes (salivary corpuscles). Amylase and maltase also are present to begin digestion of some carbohydrates. Saliva moistens the oral cavity, softens ingested materials, cleanses the oral cavity, and acts as a solvent to permit materials to be tasted. Some heavy metals are eliminated in the salivary secretions, and decreased secretion during dehydration helps initiate the sensation of thirst.

Saliva also is important in controlling the bacterial population in the mouth. In addition to producing **lysozyme,** the serous cells of the salivary glands participate in the production of immunoglobulin to suppress bacterial growth. Immunoglobulin A (**IgA**) synthesized and released by B-lymphocytes is taken up by the serous cells and complexed to a protein called the **secretory piece** before being released into the oral cavity. The secretory piece is synthesized by the epithelial cells and prevents the IgA from being broken down. The submandibular gland also secretes epidermal growth factor (EGF) and nerve growth factor (NGF) into the oral cavity.

Table 15-1 Minor Salivary Glands

Name	Location	Type of Gland
Labial glands	Upper and lower lips	Mixed
Buccal glands	Cheeks	Mixed
Anterior lingual glands	Tip of tongue	Mixed
von Ebner's glands	Near circumvallate papillae	Serous
Posterior lingual glands	Root of tongue	Mucous
Palatine glands	Palate	Mucous

Major Salivary Glands

The major salivary glands — parotid, submandibular, and sublingual — secrete only in response to nervous stimulation. The response is reflexive and can be stimulated by the smell, sight, or even thought of food.

Parotid Gland

KEY WORDS: **compound tubuloalveolar, serous, intercellular secretory canaliculi, intercalated duct, striated duct, basal striation, intralobular duct system, interlobular duct**

The parotid is the largest of the major salivary glands and is located below and in front of the external ear. The main excretory duct passes through the cheek to open into the vestibule of the mouth opposite the second molar tooth. It is a **compound tubuloalveolar** gland and in humans, most domestic mammals, and rodents is entirely **serous.** A few mucous cells are present in the parotid glands of carnivores, puppies, and lambs. The adult human parotid contains abundant, scattered fat cells.

The parotid is enclosed in a fibrous capsule and subdivided into lobes and lobules by connective tissue septae (see atlas figure 15-11). A delicate stroma surrounds the secretory units and ducts and contains numerous blood capillaries and scattered nerve fibers. Myoepithelial cells lie between the limiting basement membrane and the bases of the secretory cells and may aid in expressing secretions out of the secretory units and into the duct system. Alveoli are composed of pyramidal-shaped, serous cells with basally placed,

oval nuclei, basophilic cytoplasm, and discrete, apical secretory granules. Small channels, the **intercellular secretory canaliculi,** are found between serous cells and provide an additional route secretory products can take to reach the lumen.

The initial segment of the duct system is the **intercalated duct,** which is especially prominent in the parotid gland (see atlas figure 15-12). It is lined by a simple squamous or low cuboidal epithelium and may be associated with myoepithelial cells. Intercalated ducts are continuous with **striated ducts,** which are lined by columnar cells that show numerous **basal striations.** These elaborate infoldings of the basal plasmalemma increase the surface area, while the mitochondria associated with the infoldings provide energy at the base of the cell and play a significant role in fluid and ion transport. The intercalated and striated ducts constitute the duct system within the lobule and collectively form the **intralobular duct system** (see atlas figures 15-11 and 15-12). The remaining ducts are found in the connective tissue between lobules and are referred to as **interlobular ducts.** They are continuous with the intralobular ducts and at first are lined by a simple columnar epithelium that becomes pseudostratified and then stratified as the diameter of the duct increases. The surrounding connective tissue becomes more abundant as these ducts join to form the major excretory duct. The distal part of the duct is lined by stratified squamous epithelium that becomes continuous with the lining epithelium of the cheek.

Submandibular Gland

KEY WORDS: compound tubuloalveolar gland, mixed gland, serous demilune (crescent), intercellular canaliculi, striated duct

The submandibular gland, like the parotid, is a **compound tubuloalveolar gland** and has a fibrous capsule with septa, lobes, lobules, myoepithelial cells, and a prominent duct system. It is a **mixed gland,** with the majority of the secretory units being serous in humans, horses, and ruminants, but in dogs and cats the mucous components are more prominent. In rodents the gland is primarily serous. The mucous tubules usually show **serous demilunes (crescents)** at their blind ends (see atlas figures 15-13 through 15-15). Small channels, the **intercellular secretory canaliculi,** pass between the mucous cells and extend between the serous cells of the demilune. Thus, the secretory product of the demilunes has direct access to the lumen of the mucous tubule. Generally, the duct system is similar to that of the parotid, but the **striated ducts** are longer and hence more conspicuous in sections of the submandibular gland (see atlas figures 15-13, 15-17, and 15-18). The major excretory duct of the submandibular gland empties onto the floor of the oral cavity.

Sublingual Glands

KEY WORDS: composite gland, mixed compound tubuloalveolar gland

The sublingual is a **composite gland,** formed by a number of individual glands of variable size. Each gland opens independently onto the floor of the mouth or into the excretory ducts of the submandibular gland. The capsule is not well defined, although septa are present. It is a **mixed compound tubuloalveolar gland** with most of the secretory units being mucous in ruminants, swine, and rodents. Mixed units are present in small carnivores, humans, and horses. Serous cells are, for the most part, arranged as demilunes. Myoepithelial cells are found in relation to the secretory units. Segments of the intralobular duct system are short and not as readily seen as they are in the other two major salivary glands.

Teeth

In humans, the teeth appear as two distinct sets: primary (deciduous) and permanent. Primary teeth erupt six to eight months after birth and form a complete set of 20 by two years of age. They are shed between the sixth and thirteenth year and gradually are replaced by the permanent set of 32.

Structure

KEY WORDS: crown, root, neck, socket (alveolus), pulp cavity, apical foramen, enamel, dentin, cementum, pulp, periodontal membrane, gingiva

All teeth show the same histologic organization (Fig. 15-1). Each has a **crown** and a **root,** and the point where the two meet is called the **neck.** The root fits into a **socket** (or **alveolus**) of the mandible or maxilla. Each tooth contains a small **pulp cavity** that corresponds in shape to the external form of the tooth. The pulp cavity communicates with the alveolar cavity and periodontal membrane through the **apical foramen,** a small open-

Fig. 15-1. Structure of a tooth.

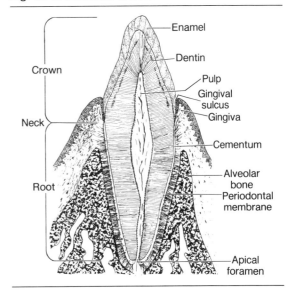

ing at the tip of the root. The hard tissues of the tooth consist of **enamel, dentin,** and **cementum.** Soft tissues associated with the tooth are the **pulp, periodontal membrane,** and **gingiva.**

Dentin

KEY WORDS: dentinal tubule, dentinal (Tomes') fibers, odontoblast, Neumann's sheath

Dentin forms the bulk of the tooth and surrounds the pulp chamber (see atlas figure 15-19). It is harder than compact bone and consists of 80 percent inorganic material and 20 percent organic substance. Most of the organic material is collagen, while the inorganic component is in the form of hydroxyapatite crystals. Dentin has a radially striated appearance due to numerous minute canals called **dentinal tubules** that pursue an S-shaped course as they extend from the pulp chamber to the dentinoenamel junction. The dentinal tubules contain fine cytoplasmic processes, called **dentinal** (or **Tomes')** **fibers,** from a cell type known as the **odontoblast** (see atlas figures 15-22 and 15-73). The thin layer of dentin that immediately surrounds each dentinal tubule shows greater refringence than the remaining dentin and is called **Neumann's sheath.** The cell body of the odontoblast lies in the pulp cavity adjacent to the dentin. The odontoblast lays down the organic matrix of dentin and is active throughout life so that there is a progressive narrowing of the pulp cavity with age. Some areas of dentin remain incompletely calcified and form the interglobular spaces. Dentin is sensitive to cold, pain, touch, and hydrogen ion concentration. Sensation is thought to be perceived by the process of odontoblast, which in turn transmits the sensory stimulation to adjacent nerves in the pulp chamber.

Enamel

KEY WORDS: enamel prism, interprismatic substance, ameloblast

Enamel covers the dentin of the crown and is the hardest substance of the body. It is acellular and consists primarily of calcium salts in the form of apatite crystals. Only 1 percent of the enamel substance is organic material. Enamel consists of thin rods called **enamel prisms** that are perpendicular to the surface of the dentin and extend from the dentinoenamel junction to the surface of the tooth. Each prism, 6 to 8 μm in diameter, follows a spiraling, irregular course to the surface of the tooth. A small amount of organic matrix surrounds each enamel prism and is called the prismatic rod sheath. Between the enamel prisms is the **interprismatic substance,** which also consists of apatite crystals in a small amount of organic matrix. Each enamel prism is the product of a single **ameloblast,** the enamel-producing cells that are lost during eruption of the tooth (see atlas figure 15-73). Thus, new enamel cannot be formed after the tooth has erupted.

Cementum

KEY WORDS: acellular cementum, cementocyte, cellular cementum, Sharpey's fibers

Cementum covers the dentin of the root of the tooth. Nearest the neck of the tooth the cementum is thin and lacks cells, forming the **acellular cementum** (see atlas figure 15-20). The remainder, which covers the apex of the tooth, contains the **cementocytes** that lie in lacunae and are surrounded by a calcified matrix similar to that of bone. This type of cementum is referred to as **cellular cementum** (see atlas figure 15-21). The organic matrix of cementum increases in thickness with age. Coarse bundles of collagen fibers penetrate the cementum as **Sharpey's fibers,** which anchor the root of the tooth to the surrounding alveolar bone of the socket (see atlas figure 15-21).

Pulp

KEY WORDS: connective tissue, apical foramen

Pulp is the **connective tissue** that fills the pulp cavity (see atlas figures 15-19, 15-22, and 15-74). It contains numerous thin, collagenous fibrils embedded in an abundant gelatinous ground substance. Stellate fibroblasts are the most prominent cells of the pulp, although mesenchymal cells, macrophages, and lymphocytes are found in limited numbers. The cell bodies of the odontoblasts also are found in the pulp, lining the perimeter of the pulp cavity immediately adjacent to the dentin. Blood vessels, lymphatics, and nerves enter and exit the pulp cavity through the **apical foramen.**

Periodontal Membrane

KEY WORDS: bundle of collagen fibers, Sharpey's fibers

The periodontal membrane consists of thick **bundles of collagen fibers** that run between the cementum covering the root of the tooth and the surrounding alveolar bone (see atlas figures 15-19 through 15-21). The fibers extend into the bone and cementum as **Sharpey's fibers.** The orientation of the fibers in the periodontal membrane varies at different levels in the alveolar socket. Although firmly attached to the surrounding alveolar bone, the fibers are not taut and the tooth is able to move slightly in each direction. The periodontal membrane forms a suspensory ligament for the tooth. In addition to typical connective tissue cells, osteoblasts and osteoclasts may be found where the periodontal membrane enters the alveolar bone. The periodontal membrane has a rich vascular supply and is sensitive to pressure changes.

Gingiva (Gum)

KEY WORDS: gingival ligament, epithelial attachment cuff

The gingiva surrounds each tooth like a collar and is attached to the periosteum of the underlying alveolar bone. Near the tooth, collagenous fibers of the gingival lamina propria blend with the uppermost fibers of the periodontal membrane. Some collagenous fibers extend from the lamina propria into the cervical (upper) cementum and constitute the **gingival ligament,** which provides a firm attachment to the tooth. The keratinized stratified squamous epithelium of the gingiva also is attached to the surface of the tooth and at this point forms the **epithelial attachment cuff.** Attachment of the cuff to the tooth is maintained by a thickened basal lamina and hemidesmosomes that seal off the dentogingival junction.

Pharynx

The oral cavity continues posteriorly into the pharynx, which extends from the base of the skull to the level of the cricoid cartilage, where it is continuous with the esophagus. The digestive and respiratory systems merge briefly in the pharynx, which is subdivided into nasal, oral, and laryngeal parts. The pharyngeal walls basically consist of three strata: a mucosa, a muscularis, and an adventitia.

Oropharynx

KEY WORDS: nonkeratinized stratified squamous epithelium, lamina propria, muscularis, skeletal muscle, adventitia

The oropharynx is lined by a **nonkeratinized stratified squamous epithelium** and a dense, fibroelastic **lamina propria.** Immediately beneath the lamina propria is a well-developed layer of elastic fibers that is continuous with the muscularis mucosae of the esophagus. Proximally, the elastic layer blends with the connective tissue between the muscle bundles of the pharyngeal wall. A submucosa is present only where the pharynx is continuous with the esophagus and in the lateral walls of the nasopharynx. The **muscularis** of the pharyngeal wall consists of the **skeletal muscle** of the pharyngeal constrictor muscles, which, in turn, are covered by connective tissue of the **adventitia.**

Tubular Digestive Tract

The tubular digestive tract consists of the esophagus, stomach, small intestine, colon, and rectum. Each region of the digestive tube consists of the four basic layers, but the components of these layers vary according to the functions of the region.

Esophagus

The esophagus is a relatively straight muscular tube about 25 cm long. It is continuous above with the pharynx at the inferior border of the cricoid cartilage and below becomes continuous with the cardia of the stomach.

Mucosa

KEY WORDS: nonkeratinized stratified squamous epithelium, lamina propria, muscularis mucosae, smooth muscle

The mucosa of the esophagus consists of a lining epithelium, a lamina propria, and a muscularis mucosae. The epithelial lining is thick and in humans consists of **nonkeratinized stratified squamous epithelium** that is continuous with the similiar epithelium of the oropharynx (see atlas figures 15-23 and 15-24). At the junction with stomach, the epithelium shows an abrupt transition to a simple columnar epithelium (see atlas figure 15-26). In species accustomed to a coarse diet, such as ruminants, the epithelium undergoes extensive keratinization. The **lamina propria** is a loose areolar connective tissue with diffuse and nodular lymphatic tissue scattered throughout its length. The **muscularis mucosae** consists of longitudinal **smooth muscle** cells in a fine, elastic network. Circularly arranged smooth muscle cells also may be present. The muscularis mucosae is continuous with the elastic layer of the pharynx at the level of the cricoid cartilage.

Submucosa

KEY WORDS: collagenous fiber, elastic fiber, longitudinal fold

The submucosa consists primarily of coarse **collagenous fibers** and **elastic fibers.** Within it are larger blood vessels, lymphatics, nerve fibers, occasional autonomic ganglia, and glands. Extensive **longitudinal folds** of the submucosa give the

mucosa of the nondistended esophagus a characteristic pleated appearance. During swallowing the bolus of food smooths out these folds and allows the lumen to increase in size temporarily, to accommodate the material swallowed.

Muscularis Externa

KEY WORDS: skeletal muscle, mixed smooth and skeletal muscle, smooth muscle

The upper one-fourth of the muscularis externa consists of **skeletal muscle** only. From the lower border of the inferior constrictor muscle of the pharynx, the muscle progressively becomes more regularly arranged into inner circular and outer longitudinal layers. In the second one-fourth of the human and opossum esophagi, **mixed skeletal and smooth muscle** is found, while in the distal one-half, only **smooth muscle** is present. In many species, including the dog, the muscularis externa consists only of skeletal muscle. Cells of autonomic ganglia are present between the inner and outer layers of smooth muscle.

Adventitia

A layer of loosely arranged connective tissue, the adventitia, covers the outer surface of the esophagus and binds it to surrounding structures. Below the diaphragm a short segment of the esophagus is covered by a serosa.

Glands

KEY WORDS: esophageal cardiac gland, lamina propria, esophageal glands proper, submucosa

Two types of glands are present in the esophagus: esophageal cardiac glands and esophageal glands proper. Two groups of **esophageal cardiac glands** are present, one group located in the proximal esophagus near the pharynx, the other in the distal esophagus near the cardia of the stomach. Both are compound tubuloalveolar glands of mucous type and occur only in the **lamina propria.** The **esophageal glands proper** also are mucous compound tubuloalveolar glands but are confined to the **submucosa** throughout the remaining length of the esophagus (see atlas figure 15-25).

Myoepithelial cells are associated with the secretory units in humans and a few other species. In the horse and cat, esophageal glands are absent.

Stomach

The stomach forms an expanded portion of the tubular digestive tract between the esophagus and small intestine. In humans and many other species, the stomach is divided into the cardia, a short region where the esophagus joins the stomach; the fundus, a dome-shaped elevation of the stomach wall above the esophagogastric junction; the corpus, the large central part; and the pylorus, a narrow region just above the gastrointestinal junction. The stomach stores and digests food, and although storage is not a prime function in humans, it is important in ruminants and other herbivorous species. The digestive functions of the stomach involve mechanical and chemical breakdown of ingested materials.

Mucosa

KEY WORDS: ruga, gastric lining epithelium, simple columnar, gastric pit (foveola)

The mucosa of the empty stomach has numerous folds or ridges called **rugae** that mostly disappear when the stomach is filled or stretched. The **gastric lining epithelium** is **simple columnar** and begins abruptly at the junction with the stratified squamous epithelium of the esophagus and ends just as abruptly at its junction with intestinal epithelium. In humans, the lining epithelium has a similar structure throughout the stomach and consists of secretory columnar cells that collectively form a secretory sheet. The neutral mucin produced by the surface epithelium is secreted continuously and forms a mucous film that helps protect the mucosa from the acid pepsin in the gastric lumen and lubricates the surface.

The apices of the columnar cells are held in close apposition by tight junctions, and the lateral cell membranes show numerous desmosomes. Scattered, stubby microvilli are present on the apical surfaces, and numerous discrete granules fill the apical cytoplasm. Granular endoplasmic reticulum is present in the basal cytoplasm, and well-developed Golgi complexes occupy the supranuclear region.

The gastric mucosa contains about three million minute tubular infoldings of the surface epithelium that form the **gastric pits** or **foveolae,** which are lined by the same simple columnar epithelium that covers the surface (see atlas figures 15-27 and 15-28). The epithelial cells on the surface are replaced every 4 to 5 days. New cells are derived from a small population of relatively undifferentiated cells located in the bottoms of the gastric pits. Cells from this region gradually migrate upward along the gastric pit to replace the cells of the surface epithelium.

A gastric lining of simple columnar cells as found in humans and some other species is not a universal condition. The gastric mucosa of several mammals (monotremes, certain kangaroos, rodents, ruminants, and several herbivorous species) is lined completely or in part by stratified squamous epithelium.

Three types of glands usually occur in the gastric mucosa: cardiac, gastric, and pyloric.

Cardiac Glands

KEY WORDS: Simple branched tubular gland, mucous cell, endocrine cell

In humans the cardiac glands begin immediately around the esophageal orifice and extend about 3.4 cm along the proximal stomach. They attain their greatest depth near the esophageal-gastric junction. Here, the tubular glands branch freely and appear to be aggregated into lobule-like complexes by the surrounding connective tissue of the lamina propria. Near the junction with the fundus, the cardiac glands show less branching, the distinct grouping disappears, and the thickness of the glandular area decreases. For the most part, cardiac glands are **simple branched tubular glands** that open into the overlying gastric pits (see atlas figure 15-29). The depth of the gastric pit and the length of the cardiac gland are approximately equal. The secretory units consist mainly of **mucous cells,** but occasional parietal cells are present and appear to be identical to those of gastric glands. A number of **endocrine cells** of undetermined nature also are present.

Gastric (Oxyntic) Glands

KEY WORDS: simple branched tubular gland, mucous neck cell, parietal cell, intracellular canaliculus, tubulovesicular system, hydrochloric acid, gastric intrinsic factor, chief (zymogen) cell, pepsinogen, pepsin, endocrine cell

The gastric (oxyntic) glands are the most abundant glands in the stomach (about 15 million) and are found along the entire corpus of the stomach. They are mainly **simple branched tubular glands** in humans, although in some species most are simple tubular (see atlas figures 15-30 and 15-31). The glands run perpendicular to the surface of the mucosa, and one or several glands may open into the bottom of each gastric pit. The gastric glands are about four times as long as the pits into which they open. Each gland contains mucous neck cells, parietal cells, chief (zymogen) cells, and endocrine cells.

Mucous neck cells occur primarily in the upper regions of the gastric glands, where the glands open into the gastric pits. The cells often appear to be sandwiched between other cell types, and their irregular shape is characteristic (see atlas figure 15-32). Some have broad apices and narrow bases, others show narrow apices and wide bases. The nucleus is confined to the base of the cell, surrounded by basophilic cytoplasm. Secretory granules fill the apical cytoplasm. Unlike the mucous cells that line the gastric surface, mucous neck cells produce an acidic mucin.

Although most numerous in the central area of the gastric glands, **parietal cells** also are scattered among mucous neck cells in the upper parts of the gland (see atlas figure 15-32). They are large, spherical cells whose bases often appear to bulge from the outer margin of the glands into the lamina propria. In routine sections, parietal cells are distinguished by their acidophilic cytoplasm. Each cell contains a large, centrally placed nucleus and numerous mitochondria and is characterized by **intracellular canaliculi.** These are invaginations of the plasmalemma that form channels near the nucleus and open at the apex of the cell into the lumen of the gland. Numerous microvilli project into the lumina of the canaliculi, their number and length varying according to the secretory activity of the cell. Immediately adjacent to each canaliculus, a series of smooth cytoplasmic membranes form small tubules and vesicles that make up the **tubulovesicular system** (see atlas figure 15-33). Secretion of **hydrochloric acid** occurs along the cell membrane that lines the canaliculi. During secretion of acid, the tubulovesicular membranes diminish and canalicular microvilli become more abundant and caniculi elongate; during acid inhibition, the reverse occurs. Parietal cells contain abundant carbonic anhydrase, which catalyzes the joining of carbon dioxide to water, forming carbonic acid (H_2CO_3). Once formed, H_2CO_3 immediately dissociates into hydrogen ions (H^+) and bicarbonate ions (HCO_3^-). Hydrogen ions are actively pumped into the lumen of the canaliculus, and bicarbonate ions pass back into the bloodstream. Simultaneously chloride ions (Cl^-) are actively transported from the blood by parietal cells into the canaliculi, where they combine with hydrogen ions to form hydrochloric acid. The increase in canalicular membrane surface area during parietal cell stimulation makes these events possible.

In addition to hydrochloric acid, parietal cells of the human stomach secrete a glycoprotein, **gastric intrinsic factor,** which complexes with dietary vitamin B_{12} in the gastric lumen; the complex is absorbed in the dista small intestine. A deficiency of intrinsic factor results in decreased absorption of vitamin B_{12}, an essential vitamin for the maturation and production of red blood cells. Lack of the vitamin results in pernicious anemia and is a condition often associated with atrophic gastritis.

Chief (zymogen) cells are present mainly in the basal half of the gastric glands and in routine sections are distinguished by their basophilia (see atlas figures 15-31 and 15-32). The cells contain abundant granular endoplasmic reticulum in the basal cytoplasm, well-developed Golgi bodies in the supranuclear cytoplasm, and apical zymogen granules, features that characterize cells involved in protein (enzyme) secretion (see atlas figure 15-34).

Chief cells secrete **pepsinogen,** a precursor of the enzyme **pepsin** that reaches its optimal activity at pH 2.0. The acid environment in the gastric lumen is created by the parietal cells. Pepsin is important in the gastric digestion of protein, hydrolyzing proteins into peptides.

Also scattered within the bases of the gastric glands are **endocrine cells,** peptide-producing cells that contain specific granules enclosed by smooth membranes (see atlas figure 15-35). The polarization of these cells suggests that they secrete into the bloodstream rather than into the lumina of gastric glands. The gastrointestinal hormones somatostatin, glucagon, and pancreatic peptide and the amine 5-hydroxytryptamine (5-HT, serotonin) have been identified in the endocrine cells of the gastric glands.

Kinetics of the Gastric (Oxyntic) Glands. Pluripotent stem cells located in the region where a gastric gland joins the bottom of a gastric pit (the isthmus) divide to maintain themselves as well as give rise to several committed cell types: pre-pit, pre-mucous neck, pre-parietal, and pre-endocrine. Chief cells are derived from mucous neck cells through a pre-zymogenic stage.

All pit cells migrate in the direction of the gastric lumen to become gastric lining epithelial cells and are eventually exfoliated into the lumen in about 5 days. Mucous neck cells, however, migrate inward toward the base of the glands and in about two weeks become pre-chief (zymogenic) cells. As fully differentiated chief cells form, they migrate to occupy the bottom of the gastric glands and remain active for up to 6 months. Thereafter, they are either lost by necrosis and shed into the lumen, or if apoptosis occurs, phagocytosed by adjacent chief cells or macrophages entering the area. Endocrine cells also arise at the isthmus and migrate toward the base of the glands where they are abundant. Their turnover time is about 3 months. In contrast, differentiating parietal cells migrate in both directions with about equal numbers migrating toward either the gastric lumen or the bottoms

of the gastric glands. They have a turnover rate of about 60 days and if they become necrotic are lost by extrusion in the lumen of the gland. If the parietal cells become apoptotic, they are phagocytosed by neighboring cells or macrophages.

Pyloric Glands

KEY WORDS: simple or branched tubular gland, mucous cell, endocrine cell, G cell, gastrin

The pyloric glands are confined to the distal 4 or 5 cm of the stomach. They are **simple or branched tubular glands** composed of **mucous cells** similar in appearance to mucous neck cells of the fundic region (see atlas figures 15-36 and 15-37). An occasional parietal cell may be present. The pyloric glands empty into pits that are about the same length as the glands. Numerous **endocrine cells,** mainly **G cells,** are present. These unicellular endocrine glands produce **gastrin,** a peptide hormone that stimulates acid secretion by the parietal cells in the remainder of the stomach. Endocrine cells that produce somatostatin and 5-HT are present in pyloric glands also. Thus, in addition to the exocrine function of mucus production, pyloric glands have important endocrine functions also.

Lamina Propria

The lamina propria of the stomach is obscured by the close approximation of the glands in the gastric mucosa. It consists of a delicate network of collagenous and reticular fibers that surround and extend between the glands and gastric pits. The lamina propria contains numerous capillaries. Numerous lymphocytes, some plasma cells, eosinophils, and mast cells are found within the lamina propria. Lymphatic nodules also may occur.

Muscularis Mucosa

The muscularis mucosa consists of an inner circular, an outer longitudinal, and, in some places, an additional outer circular layer of smooth muscle. Slips of smooth muscle extending into the lamina propria form a loose network around individual glands and extend to the gastric lining epithelium. The muscularis mucosae gives additional mobility to the gastric mucosa.

Submucosa

The submucosa consists of a coarse connective tissue rich in mast cells, eosinophils, and lymphatic cells. This layer contains lymph vessels and the larger blood vessels. Parent vessels pierce the stomach wall at the lesser and greater curvatures and supply smaller branches that run about the circumference of the stomach, in the submucosa. Smaller branches of the submucosal vessels enter the mucosa to provide its vascular supply.

Muscularis externa

The muscularis externa may consist of three layers of smooth muscle: outer longitudinal, middle circular, and sometimes an inner oblique. In the pylorus, the middle circular layer thickens to form the pyloric sphincter, which is thought to aid in controlling emptying of the stomach. Strong contractions of the muscle wall of the stomach create a churning action that contributes mechanically to the breakdown of ingested material and gastric emptying.

Serosa

A thin layer of loose connective tissue covers the muscularis externa and is covered on its outer aspect by the mesothelial lining of the peritoneal cavity, forming the serosa.

Small Intestine

The small intestine extends between the stomach and colon and is divided into the duodenum, jejunum, and ileum. Although there are minor microscopic differences among these subdivisions, all have the same basic organization as the rest of the digestive tube — mucosa, submucosa, muscularis externa, and serosa. The transition from one segment to another is gradual. The small intestine moves chyme from the stomach to the colon and completes the digestive processes by adding enzymes secreted by the intes-

tinal mucosa and accessory glands (liver and pancreas). Its primary function, however, is absorption.

Specializations For Absorption

KEY WORDS: plicae circulares, villus, microvillus, striated border, terminal web

Three specializations — plicae circulares, intestinal villi, and microvilli — markedly increase the surface area of the intestinal mucosa to enhance the absorptive process.

Plicae circulares are large, permanent folds that consist of the intestinal mucosa and a core of submucosa. These shelflike folds spiral about the lumen of the intestine for one-half to two-thirds of its circumference and may branch. Plicae begin in the upper duodenum, reach their maximum development in the proximal jejunum, and thereafter diminish in size and disappear in the distal half of the ileum.

The intestinal mucosa also presents numerous fingerlike evaginations, the **villi,** that cover the entire surface of the small intestine (see atlas figures 15-38, 15-39, 15-45, and 15-46). They consist of a core lamina propria and a covering of intestinal epithelium. Villi are 0.5 to 1.5 mm long and are best developed in the duodenum and jejunum, where they form broad, spatulate structures. In the ileum they become shorter and more fingerlike.

The surface of the intestine is increased almost 30-fold by the large numbers of closely packed **microvilli** on the luminal surfaces of the intestinal absorptive cells (see atlas figure 15-43). Microvilli make up the **striated border** seen by light microscopy. Each microvillus represents a cylindrical extension of the plasma membrane enclosing a small core of cytoplasm. Each microvillus contains numerous thin actin filaments that extend into the apical cytoplasm of the cell and contribute to the **terminal web,** a network of fine filaments that lies just beneath and parallel to the microvillus border. Near the lateral surface of the cell, the filaments merge with those associated with junctional complexes. The filaments and terminal web contribute to the cytoskeleton of the cell and also give mobility to the microvillus border.

Mucosa

KEY WORDS: simple columnar epithelium, villus, intestinal gland

The intestinal mucosa consists of a **simple columnar epithelium,** a lamina propria, and a muscularis mucosae. The numerous **villi** of the mucosal lining give a velvety appearance to the interior of the small intestine. Simple tubular **intestinal glands** empty between the bases of the villi (see atlas figures 15-39, 15-40, 15-41, 15-44, and 15-45). The glands measure 0.3 to 0.5 mm in depth and extend through the mucosa to the level of the muscularis mucosae, separated from one another by the connective tissue of the lamina propria. The intestinal glands contribute secretions that aid in the digestive process, but more important, they are the sites of renewal of intestinal epithelial cells as they are shed at the tips of the villi.

Epithelial Lining

KEY WORDS: intestinal absorptive cell, striated border, terminal bar, surface coat, goblet cell, endocrine cell, caveolated cell

The epithelium that lines the intestinal lumen contains a heterogeneous population of simple columnar cells. The principal type is the **intestinal absorptive cell,** a tall, cylindrical cell that rests on a delicate basement membrane and shows a prominent **striated border** (microvilli) at its free surface (see atlas figure 15-43). Prominent **terminal bars** unite the intestinal absorptive cells at their apices, and desmosomes scattered along the lateral surfaces help hold the cells in close apposition. The microvilli that make up the striated border are covered by a layer of glycoprotein that is elaborated by the intestinal epithelial cells. This glycoprotein has been called the **surface coat** and is resistant to mucolytic and proteolytic agents. It is believed to have a protective function and to be involved in the digestive process.

Although considerable digestion occurs in the intestinal lumen due to the presence of pancreatic enzymes and bile salts, a significant amount of digestion also occurs on the microvillus surface prior to absorption. Enzymes that take part in the breakdown of disaccharides and polypeptides are present in or along the plasma membrane of the microvilli. In addition to contributing to the digestive process, the intestinal absorptive cells are actively involved in the absorption of protein, amino acids, carbohydrates, and lipids from the intestinal lumen. Absorbed materials passing through the epithelium must enter the cell through the apical plasmalemma and are prevented from passing between the cells by the zonulae occludens, which form a tight seal around the apices of the cells. Sugars and proteins pass through the basal cell membrane to enter blood capillaries in the connective tissue cores of the villi.

Lipid absorption is peculiar in its pathway through the intestinal absorptive cells and in the fact that lipids enter lymphatic channels rather than the blood vascular system. Triglycerides are broken down to fatty acids and S-monoglycerides by pancreative lipase in the intestinal lumen. Resynthesis of triglycerides occurs in the smooth endoplasmic reticulum of the apical cytoplasm after they pass through the apical cell membrane. The reformed lipid makes its way to Golgi complexes, where it is complexed with protein to form lipoprotein droplets called chylomicrons. Chylomicrons have no limiting membranes and are discharged through the lateral cell walls of the intestinal absorptive cells into the intercellular space at the level of the nucleus, thus bypassing the basal regions (see atlas figure 15-87). The chylomicrons pass down the intercellular spaces, through the basal lamina, and enter lymphatic channels (lacteals) after passing between endothelial cells.

Goblet cells are scattered between the intestinal absorptive cells and increase in number distally in the intestinal tract. The mucus secreted by these unicellular exocrine glands lubricates and protects the mucosal surface. The apical regions of the goblet cells often are expanded by the accumulation of secretory granules; the base forms a slender region that contains the nucleus, scattered profiles of granular endoplasmic reticulum, and occasional Golgi complexes. Goblet cells lie within the lining epithelium and are united to intestinal absorptive cells by apical tight junctions and scattered desmosomes along the lateral surfaces. Goblet cells also migrate from the intestinal glands, eventually to exfoliate at the tip of the villus. In humans, the life span of goblet cells is about 4 to 5 days. They may secrete continuously but are believed to pass through only one secretory cycle.

Endocrine cells also are present in the epithelial lining, scattered within the epithelium of the villi and glands, but are far fewer in number than goblet cells. Endocrine cells secrete peptide hormones that influence gastric and intestinal secretion and motility, gallbladder contraction, and pancreatic and liver function (Table 15-2 and Fig. 15-2). They are characterized by dense secretory granules, scattered profiles of granular endoplasmic reticulum, and an electron-lucent cytoplasm. In addition to the hormones of the endocrine cell, numerous peptide hormones (neurotensin, substance P, vasoactive intestinal polypeptide, somatostatin, enkephalins) occur in the neurons of the enteric plexus. Whether these peptides serve as neurotransmitters or neuromodulators is not known.

Another cell type, the **caveolated cell,** may be seen occasionally in the epithelial lining. It is a pear-shaped cell with a wide base and narrow apex that protrudes slightly into the lumen. These cells are held in close apposition to neighboring epithelial cells by tight junctions and desmosomes. Caveolated cells have large microvilli that typically contain bundles of filaments that extend deep into the supranuclear region. Between the bundles of filaments, caveolae form small elongated channels that extend from the apical cell membrane between microvilli into the deep, apical cytoplasm. This cell type occurs elsewhere in the gastrointestinal tract and other organs of endodermal origin. They may be chemoreceptors in some regions, as in the respiratory system, but their function in the intestine is unknown.

Intestinal Glands

KEY WORDS: **undifferentiated cell, oligomucous cell, Paneth cell, intraepithelial lymphocyte**

All epithelial cells that line the intestinal surface arise from cells in the intestinal glands. The upper regions of the glands are lined by simple columnar epithelium that is similar to and continuous with that lining the intestinal lumen. It contains absorptive cells, goblet cells, scattered endocrine cells, and a few caveolated cells. **Undifferentiated cells** line the basal half of the intestinal glands and undergo frequent mitoses. Intestinal absorptive cells and **oligomucous cells,** which represent intermediate stages of goblet cell formation, lie in the mid-gland region. New intestinal epithelial cells are formed continually in the basal region of the glands, migrate by upward displacement of cells, and ultimately come to cover the villi and the entire intestinal surface. The oldest intestinal epithelial cells are shed at the tips of the villi. Complete turnover of the epithelium of the glands and lining of the intestine occurs every 4 to 5 days. As absorptive intestinal cells migrate up the villus, they increase in height and the striated border becomes more prominent.

Small groups of pyramidal-shaped cells with conspicuous granules are found at the bases of the intestinal glands. These are **Paneth cells,** which, unlike other cells of the intestinal epithelium, form a relatively stable population with a low rate of turnover (see atlas figure 15-44). Paneth cells are abundant in humans, monkeys, ruminants, and several species of rodents. Their function is unknown.

Intraepithelial lymphocytes often are seen between and within intestinal epithelial cells that cover villi or line glands.

Lamina Propria

KEY WORDS: **lymphatic nodule, Peyer's patch, M-cell, central lacteal**

The connective tissue of the lamina propria forms the cores of the villi and fills the areas between intestinal glands. The intestinal lamina propria

Table 15-2. Hormones and Related Substances of the Alimentary Canal

Hormone	Primary Location of Endocrine Cells	Primary Action
Gastrin	Antrum of stomach (G cell)	Stimulates acid secretion
Secretin	Duodenal and proximal jejunal mucosae (S cell)	Controls pancreatic H_2CO_3 secretion and biliary H_2O/ion secretion
Cholecystokinin	Mucosae of duodenum and jejunum (I cell)	Stimulates pancreatic enzyme secretion, gallbladder contraction
Enteroglucagon	Mucosa of ileum (L cell) and fundus (A cell)	Stimulates hepatic glyconeogenesis
Gastric inhibitory peptide	Mucosae of duodenum and jejunum (K cell)	Inhibits acid secretion
Motilin	Mucosa of jejunum (one type of enterochromaffin cell, EC_2)	Strong stimulator of motor activity in intestines
Vasoactive intestinal polypeptide	Gastric, small intestinal, and colonic mucosae (D_1 cell)	Stimulates intestinal motility, H_2O/ion secretion
Somatostatin	Mucosae of stomach, duodenum, and jejunum (D cell)	Inhibits the action or release of other hormones (paracrine functions)
Neurotensin	Mucosa of ileum (N cell)	Stimulates contractions of muscularis externa
Serotonin	Mucosae of small intestine and colon (enterochromaffin (EC) cells)	Stimulates intestinal motility
Histamine	Fundic mucosa of stomach (enterochromaffin-like (ECL) cell)	Stimulates secretion and intestinal motility and is a vasodilator
Bombesin-like peptide	Mucosae of stomach and jejunum (P cell)	Stimulates gastric acid secretion and exocrine pancreas secretion
Substance P	Gastric mucosa (EC_1 cell)	Stimulates intestinal motility

is rich in reticular fibers that form a delicate meshwork containing numerous reticular cells, lymphocytes, plasma cells, macrophages, and eosinophils, giving the lamina propria a very cellular appearance. The lamina propria of the intestinal tract represents a special type of lymphatic tissue and is part of the gut-associated lymphatic tissue (GALT). The free cells of the lamina propria provide a protective sleeve that encircles the intestinal lumen immediately below the epithelium. Lymphocytes are the most numerous cells present and provide a vast reserve of immunocompetent cells. Plasma cells elaborate immunoglobulin A (IgA), which is taken up by the intestinal absorptive cells and complexed to a protein (secretory piece) that is synthesized by the absorptive cell. The complex is then released from the cell and provides a protective surface for the epithelial cells — an immunologic border — against viruses and bacteria. The secretory piece acts as a carrier for the IgA and possibly protects it from lysosomal digestion while it is within the cell and from enzymatic digestion on the luminal surface. Lymphocytes often leave the lamina pro-

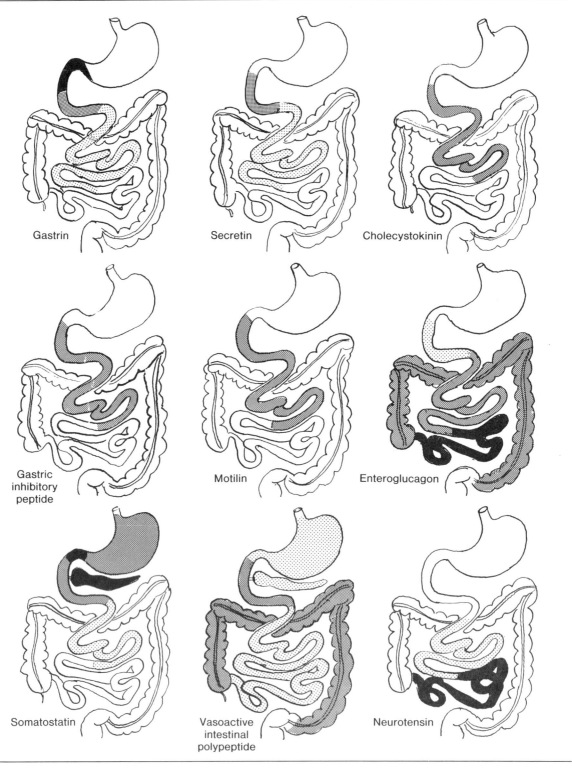

Fig. 15-2. Distribution of endocrine cells in humans.

pria to migrate through the intestinal epithelium into the lumen of the intestine.

Lymphatic nodules of variable size lie in the lamina propria, scattered along the entire intestinal tract, but become larger and more numerous distally. They are particularly numerous and well developed in the ileum and often extend the full thickness of the mucosa. The lymphatic nodules may be solitary or grouped together in aggregates called **Peyer's patches** (see atlas figure 15-47). These oval structures may be quite large — 20 mm in length — and are visible to the naked eye. Peyer's patches may occupy the full depths of the mucosa and submucosa.

A peculiar type of cell, the **M-cell,** lies in the intestinal epithelium that covers the lymphatic nodules. The cells shows characteristic microplicae on the luminal surface, rather than microvilli. M-cells sequester intact macromolecules from the intestinal lumen and transport them in membrane-bound vesicles to intraepithelial lymphocytes. The sensitized lymphocytes then migrate to various aggregates of lymphatic tissue in the lamina propria or mesenteric lymph nodes, transporting information to sites of antibody production. M-cells provide a way for the immune system to maintain immunologic surveillance of the environment in the gut lumen and to respond appropriately to any changes. M-cell monitoring of the intestinal lumen is not unique. Langerhans' cells of the epidermis perform a similar function in monitoring the external environment and relaying information to the immune system. Both are considered to be antigen-presenting cells.

Lymphatic vessels occur in the lamina propria and are important in fat absorption. Dilated lymphatic channels begin blindly in the cores of villi near their tips and form the **central lacteals.** Their walls consist of thin endothelial cells surrounded by basal lamina and reticular fibers. At the bases of the villi, the lymphatic capillaries anastomose with those coursing between intestinal glands and form a plexus before passing through the muscularis mucosae. In the submucosa they join larger lymphatic vessels. Vessels that pierce the muscularis mucosae may contain valves.

Muscularis Mucosa

KEY WORDS: inner circular layer, outer longitudinal layer

The muscularis mucosa is well defined and consists of an **inner circular layer** and an **outer longitudinal layer** of smooth muscle. It is intimately associated with thin elastic fibers. Slips of smooth muscle leave the muscularis mucosae and enter the cores of villi to provide the means by which villi contract. Contraction of villi continuously provides the intestinal epithelium covering the villi with a fresh environment for maximum absorptive efficiency. The pumplike action during contraction also aids in moving absorbed materials into the blood and lymphatic capillaries, out of vessels in the lamina propria and into the larger vessels of the submucosa, and thus further aids the absorptive process.

Small arteries run on the inner surface of the muscularis mucosae and break up into capillary networks that form a dense network of fenestrated capillaries just beneath the intestinal epithelium (see atlas figure 15-42). Near the tips of villi, the capillaries drain into small veins that run downward to anastomose with a venous plexus surrounding the intestinal glands, before joining veins in the submucosa.

Submucosa

KEY WORDS: duodenal (Brunner's) gland, branched tubular gland, urogastrone, epidermal growth factor, submucosal plexus

The submucosa consists of coarse collagenous fibers and numerous elastic fibers. It often contains lobules of adipose tissue as well as the cells normally associated with loose connective tissue. In the ileum it may contain large aggregates of lymphoid cells derived from Peyer's patches. The submucosa of the duodenum houses the **duodenal (Brunner's) glands,** the ducts of which pierce the muscularis mucosae (see atlas figure 15-48). In most marsupials, some insectivores, and several ungulates (deer, pronghorn, moose, elk, bison, sheep), the ducts empty directly into the intestinal lumen. In all other species, including humans, the ducts drain into overlying intestinal glands. These **branched tubular glands** are first encountered immediately distal to the pyloric sphincter and also may be found in the proximal jejunum in some species. They often occur in the submucosal cores of the plicae circulares. The duodenal glands are the only submucosal glands present in the gastrointestinal tract and are present only in mammals.

The duodenal glands consist of secretory cells with ultrastructural features of serous and mucous glands. In rabbits, both serous and mucous cells are present. The duodenal glands secrete a mucin-containing, alkaline fluid that protects the duodenal mucosa proximal to the entrance of the pancreatic duct from the erosive effects of acid pepsin from the stomach. Cells of the human duodenal glands show immunoreactivity for **urogastrone,** a peptide that is a potent inhibitor of gastric acid secretion, and **epidermal growth factor,** a peptide that may control proliferation and migration of intestinal epithelial cells in the proximal small intestine.

Nerve fibers and parasympathetic ganglia form a **submucosal plexus** found in the submucosa of the esophagus, stomach, and small and large intestines (see atlas figure 15-49). This plexus provides motor innervation for the muscularis mucosae and the slips of smooth muscle that enter villi or other regions of the mucosa. Large blood and lymphatic vessels also are found in the submucosa. The large mesenteric vessels pierce the muscularis externa at its attachment to the mesentery, then enter the submucosa, branch, and run around the circumference of the intestinal tube. The submucosal vessels supply and receive small tributaries from the overlying mucosa.

Muscularis Externa

KEY WORDS: **inner circular layer, outer longitudinal layer, myenteric plexus**

The muscularis externa consists of **inner circular** and **outer longitudinal layers** of smooth muscle. Both layers take a helical course around the intestinal tube. The fibers in the outer layer form a more gradual helix, giving the impression of a longitudinal arrangement. Between the two layers of smooth muscle are the nerve fibers and parasympathetic ganglia of the **myenteric plexus.** This supplies the motor innervation to the muscularis externa of the entire gastrointestinal tract.

Serosa

The muscularis externa is invested by a thin layer of loose connective tissue covered by a layer of mesothelial cells of the visceral peritoneum. Where the mesentery attaches to the intestinal wall, the serosa becomes continuous with both sides of the mesentery and encloses connective tissue elements, blood vessels, and nerves.

Ileocecal Junction

The lumen of the ileum becomes continuous with that of the large intestine at the ileocecal junction. Here the lining is thrown into anterior and posterior folds called ileocecal valves, which consist of both the mucosa and submucosa surrounded by a thickening of the inner circular layer of the muscularis externa.

Large Intestine

The large intestine is approximately 180 cm long and is divided into several regions. The cecum is continuous with the ileum at the ileocecal junction and forms a blind pouch at the proximal end of the colon. It bears the appendix, a small, slender diverticulum. The remainder of the colon is divided into ascending, transverse, and descending parts that, structurally, show the same features. The large intestine is continuous with the rectum and anal canal, the latter terminating as the anus.

Mucosa

KEY WORDS: **lacks villi, absorptive cell, goblet cell, fluid absorption, mucus secretion**

The mucosa of the large intestine **lacks villi** and has a smooth interior surface (see atlas figures 15-50 and 15-51). The lumen is lined by a simple columnar epithelium that consists of intestinal **absorptive cells** and **goblet cells.** The latter increase in number toward the rectum so that in the distal region of the colon, the epithelium consists mainly of goblet cells.

Intestinal glands of the colon are larger and more closely packed than those in the small intestine, and they increase in length distally to reach their maximum depth (0.7 mm) in the rectum (see atlas figures 15-50 and 15-51). The glands contain numerous goblet cells and, in the basal half of the glands, proliferating and undifferentiated epithelial cells and endocrine cells are present. Paneth's cells usually are absent. The turnover rate for intestinal epithelial cells in the colon is about 6 days.

The composition of the lamina propria and muscularis mucosae is the same as that of the small intestine. Scattered lymphatic nodules are present and may protrude through the muscularis mucosae to lie in the submucosa.

Ingested material enters the cecum as a semifluid and becomes semisolid in the colon. Although no digestive enzymes are secreted by the colon, some digestion does occur as a result of enzymes present in the developing fecal mass and through the action of bacterial flora normally associated with the large intestine. The primary functions of the large intestine are the **fluid absorption** and the **mucus secretion** to protect the mucosa from abrasion by the developing feces.

Submucosa

The submucosa of the colon is similar to that of the small intestine and contains the larger vessels and the submucosal plexus. Glands are not present. As in the remainder of the digestive tube, blood vessels pierce the muscularis externa and course around the circumference of the intestinal wall. The large vessels supply tributaries that penetrate the muscularis mucosae and form capillary networks in the lamina propria, around intestinal glands, and beneath the lining epithelium. The veins follow the same course as the arteries.

Muscularis Externa

KEY WORDS: taeniae coli, haustrum, plicae semilunares

The outer, longitudinal coat of the muscularis externa of the cecum and colon differs from that of the small intestine in that it forms three longitudinal bands called the **taeniae coli.** Between the taeniae the muscle coat is thinner and may be incomplete. The inner circular layer is complete and appears similar to that of the small intestine. Components of the myenteric plexus lie just external to the circular layer, as in the small intestine. Due to the tonus of the taeniae coli, the wall of the colon is gathered into outwardly bulging pockets, the **haustra.** Crescentic folds called **plicae semilunares** project into the lumen of the colon between the haustra.

Serosa

KEY WORDS: adventitia, appendices epiploicae

The serosa is incomplete in the colon, and the ascending and descending limbs are retroperitoneal. Here the muscular wall of the colon is attached to adjacent structures by an **adventitia.** Where a serosa is present, it may contain large, pendulous lobules of fat called **appendices epiploicae.**

Appendix

The structure of the appendix resembles that of the colon, but in miniature. The lumen is small and irregular in outline, and taeniae coli are absent. The lamina propria is extensively infiltrated with lymphocytes, and details of the mucosa often are obscured by the many lymphatic nodules that may fill the mucosa and submucosa.

Recto-Anal Junction

KEY WORDS: pectinate line, circumanal gland, rectal column, anal valve, hemorrhoidal plexus, internal anal sphincter, external anal sphincter

The mucosa of the first part of the rectum is similar to that of the colon except that the intestinal glands are slightly longer and the lining epithelium is composed primarily of goblet cells. The distal 2 to 3 cm of the rectum forms the anal canal, which ends at the anus. Immediately proximal to the **pectinate line,** the intestinal glands become shorter, then disappear. At the pectinate line the simple columnar epithelium makes an abrupt transition to noncornified stratified squamous epithelium (see atlas figure 15-52). After a short transition, the noncornified stratified squamous epithelium becomes continuous with the keratinized stratified squamous epithelium of the skin at the level of the external anal sphincter. Beneath the epithelium of this region are simple tubular apocrine sweat glands, the **circumanal glands,** which secrete an oily material. Circumanal glands are well developed in some species, especially during breeding cycles.

Proximal to the pectinate line, the mucosa of the anal canal forms large longitudinal folds called **rectal columns** (of Morgagni). The distal ends of the rectal columns are united by transverse mucosal folds, the **anal valves.** The recess above each valve forms an anal sinus. It is at the level of the anal valves that the muscularis mucosae becomes discontinuous, then disappears.

The submucosa of the anal canal contains numerous veins that form a large **hemorrhoidal plexus.** When distended (varicosed), these vessels protrude into the overlying mucosa and form internal hemorrhoids (piles). The inner circular layer of the muscularis externa increases in thickness and ends as the **internal anal sphincter.** The thin outer muscular layer breaks up and ends by blending with the surrounding connective tissue. Skeletal muscle fibers circumscribe the distal anal canal and form the **external anal sphincter,** which is under voluntary control.

Liver

The liver is the largest organ in the body and is both an endocrine and exocrine gland, releasing several substances directly into the bloodstream and secreting bile into a duct system.

The liver is uniquely situated with respect to the venous blood flow from the gastrointestinal tract. Blood from the portal vein, which drains the gastrointestinal tract, passes through the substance of the liver before entering the systemic circulation. The liver therefore receives all of the materials absorbed by the gastrointestinal tract except lipids, which are carried by lym-

phatics to enter the general circulation. Tributaries of the portal vein empty into hepatic sinusoids that drain into hepatic veins. The arrangement in the liver of a set of sinusoids between veins is called the *hepatic portal system.* The liver also has an arterial supply from the hepatic artery, and both the venous (portal) and arterial (hepatic) bloods percolate through the liver sinusoids and exit by way of the hepatic vein.

Structural Organization

KEY WORDS: capsule, hepatocyte, sinusoid, central vein, hepatic lobule, portal area, portal vein, hepatic artery, bile duct, lymphatic channel, liver acinus, portal lobule, subcapsular limiting plate

The liver is invested by a delicate connective tissue **capsule** that is continuous with the peritoneum. The capsule contains numerous elastic fibers and is covered by a mesothelium except for a small bare area where the liver abuts the diaphragm.

The liver is composed of epithelial cells, the **hepatocytes,** arranged in branching and anastomosing plates separated by blood **sinusoids.** Both form a radial pattern about a **central vein** that is the smallest tributary of the hepatic vein. The spokelike arrangement of hepatic plates about a central vein constitutes the basis of the classic **hepatic lobule,** which appears somewhat hexagonal in cross section, with a central vein at the center and portal areas at the corners (see atlas figure 15-53). The liver consists of about one million such units, each about 0.7 mm wide and 2.0 mm long.

A **portal area** contains a branch of the **portal vein,** a branch of the **hepatic artery,** a **bile duct,** and occasionally a **lymphatic channel** (see atlas figure 15-54). All are enclosed in a common investment of connective tissue. Blood passes from small branches of the hepatic artery and portal vein into the sinusoids that lie between plates of hepatocytes. Blood flows slowly through the sinusoids toward the center of the lobule and exits through the central vein. Hepatocytes nearest the branches of the portal vein and hepatic artery — that is, at the periphery of the lobule — receive blood with the highest nutrient and oxygen content. Both diminish as blood flows toward the central vein. Due to this arrangement, three zones can be recognized in a hepatic lobule according to the metabolic activity: a zone of permanent function at the periphery, a zone of intermittent activity near the center of the lobule, and a zone of permanent repose near the central vein. In the pig, camel, and raccoon, the classic lobule is bounded by a delicate connective tissue, but this limiting connective tissue is not present in humans. However, the boundaries of the hepatic lobule (see Fig. 15-3) can be estimated by observing the central vein and noting the portal areas at the corners of the lobule.

Also related to the blood supply is a smaller unit of liver structure called the liver acinus or functional unit (Fig. 15-3). The **liver acinus** is defined as the hepatic tissue supplied by a terminal branch of the hepatic artery and portal vein and drained by a terminal branch of the bile duct. It is represented by a diamond-shaped area with central veins at two of the opposite corners. Branches of the vessels and a branch of the bile duct lie between the two portions of adjacent hepatic lobules that they supply.

An additional lobule is related to the exocrine secretion (of bile) in the liver. This unit is the **portal lobule** and has a portal canal at its center. It consists of the hepatic tissue that is drained by a bile duct of a portal area. A portal lobule is triangular in shape and contains parts of three adjacent hepatic lobules. A central vein is located at each corner of this unit.

A single layer of small, dark hepatocytes limits the liver parenchyma beneath the capsule and is called the **subcapsular limiting plate.** A similar wall of hepatic cells surrounds the portal areas and forms the periportal limiting plate, which is pierced by tributaries of the hepatic artery, portal vein, and bile ductules.

Hepatic Sinusoids

KEY WORDS: discontinuous endothelium, fenestration, perisinusoidal space, hepatic macrophage, Kupffer cell, lipocyte

Hepatic sinusoids are larger and more irregular in shape than ordinary capillaries (see atlas figure 15-55). The sinusoidal lining consists of a simple layer of squamous epithelium supported by very little connective tissue. Three types of cells are associated with the sinusoidal lining: endothelial cells, stellate cells (Kupffer cells or hepatic macrophages), and fat-storing cells (lipocytes).

Endothelial cells constitute the major cellular element of the sinusoidal lining and in most species, including humans, form a **discontinuous endothelium.** There is no basal lamina and the cells are separated by gaps 0.2 to 0.5 μm wide. The endothelial cells also show numerous intracellular **fenestrations** or pores (see atlas figure 15-56). There are species differences in the structure of sinusoids, and in sheep, goats, and cows, the endothelium is continuous, the endothelial cells show fewer fenestrations, and there is a distinct basement membrane.

Where a discontinuous, fenestrated endothelium is present, as in humans, the sinusoidal lining is separated from the liver cells by a narrow **perisinusoidal space** (see atlas figures 15-56 and 15-58). Blood plasma flows freely through the endothelium and into the space, but the sinusoidal lining does hold back erythrocytes. Although occasional bundles of reticular fibers and fine collagenous fibers are present in the perisinusoidal space, there is no ground substance and the flow of blood plasma is unhindered. Because the plasma has direct access to the perisinusoidal space, the liver cells are constantly bathed on one surface by fluid that is rich in the nutrients absorbed by the intestinal tract. Thus, the perisinusoidal space has considerable significance in the exchange of materials between the liver and plasma. The plasmalemma of the hepatocytes that face the perisinusoidal space bear numerous well-developed microvilli that project into the

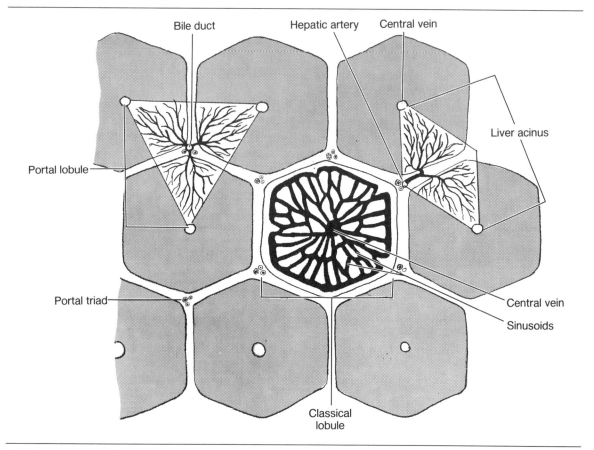

Fig. 15-3. Diagram of liver lobules.

space and greatly increase the surface area and facilitate absorption.

Also present in the sinusoidal lining are actively phagocytic cells, variously called stellate cells, **hepatic macrophages,** or **Kupffer cells** (see atlas figures 15-57 and 15-58). These form part of the sinusoidal lining and are irregularly shaped cells that expose the greater part of their cytoplasm to the blood in the sinusoid and extend processes between the endothelial cells. Unlike the neighboring endothelial cells, the cytoplasm of the hepatic phagocytes contains vacuoles, lysosomes, Golgi bodies, and short profiles of granular endoplasmic reticulum. Phagocytized material also may be present. The cells are part

of the mononuclear system of macrophages and arise from monocytes of the bone marrow.

The third type of cell is located on the side of the sinusoidal lining that faces the perisinusoidal space. This cell accumulates lipid and is most numerous in the peripheral and intermediate zones of the hepatic lobule. They have been called **lipocytes,** fat-storing, stellate, or interstitial cells, but their function is unknown.

Hepatocytes

KEY WORDS: polyploid, bile canaliculus

The parenchyma of the liver consists of large polyhedral hepatocytes arranged in plates that radiate from the region of the central vein. The surfaces of an individual hepatocyte either contact an adjacent liver cell or border on a perisinusoidal space. This latter surface bears numerous well-developed microvilli. The plates of hepatocytes are supported by a delicate stroma that consists mostly of reticular fibers.

The nuclei of hepatocytes are large and round and usually occupy the center of the cell. A single nucleus usually is present, but as many as 25 percent of hepatocytes are binucleate. There also is considerable variation in the size of nuclei from cell to cell, reflecting the **polyploid** nature of hepatocytes.

The cytoplasm of hepatocytes is rich in organelles — large arrays of granular endoplasmic reticulum, a moderate amount of smooth endoplasmic reticulum, mitochondria, Golgi complexes, peroxisomes, and lysosomes. Inclusions such as glycogen and lipid also are common. Glycogen often appears as dense rosettes (alpha particles) made up of smaller beta particles. The alpha particles measure 20 to 30 nm in diameter. The cytoplasm is variable in appearance and changes with the nutritive state of the organ.

Tiny channels, the **bile canaliculi,** course through the parenchyma between hepatocytes to end in the bile ducts of the portal areas. Bile canaliculi represent an expansion of the intercellular space, and their walls are formed by the adjacent plasmalemma of two neighboring hepatocytes (see atlas figure 15-59). Short microvilli extend from the cell membrane into the lumen. At the margins of the canaliculus, the plasma membranes are joined by occluding junctions similar to the zonula occludens in other epithelia. They form a seal to prevent bile from escaping into the intercellular spaces between hepatocytes. Golgi complexes of hepatic cells often lie adjacent to the canaliculi. The bile canaliculi show intermittent contractions.

Bile Ducts

KEY WORDS: bile ductule, interlobular bile duct, extrahepatic duct, common hepatic duct, common bile duct

Bile canaliculi unite with bile ducts in the portal canals via small, interconnecting channels called **bile ductules** (see atlas figure 15-60). They are small and have thin walls, and their small lumina are surrounded by a low cuboidal epithelium that rests on a distinct basal lamina. The terminal ductules empty into **interlobular bile ducts** of the portal areas (see atlas figure 15-61). The lumina of the bile ducts increase in diameter as they course toward the exterior, and the lining epithelium increases in height. Interlobular ducts unite to form the **extrahepatic ducts,** in which the surrounding layers of connective tissue become thicker and the lining epithelium becomes tall columnar. Two large extrahepatic ducts, the left and right hepatic ducts, unite to form the major excretory duct of the liver, the **common hepatic duct.** It is joined by the cystic duct from the gallbladder to form the **common bile duct** (ductus choledochus), which empties into the duodenum.

The major extrahepatic ducts are lined by a tall columnar, mucus-secreting epithelium. The remainder of the wall consists of a thick layer of connective tissue that is rich in elastic fibers and often contains numerous lymphocytes and occasional migrating granulocytes. Bundles of smooth muscle, running in longitudinal and oblique directions, are present in the common bile duct and form an incomplete layer that spirals around the lumen. Near the wall of the duodenum, the smooth muscle forms a complete investment and thickens to form a small sphincter, the sphincter choledochus. Distal to this region, the common bile duct and the major pancreatic duct merge as they pass through the intestinal wall and empty through a common structure, the hepatopancreatic ampulla. As the ducts pierce the duodenal wall, they are surrounded by a common sphincter of smooth muscle.

Bile is produced continuously by the liver and ultimately leaves the organ through the extrahepatic duct system. Resistance at the sphincters forces bile to enter the cystic duct and pass into the gallbladder, where it is stored. Bile formation occurs primarily at two anatomic sites: bile canaliculi and bile ductules. Secretin increases secretion of ductular bile, which is rich in bicarbonate. Glucagon increases canalicular bile secretion.

One function of the liver is to store carbohydrate in the form of glycogen. When needed, glycogen is released to the bloodstream as glucose. The liver has functions in protein metabolism; fat metabolism and storage; synthesis of fibrinogen, prothrombin, and albumin; storage of several vitamins (primarily A, D, B_2, B_3, B_4, and B_{12}); and detoxification of lipid-soluble drugs and alcohol. Detoxified materials are excreted by hepatocytes into the bile and conducted by the biliary duct system to the intestinal tract for elimination.

Bile is a complex exocrine secretion of the liver and contains bile acids, bile pigments, bile salts, cholesterol, lecithin, soaps, and neutral fats. Bile salts act as emulsifying agents and are important in the breakdown of fat in the intestinal lumen during digestion. Some bile salts may be reabsorbed in the intestinal tract to be secreted once again into the bile. This reuse of bile salts is referred to as the *enterohepatic circulatory system.*

Gallbladder

KEY WORDS: cystic duct, mucous membrane, simple columnar epithelium, lamina propria, muscularis, adventitia, serosa

The gallbladder is a saclike structure on the inferior surface of the liver, measuring about 4 cm wide and 8 cm long. It is joined to the common hepatic duct by the **cystic duct,** whose mucous membrane forms prominent spiraling folds that contain bundles of smooth muscle. These folds make up the spiral valve that prevents the collapse or distention of the cystic duct during sudden changes in pressure. The wall of the gallbladder consists of a mucous membrane, a muscularis, and a serosa or adventitia.

The **mucous membrane** of the gallbladder wall consists of a **simple columnar epithelium** and an underlying lamina propria (see atlas figures 15-62 through 15-64). The oval nuclei are located basally in the cells, and the luminal surfaces show

numerous short microvilli. The apices of adjacent cells are joined, near the lumen, by typical zonula occludens junctions. The epithelium rests on a thin basal lamina that separates it from the delicate connective tissue of the **lamina propria,** which contains numerous small blood vessels. Occasional glands are found in the lamina propria, especially where the gallbladder joins the cystic duct. These small, simple tubuloalveolar glands are thought to secrete mucus. The mucosa of the nondistended gallbladder forms large irregular folds called rugae, which flatten out as the gallbladder fills with bile (see atlas figure 15-63).

There is no submucosa in the gallbladder. The **muscularis** consists of interlacing bundles of smooth muscle that spiral around the lumen of the gallbladder. Gaps between the smooth muscle bundles are filled with collagenous, reticular, and elastic fibers. Because of the musculoelastic wall and the rugae, the gallbladder has considerable capacity for distention.

The surrounding fibroconnective tissue of the **adventitia** is fairly dense and is continuous with the connective tissue of the liver capsule. The free surface of the gallbladder (that exposed to the abdominal cavity) is covered by a **serosa.**

The gallbladder stores and concentrates bile, which is elaborated continuously by the liver. In humans the gallbladder may contain 30 to 50 ml of bile. On stimulation by cholecystokinin, the gallbladder wall contracts and the sphincters of the common bile duct and ampulla relax, allowing bile to be released into the duodenum. Some species, such as the white tailed deer and the rat, lack a gallbladder.

Pancreas

The pancreas is the second largest gland associated with the gastrointestinal tract. In humans it is a retroperitoneal organ, 20 to 25 cm long, extending transversely from the duodenum across the posterior abdominal wall to the spleen. Macroscopically it consists of a head that lies in the C-shaped curve of the duodenum, a slightly constricted neck, and a body that forms the bulk of the pancreas. It lacks a definite capsule but is covered by a thin layer of areolar connective tissue that extends delicate septae into the substance of the pancreas and subdivides it into numerous small lobules. Blood vessels, nerves, lymphatics, and excretory ducts course through the septae. The major excretory duct runs the length of the pancreas, collecting side branches along its course. The duct and its branches give some structural support to the gland.

The pancreas consists of an exocrine portion, which elaborates numerous digestive enzymes, and an endocrine portion whose secretions are important in carbohydrate metabolism. Unlike the liver, the exocrine and endocrine functions of the pancreas are performed by different groups of cells.

Exocrine Pancreas

KEY WORDS: compound tubuloacinar (alveolar) gland, pyramidal cell, zymogen granule, digestive enzyme, secretory canaliculus

The exocrine pancreas is a large, lobulated, **compound tubuloacinar (alveolar) gland** in which the secretory units are tubular or flask-shaped (see atlas figure 15-65). A delicate network of reticular fibers surrounds each secretory unit and forms the supporting stroma. Each acinus consists of a single layer of large **pyramidal cells** whose narrow apices border on a lumen, while their broad bases lie on a thin basement membrane (see atlas figure 15-66). A single, spherical nucleus is located near the base of the acinar cell, and one or more nucleoli may be present. The basal and perinuclear cytoplasm is filled with granular endoplasmic reticulum and mitochondria (see atlas figure 15-68). Extensive Golgi complexes occupy the supranuclear region and are associated with forming zymogen granules. Mature **zymogen granules** are large, spherical, homogeneous structures that are limited by a membrane and often fill the apical cytoplasm. The pancreatic acinar cell, as indicated by its morphology, is actively involved in the synthesis and release of proteins (enzymes).

Digestive enzymes of the pancreas are synthe-

sized in the granular endoplasmic reticulum of the acinar cell and pass through the cisternae of this organelle to reach the Golgi complex in small transport vesicles. Precursors of the enzymes are packaged into zymogen granules by membranes of the Golgi complex. The granules then are liberated into the apical cytoplasm, where they accumulate. When the enzymes are to be released from the cell, the granules migrate to the apical cell membrane and discharge their contents into the acinar lumen by exocytosis. The contents of the granules may also be discharged into fine **secretory canaliculi** that lie between adjacent acinar cells and are continuous with the acinar lumen. Pancreatic acinar cells secrete amylases, endopeptidases (lipases, trypsin, chymotrypsin) that cleave central peptide bonds, and exopeptidases (carboxypeptidases A and B) that cleave terminal peptide bonds. Together, these proteolytic enzymes cleave proteins in the intestinal lumen into peptide fragments that then are reduced to amino acids prior to absorption.

Deoxyribonuclease and ribonuclease also are produced by pancreatic acinar cells and digest deoxyribonucleoprotein and ribonucleoprotein, respectively. Pancreatic amylase breaks down starch and glycogen to disaccharides, and pancreatic lipase cleaves neutral fat into fatty acid and glycerol.

Duct System

KEY WORDS: centroacinar cell, intercalated duct, intralobular duct, interlobular duct, secretin, cholecystokinin, enterokinase

An extensive duct system permeates the pancreas. At their beginnings, the ducts extend into the acini and are interposed between the acinar cells and the lumen. Ductal cells within the pancreatic acini are called **centroacinar cells** and appear as flattened, light-staining cells with few organelles (see atlas figure 15-66). The wall of the short initial segment of the duct system is lined by centroacinar cells and is continuous, outside the secretory unit, with **intercalated** and **intralobular ducts** (see atlas figures 15-65 and 15-68). These ducts are tributaries of the **interlobular**

ducts found in the loose connective tissue between lobules; the transition between ducts is gradual (see atlas figure 15-67). The epithelial lining begins as simple squamous in the intercalated ducts, increases in depth to cuboidal in the intralobular ducts, and is columnar in the interlobular ducts. Scattered goblet cells and endocrine cells also are found in the ductal system. The cells lining the ducts stain lightly, and organelles are not prominent in their cytoplasm. Desmosomes are scattered along the lateral cell surfaces, and the apices of adjoining cells are united by tight junctions. The apical surfaces bear microvilli.

A scanty connective tissue consisting mainly of reticular cells supports the intercalated and intralobular ducts. The interlobular and major secretory ducts are contained within the interlobular septae and thus are surrounded by a considerable amount of fibroconnective tissue. The interlobular ducts drain into the primary and accessory pancreatic ducts.

The primary duct runs the length of the pancreas, increasing in size near the duodenum where it runs parallel to the common bile duct, with which it often shares a common opening at the greater duodenal papilla. The openings of both ducts are controlled by the sphincter of the papilla. An accessory duct may lie proximal to the main duct and opens independently into the duodenal lumen.

Secretion by the exocrine pancreas is under nervous and hormonal control. Two polypeptide hormones, secretin and cholecystokinin, are released from cells of the intestinal mucosa and influence pancreatic secretion. **Secretin,** elaborated by S-cells in the mucosae of the duodenum and proximal jejunum, stimulates the ductal system of the pancreas to secrete a large volume of fluid that is rich in bicarbonate. In the intestinal lumen, this alkaline secretion neutralizes the acid chyme from the stomach and deactivates the gastric enzyme pepsin, whose optimal activity occurs at a low pH (2.0). It also establishes the neutral to alkaline conditions needed for the optimal activity of pancreatic enzymes.

Cholecystokinin, elaborated by I-cells in the duodenal and jejunal mucosae, stimulates secretory units of the pancreas to synthesize and release digestive enzymes. The proteolytic enzymes are secreted as inactive precursors (zymogens) that, in part, are converted to their active forms by **enterokinase,** an enzyme from the intestinal mucosa. Pancreatic amylase and lipase are said to be secreted in their active forms. Cholecystokinin also stimulates the gallbladder to contract, thereby adding bile to aid in neutralizing the intestinal contents and providing bile salts that act as emulsifying agents in the breakdown of neutral fats.

Endocrine Pancreas

KEY WORDS: pancreatic islet, alpha cell, glucagon, beta cell, insulin, delta cell, somatostatin, pancreatic polypeptide, PP cell, exocytosis, fenestration

Scattered among the pancreatic acini are irregular, elongate masses of pale-staining cells called the **pancreatic islets,** which make up the endocrine portion of the pancreas (see atlas figure 15-65). In humans they number about one million. The islets are completely separated from the surrounding exocrine pancreas by a delicate investment of reticular tissue, and, as with all endocrine glands, the islets have a rich vascular supply. In ordinary tissue sections, the islets appear to be composed of a homogeneous population of pale polygonal cells, but with special stains and in electron micrographs, several distinct cell types can be identified (Table 15-3). The majority of cells are alpha and beta cells.

Alpha cells make up about 20 percent of the islets in humans and generally are located at the periphery of the islet (see atlas figure 15-70). They contain large, dense, spherical granules that are limited by a membrane. Mitochondria are long and slender with a typical internal structure. A few profiles of granular endoplasmic reticulum are scattered about the cytoplasm, and Golgi bodies usually are found near the nucleus. They contain secretory granules with diameters of about 250 nm (see atlas figure 15-71). Alpha cells produce the peptide hormone **glucagon,** which ele-

Table 15-3. Endocrine Cells of the Pancreas

Lausanne Classification of Cell Types (1977)	Hormonal Substance	Primary Function
A (alpha) cell	Glucagon	Increases blood sugar
B (beta) cell	Insulin	Decreases blood sugar
D cell	Somatostatin	Inhibitor of hormone secretion (paracrine function)[a]
PP cell	Pancreatic polypeptide	Opposes action of cholecystokinin
D$_4$ cell	Vasoactive intestinal peptide	Increases blood sugar (vasodilator)
EC cell	Serotonin	Vasoactive agent
	Substance P	Increases motility of intestines
	Motilin	Increases motility of intestines
G cell[b]	Gastrin	Increases HCl secretion in stomach

[a]Paracrine function. Secretion of somatostatin is directly into the intercellular space from which it diffuses to inhibit the secretion of adjacent endocrine cells.

[b]G cells are present only in some species or restricted to fetal life in others.

vates blood sugar. These cells have been implicated in the production of gastric inhibitory peptide, cholecystokinin, and adrenocorticotropin hormone (ACTH)-endorphin also.

Beta cells form about 78 percent of the islet cells and tend to locate near the center of the islet (see atlas figure 15-69). Their secretory granules are smaller than those in alpha cells and show species differences. In humans, bats, and dogs, beta cell granules contain small dense crystals that give them a distinctive appearance. In other species the cores of beta cells vary in shape as plates, spheres, or rosettes. The granular endoplasmic reticulum is less extensive and the Golgi complexes are more distinctive than in alpha cells. Beta cells produce **insulin,** which acts on the plasmalemma of various cell types, especially liver, muscle, and fat cells, to facilitate the entry of glucose into the cell and thus lower blood glucose. Insulin also stimulates pancreatic acinar cells.

Several other types of endocrine cells are present in small numbers in the islets. **Delta cells** secrete the hormone **somatostatin,** which inhibits hormone secretion by surrounding endocrine cells. **Pancreatic polypeptide,** secreted by **PP cells,** opposes the action of cholecystokinin and inhibits pancreatic acinar secretion. Endocrine

cells of the kind found in the islets, including alpha and beta cells, also are scattered within the ducts and acini of the exocrine pancreas. The number of different endocrine cells may vary according to their locations in the head or body of the pancreas and may relate to the different origins of these two parts. There is considerable species variation in the distribution of cells within the islets. In humans and most rodents, beta cells tend to be located centrally, while alpha, delta, and PP-cells are concentrated at the periphery of the islets. Alpha and delta cells tend to be central in the islets of the horse and monkey, whereas in teleost fishes and dogs, the various cell types are distributed randomly in the islet.

Islet cells are intimately associated with surrounding capillaries, and the secretory granules often appear to be located near the cell membrane that is adjacent to the vasculature. Secretory granules are released from islet cells by **exocytosis** into the surrounding blood vessels. The endothelium of the islet capillaries contains numerous **fenestrations** to facilitate entry of secretory products into the vasculature. In contrast, the endothelium of capillaries of the exocrine pancreas is not fenestrated.

A significant proportion of the arterial blood enters the pancreas via small interlobular and intralobular arteries that first supply the islets. Arterioles derived from these arteries give rise to capillaries at the periphery of the islets, in the region of the alpha, delta, and PP-cells. The capillaries then run centrally within the islet, after which they supply adjacent acinar cells of the exocrine pancreas. Thus, the islet cells can interact with each other and influence the function of the exocrine pancreas.

Development of the Digestive System

When the three germ layers have formed, the embryo appears as a flattened disk with the yolk sac extending from its ventral surface. This surface of the embryo and the interior of the yolk sac are covered by endoderm that forms the lining for the entire digestive tract. With further development, the embryo and gastrointestinal endoderm fold to form a cylinder. Folding begins at the ends of the embryo, creating two blind endodermal tubes, both of which are continuous with the lumen of the yolk sac at an area called the intestinal portal. The proximal endodermal tube forms the foregut, which gives rise to the oral cavity, pharynx, stomach, and proximal duodenum. The midgut communicates with the yolk sac, and from it develops the jejunum, ileum cecum, appendix, ascending colon, and part of the transverse colon. The caudal tube becomes the hindgut, which differentiates into the rest of the large intestine.

Oral Cavity

The lips begin as a thickened band, the labial lamina, that grows from the ectoderm over the primitive jaw, into the underlying mesenchyme. The labial lamina thickens, and as the central cells degenerate, splits to form the lips and gums. The cheeks arise by fusion of the upper and lower lips at their lateral angles, thus reducing the original broad mouth opening. Skeletal muscles of the lips and cheeks arise from mesenchyme that migrates from the second branchial arch to lie between mucosal and epidermal coverings.

The tongue arises from the ventral ends of the branchial arches. An ectoderm-covered oral part from the mandibular arches forms the body of the tongue; an endodermal pharyngeal part from the second branchial arch gives rise to the rest of the tongue. The junction between ectoderm and endoderm is just anterior to the sulcus terminalis. Thus, fungiform and filiform papillae are ectodermal in origin, and circumvallate papillae are endodermal in origin. At first the tongue is covered by cuboidal epithelium, which later becomes stratified squamous.

All papillae initially form as elevations of the mucosa. A thickened epithelial ring surrounds each circumvallate papilla, grows into the mesenchyme, and splits to form a trench around each papilla. Solid epithelial cords grow from the bottom of the trench and give rise to Ebner's glands. Taste buds develop on the dome of each circumvallate papilla but are replaced by the definitive buds along the sides of the papilla. Taste buds first appear as local thickenings of epithelium in which basal cells elongate, grow toward the surface, and give rise to supporting and taste cells.

The major and minor salivary glands are considered to arise from ectoderm. All begin from the epithelial surface as buds that grow and branch, treelike, to form a system of solid ducts (see atlas figure 15-76). Terminal twigs, which eventually form intercalated ducts, round out at their ends to form secretory tubules and acini. Canalization of the duct follows. The sublingual gland differs slightly in that buds form from the oral epithelium and each remains a discrete gland. In most species, the parotid appears first, followed by the submandibular, sublingual, and, later still, minor glands. Mesenchyme surrounding the epithelial primordia provides the capsule and septae of the larger glands.

At birth, the submandibular gland of the cat is not fully differentiated, and in mice, rats, and hamsters acini are lacking and glandular development is not complete until maturity. In the submandibular of the opossum and parotid glands of the pig, maturation of ducts precedes that of acinar cells, whereas in the submandibular glands of rats and mice, the opposite is true.

Teeth have a dual origin: Enamel arises from ectoderm; dentin, pulp, and cementum arise from mesoderm. Tooth development begins with the appearance of the dental lamina, a plate of epithelium on which knoblike swellings (enamel organs) appear at intervals. These give rise to enamel and also act as molds for tooth development. The enamel organs grow into the mesenchyme to form inverted, cuplike structures invaginated at the bases by dental papillae. The latter are condensations of mesenchyme that give rise to the dentin and pulp of the teeth. The enamel organ forms a double-walled sac, of which the outer and inner walls differentiate into outer and inner enamel layers, respectively. Loosely arranged cells lie between the two layers and form the enamel pulp. Cells of the inner layer become ameloblasts and produce enamel prisms, beginning at the interface with the dental papillae. Mesenchymal cells of the papillae next to the inner dental layer enlarge and differentiate into odontoblasts. These form a single layer of columnar cells whose apices face the ameloblasts. Odontoblasts produce predentin that soon calcifies to become definitive dentin. Mesenchyme central to the odontoblasts forms the dental pulp (see atlas figure 15-74).

Dentin is the first of the hard tissues to appear in the tooth. Thereafter, both enamel and dentin are laid down, beginning at the apex and progressing toward the root. As the enamel and dentin layers thicken, the odontoblasts and ameloblasts gradually move away from each other. Ameloblasts migrate peripherally, remaining at the outer surface of the enamel, and eventually are lost from the tooth at eruption (see atlas figures 15-72 and 15-73). Before they are lost, ameloblasts lay down an acellular layer called the enamel cuticle that covers the enamel, adhering tightly to it. This cuticle may persist for a considerable time after the teeth erupt and the ameloblasts are lost. Odontoblasts progress centrally into the pulp cavity where they persist. As they retreat, the odontoblasts trail fine processes that extend through the dentin to the dentinoenamel junction. The entrapped processes form the dentinal fibers contained in fine dentinal tubules.

Mesenchyme around the developing enamel organ differentiates into the loose connective tissue of the dentinal sac. Near the root, the inner cells of the sac become cementoblasts and cover the dentin with cementum. Cells at the exterior of the sac differentiate to produce the alveolar bone that surrounds each tooth. The connective tissue between the external and internal layers of the dental sac gives rise to the peridontal membrane. Before the tooth erupts, a small crater appears in the gingival epithelium and connective tissue, immediately above the crown. The crater, which expands to accommodate the tooth as it emerges, develops from focal pressure necrosis as the tooth grows upward, by means of lytic activity of enzymes produced by the dental epithelium, or both (see atlas figure 15-75).

Alimentary Canal

The esophagus, stomach, small intestine, and colon initially consist of an endodermal tube surrounded by a layer of splanchnic mesoderm. The endoderm gives rise to the lining epithelium and all associated glands of the digestive tube; mesoderm differentiates into the supporting layers of the gastrointestinal tube.

The esophagus begins as a short tube connecting the pharynx and stomach. As the neck region and thorax develop, the tube elongates. Initially, the esophagus is lined by simple columnar epithelium, which gradually becomes stratified and thickened. Unlike birds and reptiles, however, in humans the esophagus does not become occluded (see atlas figures 15-77 and 15-78). Ciliated columnar and occasional goblet cells appear among the squamous cells. In chickens, turkeys, guinea fowl, pigeons, opossum, rats, and humans, ciliated cells persist only until hatching or birth, whereas in frogs and other amphibians, cilia are retained even in the adult. In humans, opossums, and carnivores the lining remains a wet stratified squamous epithelium, but in rodents and ruminants it becomes cornified.

The first glands to appear are the esophageal cardiac glands, followed by the esophageal glands proper, which continue to develop postnatally. Outgrowths at the base of the epithelium give rise to the ductal system of the glands; the secreting units arise as terminal branches of the ducts (see atlas figure 15-78).

The stomach begins as a fusiform expansion of the foregut, lined by a simple or pseudostratified columnar epithelium of endodermal origin (see atlas figure 15-79). It may remain simple or, as in rodents, regions may become stratified. Gastric pits arise as simple invaginations of the surface epithelium into underlying mesenchyme. In humans, the pits form first along the lesser curvature, then gradually in other regions. About 3 weeks later, they appear in the pyloric and cardiac areas. Soon after the pits form, oxyntic glands develop, arising from epithelial buds at the base of the pits (see atlas figures 15-80 and 15-81). Pyloric and cardiac glands develop similarly, but later than the oxyntic glands (see atlas figure 15-82). In species with a forestomach (rodents) or a ruminant type of stomach, cornification of the lining epithelium usually occurs before birth.

Development of the intestine and the appearance of villi, glands, and the various cell types usually follow a proximal to distal progression. The intestinal tract begins as a simple endodermal tube extending from stomach to cloaca. As the tube elongates, a caudal growth indicates the initial development of the cecum from which the appendix arises as the result of extremely rapid growth at the blind end. In the duodenum, a rapid proliferation of cells in the epithelial lining temporarily occludes the lumen. Vacuoles later appear in the epithelium, coalesce, and restore patency to the lumen. To a lesser degree, similar events occur in the remainder of the small intestine and colon. The lining epithelium now is four to five cells thick, has smooth luminal and basal surfaces, and lies on a distinct basement membrane. The underlying mesenchyme has not separated into lamina propria and submucosa (see atlas figure 15-83).

Proliferation of the epithelium, together with invaginations of the mesenchyme, produce folds or ridges in the mucosa, and as they increase in number, the luminal border becomes irregular. The first villi arise from the breakup of the mucosal ridges, and since some folds are covered by stratified cuboidal and others by simple columnar epithelium, these villi vary in thickness (see atlas figures 15-83B and 15-84). Subsequently, new generations of villi form as simple evaginations of epithelium and connective tissue, without the prior development of mucosal folds. Villi that develop in the colon, cecum, and appendix disappear in the second half of fetal life (see atlas figures 15-88 and 15-89).

Intestinal glands develop as simple tubular downgrowths of the epithelium between villi. Depending on the species, duodenal glands arise from outgrowths of epithelium on the intestinal floor between villi, or from intestinal glands.

As villi form, myoblasts differentiate in the mesenchyme to establish the muscularis mucosae. At this time, the epithelium is simple columnar, and goblet and enteroendocrine cells develop in a cranial-caudal progression. Paneth cells are among the last to appear. The muscularis externa arises before the muscularis mucosae with the inner coat being the first to form (see atlas figure 15-84). Its formation involves differentiation and proliferation of smooth muscle from mesenchyme, followed by hypertrophy, which accounts for most of the final thickness of the muscle coat. Plicae circulares form late in humans, long after villi have developed.

In most postnatal animals, a well-developed endocytic complex is present in the epithelial cells that cover the villi in the distal ileum. The complex usually persists until weaning and consists of numerous vesicles and tubules formed by invaginations of the cell membrane between microvilli (see atlas figures 15-85 and 15-86). These join with inclusion-containing vacuoles of various sizes in the supranuclear cytoplasm. The complex is implicated in the absorption of macromolecules.

The liver primordium begins as a thickening of endodermal epithelium in the anterior intestinal portal (future duodenum) of the developing gastrointestinal tube. A hollow ventral outgrowth appears, lined by simple columnar epithelium that is continuous with the duodenal lining. This hepatic diverticulum enlarges, grows into the vascular mesenchyme of the septum transversum, and then divides. A large cranial portion differentiates into the hepatic parenchyma and associated intrahepatic bile ducts; a small caudal part forms the common bile duct, cystic duct, gallbladder, and interhepatic bile ducts. The surrounding mesenchyme forms the capsule and stroma.

At first the hepatic cells are small and irregular in shape and usually contain numerous lipid droplets. They may form an irregular network of cords separated by islands of hemopoietic cells, but there is little organization into plates and sinusoids that are clearly defined (see atlas figure 15-98). As differentiation proceeds, irregular plates of cells form, extending from the central veins toward the periphery of each developing lobule, and sinusoids become apparent. The lobulation seen in the adult is not present in developing embryos or lower vertebrates and is thought to result from the hemodynamics of blood flow through the liver. Early liver growth results mainly from hyperplasia, but in some species, hypertrophy also occurs. Lipid is lost from hepatocytes, and hemopoietic activity wanes and ceases before or shortly after birth.

Bile canaliculi first appear at 6 weeks in the human embryo, before bile secretion begins. During the next 3 or 4 weeks, the rest of the intrahepatic biliary system forms from hepatocytes near the limiting plate of the lobules and then joins with interlobular ducts in the portal areas.

The caudal hepatic diverticulum soon becomes a solid cord of cells that gives rise to the cystic duct and gallbladder. Epithelial cords and blood vessels grow into the connective tissue between lobules and differentiate into hepatic ducts that unite with bile ducts. How the two join is unknown.

The pancreas develops from endodermal eva-

ginations of the gastrointestinal tract wall in two sites on opposite sides of the duodenum. These form ventral and dorsal pancreatic buds, which fuse after the ventral bud has migrated dorsally. The major execretory ducts develop in the ventral bud; the accessory duct arises in the dorsal bud. The parenchyma at first consists of a series of blind tubes of simple columnar epithelium that branch and expand into the surrounding mesenchyme (see atlas figures 15-90 and 15-91A). Acini form at the ends of the smallest ducts, but some also arise as paratubular buds from larger ducts. As ducts and acini form, lobes and lobules gradually take shape outlined by the surrounding connective tissue (see atlas figures 15-92 through 15-94). Some acinar cells expand proximally along the ducts, and some of the terminal ductal cells become incorporated into the acini as centroacinar cells. Further increase in acinar cells occurs mainly by division of differentiated cells and may extend into late postnatal life (see atlas figure 15-97).

Simultaneously, islet cells differentiate from endodermally derived progenitor cells within the duct system (see atlas figure 15-94B). Most islets develop at the ends of ducts, but paratubular outgrowths also occur. As ducts and acini continue to develop near the periphery of the lobules, the previously formed islets come to be more centrally placed in the lobule; these are the secondary islets (see atlas figures 15-95 and 15-96). Many islets retain their connections with the ductal epithelium from which they arose, but as the exocrine parenchyma increases, continuity of islet and duct is obscured. A few primary islets are found outside the lobule, within the interlobular connective tissue. These represent the first endocrine cells to develop from the first tubules, prior to formation of smaller ducts and acini. Isolated cells or small groups of endocrine cells remain scattered along the ductal system or occur between acinar cells, even in the adult.

Functional Summary

The digestive system is designed for breaking down ingested materials to their basic constituents, which then are absorbed and used by the organism. The process of mechanical and chemical breakdown of food substances is called digestion.

The oral cavity is specialized to take in and mechanically break down food through the cutting and grinding action of the teeth. The pulverized food is moistened and softened by secretions of the major and minor salivary glands. Digestion of carbohydrates is initiated in the oral cavity by the enzymes amylase and maltase, which are secreted by the major salivary glands. This chemical digestion of carbohydrates is short-lived, however, as both enzymes are destroyed by the acid environment of the stomach. Epidermal growth factor (EGF) and nerve growth factors from the submandibular glands influence the kinetics of epithelial tissues and other tissues lining the alimentary canal. Salivary gland secretions also moisten and clean the mouth, provide a proper environment for taste, and act as vehicles to transport heavy metals out of the body. When salivary gland secretion decreases during dehydration, it initiates the sensation of thirst and thus is a factor in maintaining fluid balance. The stratified squamous epithelium that lines the oral cavity protects the underlying structures from abrasion during eating. In regions subjected to excessive abrasion (gingiva and palate), the epithelium is cornified.

The tongue is important for chewing and swallowing, and in cows and antelopes it serves in the gathering of food. The interior of the tongue, cheek, and lips consists of skeletal muscle and is under voluntary control. The three structures serve to direct food to the teeth during mastication, direct it to the back of the throat for swallowing, and provide the voluntary control for suckling and speech.

The mixture of saliva and ground food is formed into a semisolid bolus that, when of the right consistency, is swallowed. Saliva is important for this activity also; swallowing is impossible if the mouth is parched. During the initial stage of swallowing, the bolus is directed to the oropharynx by several simultaneous, coordinated events. The anterior part of the tongue is pressed firmly against the hard palate and at the same time, the base of the tongue is retracted. Bone in the hard palate provides a rigid platform against which the tongue can press and prevents collapse of the palate due to the pressure exerted against it during swallowing. Formation of a mucoperiosteum prevents sliding and tearing of the mucosa that covers the palate. As these events occur, the larynx and pharynx are elevated to receive the bolus. Skeletal muscles associated with the soft palate contract, moving the soft palate upward to seal off the oropharynx and prevent food from entering the nasopharynx and nose. As the pharynx is elevated, its lumen dilates to receive the bolus from the oral cavity. Simultaneously, the musculature of the larynx contracts, closing the entrance to the respiratory tree. Skeletal muscle fibers of the three pharyngeal constrictor muscles contract about the entering bolus and quickly force it into the esophagus.

Skeletal muscle fibers in the muscularis externa of the upper esophagus are fast-acting, and their constriction carries the bolus of food into the central region of the esophagus, where there is a gradual transition to slow-acting smooth muscle. Peristaltic waves are formed by the smooth muscle in the lower half of the esophagus and move the bolus into the stomach. Because of peristalsis, materials from the esophagus enter the stomach in spurts. The lumen of the esophagus in humans is lined by a wet stratified squamous epithelium that, as in the oral cavity, protects the surrounding structures from the abrasive action of materials as they pass through the lumen. The esophageal glands provide a lubricant for passage of material. The main function of the esophagus is to transport food from the oral cavity to the stomach. It secondarily serves to warm or cool ingested materials.

In the stomach the arrangement of the muscle layers provides a churning action that promotes mixing with gastric secretions and mechanical breakdown of foodstuff. Protein is degraded by pepsin, an endopeptidase that splits peptide linkages near the center of the molecule. In addition to secreting hydrochloric acid and pepsin, the gastric mucosa secretes a considerable amount of fluid (about 1000 ml of gastric juice after each meal in humans), most of which is reabsorbed in the intestinal tract. In humans the parietal cells also secrete gastric intrinsic factor, which binds to vitamin B_{12}, important in erythropoiesis. The complex is absorbed in the intestine. If gastric intrinsic factor is not produced or is present in insufficient amount, much of the vitamin passes through the intestinal tract and is lost in the feces, resulting in development of pernicious anemia. The gastric mucosa of many suckling mammals contains rennin, an enzyme that curdles milk, and a lipase that begins the digestion of fat.

The contents of the proximal stomach are semisolid, whereas those in the distal region form a pulplike, fluid mass called chyme. After reaching the proper consistency, chyme enters the duodenum in small portions. The smooth muscle of the pyloric sphincter helps to control the evacuation of the stomach.

The simple columnar epithelium that lines the stomach forms a glandular sheet that secretes a neutral mucin. The epithelium and it secretions protect the stomach from the erosive effect of pepsin in the gastric lumen. The mucus secreted by the cardiac and pyloric glands helps to protect the mucosa where the stomach joins the esophagus and duodenum, respectively. Gastrin-producing endocrine cells are present in large numbers in the pyloric glands; gastrin stimulates acid secretion and gastric motility. Because of the large population of G cells, the pyloric region is not merely a mucus-secreting area but also assumes the status of an endocrine organ.

As the acid chyme enters the duodenum it is subjected to a change of pH. Duodenal glands secrete an alkaline fluid that protects the proximal duodenal mucosa from the acid pepsin from the stomach. The duodenal glands, like the submandibular glands, are involved in the secretion of EGF. The alkaline secretions of the pancreas and liver elevate the pH to neutral or alkaline and provide an environment optimal for the activities of digestive enzymes secreted by the pancreas; the proteolytic enzyme of the stomach, pepsin, is deactivated. Bile salts also are added to the intestinal contents and act as detergents or emulsifying agents to aid in the digestion of fats by pancreatic lipase.

Most of the digestive process takes place in the intestinal lumen. The final degradation of materials to their basic components (amino acids, monosugars, monoglycerides, fatty acids) occurs on the luminal surface of the intestinal epithelial cells just prior to absorption.

The intestinal wall is specialized for absorption of digested materials, and the surface area available is greatly increased by the plicae circulares, villi, and microvilli. The efficiency of absorption is further increased by movement of the villi and by segmental movement of the luminal contents by contractions of the muscularis externa, which move the intestinal contents back and forth. Peristaltic waves of the muscularis externa move the content through the intestine and along the remainder of the tract. As materials are absorbed, the luminal contents become more concentrated. Correspondingly, there is an increase in the number of goblet cells distally in the small intestine to provide mucus for lubrication.

Goblet cells are among the most numerous cells in the colon, and they increase in number toward the rectum. Villi are absent in the colon, but intestinal glands remain a prominent feature of the mucosa. The primary function of the colon is to absorb fluid that remains in the luminal contents. As the fecal mass develops, secretions from the large population of goblet cells provide the lubrication necessary to prevent damage to the colonic mucosa. In the upper rectum, the lining epithelium is made up primarily of goblet cells.

The anal canal is lined by a wet stratified squamous epithelium that protects this area from abrasion by the feces during defecation. Smooth muscle of the inner circular layer of the muscularis externa forms the internal anal sphincter. The surrounding skeletal muscle fibers adjacent to the anal orifice form the external sphincter, which is under voluntary control.

The organism is protected from a vast, ever present population of microorganisms in the digestive system by immunoglobulins (mainly IgA) that form a barrier against fungal, bacterial, and viral invasions. The immunologic barrier extends throughout the digestive tract and is the joint product of epithelial and lymphatic cells. The epithelial component, the secretory piece, is thought to protect the immunoglobulin from digestion both within and outside the cell. In the small intestine and colon, this barrier together with phagocytes forms a protective sleeve around the intestinal lumen. Large amounts of IgA also enter the intestinal lumen from the liver via the hepatobiliary pathway and play an important role in keeping the population of microorganisms in check.

From its exocrine portion, the pancreas provides enzymes that digest carbohydrates, proteins, and lipids. The endocrine portion secretes insulin and glycogen, hormones that are instrumental in regulating blood glucose levels, the flow of glucose across cell membranes, and glyconeogenesis in the liver. Carbohydrate is stored by the liver as glycogen, which can be released into the bloodstream as glucose. The liver contributes bile salts for the emulsification of fats during digestion, plays a vital role in detoxification, and supplies proteins that are important in blood coagulation. The liver functions in lipid transport and maintains lipid levels in blood. Lipid is complexed to protein in the hepatocytes, secreted into the perisinusoidal space, and transported in the blood as plasma lipoprotein.

The endocrine cells of the gastrointestinal tract and pancreatic islets produce hormones that influence or control gastric secretions, gastrointestinal motility, gastric emptying, gallbladder contraction, and pancreatic and liver secretion. How the specific hormones interact with one another or are influenced by other major endocrine organs is unknown.

Clinical Correlations

A common inflammatory lesion of the oral mucosa is caused by the herpes simplex virus, resulting in "cold sores" or "fever blisters." These lesions frequently occur at the vermillion border of the lips as groups of small vesicles (blisters) that rupture and form small shallow ulcers with red margins and necrotic centers.

Although various tumors occur in major and minor salivary glands, the parotid is the most commonly affected. The tumors usually are be-

nign, mixed tumors believed to arise from intercalated ducts and involve both epithelial and connective tissue elements. The epithelial cells may be low columnar and arranged in acini lined by two layers of cells, but there may be transitions to stratified squamous epithelium. The epithelial cells may extend into and merge with the connective tissue stroma and often appear to secrete mucinous material into the stroma. Cartilage and even bone may develop in the stroma.

Chronic inflammation of the salivary glands may result in loss of secretion followed by a dry mouth, difficulty in swallowing, and extensive dental caries. In this case the salivary glands often are swollen and infiltrated by lymphocytes and plasma cells, and secretory acini become atrophic and eventually disappear. The ducts show proliferation of the lining epithelium to form masses of cells.

The most common pathologies of teeth are dental caries, abnormal tooth eruptions, and periodontal disease. The latter is the result of inflammation of the gingiva and periodontal membrane caused by the invasion and proliferation of bacteria. With the destruction of the periodontal membranes, teeth become loose in the socket and eventually are lost.

Esophageal inflammations usually occur as the result of irritation by ingested material or reflux of gastric contents rather than from microorganisms. When the lower esophagus is chronically subjected to gastric acid, a chemically induced chronic esophagitis results. The esophageal epithelium undergoes metaplasia, changing from wet stratified squamous to simple columnar, similar to that of the gastric mucosa, and ulceration may occur.

Most bacteria entering the stomach are soon killed by the acid gastric juice, but salmonella, staphylococci, and dysentery bacilli can tolerate the gastric environment and induce an acute inflammation (gastritis). Acute gastritis also can occur from irritants such as alcohol, hot fluids, and aspirin or other analgesics. Alcohol and aspirin permit back-diffusion of hydrogen ions through the protective mucous layer and into the gastric mucosa. In the most severe form of gastritis — acute hemorrhagic gastritis — focal erosion and edema of the mucosa occur, associated with mucosal or submucosal bleeding. Chronic gastritis is associated with variable loss of glandular tissue, especially parietal cells. Often there is an associated decrease in the production of hydrochloric acid, intrinsic factor, and enzymes. The gastric epithelial cells appear altered in shape and arrangement. In severe cases (atrophic gastritis), parietal and chief cells are lost to a variable degree and the glands are reduced in number and consist of an epithelium that is similar in appearance to that of the gastric lining. The lamina

propria is widened in areas and heavily infiltrated by plasma cells and lymphocytes, but the total mucosa may be thinned and rugae are not prominent. The gastric glands may atrophy, with complete replacement of parietal and chief cells by mucus-secreting cells. Metaplasia is common, and the glands come to resemble those of the intestine, complete with intestinal epithelial, goblet, and Paneth cells.

Peptic ulcers can be found not only in the stomach but also in other parts of the digestive tract. Peptic ulceration is especially common in areas exposed to acid gastric juice. Stomach ulcers are thought to develop when the mucous layer on the gastric mucosa is defective, whereas duodenal ulcers are considered to arise because of hypersecretion of gastric acid. Acute peptic ulcers usually involve only the mucosa and submucosa; subacute ulcers extend to the muscularis externa; and chronic ulcers are defined as those that have penetrated the muscle wall. The ulcer crater is lined by a thin layer of necrotic tissue infiltrated by leukocytes and overlying a bed of granulation tissue. In chronic ulcers the muscle coats are interrupted and merge into the fibrous tissue in the outer layers of the ulcer lining. The mucosal epithelium at the margins may show signs of regeneration. Healing with scar formation may occur and may result in puckering of the mucous membrane. It has been demonstrated that a large number of peptic ulcers are the result of an infectious disease caused by chronic infection of *Helicobacter pylori. Helicobacter* colonizes only the mucus film on the gastric mucosa but elicits an immune response. As a result an inflammation (gastritis) occurs but the bacteria remain unharmed due to their location.

Regional enteritis (Crohn's disease) is a relatively uncommon disease that can involve the small and large bowel but most commonly affects the terminal ileum. Nonspecific inflammatory changes extend through the entire thickness of the wall but are most marked in the submucosa, which shows focal accumulations of lymphocytes. The lumen is markedly narrowed. The swollen mucosa becomes ulcerated and often shows metaplastic changes to resemble pyloric glands. Ulcerative colitis is an inflammatory lesion of the large intestine that mainly involves the mucosa. The mucosa shows dense infiltration by plasma cells. Intestinal glands are infiltrated by leukocytes and red cells and contain much mucus. The epithelium breaks down, releasing material into the lamina propria and precipitating frank ulceration that rarely extends beyond the submucosa.

The products of digestion are absorbed mainly by the small intestine, and any disease of the small intestine can interfere with absorptive activities. Absorption of different materials may occur at specific sites: Vitamin B_{12} is absorbed in the distal ileum, and iron is absorbed in the duodenum. Diseases in these areas can cause a corresponding dietary deficiency. In severe disease, protein, carbohydrate, fat, mineral, vitamins, and so forth may be poorly absorbed. The primary malabsorption disorders are tropical sprue and celiac disease, both of which are associated with villous atrophy. The villi may show extensive fusion and appear shorter and broader than normal. The villous epithelium often shows degenerative changes and the crypts are enlarged and hyperplastic. These changes have been interpreted as indicating a decreased life span of the epithelial cells with a compensatory increase in production (hyperplasia) of cells in the glands.

Benign and malignant tumors are common in the large intestine. Polyploid adenomas are benign tumors that consist of neoplastic glands whose cells show variable changes, including nuclear hyperchromatism (indicative of polyploid change) and loss of polarity. Villous papilloma are especially common in the rectum and represent benign tumors consisting of fronds of connective tissue covered by mucin-secreting epithelium. In spite of the designation benign, the tumors are apt to become malignant.

Hirschsprung's disease is a rare congenital absence of parasympathetic neurons of the myenteric and submucosal plexuses in the distal sigmoid colon. This results in excessive activity of the sympathetics with inhibition of propulsive action of the affected intestinal wall, and stimulation of the smooth muscle contractions in the internal anal sphincter. Gross distention of the colon results, extending as far back as the cecum and tapering abruptly into a narrow rectal segment. Enormous accumulation of fecal material and repeated attacks of obstruction occur.

Hepatitis is any widespread inflammatory lesion of the liver and may result from alcohol and drug use, viruses, and biliary disease. Acute viral hepatitis is characterized by a diffuse inflammation of the liver and widespread, scattered necrosis of hepatocytes, accompanied by lymphocytic infiltration of portal areas and parenchyma. Hepatocytes, especially in the centrilobular region, may be swollen and show an eosinophilia and an increased granularity of the cytoplasm, which is condensed around the nuclei. Kupffer cells increase in size, and the sinusoids are infiltrated by lymphocytes also. As the hepatocytes become necrotic and eventually lyse, the liver plates are disrupted. The injury is brief, and hypertrophy and hyperplasia of the hepatocytes occur with formation of binucleate cells.

In cirrhosis, the liver substance is marked by an excess of fibrous connective tissue that separates the parenchyma into a succession of isolated nodules. It results from chronic damage to liver cells with persistent inflammation and fiber formation. The condition is irreversible, even when the causal agent is removed. The nodules of liver tissue generally do not show the usual lobular pattern, and the portal areas and central veins lack their normal relationship and spacing. The hepatocytes show evidence of atrophy with foci of hypertrophic and hyperplastic cells, so that in some areas the cells are large while in others they are small. The fibrous septae that separate the nodules may contain fine fibrils or coarse fibers of collagen. The fibrosis involves the portal areas and also entraps the central veins. The fibrous tissue appears to arise near damaged liver cells.

Pancreatitis can result from several causes, including alcohol abuse, trauma, and biliary tract disease, and may occur in acute or chronic forms. Acute pancreatitis essentially consists of an acute necrosis of pancreatic acinar cells with greater or lesser hemorrhage followed by suppuration and even gangrene. The tissue shows hemorrhage, tissue destruction, and inflammation, the proportions of which vary from area to area. Hemorrhage may be the main feature, with the tissue suffused with blood. Small veins and capillaries may be packed with blood, and their walls later become necrotic. In other areas there may be well-defined necrosis of glandular and interstitial tissue with marked infiltration of leukocytes. Secondary infection is common and may lead to an outpouring of leukocytes and abscess formation. In chronic pancreatitis the gland usually is shrunken and atrophic. Fibrosis occurs chiefly between lobules but may be more diffuse and occur between the acini. The islets usually are less involved than the acinar tissue but may become involved later. The acini and ducts often appear compressed and distorted.

Tumors arising from endocrine cells within the gastrointestinal mucosa or endocrine pancreas also can occur. These are classified as gastrinomas, VIPomas, somatostatinomas, insulinomas, or glucagonomas, the name determined according to the most abundant secretory product produced. The term *carcinoid* generally is used for a similar neuroendocrine tumor of slightly different morphology that usually is involved in the hypersecretion of serotonin.

Atlas and Table of Key Features

Key Features of the Alimentary Tract

	Epithelium	Muscularis Mucosae	Muscularis Externa	Lymphatic Tissue	Glands
Esophagus	Stratified squamous nonkeratinizing	Prominent; longitudinal smooth muscle	Outer longitudinal, inner circular layers. Skeletal in upper one-fourth, mixed in middle one-fourth, smooth in lower one-half	Few nodules, diffuse in lamina propria	1. Esophageal proper, scattered along length of esophagus in submucosa. compound tubuloalveolar, mucus-secreting 2. Esophageal cardiac, proximal and distal ends in lamina propria. Compound tubuloalveolar, mucus-secreting
Stomach Cardia	Simple columnar	Smooth muscle; inner circular, outer longitudinal; a third outer circular layer in some areas	Outer longitudinal, middle circular, inner oblique smooth muscle	Small patches of diffuse lymphatic tissue; rare nodules	Long pits (one-half the depth of mucosa); simple branched tubular; mucous, endocrine, and occasional parietal cells
Fundus	Simple columnar	Same	Same	Same	Short pits (one-fourth the depth of the mucosa); simple branched tubular; mucous neck, parietal, chief, and endocrine cells
Pylorus	Simple columnar	Inner circular, outer longitudinal smooth muscle	Same	Occasional small lymphatic nodules in lamina propria	Long pits (one-half the depth of mucosa); simple branched tubular; mucous, occasional parietal and numerous endocrine cells (G cells)

Key Features of the Alimentary Tract (continued)

	Epithelium	Muscularis Mucosae	Muscularis Externa	Lymphatic Tissue	Glands
Duodenum	Villi covered by simple columnar absorptive cells with microvillus border; goblet and endocrine cells	Inner circular, outer longitudinal smooth muscle	Inner circular, outer longitudinal smooth muscle. Myenteric plexus between layers	Solitary nodules and diffuse lymphatic tissue	1. Intestinal glands in lamina propria. Simple tubular; absorptive; goblet cells; endocrine and Paneth cells 2. Brunner's glands in submucosa; branched tubular
Small intestine	Villi covered by simple columnar absorptive cells; goblet cells increase in number from upper to lower; endocrine cells present	Same	Same	Nodular lymphatic tissue forms aggregates (Peyer's patches) in ileum	Intestinal glands; same as for duodenum
Colon	Villi absent; simple columnar absorptive cells; goblet cells increase in number	Same	Outer longitudinal layer condensed into 3 bands — taeniae coli	Solitary nodules and diffuse lymphatic tissue	Intestinal glands; goblet, endocrine, and absorptive cells; Paneth cells absent
Rectum	Simple columnar; mainly goblet cells	Same	Inner circular and outer longitudinal	Solitary nodules	Intestinal glands; goblet cells more abundant
Anal canal	At pectinate line becomes stratified squamous, noncornified, then stratified squamous cornified at orifice	Disappears at level of anal columns	Inner circular layer thickens to form internal sphincter, outer longitudinal layer disappears	Solitary lymphatic nodules	1. Intestinal glands disappear at pectinate line 2. Apocrine sweat glands (circumanal glands)

Oral Cavity

Junction with vermillion border

Keratinized stratified squamous epithelium

Nonkeratinized stratified squamous epithelium

Fig. 15-4. A section of lip from an infant that illustrates the vermillion border. (LM, ×100.)

Fungiform papilla

Filiform papillae

Fig. 15-5. Dorsal surface of tongue demonstrating the surface features of filiform papillae. (LM, ×100.)

Fig. 15-6. The interwoven nature of intrinsic musculature characteristic of the tongue. (LM, ×100.)

Fig. 15-7. A fungiform papilla of human tongue. (LM, ×250.)

Fig. 15-8. A circumvallate papilla. Note its position relative to the dorsal surface of the tongue and the position of von Ebner's glands. (LM, ×10.)

Fig. 15-9. Taste buds from the lateral surface of a circumvallate papilla. (LM, ×250.)

Fig. 15-10. The epithelial lining of a human hard palate. (LM, ×250.)

Salivary Glands

Fig. 15-11. Lobules comprising a parotid gland. (LM, ×75.)

Capillaries

Intralobular duct

Intercalated duct

Serous acini

Serous acinus

Fig. 15-12. A region of a parotid gland showing several serous acini, an intercalated duct, and an intralobular (striated) duct. Note the abundance of capillaries adjacent to the intralobular duct. (LM, ×250.)

Intralobular duct

Mucous tubule

Serous acini

Intralobular ducts

Intralobular ducts

Mucous tubule

Intralobular ducts

Fig. 15-13. A section of a submandibular gland showing abundant profiles of the intralobular ducts. (LM, ×160.)

Intralobular duct

Mucous cells

Serous demilunes

Serous acinus

Striated duct

Serous acini

Fig. 15-14. A region from a submandibular gland that demonstrates serous and mucous cells as well as ductal elements. (LM, ×250.)

Nucleus

Granular endoplasmic reticulum

Mitochondrion

Tight junction

Secretory granules

Fig. 15-15. Serous acinar cells from the submandibular gland. (TEM, ×3,000.)

Nucleus of
serous
acinar cell

Granular
endoplasmic
reticulum

Desmosome

Process of
myoepithelial
cell

Fig. 15-16. The process of a myoepithelial cell adjacent to a serous cell of a submandibular gland. (TEM, ×4,000.)

Golgi
complex

Tight
junction

Fig. 15-17. An intercalated duct of a submandibular gland. (TEM, ×4,000.)

Fig. 15-18. A region of intralobular duct from a submandibular gland. Compare with the intercalated duct shown in 15-17. (TEM, ×3,000.)

Tooth

Fig. 15-19. The root of a molar tooth within the alveolar bone of a jaw. Note the periodontal membrane and gingiva. (LM, ×30.)

Dentine

Acellular cementum

Periodontal membrane

Alveolar bone

Fig. 15-20. Periodontal membrane uniting tooth root to an alveolar bone. (LM, ×250.)

Alveolar bone

Periodontal membrane

Sharpey's fibers

Cementodentinal junction

Cellular cementum

Dentine

Fig. 15-21. Tooth root deep within a jaw shows cellular cementum as well as Sharpey's fibers (compare with 15-20). (LM, ×250.)

Fig. 15-22. The interior of a tooth root demonstrates the elements of the pulp as well as the position of odontoblasts, predentin, and dentine. (LM, ×250.)

Esophagus

Fig. 15-23. Surface features of the nonkeratinized stratified squamous epithelium of a human esophagus (compare with 15-24). (SEM, ×200.)

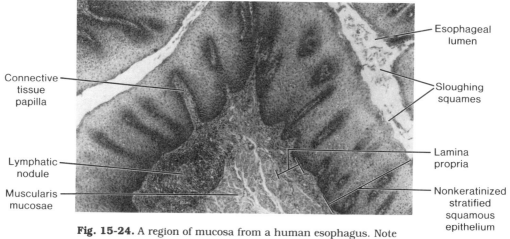

Connective tissue papilla

Lymphatic nodule

Muscularis mucosae

Esophageal lumen

Sloughing squames

Lamina propria

Nonkeratinized stratified squamous epithelium

Fig. 15-24. A region of mucosa from a human esophagus. Note the lymphatic nodule. (LM, ×100.)

Submucosa

Esophageal glands proper

Stratified squamous epithelium

Lamina propria

Muscularis mucosae

Duct of esophageal gland

Fig. 15-25. Distal esophagus containing esophageal glands. (LM, ×40.)

Simple columnar epithelium of stomach

Lamina propria

Esophageal gastric junction

Nonkeratinized stratified squamous epithelium of esophagus

Fig. 15-26. The abrupt transition of simple columnar to nonkeratinized stratified squamous epithelium at the esophageal gastric junction. (LM, ×250.)

Stomach

Surface of gastric lining epithelium

Gastric pits

Fig. 15-27. The surface of a human fundic stomach exhibiting numerous gastric pits. (SEM, ×200.)

Lumen

Simple columnar epithelium

Mucous granules

Basement membrane

Lamina propria

Fig. 15-28. Surface lining epithelium of a human stomach. (LM, ×500.)

Mucous cells

Parietal cells

Endocrine cell

Duct of cardiac gland

Endocrine cell

Parietal cells

Fig. 15-29. Cardiac glands from a human stomach. (LM, ×400.)

Branching gastric gland

Branching gastric gland

Fig. 15-30. A dissected preparation illustrating the tubular nature of the gastric (oxyntic) glands from a human stomach. Note that several of the glands branch. (SEM, ×250.)

Artery

Submucosa

Muscularis mucosae

Muscularis externa

Chief cells

Gastric pits

Fundic glands

Fig. 15-31. The appearance of fundic (oxyntic) glands from a human stomach as they appear in section (compare to 15-30). Note the position of the chief cells at the bases of the oxyntic glands. (LM, ×50.)

Chief
cells

Zymogen
granules

Endocrine
cells

Parietal
cell

Endocrine
cell

Parietal
cells

Mucous neck
cells

Fig. 15-32. A region of gastric mucosa showing chief, parietal, endocrine, and mucous neck cells, which together make up the oxyntic glands. (LM, ×250.)

Tubulovesicular
system

Intracellular
canaliculus

Nucleus

Microvilli

Lysosome

Intracellular
canaliculi

Fig. 15-33. The ultrastructural features of a human parietal cell. (TEM, ×10,000.)

Nucleolus

Nucleus

Granular endoplasmic reticulum

Golgi complex

Zymogen granules

Fig. 15-34. The ultrastructural features of a human chief cell. (TEM, ×2,000.)

Parietal cell nucleus

D cell nucleus

Intracellular canaliculus

Lamina propria

D_1 cell nucleus

Fig. 15-35. The ultrastructural features of two endocrine cell types in a human oxyntic gland. (TEM, ×2,000.)

Lamina propria

Muscularis mucosae

Gastric pits

Pyloric glands

Fig. 15-36. Pyloric glands from a segment of human pyloric stomach. Note that these glands are confined to the mucosa. (LM, ×250.)

Golgi complex

Nucleus of mucous cell

Lumen of pyloric gland

Secretory granules

Fig. 15-37. Mucous cells from a human pyloric gland. (TEM, ×3,000.)

Small Intestine

Fig. 15-38. Duodenal villi from a segment of human small intestine. (SEM, ×100.)

Fig. 15-39. A section of human jejunum illustrating intestinal villi and glands (crypts). (LM, ×40.)

Fig. 15-40. Isolated villi and intestinal glands from a duodenum. (SEM, ×200.)

Fig. 15-41. Isolated intestinal glands from a jejunum as viewed from the external surface. (SEM, ×350.)

Fig. 15-42. Corrosion cast of vasculature from the duodenal mucosa. Note the vascular bed within the villi. (SEM, ×100.)

Fig. 15-43. Apices of three intestinal epithelial cells as shown by a freeze-fracture replica. Note the border of microvilli. (×25,000.)

Goblet cell

Paneth cell

Intestinal glands

Muscularis mucosae

Paneth cells

Collagen bundle

Meissner's plexus

Venule

Fig. 15-44. The bases of human intestinal glands exhibit scattered Paneth cells. Note the underlying muscularis mucosae. (LM, ×250.)

Inner circular layer of muscularis externa

Vein

Submucosa

Artery

Muscularis mucosae

Villi

Lamina propria

Intestinal gland

Fig. 15-45. A segment of ileum from a child. Note the concentration of goblet cells. (LM, ×40.)

Villus

Villi

Fig. 15-46. Villi from adult human ileum. (SEM, ×200.)

Intestinal glands

Muscularis mucosae

Lymphatic nodule

Germinal center

Submucosa

Fig. 15-47. A portion of human ileum illustrating a Peyer's patch. (LM, ×100.)

Fig. 15-48. A region of human duodenum illustrating the duodenal glands. Note that these glands empty into intestinal glands shown at the right. (LM, ×250.)

Fig. 15-49. The submucosa (Meissner's) plexus within the submucosa of human jejunum. Note the adjacent nerve fibers. (LM, ×400.)

Colon

Muscularis mucosae

Goblet cells

Intestinal glands

Diffuse lymphatic tissue

Lamina propria

Lumen

Submucosa

Fig. 15-50. A region of mucosa from the human colon. Note the absence of villi. (LM, × 100.)

Fig. 15-51. A region of isolated colonic mucosa showing intestinal glands and their openings on the mucosal surface. Note that villi are absent. (SEM, ×120.)

Anal Canal

Nonkeratinized stratified squamous epithelium

Connective tissue papilla

Lamina propria

Fig. 15-52. The epithelium lining the anal canal. (LM, ×250.)

Liver

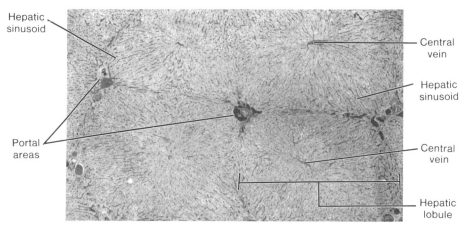

Hepatic sinusoid

Central vein

Hepatic sinusoid

Portal areas

Central vein

Hepatic lobule

Fig. 15-53. A section of the pig liver showing four adjacent hepatic lobules. (LM, ×40.)

Portal triad

Portal vein

Hepatic artery

Bile duct

Hepatic artery

Bile duct

Portal vein

Fig. 15-54. A region of human liver showing two portal triads. (LM, ×40.)

Binucleate
hepatocyte

Kupffer
cell

Endothelial
cell

Plates of
hepatocytes

Hepatic
sinusoids

Fig. 15-55. Hepatic cords and sinusoids of the liver. Note the
Kupffer cell near the center of the photomicrograph. (LM, ×300.)

Hepatocyte

Space
of Disse

Outer
surface of
sinusoidal en-
dothelium

Reticular
fibers

Fenestrations
of endothelial
cell

Microvilli of
hepatocyte
projecting
into the
space of Disse

Hepatocyte

Fig. 15-56. A portion of a hepatic sinusoid. Note the
surrounding hepatocytes and the perisinusoidal
space of Disse. (SEM, ×6,000.)

Fig. 15-57. A region of a hepatic lobule from a liver that had been injected with India ink to demonstrate Kupffer cells. (LM, ×250.)

Fig. 15-58. A Kupffer cell within a hepatic sinusoid. (TEM, ×10,000.)

Plasmalemma

Mitochondria

Nucleus

Tight junction

Lumen of bile canaliculus

Golgi complex

Glycogen

Granular endoplasmic reticulum

Fig. 15-59. A bile canaliculus between two adjacent hepatocytes. (TEM, ×6,000.)

Hepatocyte

Lumen of bile ductule

Tight junction

Fig. 15-60. A bile ductule (canal of Hering) of the liver. Note the adjacent hepatocytes. (TEM <×3,500.)

Fig. 15-61. An interlobular bile duct from a portal triad of the liver (compare with 15-54). (TEM, ×2,000.)

Gallbladder

Fig. 15-62. Apices of surface cells lining a human gallbladder. (SEM, ×500.)

Simple columnar epithelium

Bundles of smooth muscle (muscularis)

Adventitia

Fig. 15-63. A section through the wall of a human gallbladder shows the elaborately folded mucosa. (LM, ×40.)

Nucleus

Simple columnar epithelium

Lamina propria

Fig. 15-64. The simple columnar epithelium lining a human gallbladder. (LM, ×250.)

Pancreas

Acinus

Islet

Intralobular
duct

Pancreatic
acini

Intralobular
ducts

Fig. 15-65. A section of pancreas showing both exocrine and endocrine components. (LM, ×100.)

Zymogen
granules

Centroacinar
cell

Acinus

Fig. 15-66. A section through a pancreatic acinus. Note the zymogen granules within acinar cells and the centroacinar cell. (LM, ×1,000.)

Pancreatic lobule

Pancreatic acini

Arteriole

Lumen of interlobular duct

Fig. 15-67. An interlobular duct within a human pancreas. (LM, ×100.)

Lumen of acinus

Zymogen granules

Granular endoplasmic reticulum

Nucleus of pancreatic acinar cell

Lumen of intralobular duct

Tight junction

Fig. 15-68. A region of pancreas showing the ultrastructural details of an acinar cell and an intralobular duct. (TEM, ×2,000.)

Pancreatic
acini

Capillaries

Insulin-
containing
cells
(stained black)

Fig. 15-69. A pancreatic islet stained by immunohistochemical means to demonstrate insulin. Note that the insulin immunoreactivity is concentrated near the cell surfaces facing capillaries. (LM, ×250.)

Glucagon-
containing
cells

Fig. 15-70. A pancreatic islet stained by immunohistochemical means to demonstrate glucagon. Note that glucagon-immunoreactive cells are concentrated at the periphery of the islet. (LM, ×250.)

Granular
endoplasmic
reticulum

Portion of
pancreatic
acinar cell

Alpha (*A*)
cells of
islet

Secretory
granules

Fig. 15-71. Ultrastructural features of two alpha cells in a pancreatic islet. (TEM, ×3,000.)

Development — Tooth

Stellate
reticulum

Alveolar
bone

Wall of
dental sac

Marrow
cavity

Dentine

Enamel

Pulp

Stratified
squamous
epithelium

Fig. 15-72. A developing human tooth within a jaw prior to its emergence into the oral cavity. (LM, ×10.)

Dentine

Dentoenamel junction

Odontoblasts

Tomes' fibers

Ameloblasts

Enamel prism

Enamel

Fig. 15-73. A section through the wall of a developing human tooth illustrating odontoblasts, dentine, enamel, and ameloblasts. (LM, ×250.)

Capillary

Fibroblast nuclei

Venules

Fig. 15-74. Pulp of a developing human tooth. (LM, ×250.)

Developing crater

Emerging crown

Gingival surface

A   B

Fig. 15-75. A sequence of scanning electron micrographs illustrating tooth eruption. (×40.)

Submandibular Gland

Epidermis

Interlobular duct

Excretory duct

Intralobular ducts

Fig. 15-76. The submandibular in the initial steps of development. Note that only the ductal elements are present at this stage of development. (LM, ×35.)

Esophagus

Lumen of esophagus

Esophageal epithelium

Lamina propria

Fig. 15-77. The epithelial lining of a developing esophagus. (LM, ×250.)

Developing gland

Esophageal epithelium

Developing gland

Fig. 15-78. A region of esophageal mucosa that shows the differentiation of esophageal glands. (LM, ×250.)

Stomach

Developing mucosa

Serosa

Muscularis externa

Fig. 15-79. The oxyntic mucosa from the fundus of the developing stomach prior to the formation of glands. (LM, ×400.)

Circular layer of muscularis externa

Serosa

Surface epithelium

Developing gastric glands

Fig. 15-80. Mucosa from the fundic stomach showing the early development of the gastric (oxyntic) glands. (LM, ×100.)

Surface epithelium

Fundic glands

Muscularis mucosae

Gastric pit

Submucosa

Muscularis externa { Inner circular / Outer longitudinal

Serosa

Fig. 15-81. A section through the wall of a developing stomach showing the developing fundic (oxyntic) glands. Compare with the earlier stage of development shown in 15-80. (LM, ×100.)

Gastric pit

Surface epithelium

Developing pyloric glands

Lamina propria

Muscularis mucosae

Fig. 15-82. A region of pyloric stomach shows the early stages of pyloric gland development. (LM, ×400.)

Small Intestine

Stratified epithelium

Mesenchyme

Circular layer of muscle

Initial villus formation

A   B

Fig. 15-83. Cross section of small intestine early in fetal development. B. Small intestine from a fetus slightly older than that shown in A. Note the formation of ridges within the mucosa, which signals the initial formation of villi. (LM, ×250.)

Circular layer of muscularis externa

Cells in mitosis

Villi

Developing pancreatic lobule

Fig. 15-84. The formation of villi in the small intestine from a fetus older than that shown in 15-83. (LM, ×250.)

Vacuoles

Endocytic
complex

Intestinal villus
in cross section

Fig. 15-85. Cross section of an intestinal villus from a suckling mammal. Note the endocytic complex and the numerous vacuoles that fill the apical and basal cytoplasm of each absorptive cell. (LM, ×500.)

Microvilli

Endocytic
complex

Fig. 15-86. An electron micrograph of the apical endocytic complex demonstrates that it consists of invaginations, tubules, and vacuoles (compare with 15-85). (TEM, ×15,000.)

Mitochondrion

Chylomicra
in dilated
intercellular
space

Nucleus of
intestinal
epithelial
cell

Desmosome

Nucleus of
intestinal
epithelial
cell

Fig. 15-87. The intercellular space between the bases of two adjacent intestinal epithelial cells from a suckling mammal expanded by the accumulation of chylomicra. (TEM, ×8,000.)

Colon

Mesenchyme

Lumen

Circular
layer of
muscularis
externa

Fig. 15-88. The early development of colon from a young fetus. Note that the circular layer of the muscularis externa consists only of a single layer of smooth muscle cells. (LM, ×200.)

Circular
layer of
muscularis
externa

Developing
intestinal
glands

Serosa

Fig. 15-89. A region through the wall of colon illustrating the initial appearance of the intestinal glands during development. (LM, ×350.)

Pancreas

Mitotic figure

Zymogen
granules

Proacinar
cell

Mitotic figure

A   B

Fig. 15-90. Expanding exocrine tubules from a pancreas early in development. Note mitotic figures and zymogen granules in scattered cells. (LM, ×1,000.)

Proacinar cells

Endocrine cell

Developing islet

Pancreatic tubule

A   B

Fig. 15-91. Expanding exocrine tubules of pancreas early in development. A. Note endocrine cell. B. Note developing islet. (LM, ×1,000.)

Intralobular ducts

Developing acinus

Developing lobule

A   B

Fig. 15-92. Pancreatic lobules in the initial stages of development. Note the branched intralobular duct system. (LM, ×250.)

Developing lobule

Intralobular ducts

Developing acini

Fig. 15-93. A developing pancreatic lobule at a later stage of development than shown in 15-92. (LM, ×250.)

Interlobular duct

Intralobular duct

Acinus

Islet

Intralobular duct

Islet

A   B

Fig. 15-94. Two regions of developing pancreas. A. Note continued expansion of the exocrine component. (LM, ×250.) B. Note development of the endocrine component (islets). (LM, ×100.)

Fig. 15-95. A region of developing pancreas showing both primary and secondary islets. (LM, ×250.)

A   B

Fig. 15-96. Established lobules within a developing pancreas. Note position of the islets. Compare to 15-94 and 15-95. (LM, ×100.)

Endocrine cells within acinus

Acinus

Acinar cell in mitosis

A   B

Fig. 15-97. The differentiation of mature-appearing acinar cells within a developing pancreas. Note the two endocrine cells shown in A. (LM, ×400.)

Liver

Hepatocyte

Hepatic cords

Island of hemopoietic cells

Fig. 15-98. A region of liver early in development that shows active hemopoiesis. (LM, ×250.)

Review Questions and Answers

Questions

77. List in order the different types of surface lining epithelium encountered in the digestive tract beginning with the oral cavity and ending with the anal canal. Briefly discuss the functional significance of each type listed.
78. List and briefly discuss three morphologic adaptations for absorption found in the small intestine.
79. Discuss the classic and portal hepatic lobules in relation to blood and bile flow of the liver lobule.
80. Discuss the morphology and functional significance of the perisinusoidal space.
81. Briefly discuss the relationship of two endocrine cells in the gastrointestinal mucosa to the exocrine pancreas and its function.
82. Briefly discuss the ultrastructure of a pancreatic acinar cell as related to its function.

Answers

77. The oral cavity is lined thoroughout by a wet stratified squamous epithelium that provides a protective surface resistant to abrasion. The dorsum of the tongue, the hard palate, and the gingiva are subjected to a greater degree of abrasion by foodstuff, and in these regions the lining epithelium may become cornified. The esophagus also is lined by stratified squamous epithelium, which in humans is noncornified. As in the oral cavity, it provides protection against the abrasive action of materials that pass through the esophagus to the stomach. At the esophageal-gastric junction there is an abrupt transition from nonkeratinized stratified squamous epithelium to the simple columnar epithelium of the stomach.

    The epithelial lining of the stomach is organized into a secretory sheet that secretes continuously. The neutral mucin produced by the surface epithelium of the stomach forms a mucous film that protects the gastric mucosa chemically from the acid pepsin in the lumen. The mucus secretion also lubricates the mucosal surface. This type of lining epithelium ends abruptly at the gastrointestinal junction.

    The small intestine is lined by a heterogeneous population of simple columnar cells. The principal cell type is the intestinal absorptive cell, which shows a prominent microvillus border on its apical (luminal) surface. This cell serves primarily in the absorption of digested materials from the intestinal lumen. Goblet cells within the lining epithelium represent unicellular exocrine glands that secrete mucus to lubricate and protect the mucosal surface. As materials pass through the intestinal tract, fluids are absorbed and the luminal contents become firmer and more abrasive. Thus, the number of goblet cells increases distally in the intestinal canal, and in the distal colon they become the most prominent cell type. A variety of endocrine cells (unicellular endocrine glands) are found in limited numbers, scattered throughout the lining epithelium of the small intestine and colon. They secrete a number of peptide hormones that influence gastric secretion, motility, gallbladder contraction, and hepatic and pancreatic activity.

    An abrupt transition from simple columnar to noncornified stratified squamous epithelium occurs at the junction between the rectum and anal canal. The wet stratified squamous epithelium of the anal canal protects this region from the abrasive effects of the fecal mass during defecation.

78. Three morphologic adaptations for absorption are found in the small intestine: plicae circulares, villi, and microvilli. The plicae

circulares are large, permanent, shelflike folds that may branch and that spiral about the lumen of the intestine for one-half to two-thirds of its circumference. They consist of intestinal mucosa with a central core of submucosa. Plicae begin in the duodenum, reach their maximum development in the proximal jejunum, and diminish in size and disappear in the distal half of the ileum.

Villi are best developed in the duodenum and jejunum, where they form broad, spatulate structures; in the ilium they are shorter and more fingerlike. Villi consist of a central core of lamina propria covered by intestinal epithelium. They are mobile structures and contract four to five times a minute, extending and retracting from the intestinal lumen.

Microvilli are fingerlike evaginations of the apical plasmalemma that extend from the intestinal absorptive cells. They are closely packed and form the striated border of light microscopy.

All three structures greatly increase the surface area of the intestinal mucosa and increase its absorptive capacity.

79. A classic liver lobule is related to the blood flow through the liver. It consists of a central vein about which radiate branching and anastomosing plates of hepatocytes. The plates are separated by blood sinusoids and thus assume a spokelike arrangement. The hepatic lobule itself is somewhat hexagonal in cross section, with a central vein at the center and portal areas at the corners. Blood passes from small branches of the hepatic artery and portal vein into the sinusoids that lie between the plates of hepatocytes. Blood flows slowly through the hepatic sinusoids toward the center of the lobule and leaves through the central vein.

The lobule associated with the exocrine secretion of the liver (bile) is termed the portal lobule and has at its center a portal canal. A portal lobule consists of the surrounding hepatic tissue that is drained by a bile duct of a portal area. It is triangular in shape and contains portions of three adjacent hepatic lobules. A central vein is located at each corner of a portal lobule.

Thus, blood flow in the liver is directed toward the central vein of the classic lobule, whereas bile flows in the opposite direction — that is, toward the periphery of the lobule to bile ducts in surrounding portal areas.

80. Hepatic sinusoids are wider and have a more irregular shape than most capillaries. In those species where a discontinuous, fenestrated type of endothelium is present, the sinusoidal lining is separate from hepatocytes by a narrow space called the perisinusoidal (Disse's) space. It is devoid of ground substance and most connective tissue elements. Blood plasma flows freely through the endothelium and into and through the perisinusoidal space. Because the blood plasma has direct access to it, liver cells are constantly bathed on one surface by plasma that is rich in nutrients absorbed by the gastrointestinal tract. The plasmalemma of hepatocytes adjacent to the perisinusoidal space exhibits numerous well-developed microvilli that increase its surface area and facilitate absorption. The perisinusoidal space has considerable functional significance in the active exchange of nutrients between the blood plasma and hepatocytes.

81. Two distinct polypeptide hormones, secretin and cholecystokinin, are released from endocrine cells in the intestinal mucosa. These hormones influence secretion by the exocrine pancreas. Secretin, produced by the S cells of the duodenal and proximal jejunal mucosae, stimulates the ductal system of the exocrine pancreas to secrete a large volume of fluid that is rich in bicarbonate. Cholecystokinin, produced by the I cells of the duodenal and jejunal mucosa, stimulates the synthesis and release of digestive enzymes by the pancreatic acinar cells.

82. The pancreatic acinar cell is actively involved in the synthesis and release of digestive enzymes. Ultrastructurally, the acinar cell is characterized by an abundance of granular endoplasmic reticulum, which fills the basal and perinuclear cytoplasm. Extensive Golgi complexes occupy the supranuclear region and are associated with forming zymogen granules that accumulate in and often fill the apical cytoplasm. An acinar cell contains a single, spherical nucleus located at its base, and one or more nucleoli may be present. A variety of digestive enzymes (proteins) are synthesized in the granular endoplasmic reticulum and pass through the cisternae of this organelle to reach the Golgi complex via small transport vesicles. These precursors of the active digestive enzymes are packaged into membrane-bound zymogen granules by the Golgi complex and then are released into the apical cytoplasm. The zymogen granules migrate to the apical cell membrane, fuse with it, and discharge their contents into the acinar lumen by the process of exocytosis.

16 Urinary System

The urinary system consists of the kidneys, ureters, urinary bladder, and urethra. The kidneys constitute the glandular component; the remainder of the urinary system forms the excretory passages. The ureters conduct urine from the kidneys to the bladder, where it is stored temporarily. In turn, the bladder is drained by the urethra, through which the urine ultimately is voided from the body.

Kidneys

The kidneys are a pair of compound tubular glands that clear the blood plasma of metabolic wastes, regulate the fluid and salt concentrations of the body, eliminate foreign chemicals, and help maintain the acid-base balance of the body. In addition to excretory functions, the kidneys have properties of endocrine organs and release two substances, renin and erythropoietin, directly into the bloodstream. Renin is important in regulating blood pressure and sodium ion concentration; erythropoietin influences hemopoietic activity.

Macroscopic Features

KEY WORDS: hilum, renal sinus, renal pelvis, major calyx, minor calyx, renal papilla, cortex, medulla, medullary pyramid, renal column, medullary ray, renal lobe, renal lobule, multilobular kidney

Human kidneys are bean-shaped organs that lie in a retroperitoneal position against the posterior abdominal wall, one on either side of the upper lumbar vertebrae. Each is contained within a thin but strong connective tissue capsule that contains much fat. The renal artery and nerves enter the kidney on the medial border at the **hilum,** a concavity that also serves as the point of exit for the renal vein, lymphatics, and ureter. The hilum is continuous with the **renal sinus,** a large, central cavity surrounded by the parenchyma of the kidney and filled with loose areolar connective tissue that normally contains much fat. Nerves, lymphatics, and branches of the renal artery and vein run through the sinus. The **renal pelvis** is a funnel-shaped expansion of the ureter where it joins the kidney; it also passes through the sinus, dividing into two or three short tubular structures called the **major calyces.** These in turn divide into eight to twelve smaller units called **minor calyces.** Each minor calyx forms a cylindrical attachment around a conical projection of renal tissue called a **renal papilla.**

When a hemisection of the kidney is examined macroscopically, the organization of the parenchyma into two distinct regions can be seen readily. The darker, granular-appearing outer region is the **cortex,** which forms a continuous layer beneath the capsule. The inner region or **medulla** is paler and smoother and consists of 8 to 20 cone-shaped structures called **medullary pyramids,** which are separated from each other by inward extensions of cortical tissue (see atlas figure 16-3). The cortex that separates adjacent pyramids makes up a **renal column.** The bases of the pyramids are directed toward the overlying cortex, while their apices are oriented toward the renal sinus and form the renal papillae. From the bases of the pyramids, groups of tubules extend into the cortex, giving it a striated appearance. These striations represent a continuation of medullary tissue into the cortex and constitute the **medullary rays.**

The arrangement of cortex and medulla allows subdivision of the kidney into smaller units, the lobes and lobules. A medullary pyramid, together with its closely associated cortical tissue, forms a **renal lobe,** while a medullary ray, together with its associated cortical tissue, forms a **renal lobule.** When the kidney consists of several lobes, it is referred to as a **multilobular kidney;** the kidneys of humans are this type. In several species (rat, mouse, and rabbit) the kidneys are unilobular and consist of a single pyramid and its associated cortex.

Microscopic Features

KEY WORDS: **uriniferous tubule, nephron, collecting duct**

Each renal lobule is made up of numerous epithelial tubules called **urinferous tubules** (Fig. 16-1) that collectively form the parenchyma of the kidney. Each uriniferous tubule can be divided into a **nephron,** which is the secretory portion, and a **collecting duct,** which is the excretory portion that carries urine to the renal pelvis.

Nephron

KEY WORDS: **renal corpuscle, proximal tubule, thin segment, distal tubule, loop of Henle**

There are one to two million nephrons in the human kidney, each representing a functional unit of the kidney. A nephron is a blindly ending epithelial tubule that can be subdivided into several components, each differing in structure, function, and position in the kidney. During urine formation the various segments of a nephron take part in filtration, secretion, and resorption. A typical nephron consists of a **renal corpuscle,** a **proximal tubule** with convoluted and straight portions, a **thin segment,** and a **dis-**

tal tubule that also has convoluted and straight parts. Those segments of the nephron between the proximal and distal convoluted tubules (i.e., the straight descending part of the proximal tubule, the thin segment, and the straight ascending portion of the distal tubule) are collectively referred to as the **loop of Henle.**

The renal corpuscle and the proximal and distal convoluted tubules occur only in the cortex, whereas Henle's loop generally is confined to the medulla or to a medullary ray. The size of the nephrons and the length of their various segments vary according to the position of the parent renal corpuscle in the cortex. Renal corpuscles near the medulla are larger and the tubules are longer than are those of nephrons whose renal corpuscles are located in the periphery of the cortex. Nephrons from the subcapsular region have small renal corpuscles, and their thin segments of the **loop of Henle** extend for only a short distance into the medulla. Nephrons whose renal corpuscles occupy an intermediate position in the cortex show intermediate features.

Renal Corpuscle

KEY WORDS: **glomerulus, glomerular capsule, parietal layer, visceral layer, capsular epithelium, glomerular epithelium, capsular space, vascular pole, urinary pole, podocyte, primary process, secondary (foot) process (pedicle), slit pore (filtration slit), slit membrane, common basal lamina, fenestrated glomerular endothelium, mesangial cell, extraglomerular mesangium, intraglomerular mesangial cells, filtration barrier**

A renal corpuscle is roughly spherical and measures 150 to 250 μm in diameter. It consists of a capillary tuft, the **glomerulus,** which projects into a blind expansion of the uriniferous tubule called the **glomerular capsule** (see atlas figures 16-4 through 16-6). The outer layer of the capsule surrounds the glomerulus as the **parietal layer,** which then reflects onto the glomerulus where it is intimately applied to the glomerular capillaries to form a complete covering called the **visceral layer** of the glomerular capsule. The parietal layer

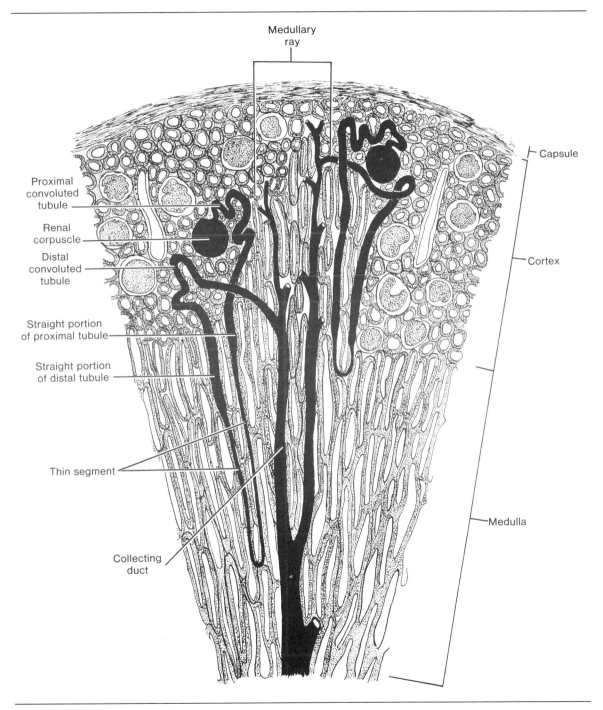

Medullary ray

Capsule

Proximal convoluted tubule

Renal corpuscle

Distal convoluted tubule

Cortex

Straight portion of proximal tubule

Straight portion of distal tubule

Thin segment

Medulla

Collecting duct

Fig. 16-1. Diagram of uriniferous tubules.

also is known as the **capsular epithelium,** while the visceral layer frequently is referred to as the **glomerular epithelium.** The visceral and parietal layers of the capsule are separated only by a narrow **capsular space.**

The **vascular pole** is that area of the renal corpuscle at which the afferent and efferent arterioles enter and leave. As the afferent arteriole enters the renal corpuscle, it immediately divides into several primary branches, each of which forms a complex of capillaries (a capillary lobule) that then reunite to form the efferent arteriole. Each glomerulus is made up of several such capillary lobules. On the side opposite the vascular pole, the capsular space becomes continuous with the lumen of the proximal convoluted tubule; this region is known as the **urinary pole** (see atlas figures 16-5 and 16-14).

The parietal layer of the glomerular capsule consists of a single layer of tightly adherent squamous cells that contain few organelles (see atlas figures 16-5 and 16-14). Near the urinary pole there is an abrupt transition from this simple squamous form to the large pyramidal cells that line the proximal convoluted tubule. At the vascular pole, the simple squamous capsular epithelium changes to a specialized cell type called the podocyte.

Podocytes are large, stellate cells whose bodies lie some distance from the underlying capillaries, separated from them by several cytoplasmic extensions called the **primary processes** (see atlas figures 16-7 and 16-8). These processes wrap around the glomerular capillaries and give rise to numerous **secondary (foot) processes (pedicles)** that interdigitate with similar processes from adjacent podocytes to completely invest the capillary loops of the glomerulus. The narrow clefts between the interdigitating processes form the **slit pores (filtration slits),** which measure about 25 nm in width (see atlas figures 16-8 and 16-10). The gaps may be bridged by a thin **slit membrane.**

The foot processes of the podocytes and the endothelial cells of the glomerular capillaries share a continuous **common basal lamina** that measures 0.1 to 0.5 μm thick (see atlas figure 16-10). The basal lamina consists of a proteoglycan matrix that is rich in heparan sulfate and contains type IV collagen and sialic acid. Although the initial contact between glomerular epithelium and vascular endothelium is essential to establish the common basal lamina, thereafter it is laid down and maintained by the podocytes themselves.

The glomerular capillaries are lined by a **fenestrated glomerular endothelium** (see atlas figures 16-9 and 16-10). The attenuated squamous cells show numerous large pores (fenestrae) that measure 50 to 100 nm in diameter.

The renal corpuscle also shows stellate cells with long cytoplasmic processes that contain numerous filaments. These are **mesangial cells,** which occupy the area between the afferent and efferent arterioles at the vascular pole, where they lie in a matrix of amorphous material. The cells constitute the **extraglomerular mesangium** and are continuous with cells of similar appearance, the **intraglomerular mesangial cells,** that lie between the glomerular endothelium and the basal lamina. The latter cells are thought to clear away large protein molecules that become lodged on the common basal lamina during filtration of blood plasma. Mesangial cells may participate in the removal of older portions of the basal lamina from the endothelial side as it is added to by the podocytes. Mesangial cells are of clinical importance in some kidney disease because of their tendency to proliferate.

The renal corpuscle is the filter of the nephron. The fenestrated glomerular endothelium, the common basal lamina, and the foot processes of the glomerular epithelium form the **filtration barrier** of the renal corpuscle (Fig. 16-2 and see atlas figure 16-10). This barrier permits passage of water, ions, and small molecules from the capillaries into the capsular space, but larger structures such as the formed elements of the blood and large irregular molecules are retained. The capillary endothelial cells prevent passage of formed elements; the common basal lamina restricts passage of molecules with a molecular weight greater than 400,000. Substances of small molecular weight (40,000 or less) cross the basal lamina and pass through the filtration slits and the surrounding glomerular epithelium to enter

Primary process
of podocyte

Pedicles
of podocyte

Basal
lamina

Fenestrated
endothelium

Fig. 16-2. Diagram of the filtration barrier.

the capsular space. Material that collects in the capsular space is not urine but a filtrate of blood plasma.

Although materials with molecular weights larger than 45,000 or that have highly irregular shapes may pass through the endothelium and common basal lamina, they are unable to traverse the barrier provided by the foot processes of the podocytes. The filtration barrier limits passage of materials not only on the basis of size and shape but also with respect to their charge. Anionic molecules are more restricted in their passage through the filtration barrier than are neutral molecules of similar size. Heparan sulfate is a negatively charged (polyanionic) molecule of the glomerular basal lamina. The sialoprotein (podocalyxin) coats the podocyte foot processes and together with heparan sulfate gives the filtration barrier a net negative charge. Thus, the glomerular epithelium as well as the common basal lamina are important in limiting the kinds of materials that pass from the blood into the capsular space.

The energy for the filtration process is supplied by the hydrostatic pressure of the blood in the glomerular capillaries. The pressure (about 70 mm Hg) provides sufficient force to overcome the colloidal osmotic pressure of substances in the blood (approximately 33 mm Hg) and the capsular pressure of the filtration membrane (about 20 mm Hg). The resulting filtration pressure (approximately 18 mm Hg) is great enough to force filtrable materials through all three layers of the filtration barrier and into the capsular space.

The hydrostatic pressure exerted within the glomerular capillaries results from the unusual vascular arrangement of the glomerulus. Most vascular areas of the body are supplied by arterioles that form capillaries that then reunite into venules, but the glomerular capillaries are interposed between an afferent arteriole that conducts blood to the glomerulus and an efferent arteriole that conducts blood away from the glomerulus. This arrangement results in considerable pressure being exerted on the capillary walls and can be regulated by contraction of either arteriole.

As more filtrate from the blood enter the capsular space, the rise in pressure forces the filtrate into the lumen of the proximal convoluted tubule. The capsular epithelium forms a tight seal around each renal corpuscle, preventing leakage of filtrate into the cortical tissue.

Proximal Tubule

KEY WORDS: proximal convoluted tubule, microvillus (brush) border, straight portion, apical canaliculus, endocytic complex

The proximal tubule begins at the urinary pole of the renal corpuscle and is the largest segment of the mammalian nephron. It is about 17 mm long and makes up most of the cortex. The proximal tubule is divided into a convoluted portion (pars convoluta) and a straight portion (pars recta). The convoluted portion is the longer of the two parts and is the one most frequently seen in sections of the cortex. After a tortuous course through the cortex in the region of its parent renal corpuscle, the proximal tubule takes a more direct route through the cortex to become the straight portion of the proximal tubule. It then enters the medulla or a medullary ray, where it turns toward a renal papilla as the first part of the loop of Henle.

The **proximal convoluted tubule** consists of a single layer of large, pyramidal cells that have a well-developed **microvillus (brush) border** (see atlas figures 16-11, 16-14, and 16-15). The lateral surfaces of the cells form an intricate system of interdigitating processes and ridges that often extend beneath neighboring cells to interdigitate with similar processes of adjacent cells. Tight junctions fuse the apices of the adjacent cells together around the tubular lumen and clearly delineate apical and basolateral cell membrane domains. Thus, a complex labyrinth of cell membranes extends into the basal region of the epithelium. Compartmentalization of the lateral and basal regions results in a greater surface area of cell membrane, which facilitates the transport of ions (see atlas figure 16-16).

In typical tissue sections, profiles of proximal convoluted tubules are the most common structures seen in the cortex and usually show a stellate lumen bounded by a distinct brush border. Each cell of the proximal tubule has a large spherical nucleus, but not all cells show a nucleus be-

cause of the large size of the cells. The cells contain a supranuclear Golgi complex and numerous rod-shaped mitochondria parallel to the long axis of the cell, closely associated with the lateral ridges and processes. The cytoplasm usually is darkly staining and granular.

Structurally, the convoluted and straight parts of the proximal tubule are similar, but the cells of the **straight portion** are shorter, and the brush border and lateral interdigitations are less well defined than in the convoluted part. Mitochondria are abundant but are smaller and more randomly scattered.

One of the main functions of the proximal tubule is absorption of the glomerular filtrate. The brush border, which consists of closely packed, elongated microvilli, increases the surface area available for absorption by about 30-fold (see atlas figures 16-15 and 16-16). The microvilli are embedded in a coat of extracellular proteoglycan (glycocalyx) that may contain enzymes that facilitate the absorptive process. The apical surfaces of cells absorb sugars and amino acids from the luminal contents in a manner similar to that of intestinal epithelial cells. Normally, all the glucose in the glomerular filtrate is absorbed in the proximal convoluted tubule. If blood glucose levels exceed the absorptive capacity of the enzymes that control the absorption of glucose, the excess spills into the urine (glycosuria).

Protein is absorbed in the proximal tubule by a system of invaginations called **apical canaliculi** that give rise to a series of small vesicles containing protein sequestered from the lumen. The tubular invaginations, the vesicles, and the vacuoles together make up the **endocytic complex,** which is actively involved in protein absorption (see atlas figure 16-15). The vesicles coalesce to form large vacuoles that condense and ultimately fuse with lysosomes whose acid hydrolases reduce the protein to amino acids that are released back into the bloodstream.

Over 80 percent of the sodium chloride and water of the glomerular filtrate is absorbed in the proximal tubule. Sodium ion is actively transported from the lumen, and chloride ion and water follow passively with no expenditure of energy by the cell to maintain the osmotic balance. The force that moves sodium ion is an active adenosinetriphosphatase (ATPase)-sodium pump located along the lateral cell membranes that form the complex intercellular space. Other inorganic ions and vitamin C also are absorbed by the proximal convoluted tubule.

In addition to absorption, the proximal convoluted tubule secretes organic acids and bases that are destined to be eliminated in the urine. Hence, this region of the nephron serves as an exocrine gland. Hydrogen ion also is secreted into the lumen in exchange for bicarbonate ions. Parathyroid hormone acts to decrease phosphate resorption in the proximal convoluted tubule.

Thin Segment

KEY WORDS: simple squamous epithelium

The simple cuboidal epithelium of the straight descending part of the proximal tubule (the initial segment of the loop of Henle) changes abruptly in the thin segment to an attenuated **simple squamous epithelium** (see atlas figures 16-17 and 16-18). The luminal diameter of the nephron also decreases markedly, from 65 μm in the descending portion to about 20 μm in the thin segment. The thin segment is confined largely to the medulla of the kidney and forms the thin limb of the loop of Henle.

The nuclei of the lining epithelial cells are centrally placed and cause this area of the cell to bulge into the lumen of the tubule. At the luminal surface, the brush border of the proximal tubule is replaced by short, scattered microvilli. Ultrastructurally, the cytoplasm shows fewer organelles, the lateral cell membranes have elaborate folds that interdigitate with those of adjacent cells. The cells are united at their apices by typical junctional complexes. The lateral interdigitations are less well developed near the hairpin loops. The cells rest on a relatively smooth basal lamina of moderate thickness. The length of the thin segment varies with each nephron and depends on the position of the parent renal corpuscle in the cortex. Thin segments are short or even absent

from nephrons whose renal corpuscle is located near the capsule and are longest when the renal corpuscle is located near the medulla. In these nephrons, the thin segments may extend almost to the tip of a renal papilla.

Distal Tubule

KEY WORDS: straight portion, macula densa, pars maculata, juxtaglomerular cell, convoluted portion, basal striation

The distal tubule is divided into a straight part (pars recta), a portion that contains the macula densa (pars maculata), and a convoluted portion (pars convoluta).

The **straight portion** of the distal tubule begins as a transition from the thin segment of the nephron. In several species the transition is abrupt, but in humans it occurs more gradually. The epithelium becomes cuboidal, and while a few microvilli are present, the cells lack the brush border and apical canaliculi of the proximal tubule. Interdigitating processes are present along the basolateral surfaces of the cells, and these contain numerous mitochondria (see atlas figures 16-19 and 16-20). The straight part of the distal tubule constitutes the thick ascending limb of the loop of Henle and completes the looping course of this structure as it ascends through the medulla. It then reenters the cortex to return to the parent renal corpuscle.

As it reaches the renal corpuscle, the distal tubule assumes a close relationship with the afferent arteriole, and where it contacts the arteriole, the tubule contains a group of specialized cells that form the **macula densa** (dense spot) (see atlas figures 16-11 and 16-13). This segment of the tube is called the **pars maculata.** The cells are taller and narrower than in adjacent tubules, so that their nuclei are closer together and are more prominent. Cells of the macula densa are polarized toward the basal surface — that is, the Golgi membranes and occasional granules are found basal to the nucleus, facing the basal cell membrane. The macula densa is related to a modified region of the afferent arteriole that contains the **juxtaglomerular cells** and is considered to represent an endocrine portion of the kidney (see atlas figures 16-11 and 16-12). This feature and the polarization of the cell suggest that the macula densa monitors the luminal fluid in the distal tubule. Cells of the macula densa produce the enzyme nitric oxide synthase. The nitric oxide released by the macula densa is thought to control vascular tone of the afferent and/or efferent arterioles, thereby influencing kidney function.

The macula densa marks the division between the ascending and **convoluted portion** of the distal tubule. The convoluted portion runs a tortuous course in the cortex near the renal corpuscle of its origin. The distal convoluted tubule is shorter than the proximal convoluted tubule, so fewer sections of the distal tubule are seen in histologic preparations. The lumen of the distal tubule generally is wider than that of the proximal tubules, the cells are shorter and lighter staining, and nuclear profiles usually are seen in each cell, partly because many are binucleate. A brush border is lacking.

Electron micrographs show deep, elaborate infoldings of the basal cell membrane associated with numerous elongated mitochondria that lie parallel to the long axis of the cell, producing the prominent **basal striations** of light microscopy (see atlas figure 16-19). The cells of the distal tubules show a few luminal microvilli.

The distal tubule is the main site for acidification of urine, and it is here that further absorption of bicarbonate occurs in exchange for hydrogen ions. About one-half of the bicarbonate in the glomerular filtrate has already been absorbed in the proximal tubule. The distal tubule also is the site where ammonia is converted to ammonium ion. Thus, this segment of the nephron plays an important role in maintaining the acid-base balance of the body. Aldosterone, a steroid hormone, promotes transport of sodium ion from the distal tubule in exchange for potassium ion. Inadequate concentrations of aldosterone result in a serious loss of sodium in the urine. The last portion of the distal tubule can become permeable to water under the influence of antidiuretic hormone (ADH).

Loop of Henle

KEY WORDS: straight portion of proximal tubule, thin segment, straight portion of distal tubule, countercurrent multiplier system

The loop of Henle is interposed between the proximal and distal convoluted tubules and consists of the **straight portion of the proximal tubule,** the **thin segment,** and the **straight portion of the distal tubule.** Only the kidneys of mammals and birds have well-established loops of Henle. In desert animals the loops and renal papillae are long, whereas in aquatic species the loops are less developed and the renal papillae are short. The loops descend in the medulla for variable distances, form hairpin loops, then ascend through the medulla, parallel to the descending limb, to the cortex.

The loop of Henle is essential for the production of hypertonic urine and is important in the conservation of body water. The loop acts as a **countercurrent multiplier system** to aid in the concentration of urine. The descending thin segment is permeable to sodium ions and water, whereas cells in the ascending limb possess a "sodium pump" that moves sodium from the tubular lumen into the surrounding interstitium. However, there is evidence that the ion actively being pumped is chloride and that sodium follows passively. The ascending limb is relatively impermeable to water, so sodium ions are trapped in the interstitial substance of the medulla, resulting in an increase in the osmotic concentration around the tubules in the medulla. Sodium ions may passively diffuse into the descending limb but are pumped out again by the ascending limb as the cycle repeats itself over and over. The sodium trap thus formed establishes an osmotic gradient that increases in strength toward the renal papillae. This gradient is important for the conservation of water and formation of hypertonic urine by the distal tubules and collecting ducts.

Collecting Ducts

KEY WORDS: initial segment, arched portion, medullary collecting duct, papillary duct, area cribrosa, principal (light) cell, intercalated (dark) cell, renal interstitium

The collecting ducts can be subdivided according to their location in the kidney. The **initial segment** is found in the cortex and includes short connecting portions that unite the distal tubules of cortical nephrons to collecting ducts and **arched portions** that are formed by the confluence of several connecting portions from juxtamedullary nephrons. The arched portions originate deep in the cortex, which they ascend through before arching to descend within a medullary ray.

Medullary collecting ducts occur primarily in the medulla. As the ducts pass through the medulla they converge to form larger, straight collecting ducts called **papillary ducts,** which end at the tip of a renal papilla (see atlas figures 16-17 and 16-23). The numerous openings of the papillary ducts give a sieve-like appearance to the external surface of the papillae; the area has been called the **area cribrosa.** The external surfaces of the papillae are covered by transitional epithelium.

The lining epithelium of the collecting ducts contains principal and intercalated cells. The **principal (light) cells** generally are cuboidal with centrally placed, round nuclei and lightly staining cytoplasm with characteristic, distinct cell boundaries (see atlas figure 16-17). Ultrastructurally, the light cells show scattered, short microvilli on their apical surfaces, scattered mitochondria, and some infolding of the basal plasmalemma (see atlas figure 16-22). They also possess a single, centrally located cilium (see atlas figure 16-21).

Scattered between the light cells are the **intercalated (dark) cells,** which have more mitochondria, stain more deeply, and show a large number of vesicles in the apical cytoplasm. The cells lack central cilia, but the apical plasmalemma shows microplicae. The function of these cells is unknown. As the collecting tubules pass through the medulla, the cells increase in height to become tall columnar in the papillary ducts.

The collecting ducts conserve water and produce hypertonic urine. As the ducts traverse the medulla to the tips of the pyramids, they pass through the increasingly hypertonic environ-

ment established by the loop of Henle. The permeability of the collecting ducts to water is controlled by ADH. In the presence of ADH, water is drawn from the collecting ducts by osmosis because of the hypertonic environment maintained in the medullary interstitium. The loss of water from the tubular contents results in a concentrated, hypertonic urine. If ADH is lacking due to injury or disease, the kidney is unable to concentrate urine and copious amounts of dilute urine are produced, resulting in severe dehydration. This condition is known as diabetes insipidus.

The **renal interstitium** fills the spaces between the tubular elements of the kidney. The cortical interstitium is relatively scant except around blood vessels and consists of fine bundles of collagen, fibroblasts, and scattered phagocytes. The medullary interstitium is more plentiful, and its cells are parallel to the long axis of the tubules. These interstitial cells possess long, branching processes that encircle adjacent tubules and blood vessels. Pleomorphic interstitial cells filled with small lipid droplets also occur in the medullary interstitium at regular intervals between the epithelial tubules and vessels. The cells are suspected to be endocrine cells and may secrete an antihypertension factor. The medullary interstitium contains abundant intercellular matrix and small bundles of collagen.

Juxtaglomerular Apparatus

KEY WORDS: juxtaglomerular (JG) cell, renin, angiotensinogen, angiotensin I, angiotensin II, aldosterone, erythropoietin, extraglomerular mesangium

The juxtaglomerular apparatus consists of the macula densa of the distal tubule, the extraglomerular mesangium, and the juxtaglomerular cells in the wall of the afferent arteriole. The **juxtaglomerular (JG) cells** appear to be highly modified smooth muscle cells in the wall of the afferent arteriole as it enters the renal corpuscle. The cells contain a number of secretory granules, well-developed Golgi complexes, and abundant granular endoplasmic reticulum. The JG cells produce **renin,** which, when released into blood, converts the plasma protein **angiotensinogen** to **angiotensin I.** A converting enzyme in the blood converts angiotensin I to the polypeptide **angiotensin II,** which acts on the zona glomerulosa of the adrenal cortex, stimulating it to release aldosterone. **Aldosterone** influences the distal tubule to transport sodium ion from the lumen in exchange for potassium ion. Angiotensin II also is a potent vasoconstrictor and elevates blood pressure. The juxtaglomerular apparatus of some species produces **erythropoietin,** an agent that stimulates erythropoiesis in the bone marrow.

The location of the macula densa, its basal polarization, and its orientation toward adjacent JG cells suggest that the two groups of cells may interact. The macular densa may "sense" the sodium ion concentration in the distal tubule and thereby influence the activity of JG cells.

The **extragomerular mesangium** forms a loose mass of cells between the afferent and efferent arterioles. Component cells may contain granules, but their exact role in the function of the juxtaglomerular apparatus is unknown.

Vascular Supply

KEY WORDS: renal artery, segmental artery, interlobar artery, arcuate artery, interlobular artery, intralobular artery, afferent arteriole, efferent arteriole, peritubular capillary network, vasa recta, vascular countercurrent exchange

The vascular pattern of the kidneys is complex and shows regional specializations related to the organization and function of the various parts of the nephron. The **renal arteries** arise from the abdominal aorta and before reaching the renal sinus usually divide into branches that pass anterior and posterior to the renal pelvis to enter the renal sinus. Here they give rise to **segmental arteries,** which also divide to form **interlobar arteries** that run between renal lobes. At the corticomedullary junction, these arteries divide into several **arcuate arteries** that arch across the base of each medullary pyramid and give off **interlobular arteries** that pass into the cortex between lobules. The interlobular arteries run peripherally in the cortex, giving rise to a system of **in-**tralobular arteries** that enter renal lobules and provide **afferent arterioles,** which supply the glomeruli of renal corpuscles. As the **efferent arteriole** leaves the renal corpuscle of a cortical nephron, it immediately breaks up into a **peritubular capillary network** that supplies the convoluted tubules.

The main circulation of the renal cortex is unique in that the same arterioles give rise to two distinct, sequential capillary beds: the glomerular and peritubular capillaries. Efferent arterioles from juxtamedullary nephrons, on the other hand, form several long, straight vessels, the **vasa recta,** that descend into the medullary pyramid and form hairpin loops. Like the loop of Henle, the loops of the vasa recta are staggered throughout the medulla. The walls of the vasa recta are thin, and the endothelium of the ascending (venous) limb is fenestrated. The vasa recta pass in close proximity to the loop of Henle, permitting interchange between the two elements. The vasa recta form a **vascular countercurrent exchange** system that removes excess water and ions. The osmotic gradient is not disrupted due to the slower flow rate and the smaller volume in the vasa recta. Blood flow through the vasa recta is in the opposite direction to the flow of fluid through the loops of Henle and also helps prevent disruption of the osmotic gradient.

The venous drainage of the kidney is similar to and follows the same course as the arterial supply. However, there is no venous equivalent of the glomerulus or the afferent and efferent arterioles. The venous system of the medulla begins in the ascending limb of the vasa recta, which drains into interlobular or arcuate veins. In the peripheral cortex, capillaries unite to form small veins that assume a starlike pattern as they drain into interlobular veins. The renal veins drain into the inferior vena cava. The left renal vein differs in that it is much longer and receives venous drainage from the left gonad.

Extrarenal Passages

The extrarenal passages consist of the minor and major calyces, renal pelvis, ureter, urinary bladder, and urethra. They convey urine to the outside of the body or, in the case of the bladder, store it temporarily. Except for the urethra, all have a similar basic structure with a mucosa, muscularis, and adventitia. The layers are thinnest in the minor calyces and increase in depth distally to reach their maximum development in the bladder.

Calyces, Renal Pelvis, Ureters, and Bladder

KEY WORDS: mucosa, transitional epithelium, lamina propria, muscularis, adventitia

The thickness of the wall of the excretory passage gradually increases from the upper to lower parts; except for this, all parts of the extrarenal passages show a similar structure. The lumen is lined by a **mucosa** consisting of **transitional epithelium** that rests on a lamina propria. There is no submucosa, and the lamina propria blends with the connective tissue of the well-developed muscular coat.

Transitional epithelium covers the external surfaces of the renal papillae and reflects onto the internal surfaces of the surrounding minor calyces (see atlas figure 16-23). It also is continuous with the epithelium of the papillary ducts, thus providing a complete epithelial lining that prevents escape of urine into the neighboring tissues. Transitional epithelium forms a barrier to the diffusion of salts and water into and out of the urine. In the major and minor calyces, the epithelium is two to three cells thick, increasing in the ureter to four or five layers and to six, eight, or more layers in the bladder (see atlas figures 16-23 through 16-27). The surface cells are large and rounded and in the relaxed bladder have convex or dome-shaped borders that bulge into the lumen. The superficial cells sometimes contain large polyploid nuclei. The epithelium in the distended organ shows considerable changes in morphology. In the filled bladder, or as urine is propelled down the ureter, the epithelium is stretched and flattened and temporarily assumes the appearance of a thin stratified squamous epithelium. When the intraluminal pressure is re-

lieved, the epithelium again assumes its nondistended appearance. In the relaxed bladder the apical cytoplasm of the superficial cells contains fine filaments and fusiform vesicles that are limited by a membrane of the same thickness as the cell membrane. These vesicles are thought to represent reserve surface membrane for use during distention. Transitional epithelium lies on a very thin basement membrane that usually is not seen with the light microscope.

The epithelium lies on a **lamina propria** that consists of a compact layer of fibroelastic connective tissue. Some diffuse lymphatic tissue also may be present.

The **muscularis** of the urinary passageways consists of bundles of smooth muscle separated by abundant fibroconnective tissue and begins in the minor calyces as two thin layers of smooth muscle. The inner, longitudinal layer begins at the attachment of the minor calyces to the renal papillae; the outer layer of muscle spirals around the renal papilla forming a thin coat. The walls of the minor calyces contract periodically around the renal papillae and aid in moving urine from the papillary ducts to the calyces and into the renal pelvis. The muscularis of the renal pelvis and upper two-thirds of the ureter consist of the same two layers and differ only in thickness (see atlas figure 16-24). An additional outer, longitudinal layer of smooth muscle is added in the lower one-third of the ureter.

The distal ends of the ureters, the intramural portions, pass obliquely through the wall of the bladder to empty into its lumen. The circular layer of smooth muscle disappears and the contractions of the longitudinal layers help dilate the lumen of the distal ureter so that urine can enter the bladder. Peristaltic waves periodically pass along the ureter to convey urine to the bladder, into which it empties in small spurts. As the bladder fills, the pressure of its contents keeps the intramural portions of the ureters closed due to their oblique course in the bladder wall. The ureters open only when urine is forced through them. Reflux of urine into the ureters is prevented by a valvelike flap of bladder mucosa that lies over the ureteral openings.

The muscularis of the urinary bladder is moderately thick and consists of inner longitudinal, middle circular, and outer longitudinal layers of smooth muscle (see atlas figure 16-26). The middle layer is the most prominent and spirals around each ureteral opening. Around the internal urethral orifice the muscle increases in thickness to form the internal sphincter of the bladder.

A coat of fibroelastic tissue, the **adventitia,** surrounds the muscularis and attaches the extrarenal passages to surrounding structures. In the renal pelvis it blends with the capsule of the kidney. On the superior surface of the bladder the fibroelastic coat is covered by peritoneum. The adventitia contains numerous blood vessels, lymphatics, and nerves. Blood vessels pierce the muscularis, provide it with capillaries, and then form a plexus of small vessels in the lamina propria. A rich capillary layer lies immediately beneath the epithelium. Nerve fibers and small ganglia also occur in the adventitia and represent the sympathetic and parasympathetic divisions of the autonomic nervous system. Parasympathetic fibers are important for control of micturition.

Male Urethra

KEY WORDS: prostatic urethra, membranous urethra, sphincter urethrae, penile urethra (pars cavernosa), fossa navicularis, glands of Littre, intraepithelial nests

In the male, the urethra conveys urine from the bladder to the exterior and serves for the passage of seminal fluid during ejaculation. The male urethra is 18 to 20 cm long and has three segments. The first segment is 3 to 4 cm long and lies within the prostate, an accessory sex gland. This part forms the **prostatic urethra** (pars prostatica) and is lined by transitional epithelium similar to that of the bladder. The **membranous urethra** (pars membranacea) is very short (1.5 cm) and extends from the apex of the prostate to the root of the penis. The membranous urethra pierces the skeletal muscle of the urogenital diaphragm immediately before it enters the penis. Skeletal muscle surrounding this part of the urethra forms the external sphincter (**sphincter urethrae**) and is under voluntary control during micturition.

The third and longest segment, about 15 cm, is the **penile urethra (pars cavernosa),** which runs longitudinally through the corpus cavernosa urethrae to end at the tip of the glans penis. The membranous and penile parts of the urethra are lined by stratified or pseudostratified columnar epithelium. Stratified squamous epithelium often occurs in patches in the penile portion and also lines a distal enlargement, the **fossa navicularis.** The mucous membrane of the urethra shows small depressions or invaginations called the lacunae of Morgagni, which are continuous with the branched tubular **glands of Littre** (see atlas figure 16-28). The epithelium lining these glands is the same as that of the luminal surface which contains **intraepithelial nests** of clear, mucus-secreting cells. The lamina propria beneath the urethral epithelium is a highly vascular, loose fibroconnective tissue rich in elastic fibers. The mucosa is bounded by inner longitudinal and outer circular layers of smooth muscle.

Female Urethra

The female urethra is shorter than the male (3 to 5 cm long) and is lined by stratified squamous epithelium, although patches of stratified or pseudostratified columnar may be found. Glands of Littre are present throughout its length. As in the male, the lamina propria is a vascular, fibroelastic connective tissue that contains numerous venous sinuses. The surrounding muscularis consists of an inner longitudinal layer of smooth muscle bundles and an outer circular layer. The female urethra is surrounded by skeletal muscle of the urogenital diaphragm that forms the sphincter urethrae at its orifice.

Development of the Urinary System

The urinary and reproductive systems arise in common from mesoderm of the urogenital ridge.

In reptiles, birds, and mammals, a nonfunctional pronephros, a mesonephros functional in the fetus, and a metanephros (the definitive kidney) arise successively each caudal to the last with some overlapping. A functional pronephros occurs only in chordates such as *Amphioxus* and myxinoid fishes. Except for lacking loops of Henle, pronephric and mesonephric nephrons resemble those of the metanephros (see atlas figures 16-29 and 16-30). Although the nephron and collecting tubules form continuous structures in the definitive kidney, each has a separate origin, unlike other exocrine glands in which secretory and ductal units arise from the same primordium. Mesonephroi are drained by mesonephric ducts that regress in the female but in the male are incorporated into the reproductive tract. By a series of subdivisions, an outgrowth of the duct, the ureteric bud, gives rise to ureters, renal pelvis, major and minor calyces, papillary ducts, and collecting tubules. The ureteric bud extends into the metanephric blastema, a mass of mesoderm that gives rise to nephrons (see atlas figure 16-31). The looser, more external layer of mesoderm forms the interstitial tissue and capsule of the kidney.

Proliferation of mesoderm in the subcapsular nephrogenic zone results in solid ovoid masses in which the mesenchymal cells that lie adjacent to collecting tubules form double-layered caps (see atlas figures 16-32 and 16-33). The rest of the cell mass forms a primitive renal vesicle located betewen a main collecting tubule and one of its branches. Cells of the renal vesicle and collecting tube do not make contact.

Each renal vesicle gives rise to a nephron unit. The single-layered vesicle lengthens and two indentations appear, transforming it into an S-shaped tubule. The space between the middle and low limbs of the S fills with mesodermal cells and a capillary. Together, the vessel and lower limb of the tubule evolve into a renal corpuscle. The capillaries lie immediately adjacent to the concave, external surface of the lower limb and as they expand into the tubule, they acquire an epithelial covering and form the glomerular capillaries. The parietal layer of the glomerular capsule, which originates from the opposite side of the tubule, constricts around the point of entry of the capillary loops and establishes the vascular pole. Where the tubule surrounds the developing capillaries, the columnar cells and endothelial cells share a basal lamina (see atlas figures 16-33 through 16-38).

The provisional glomerular epithelial cells show numerous desmosomes and zonula adherens—like structures that maintain contact between the epithelial cells as the capillary loops expand. The attachments occur mainly along the central, lateral regions of the cells, rather than at their apices, thus maintaining cell-to-cell union as the glomerular epithelium changes from simple cuboidal to a layer of podocytes. The attachments are transitory and are lost as the podocytes evolve. With development, podocytes become cuboidal and extend fingerlike processes from their basal surfaces toward adjacent cells (see atlas figure 16-39). The cells begin to separate from one another, and their foot processes increase in size and mingle with others to cover the expanding capillaries.

The opposite end of the S-shaped tubules unite with nearby collecting tubules, and the lumina become continuous. The tubules elongate, become U-shaped, and give rise to proximal and distal tubules and loops of Henle. The latter are the last segments to form and are not numerous until late in development.

Initially, development of the kidney is concerned with formation of nephrons; this is followed by a period of growth and differentiation of established nephrons. In humans, nephrogenesis is complete by the thirty-fifth week, but there is much species variation. In the guinea pig, it is not complete until birth and in marsupials, not until late in postnatal life. In humans, renin-immunoreactive cells appear in the mesonephros by the sixth week of gestation and in the metanephros by the eighth week, suggesting that the renin-angiotensin system may be active even during early fetal life.

Early in development, the digestive and urogenital systems open into a common space, the cloaca. Later, a wedge of mesenchyme, the urorectal septum, divides the cloaca into a dorsal rectum and a ventral bladder and urogenital sinus. The endodermal lining of the newly formed bladder becomes stratified and the surrounding mesenchyme differentiates into the muscular wall of the bladder.

Functional Summary

The kidney serves as an organ of excretion, is both an endocrine and exocrine gland, is a target organ of other endocrine glands, and plays an important role in the acid-base balance of the organism.

The uriniferous tubules perform three separate functions in the formation of urine: filtration, secretion, and selective absorption. The tubules do not synthesize and release new material in significant amounts but eliminate excess water and waste products of metabolism that are being transported in the blood plasma. After filtration of the plasma, metabolic wastes such as urea, uric acid, and creatinine are not absorbed but remain in the tubular lumen and form constituents of the urine that will be eliminated.

The renal corpuscles filter blood plasma and in humans, the kidneys produce about 125 ml of glomerular filtrate each minute. About 124 ml of this is absorbed by the rest of the uriniferous tubule, resulting in the formation of approximately 1 ml of urine. The total glomerular filtrate in humans during a 24-hour period is 170 to 200 liters, of which about 99 percent is absorbed. The filtration process is driven by the hydrostatic pressure of blood, which is sufficient to overcome the colloidal osmotic pressure of plasma and the capsular pressure at the filtration membrane. The resulting filtrate contains ions, glucose, amino acids, small proteins, and the nitrogenous wastes of metabolism. Blood cells and proteins of large molecular weight are prevented from entering the capsular space by the filtration barrier.

The glomerular filtrate is reduced to about 15 percent of its original volume in the proximal convoluted tubule. In addition to the obligatory absorption of sodium chloride and water, glucose, amino acids, proteins, and ascorbic acid are actively absorbed in the proximal convoluted tubules. Bicarbonate also is absorbed here in exchange for the secretion of hydrogen ions. Exogenous organic bases and acids are actively secreted into the lumen by the epithelium of the proximal convoluted tubule, thus fulfilling the requirements of an exocrine gland. Most of the materials that have passed through the filtration barrier are immediately resorbed by the epithelium of the uriniferous tubules and put back into the circulation. Materials in excess of the body's needs as well as any metabolic wastes (urea, uric acid, creatinine) pass along the tubular lumen and are excreted in the urine.

The loop of Henle is essential for the conservation of water and production of hypertonic urine. An active sodium pump mechanism resides in the cells of the ascending limb of the loop and creates and maintains a gradient of osmotic pressure that increases from the base of the medulla to the papillary tip. Henle's loops, with their hairpin loops, act as a countercurrent multiplier system to maintain the gradient.

The distal tubule is the principal site for acidification of urine and is the site for further absorption of bicarbonate in exchange for secretion of hydrogen ions. It therefore plays an important role in acid-base balance. The conversion of ammonia to ammonium ions also occurs in the distal tubule. Absorption of sodium ions in the distal tubule is referred to as facultative absorption and is controlled by the steroid hormone aldosterone, which increases the rate of absorption of sodium ion and excretion of potassium ion. If aldosterone is absent, large amounts of sodium are lost in the urine. Parathyroid hormone also acts on the distal convoluted tubule of the nephron to promote absorption of calcium ion and inhibit absorption of phosphate ion from the developing urine.

Collecting ducts pass through the hypertonic environment of the medulla. The permeability of the collecting ducts as well as the last portion of the distal tubule to water is controlled by ADH. In the presence of ADH, the collecting ducts and the last segment of the distal tubule become permeable to water, which, by osmosis, leaves the lumen to enter the surrounding interstitium. The flow of water out of the tubular fluid thus produces a hypertonic urine. If the concentration of ADH in the blood is low, a larger volume of dilute urine results because the permeabilty of the collecting ducts to water is decreased.

Atrial natriuretic factor (ANF) belongs to a family of atrial peptides stored in atrial-specific granules within atrial cardiac myocytes. When released, ANF acts on the kidney to increase sodium excretion and to increase the glomerular filtration rate. Its precise mode of action is unknown.

The endocrine part of the kidney, the juxtaglomerular apparatus, elaborates renin, an enzyme that acts on angiotensinogen in the blood plasma, converting it to an inactive protein called angiotensin I. A converting enzyme in the blood converts angiotensin I to the angiotensin II that stimulates the zona glomerulosa of the adrenal to release aldosterone. Aldosterone stimulates the distal tubule of the nephron to absorb sodium ions in exchange for potassium ions. Angiotensin II is a potent vasoconstrictor also and raises blood pressure. The renin-angiotensin system is influenced by blood flow through the kidney and is an important factor in hypertension. In some species the juxtaglomerular apparatus also produces a blood-borne factor called erythropoietin, which stimulates erythropoiesis in the bone marrow.

A minor calyx is attached around each renal papilla and represents the beginning of the extrarenal passageways. Minor calyces undergo periodic rhythmic contractions that aid in moving urine from the papillary ducts into the extarenal system. The walls gently contract around each renal papillae and transport the urine to the renal pelvis. Periodic contractions of the muscular walls propel small amounts of urine from the renal pelvis through the ureter to the urinary bladder, where it is temporarily stored until a sufficient volume is obtained for urine to be evacuated through the urethra. Contraction of the muscularis of the bladder wall together with voluntary relaxation of the skeletal muscle that forms the sphincter urethrae accomplishes this process during micturition.

Clinical Correlations

The most extreme abnormality of the urinary system is renal agenesis, the complete absence of renal tissue, which occurs when the two primordia of the urinary system (ureteric bud and metanephric blastema) fail to unite during development. Cysts may occur in the otherwise normal kidneys because of incomplete development of several nephrons. Some cysts may appear relatively late in infancy and represent a failure of the developing collecting duct (the distal-most branch of the ureteric bud) to unite with the developing nephrons that it drains. These then degenerate to form cystlike structures.

Glomerular disease may involve changes in the number of cells making up the glomerulus, infiltration by leukocytes, increase in the amount of extracellular material, or accumulation of foreign deposits in the filtration barrier. Cellular and extracellular changes may involve each glomerulus completely, a few glomeruli completely, or portions of a few glomeruli.

Glomerulonephritis refers to disease in which the lesions mainly involve the glomerulus but other parts of nephron are involved including the surrounding interstitium. Many forms of glomerulonephritis are related to interacting, host-produced proteins that are active in immune reactions. Glomeruli sometimes are the only site where immune complexes are deposited and persist for long periods. The deposition of such materials on the filtration membrane may be due to the high filtration pressures and the thickness of the basal lamina. Immune complexes deposited in the filtration barrier reduce the rate of glomerular filtration and initiate destruction of the plugged glomeruli. The glomerular basement membrane may become coarse and thick.

An acute diffuse glomerulonephritis may follow streptococcal infections of the throat, ears, or skin. In adults the disease may be severe and even fatal. The cortex of the kidney is pale and swollen by edema, the glomeruli are diffusely enlarged due to increased cellularity, and the capsular space is decreased or obliterated. Capillary lumina are narrowed, and uniform thickening of the basement membrane may occur (membranous glomerulonephritis). The cells comprising the filtration barrier are increased in number (proliferative glomerulitis), and the kidney is then characterized by large, cellular glomeruli. Initially, endothelial proliferation predominates but

is followed by proliferation of mesangial cells. Subendothelial immune complexes often are present in the glomerular basement membrane, and the deposits of fibrin and the excess protein and red cells that enter the capsular space contribute to blockage of normal filtration. Podocytes may show some focal fusion of foot processes. Changes in the rest of the kidney are secondary to the glomerular damage. The interstitial tissue is swollen (edematous) and may contain leukocytes. The tubules contain protein and red cell casts and the lining cells contain hyaline droplets.

The disease can be progressive (chronic glomerulonephritis), leading to hypertension, uremia, and death. The kidneys are reduced in size and the capsule can be firmly adherent. Microscopically, a few of the glomeruli are normal or nearly so, some may be hypertrophic, and the rest are replaced by scar tissue. The tubules are extensively atrophic and many are completely lost. The interstitial tissue is infiltrated by lymphocytes.

The cells of the kidney tubules show a high metabolic turnover and thus are sensitive to low oxygen levels and toxic agents. Acute tubular necrosis can occur as a result of crushing injuries or other trauma that induces myoglobinuria. Focal damage to various segments of the renal tubules occurs but is especially marked in the distal tubules. Toxic damage to tubules occurs from chemicals, bacterial toxins, metals, or drugs. Coagulative necrosis of the proximal tubules occurs, especially after copper or mercury poisoning. Fatty degeneration of tubules occurs after carbon tetrachloride poisoning.

Atlas and Tables of Key Features

Key Features of the Kidney

	Primary Location	Features of Epithelium	Other Features
Proximal convoluted tubule	Cortex	Large granular, dark-staining cells; brush border; not all cells show a nuclear profile	Stellate or irregular lumen
Distal convoluted tubule	Cortex	Light-staining columnar cells; each cell shows nuclear profile	Smooth luminal surface, large, circular in outline
Renal corpuscle (Bowman's capsule, glomerulus)	Cortex	Glomerular epithelium — light staining nuclei; glomerular endothelium — dark staining nuclei	Vascular and urinary poles, thick basal lamina
Thin segment (loop of Henle)	Medulla	Light-staining tubule lined by simple squamous epithelium	Narrow lumen
Thick segment (loop of Henle)	Medulla	Light-staining cuboidal cells	Wider lumen
Collecting tubule	Medulla	Light-staining columnar cells, distinct cell boundaries	

Key Features of Extrarenal Passages

	Epithelium	Supporting Wall
Ureter (proximal two-thirds)	Transitional (4–5 cell layers)	Inner longitudinal and outer circular smooth muscle
Ureter (distal one-third)	Transitional (4–5 cell layers)	Inner longitudinal, middle circular, and outer longitudinal smooth muscle
Male urethra		
Pars prostatica	Transitional	Prostate
Pars membranacea	Transitional	Skeletal muscle (sphincter urethrae)
Pars cavernosa	Stratified and/or pseudostratified columnar; patches of wet stratified squamous in fossa navicularis	Erectile tissue of corpus cavernosum urethrae
Female urethra	Stratified columnar; stratified squamous	Inner longitudinal, outer circular smooth muscle

Kidney

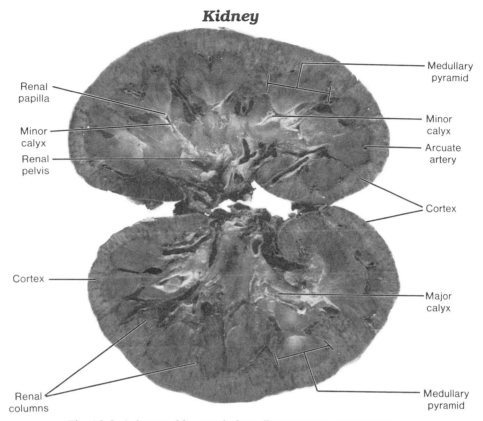

Renal papilla

Minor calyx

Renal pelvis

Medullary pyramid

Minor calyx

Arcuate artery

Cortex

Cortex

Major calyx

Renal columns

Medullary pyramid

Fig. 16-3. A dissected human kidney illustrating its anatomical features (actual size).

Afferent arteriole

Glomeruli

Afferent arterioles

Intralobular artery

Fig. 16-4. A region of renal cortex from a kidney injected with colored gelatin to demonstrate the vasculature. (LM, ×100.)

Glomerulus

Proximal convoluted tubule

Proximal convoluted tubules

Lumen of proximal convoluted tubule (urinary pole)

Capsular epithelium

Fig. 16-5. A region of renal cortex showing a renal corpuscle and several proximal convoluted tubules. (SEM, ×250.)

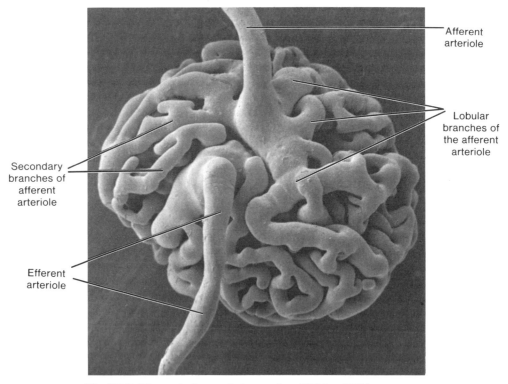

Secondary branches of afferent arteriole

Efferent arteriole

Afferent arteriole

Lobular branches of the afferent arteriole

Fig. 16-6. The cast of a renal glomerulus. (SEM, ×800.)

Podocytic investment of glomerular capillary

Cell bodies of podocytes

Primary process

Podocyte cell body

Pedicles

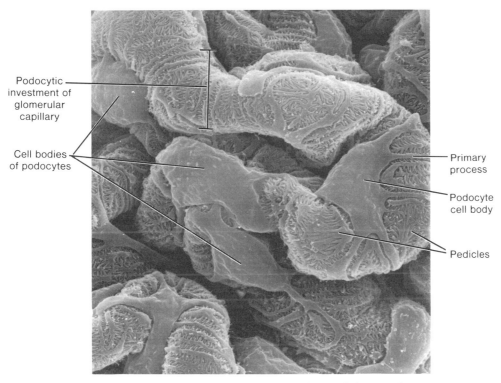

Fig. 16-7. Podocytes comprise the glomerular epithelium and form a complete investment around glomerular capillaries. (SEM, ×2,300.)

Primary processes

Primary processes

Pedicles

Primary processes

Primary process

Pedicles

Cell body of podocyte

Microprojections

Fig. 16-8. Details of podocytes forming the glomerular epithelium. Note the uniformity of the interdigitating pedicles. (SEM, ×7,600.)

Fenestrations

Fenestrations

Fig. 16-9. A portion of a fenestrated glomerular endothelial cell viewed from the capillary lumen. (SEM, ×35,000.)

Capsular space —
Slit diaphragm —
Glomerular basement membrane —
Endothelium —
Fenestrations —

Pedicles —
Slit pore —
Capillary lumen —

Fig. 16-10. A section through the renal filtration barrier. (TEM, ×80,000.)

Afferent arteriole —
Macula densa —
Juxtaglomerular cells —
Proximal convoluted tubule —

Arteriole —
Distal convoluted tubule —
Glomerulus —

Fig. 16-11. A renal corpuscle from the outer kidney cortex. (LM, ×250.)

Erythrocytes

Endothelial
cells

Granules in
juxtaglomerular
cells

Granules in
juxtaglomerular
cells

Distal
convoluted
tubule

Fig. 16-12. Juxtaglomerular cells within the wall of an afferent arteriole. (LM, × 1,000.)

Granules of
juxtaglomerular
cells

Macula
densa

Endothelial
cells

Distal
convoluted
tubule

Fig. 16-13. A macula densa lying immediately adjacent to an afferent arteriole, the wall of which contains juxtaglomerular cells. (LM, × 1,000.)

Distal convoluted tubule

Urinary pole

Proximal convoluted tubule

Parietal layer of Bowman's capsule

Glomerulus

Parietal layer of Bowman's capsule

Fig. 16-14. A renal corpuscle showing a urinary pole (compare with 16-5). (LM, ×250.)

Lumen of proximal convoluted tubule

Invaginating tubules of endocytic complex

Vacuole

Microvilli of brush border

Invaginating vesicles of endocytic complex

Fig. 16-15. The brush (microvillus) border and apical endocytic complex of a cell lining the proximal convoluted tubule. (TEM, ×10,000.)

Microvilli of brush border

Vacuole

Microvilli

Nucleus

Basal interdigitations

Fig. 16-16. A fractured preparation of proximal convoluted tubule illustrating microvilli forming the brush border and infoldings of the basolateral membrane. (SEM, ×7,000.)

Fig. 16-17. Epithelial tubules forming the renal medulla. (LM, ×250.)

Fig. 16-18. Epithelial cells lining a thin segment of the loop of Henle. (TEM, ×3,000.)

Lumen of distal convoluted tubule

Basal striations

Fig. 16-19. Two distal convoluted tubules stained with iron hematoxylin to demonstrate mitochondria of the basal striations. (LM, ×400.)

Basal infoldings of plasmalemma

Plasmalemma

Mitochondria

Nucleus

Lumen

Fig. 16-20. Basal striations of cells lining the distal convoluted tubule consist of basolateral infoldings of the plasmalemma and their associated mitochondria (compare with 16-19). (TEM, ×3,000.)

Cilium of
light cell

Apical
surface of
dark cell

Microplicae

Cilium of
light cell

Light cell

Fig. 16-21. Surface features of apices of light and dark cells in a
human collecting tubule. (SEM, ×8,000.)

Nucleus

Basal lamina

Lumen

Apical tight junction

Fig. 16-22. Two cells from the wall of a collecting tubule. (TEM, ×2,000.)

Renal papilla

Papillary ducts of Bellini

Transitional epithelium

Smooth muscle

Lumen

Fig. 16-23. A renal papilla together with its surrounding minor calyx from a human kidney. (LM, ×40.)

Ureter

Fat cells

Outer circular layer of smooth muscle

Adventitia

Inner longitudinal layer of smooth muscle

Lumen

Transitional epithelium

Lamina propria

Fig. 16-24. A portion of the wall of a human ureter. (LM, ×100.)

Urinary Bladder

Mucosal folds

Fig. 16-25. The mucosal surface of the urinary bladder. (SEM, ×20.)

Transitional epithelium

Lamina propria

Bundles of smooth muscle

Muscularis

Fig. 16-26. A section through the urinary bladder wall. (LM, ×100.)

Transitional epithelium

Lamina propria

Fig. 16-27. Transitional epithelium lining a urinary bladder. (LM, ×250.)

Urethra

Lumen of penile urethra

Diffuse lymphatic tissue

Lamina propria

Glands of Littre

Fig. 16-28. A region of human penile urethra illustrating the glands of Littre. (LM, ×100.)

Development

Developing gonad

Mesonephros

Müllerian duct

Mesonephric duct

Fig. 16-29. Surface features of the mesonephros showing both the mesonephric and müllerian ducts. Note the position of the developing gonad. (SEM, ×50.)

Fig. 16-30. A section through the length of a mesonephros demonstrates that the renal corpuscles are concentrated along the medial surface. (LM, ×20.)

Fig. 16-31. The metanephros in the initial stage of development. Note that only collecting tubules and early differentiating nephrons are present. (LM, ×400.)

Mesodermal (nephronogenic) cells

Collecting tubule

Collecting tubule

Fig. 16-32. A region of the metanephros illustrating a group of nephronogenic mesodermal cells in close association with a collecting tubule. (LM, ×400.)

Collecting tubule

Developing proximal tubule

Developing renal corpuscle

Fig. 16-33. A differentiating nephron in the cortex of the metanephros. (LM, ×400.)

Fig. 16-34. A differentiating nephron showing the initial development of the components of a renal corpuscle. (LM, ×400.)

Collecting tubule

Invading glomerular capillaries

Parietal layer

Developing glomerular epithelium

Proximal convoluted tubule

Fig. 16-35. A developing glomerulus within the expanding cortex of the metanephros (LM, ×400.)

Developing glomerular capillaries

Collecting tubule

Layer of developing podocytes

Proximal convoluted tubule

Podocytes

Developing glomerular capillaries

Parietal layer

Renal corpuscle

Proximal convoluted tubule

Fig. 16-36. Recently differentiated podocytes within a forming renal corpuscle. (LM, ×400.)

Parietal layer

Podocytes

Glomerular capillaries

Capsular space

Urinary pole

Collecting tubule

Proximal convoluted tubule

Fig. 16-37. A recently differentiated nephron in the metanephros. Compare the well-defined renal corpuscle with 16-33, 16-34, 16-35, and 16-36, which illustrate its differentiation and development. (LM, ×400.)

Capsule

Developing 2nd generation nephron

Collecting tubule

Juxtamedullary (1st generation) renal corpuscles

Fig. 16-38. The cortex of a developing kidney (metanephros), illustrating the differentiation of a second generation of nephrons. (LM, ×250.)

Parietal layer

Podocytes

A   B

Podocyte

Developing foot processes (pedicles)

Fig. 16-39. A fracture preparation of renal corpuscles showing the differentiating podocytes that cover underlying glomerular capillaries. The foot processes are only in the initial stages of development (compare to 16-37). (A. SEM, ×1,200. B. SEM, ×4,000.)

Review Questions and Answers

83. Describe the morphology of a renal corpuscle.
84. List the components of the filtration barrier and briefly discuss the functional significance of each.
85. List three hormones that influence the function of the uriniferous tubule and briefly discuss the effect of each.
86. Briefly discuss the morphology and function of the juxtaglomerular apparatus.
87. Discuss the morphology and function of the loop of Henle.

Answers

83. A renal corpuscle consists of a capillary tuft, the glomerulus, which projects into a blindly ending expansion of the uriniferous tubule called Bowman's capsule. Each renal corpuscle has a vascular pole, where afferent and efferent arterioles enter and leave the glomerulus, and a urinary pole, where the capsular space becomes continuous with the lumen of the proximal convoluted tubule.

    The epithelium of the parietal layer of Bowman's capsule consists of a single layer of tightly adherent squamous cells that prevent the leakage of glomerular filtrate into surrounding cortical tissue. At the vascular pole, component cells of the investing glomerular epithelium dramatically change their morphology from the simple squamous cells of the capsular epithelium to large, stellate-shaped podocytes. Cytoplasmic extensions from the podocytes, the primary processes, wrap around the underlying glomerular capillaries and give rise to numerous secondary processes that interdigitate with similar processes from adjacent podocytes to completely surround the capillary loops of the glomerulus. Narrow clefts called filtration slits lie between the interdigitating secondary process. The secondary processes of the podocytes and the heavily fenestrated endothelium share a continuous, common basal lamina. The renal corpuscle is that portion of the nephron that functions in filtration.

84. The filtration barrier of a renal corpuscle consists of three entities: a fenestrated glomerular endothelium, a common basal lamina, and foot processes of the glomerular epithelium. The glomerular endothelium prevents the passage of formed blood elements (blood cells and platelets) while the common basal lamina restricts the passage of substances with a molecular weight greater than 400,000 or highly charged molecules. Substances of smaller molecular weight (40,000 or less) traverse the endothelial barriers and the common basal lamina and pass through the filtration slits of the surrounding glomerular epithelium to enter the capsular space. Although materials with a molecular weight larger than 45,000 or that have a highly irregular shape may pass through the fenestrated endothelium and common basal lamina, they are unable to traverse the barrier provided by the foot processes of the podocytes. The barrier also limits passage of materials with respect to charge. Heparan sulfate and podocalyxin give the barrier a net negative charge; therefore anionic molecules are more restricted in their passage through the basal lamina of the barrier than are neutral molecules of similar size. Hydrostatic pressure of blood in the glomerular capillaries is sufficient to overcome the colloidal osmotic pressure of substances in the blood and the capsular pressure of the filtration membrane.

85. Three hormones that influence the function of the uriniferous tubule are aldosterone, parathyroid hormone, and anti-

diuretic hormone (ADH). Aldosterone, a steroid hormone from the adrenal cortex, promotes sodium ion transport from the lumen of the distal tubule in exchange for potassium ion. Inadequate concentrations of aldosterone result in a serious loss of sodium in the urine. The presence of parathyroid hormone also acts on the tubular components of the nephron to promote absorption of calcium ion and to inhibit the absorption of phosphate ion from the forming urine. Antidiuretic hormone acts primarily on distal tubules and collecting ducts and increases their permeability to water. In the presence of ADH water leaves the lumen of the tubules by osmosis, being drawn by the hypertonic environment of the surrounding interstitium. The flow of water out of the tubular fluid and into the interstitium produces a hypertonic urine. If the concentration of ADH in the blood is low, the permeability of the collecting ducts to water is decreased, resulting in a larger volume of dilute urine.

86. The juxtaglomerular apparatus is the endocrine portion of the kidney and consists of the juxtaglomerular (JG) cells, the macula densa, and the extraglomerular mesangium. The JG cells are found within the wall of the afferent arteriole and are thought to be modified smooth muscle cells. They are cuboidal in shape and contain secretory granules, well-developed Golgi complexes, and numerous profiles of granular endoplasmic reticulum. The JG cells synthesize, at least in part, an enzyme called renin that activates the angiotensin-aldosterone system. The location of the macula densa and its basal polarization and orientation toward the JG cells suggest a functional relationship between these two cell groups. The macula densa is thought to sense the sodium ion concentration in the distal tubule and may influence the activity of the JG cells. The extraglomerular mesangium forms a loose mass of cells between the afferent and efferent arterioles. Component cells may contain granules, but their exact role in the function of the juxtaglomerular apparatus is unknown. The juxtaglomerular apparatus in some species also produces a blood-borne factor called erythropoietin, which stimulates erythropoiesis in the bone marrow.

87. The loop of Henle is that part of the nephron that is interposed between the proximal and distal convoluted tubules and consists of the straight portion of the proximal tubule, the thin segment, and the straight portion of the distal tubule (the ascending thick limb). The loops of Henle descend in the medulla for variable distances, form a hairpin loop, and then ascend parallel to the descending limb, back through the medulla to the cortex. The loop of Henle is essential for the conservation of water and the production of hypertonic urine. An active sodium pump mechanism resides in the cells of the ascending limb and provides and maintains a gradient of osmotic pressure that increases from the base of the medulla to the papillary tip. The loops of Henle with their hairpin turns play an important role by serving as a countercurrent multiplier system to maintain this osmotic gradient.

17 Meiosis and Male Reproductive Organs

In mammals the male and female reproductive organs produce the gametes, provide a mechanism by which the gametes can be brought together to yield a new individual, and in the female, house and nourish the zygote until birth of that new individual.

The generative organs for the production of male gametes (sperm) are the testes, while in the female the ovary is the site of the female gametes, the ova. Gametes cannot contain the diploid (somatic) number of chromosomes since their fusion would result in a doubling of the chromosomes with each new generation. Thus, the gametes can contain only half the somatic number of chromosomes, and reduction to the haploid number occurs through a special form of cell division called meiosis.

Meiosis

KEY WORDS: two cell divisions, one DNA replication, first meiotic division, separation of homologous chromosomes, second meiotic division, separation of chromatids

Meiosis is characterized by **two cell divisions** but only **one replication of deoxyribonucleic acid (DNA).** Chromosomal DNA is duplicated during interphase, prior to the first division, and results in a double or tetraploid amount of DNA within the diploid number of chromosomes. This is no different from what occurs during replication of DNA prior to ordinary mitosis. The **first meiotic division** brings about **separation of homologous chromosomes,** and while this results in halving the number of chromosomes, each chromosome contains a double amount of DNA so that the total content of DNA within the resulting cells remains diploid. A **second meiotic division** then occurs without a period of DNA replication. Sister **chromatids are separated** at this time to yield cells with the haploid number of chromosomes and the haploid amount of DNA.

The stages of meiotic division are the same as those of mitosis, namely prophase, anaphase, metaphase, and telophase.

Prophase I

KEY WORDS: leptotene, zygotene, synapsis (conjugation), bivalent, pachytene, tetrad, diplotene, crossing over, chiasma, recombination, diakinesis

The first meiotic prophase is long and complex and varies markedly from that of mitosis. It customarily is divided into five stages: leptotene, zygotene, pachytene, diplotene, and diakinesis.

In **leptotene** the chromosomes begin to condense and become visible as individual, slender threads that resemble those of early prophase of mitosis. In many animals the ends of the chromosomes become oriented to the side of the nucleus nearest the centrosome, with the bodies of the chromosomes extending in loops into the interior of the nucleus.

During **zygotene,** the homologous chromosomes come together in pairs in which the chromosomes lie side by side, aligned point-for-point along their lengths. Because of the close apposition of the homologous chromosomes at this stage, they appear to be present in the haploid number. This pairing is called **synapsis** (or **conjugation**), and each pair of homologous chromosomes forms a **bivalent.**

The chromosomes continue to contract and at **pachytene** are short and thick. Each chromosome of the bivalent begins to split lengthwise and then can be seen to consist of two chromatids; the bivalent therefore consists of four chromatids and is frequently called a **tetrad.**

In the **diplotene** stage, each chromosome splits into its constituent chromatids, which remain attached only at their centromeres (kinetochores). The homologous chromatids move apart slightly and the tetrad formation becomes more obvious. At points along their lengths, the homologous chromatids make contact with each other and exchange segments; this exchange constitutes **crossing over.** The physical regions where the contacts are made are called **chiasmata.** The exchange of segments between homologous chromatids results in reassortment or **recombination** of the genetic material. The chromosomes continue to shorten and thicken and the nucleolus begins to fragment and disappear.

Diakinesis is marked by an even greater contraction of the chromosomes that are scattered throughout the cell. The homologous chromosomes still are paired but are joined only at the chiasmata. At the end of prophase I, the nuclear envelope and nucleoli have disappeared and the tetrads have begun their migration to the equator of the cell.

Metaphase I

Metaphase I is similar to the metaphase of mitotic division except that pairs of chromosomes (bivalents), not single chromosomes, are arranged about the spindle. The homologous pairs are aligned so that the members of each pair lie at either side of the equatorial plate, with the centromeres of homologous chromosomes facing opposite poles.

Anaphase I and Telophase I

Anaphase I and telophase I also are similar to those of mitotic cell division. However, at anaphase I of meiosis, the centromeres have not split so that rather than chromatids separating and moving to opposite poles, whole chromosomes, each consisting of two chromatids, are separated. Reconstruction of the nuclei and cytoplasmic separation occur at telophase I to yield two new cells. However, since the orientation of the bivalents on the equatorial plate is random, there is a random assortment of maternal and paternal chromosomes in each of the telophase nuclei.

Meiotic Division II

KEY WORDS: **no DNA synthesis, splitting of centromeres, separation of chromatids**

The second meiotic division is more like that of mitosis and occurs after a brief interphase during which there is **no synthesis of DNA.** In some species, the cells produced at the end of the first division enter directly into metaphase II and bypass a second prophase. The **centromeres split** at metaphase and the **chromatids separate** during anaphase. Unlike mitosis, the sister chromatids are not identical, due to the crossing over that occurred during the first meiotic prophase and to the random alignment of the homologous chromosomes at the first division. Following telophase and cytokinesis, four haploid cells result.

Differences in Meiosis of Male and Female Germ Cells

The mechanics of meiosis are the same regardless of whether sperm or ova are produced, but there are marked differences in the net yield of the two types of gametes and in the times at which meiosis is initiated. In the male, four viable, functioning sperm are produced from each germ cell that enters meiosis, whereas the same events in the female yield only a single functioning ovum. After the first and second meiotic divisions, the cytoplasm is distributed evenly among the developing sperm, but in the formation of ova the bulk of the cytoplasm is passed to only one cell. The remaining ova, called polar bodies, receive so little cytoplasm that they are unable to survive.

The time at which meiotic division is initiated in the male and female germ cells is remarkably different. In the human female, the germ cells begin their meiotic divisions in the embryo, and by the fifth month of intrauterine life, the developing ova are in the diplotene stage of the first meiotic division but the division is not complete until just before ovulation. Hence, many of the ova remain suspended in the diplotene stage for several decades. The second meiotic division and the formation of the second polar body occur only after fertilization. In contrast, meiotic division in the male germ cells is not initiated until puberty, and once the cell has entered meiosis, the process is carried to completion with no prolonged interruption. A diagrammatic representation of meiosis is given in Figure 17-1.

Male Reproductive System

The male reproductive system consists of the gonads (testes), their excretory ducts, the accessory glands, and the penis. The gonads supply the male germ cells or gametes (sperm), which are conducted to the exterior by the excretory system, which includes the penis. The accessory glands contribute secretions that, together with the sperm, form the semen.

Testes

KEY WORDS: tunica vaginalis, tunica albuginea, mediastinum testis, septula testis, lobuli testis, seminiferous tubules, tunica vasculosa, interstitial tissue, interstitial cells (of Leydig)

The testes are compound tubular glands that in most mammals, including humans, lie within a scrotal sac, suspended from the body by a spermatic cord. The testes are dual organs that act as exocrine glands producing a holocrine secre-

tion, the sperm, and as endocrine organs that secrete male sex hormone, testosterone.

Each testis is covered anteriorly and laterally by a simple squamous epithelium (mesothelium) called the visceral layer of **tunica vaginalis.** On the posterior aspect of the testis, this mesothelium reflects onto the scrotal sac and lines it as the parietal layer of the tunica vaginalis. The serous cavity between visceral and parietal layers allows the testes to move freely and reduces the chance of injury from increased pressure on the exterior of the scrotum.

A thick, fibrous capsule, the **tunica albuginea,** lies beneath the visceral layer of tunica vaginalis, separated from it only by a basal lamina. Tunica albuginea consists of a dense fibroelastic connective tissue that contains scattered smooth muscle cells. In humans, the muscle cells are concentrated in the posterior region, where the tunica albuginea thickens and projects into the testis to form the **mediastinum testis.** Connective tissue partitions, the **septula testis,** extend from the mediastinum into the interior of the testis and subdivide it into approximately 250 pyramid-shaped compartments called **lobuli testis.** The apices of the compartments are directed toward the mediastinum, and each lobule contains one to four convoluted **seminiferous tubules** that represent the exocrine portion of the testis. Their product is whole cells (spermatozoa).

The inner region of the tunica albuginea, the **tunica vasculosa,** consists of loose connective tissue and contains numerous small blood vessels that supply the testis. The connective tissue extends into each lobule and fills the spaces between the seminiferous tubules, forming the **interstitial tissue** of the testis. The interstitial tissue is rich in extracellular fluid and contains abundant small blood vessels and lymphatics that form a plexus around the seminiferous tubules. In addition to fibroblasts, the interstitial tissue contains macrophages, mast cells, mesenchymal cells, and large polyhedral cells 15 to 20 μm in diameter. These are the **interstitial cells (of Leydig),** which commonly occur in groups and make up the endocrine portion of the testis. They

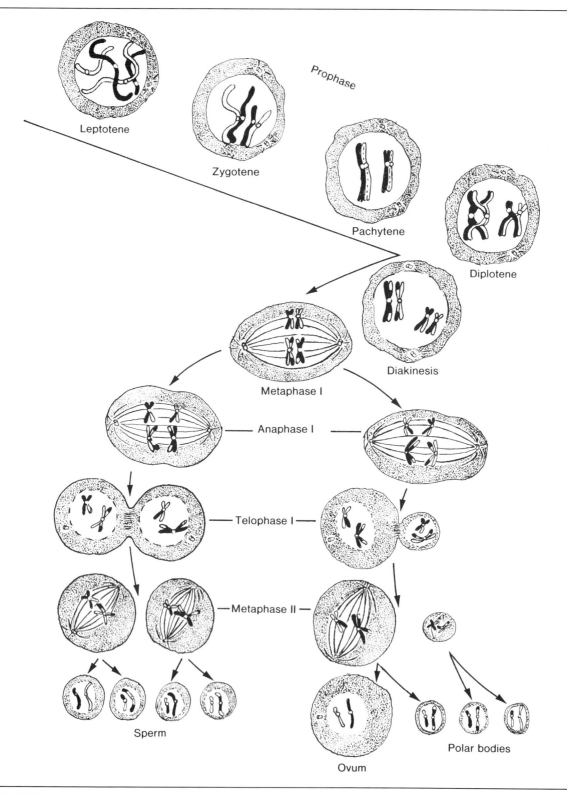

Fig. 17-1. Diagrammatic representation of meiotic division.

secrete the male steroid hormone testosterone. Interstitial cells usually contain single, large, spherical nuclei, but binucleate cells are not uncommon. In electron micrographs, the cytoplasm shows abundant smooth endoplasmic reticulum, well-developed Golgi complexes, and numerous mitochondria, which, in many species, contain tubular rather than lamellar cristae.

Testosterone and its metabolites are essential for the proliferation and the differentiation of excretory ducts and male accessory sex glands and for maintaining these structures in a functional state. Testosterone influences other tissues and is responsible for beard growth, low pitch of the voice, muscular build, and male distribution of hair. Production of testosterone by the interstitial cells is controlled by a gonadotropic hormone called interstitial cell–stimulating hormone (ICSH), which is secreted by cells in the anterior pituitary.

Most of the enzymes involved in the synthesis of testosterone are located in the smooth endoplasmic reticulum, although the enzymes for one step (conversion of cholesterol to pregnenolone) are found in the mitochondria of interstitial cells. In humans, interstitial cells are characterized by large cytoplasmic crystals called the crystals of Reinke. These proteinaceous bodies are highly variable in shape and size but are readily seen with the light microscope (see atlas figure 17-12). In electron micrographs they show a highly ordered structure. The crystals appear in the testes of most postpubertal males and vary considerably in number. Their significance is unknown.

Seminiferous Tubules

KEY WORDS: peritubular tissue, myoid (peritubular contractile) cell, germinal epithelium, supporting (Sertoli) cell, spermatogenic cell

Each testicular lobule contains one to four highly convoluted seminiferous tubules that measure 150 to 250 μm in diameter and 30 to 70 mm long. A seminiferous tubule consists of a complex stratified germinal (seminiferous) epithelium surrounded by a layer of peritubular tissue (see atlas figures 17-6 and 17-7).

The **peritubular tissue** is separated from the germinal epithelium by a basal lamina and consists of collagenous fibers and flattened cells that, depending on the species, may contain numerous actin filaments. These are the **myoid (peritubular contractile) cells.** In some primates and several other species (bull, ram, boar), the peritubular tissue contains three to five layers of myoid cells that are said to be contractile and may be responsible for the rhythmic contractions seen in the seminiferous tubules. This propulsive action helps to move sperm and testicular fluid from the seminiferous tubules into the excretory ducts.

The **germinal epithelium** of the adult is unique among epithelia in that it consists of a fixed, stable population of **supporting (Sertoli) cells** and a proliferating population of differentiating **spermatogenic cells.** Developing germ cells slowly migrate upward along the lateral surfaces of the supporting cells to be released at the free surface into the lumen of the seminiferous tubule.

Sertoli Cells

KEY WORDS: tall columnar, basal compartment, adluminal compartment, blood-testis barrier, androgen-binding protein, inhibin

The Sertoli cell is a **tall columnar** cell that spans the germinal epithelium from the basal lamina to the luminal surface (see atlas figures 17-7, 17-9, and 17-10). The cell has an elaborate shape with numerous lateral processes with recesses or concavities that surround differentiating spermatogenic cells. The apical portion of the cells also envelops developing germ cells and releases them into the lumen of the seminiferous tubule. The expanded portion of the cell contains an irregularly shaped nucleus distinguished by a large, prominent nucleolus that is readily seen with the light microscope. The basal cytoplasm contains abundant smooth endoplasmic reticulum, and a large, well-developed Golgi complex occupies the supranuclear region. The cytoplasm contains many lipid droplets, lysosomes, thin elongated mitochondria, scattered profiles of granular endoplasmic reticulum, and a sheath of fine filaments that envelops the nucleus and separates it from the organelles. Microtubules are present also, their numbers depending on the state of activity of the cell. Human Sertoli cells feature membrane-bound inclusions called the crystalloids of Charcot-Böttcher; their function is unknown.

Tight junctions occur between adjacent Sertoli cells near their bases and subdivide the germinal epithelium into basal and adluminal compartments, each of which has a separate, distinct population of spermatogenic cells. The **basal compartment** extends from the basal lamina of the germinal epithelium to the tight junctions; the **adluminal compartment** lies between the tight junctions and the lumen of the tubule. The tight junctions between the Sertoli cells appears to form, at least in part, a **blood-testis barrier** (Fig. 17-2). Germ cells in the basal compartment are contained within an environment that has access to substances in the blood, while the germ cells in the adluminal compartment reside in a specialized milieu that is maintained and controlled by the Sertoli cells. A number of plasma proteins are present in the basal compartment that are not found in the luminal contents of the seminiferous tubule that, however, are rich in other amino acids and ions. Sertoli cells are thought to provide all the nutrients for the avascular germinal epithelium.

In addition to secreting testicular fluid, Sertoli cells release **androgen-binding protein,** whose synthesis is thought to be stimulated by a pituitary gonadotropin, follicle-stimulating hormone (FSH) (Fig. 17-3). The protein binds testosterone, thus providing the adluminal compartment with the level of hormone needed for the normal differentiation and development of germ cells. The blood-testis barrier helps to confine the high concentration of testosterone to the adluminal compartment and thus allows a different environment to be established in the basal compartment. Many of the developing germ cells in

Fig. 17-2. Germinal epithelium.

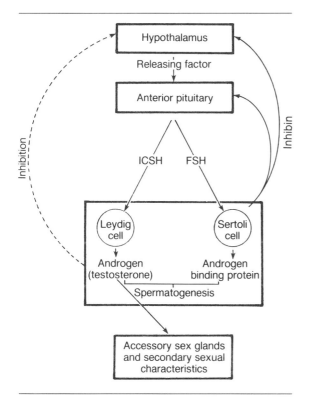

Fig. 17-3. Endocrine control of testicular functions. (ICSH = interstitial cell–stimulating hormone; FSH = follicle-stimulating hormone.)

portant in the release of germ cells into the lumen. The microtubules and actin filaments in the cytoplasmic processes of the Sertoli cells may provide these processes with the mobility they need to carry out their functions. The numerous gap junctions that occur between adjacent Sertoli cells facilitate communication between cells along specific segments of a seminiferous tubule during migration and release of germ cells. Sertoli cells also secrete a glycoprotein known as **inhibin.** Inhibin suppresses the secretion of FSH by the anterior pituitary and via this feedback loop acts to control the rate of spermatogenesis.

Spermatogenic Cells

KEY WORDS: **spermatogenesis, type A spermatogonia, type B spermatogonia, primary spermatocyte, secondary spermatocyte, spermatid**

The spermatogenic cells of the germinal epithelium consist of spermatogonia, primary and secondary spermatocytes, and spermatids. These are not separate cell types but represent stages in a continuous process of differentiation called **spermatogenesis.** The term includes the entire sequence of events in the transformation of diploid spermatogonia at the base of the germinal epithelium into haploid spermatozoa that are released into the lumen of the seminiferous tubule.

Spermatogonia lie in the basal compartment of the germinal epithelium, immediately adjacent to the basal lamina (see atlas figures 17-7, 17-9, and 17-10). The cells are 10 to 20 μm in diameter and round or ellipsoidal in shape, and the nucleus of each cell contains the diploid number of chromosomes. Two types of spermatogonia can be differentiated. **Type A spermatogonia** replicate by mitosis and provide a reservoir of stem cells for the formation of future germ cells. During mitotic division, some type A spermatogonia give rise to intermediate forms that eventually produce **type B spermatogonia;** these are committed to the production of primary spermatocytes. The two types of spermatogonia can be differentiated by their nuclei. Type A spermatogonia have spherical or elliptical nuclei with fine chromatin gran-

the adluminal compartment are haploid and might be regarded as foreign material by the body if released into surrounding tissues. The tight junctions between Sertoli cells may prevent haploid germ cells from contacting general body tissues and thus prevent an antibody response to the organism's own germ cells. Although tight junctions probably contribute to the barrier, there may be other factors involved.

Sertoli cells phagocytize any degenerating germ cells and take up the residual cytoplasm that normally is shed during release of mature germ cells into the seminiferous tubule. In addition to providing mechanical and nutritional support for developing sperm, Sertoli cells also control the movement of germ cells from the basal lamina through the epithelium to the lumen and are imules and one or two nucleoli near the nuclear envelope. The lighter-stained, spherical nuclei of type B spermatogonia contain variably sized clumps of chromatin, most of which are arranged along the nuclear envelope. Only a single, centrally placed nucleolus is found.

Primary spermatocytes at first resemble type B spermatogonia, but as they migrate from the basal lamina of the germinal epithelium, they become larger and more spherical and the nucleus enters the initial stages of division (see atlas figures 17-7 through 17-10). Primary spermatocytes usually are found in the central zone of the germinal epithelium. How these large cells pass from the basal to the adluminal compartment is unknown.

The primary spermatocyte undergoes the first meiotic division to produce **secondary spermatocytes.** The homologous chromosomes have separated and the number is reduced by half, but the cells contain the diploid amount of DNA. Secondary spermatocytes lie nearer the lumen than the primary forms and are about half their size. Unlike the extended division of primary spermatocytes, secondary spermatocytes divide quickly in the second meiotic division to produce **spermatids,** which contain the haploid number of cells and the haploid amount of DNA. Because they divide so quickly after being formed, secondary spermatocytes are seen only rarely in the germinal epithelium. Spermatids are about half the size of secondary spermatocytes. Numerous spermatids in different stages of maturation border the lumen of the seminiferous tubule (see atlas figures 17-7 through 17-11).

The cell divisions that take place during formation of male germ cells are unique in that not only is the genetic material reduced by one half, the division of the cytoplasm is incomplete. Thus, the cells resulting from a single spermatogonium remain in cytoplasmic continuity throughout the different stages of differentiation. The continuity is broken only when the sperm are finally released by the Sertoli cell.

Spermiogenesis

KEY WORDS: acrosome, acrosomal vesicle, head cap, axoneme, implantation fossa, connecting piece, annulus, middle piece, head

The elaborate events by which spermatids differentiate into slender, motile sperm are called spermiogenesis. Newly formed spermatids are round cells with central, spherical nuclei, prominent Golgi complexes, numerous mitochondria, and a pair of centrioles. Each of these components undergoes changes during spermiogenesis.

At the onset of spermiogenesis, many small granules appear in the Golgi membranes and eventually coalesce to form a single structure called the **acrosome.** The developing acrosome is bounded by a membrane, the **acrosomal vesicle,** which also is derived from the Golgi complex and is closely associated with the outer layer of the nuclear envelope. The acrosomal vesicle expands, then collapses over the anterior half of the nucleus to form the **head cap.** The acrosome, which contains hydrolytic enzymes, remains within the acrosomal membrane. As these events occur, the two centrioles migrate to a position near the nucleus on the side opposite the forming acrosome. Nine peripheral doublets plus a central pair of microtubules develop from the distal centriole and begin to form the **axoneme** of the tail. The proximal centriole becomes closely associated with a caudal region of the nucleus called the **implantation fossa.**

As the axoneme continues to develop, nine longitudinal coarse fibers extend around it and blend with nine short, segmented columns that form the **connecting piece,** which unites the nucleus (head) with the tail of the spermatozoon. The **annulus,** a ringlike structure, forms near the centrioles and migrates down the developing flagellum. Randomly distributed mitochondria migrate to the flagellum and become aligned in a tight helix between the centrioles and the annulus. This spirally arranged mitochondrial sheath characterizes the **middle piece** of the tail of a mature spermatozoon.

Simultaneously, marked changes occur in the nucleus: It becomes condensed, elongated, and slightly flattened. Together with the acrosome, it forms the sperm **head.** The bulk of the cytoplasm now is associated with the middle piece of the evolving spermatid, and as differentiation nears completion, the excess cytoplasm is shed as the residual body, leaving only a thin layer of cytoplasm to cover the spermatozoon. The residual cytoplasm is phagocytized by Sertoli cells as the spermatozoa are released into the lumen of the seminiferous tubule. Although morphologically the spermatozoa appear mature, they are nonmotile and incapable of fertilization at this time.

In most species, spermatids at specific stages of differentiation always are associated with spermatocytes and spermatogonia, which also are at specific stages of development. A series of such associations occur along the length of the same seminiferous tubule, and the distance between two identical germ cell associations is called a "wave" of seminiferous epithelium. Although waves of activity are not seen in humans, the fundamental pattern of cycling of the germinal epithelium is the same as in other mammals. The time taken for spermatogonia to become spermatozoa is relatively constant and species-specific: In humans it is about 64 days. If germ cells fail to develop at their normal rate, they degenerate and are phagocytosed by adjacent Sertoli cells.

Spermatozoa

KEY WORDS: head, tail, acrosomal cap, neck, capitulum, middle piece, principal piece, end piece, capacitation

Spermatozoa that lie free in the lumina of seminiferous tubules consist of a **head** containing the nucleus and a **tail,** which eventually gives motility to the free cell (see atlas figures 17-25 and 17-26). The chromatin of the nucleus is very condensed and reduced in volume, providing the functionally mature sperm with greater mobility. The condensed form of chromatin also protects the genome while the spermatozoon is en route to fertilize the ovum. The **acrosomal cap** covers the anterior two-thirds of the nucleus and contains lysosomes that are important for penetra-

tion of the ovum at fertilization. The size and shape of the nucleus vary tremendously in different species.

The sperm tail is about 55 μm long and consists of a neck, middle piece, principal piece, and end piece. The structural details of the different segments are best seen with the electron microscope (Fig. 17-4).

The **neck** is the region where the head and tail unite. It contains the connecting piece that joins the nine outer dense fibers of the tail to the implantation fossa of the nucleus. The region of the connecting piece that joins the implantation fossa is expanded slightly to form the **capitulum.** The **middle piece** extends from the neck to the annulus and consists of the axoneme, the nine coarse fibers, and the helical sheath of mitochondria (see atlas figures 17-25 and 17-26). The **principal piece** is the longest part of the tail and consists of the axoneme and the nine coarse fibers $(2 + 9 + 9)$ enclosed by a sheath of circumferential fibers. The circumferential fibers join two longitudinal thickenings of this sheath located on opposite sides. The **end piece** is the shortest segment of the tail and consists only of the axoneme surrounded by the cell membrane.

The last step in the physiologic maturation of spermatozoa takes place in the female reproductive tract and is called **capacitation.** This final activation requires 1 to 66 hours to complete, depending on the species, and is characterized by changes in the acrosomal cap and the respiratory metabolism of the spermatozoa. Capacitation substantially increases the number of spermatozoa capable of fertilization, but the mechanism of this activation is unknown.

Excretory Ducts

The excretory ducts consist of a complex system of tubules that link each testis to the urethra, through which the exocrine secretion, semen, is conducted to the exterior. The duct system consists of the tubuli recti (straight tubules), rete testis, ductus efferentes, ductus epididymis, ductus deferens, ejaculatory ducts, and prostatic, membranous, and penile urethra.

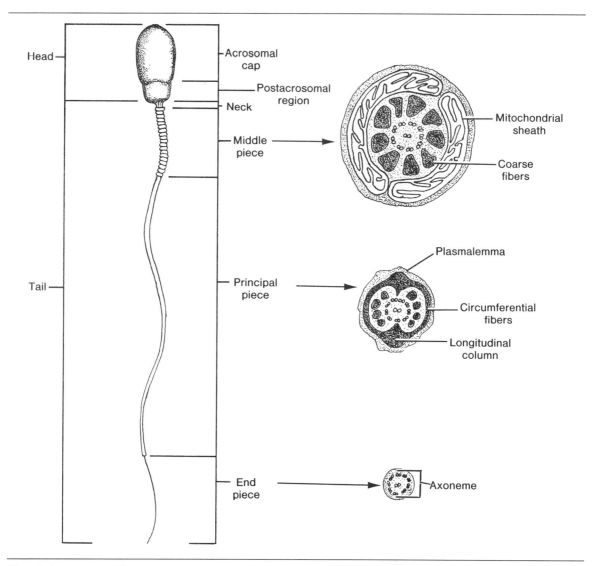

Fig. 17-4. Structure of a spermatozoon.

Tubuli Recti

KEY WORDS: simple columnar epithelium

Near the apex of each testicular lobule, the seminiferous tubules join to form short, straight tubules called the tubuli recti. The lining epithelium has no germ cells and consists only of Sertoli cells. This **simple columnar epithelium** lies on a thin basal lamina and is surrounded by loose connective tissue. The lumina of the tubuli recti are continuous with a network of anastomosing channels in the mediastinum, the rete testis.

Rete Testis

KEY WORDS: simple cuboidal epithelium

The rete testis is lined by **simple cuboidal epithelium** in which each of the component cells bears short microvilli and a single cilium on the apical surface. The epithelium lies on a delicate basal lamina. The channels of the rete testis are surrounded by a dense bed of vascular tissue (see atlas figure 17-13). The rete testis of some species may lie axially in the testis and drain surrounding seminiferous tubules along its entire length.

Ductuli Efferentes

KEY WORDS: initial segment, head of epididymis, tall and short columnar, ciliated and nonciliated cells

In humans, 10 to 15 ductuli efferentes emerge from the mediastinum on the posterior-superior surface of the testis and unite the channels of the rete testis with the ductus epididymis. The ductules follow a convoluted course and, with their supporting tissue, make up the **initial segment** of the **head of the epididymis.** The luminal border of the efferent ductules shows a characteristic irregular contour due to the presence of alternating groups of **tall and short columnar** cells (see atlas figure 17-14). **Ciliated and nonciliated cells** are present. Each contains the organelles normally associated with epithelia as well as supranuclear granules that are lysosomal in nature. The nonciliated cells show numerous microvilli on their apical surfaces and are thought to absorb much of the testicular fluid that is present in this part of the ductal system. Cilia on the other cell type beat toward the epididymis and help move the nonmotile sperm and testicular fluid in that direction.

The epithelium lies on a basal lamina and is bounded by a layer of circularly arranged smooth muscle that thickens toward the duct of the epididymis. Cilia are not found beyond the ductuli efferentes, and the movement of sperm through the remainder of the duct system depends on the contractions of the muscular wall.

Ductus Epididymidis

KEY WORDS: pseudostratified columnar, principal cell, stereocilia, basal cell, smooth muscle, three-layered coat

The efferent ductules gradually unite to form a single ductus epididymidis that measures 5 to 7 M long. This highly coiled duct and its associated vascular connective tissue form the rest of the head and the body and tail of the epididymis. The epithelial lining is **pseudostratified columnar** and consists of principal and basal cells (see atlas figure 17-15).

Principal cells are the most numerous and are very tall (80 μm) in the proximal segment, but gradually decrease in height distally to measure only 40 μm near the junction with the ductus deferens. Long microvilli, inappropriately called **stereocilia,** extend from the apical surfaces of the principal cells. A very large Golgi complex takes up a supranuclear position in the cell, and the basal region is filled by an abundance of endoplasmic reticulum. Lysosomes, multivesicular bodies, and numerous coated vesicles also are present. One of the functions of the principal cell is absorption; together, the proximal portion of the ductus epididymidis and the ductuli efferentes absorb over 90 percent of the fluid produced by the seminiferous epithelium.

Basal cells are small, round cells that lie on the basal lamina, interposed between the principal cells. They have a lightly staining cytoplasm with few organelles. Scattered intraepithelial lymphocytes often are present in the epithelium of the ductus epididymidis.

The epididymal epithelium lies on a basal lamina and is surrounded by a thin lamina propria and a thin layer of circularly arranged **smooth muscle** cells. Near the ductus deferens, the muscle layer thickens and becomes **three layered** (inner longitudinal, middle circular, outer longitudinal); it is continuous with that of the ductus deferens. The regional differences reflect differences in the mobility of the ductus epididymidis. Proximally, the duct shows spontaneous peristaltic contractions that slowly move spermatozoa through the epididymis; distally, the peristaltic contractions are reduced and this region serves to store sperm. Spermatozoa become physiologically mature as they pass through the epididymis. Those entering the proximal part of the duct mostly are incapable of fertilization and swim in a weak, random fashion. Spermatozoa from the distal portion are capable of fertilizing ova and show strong, unidirectional motility. How the ductus epididymidis contributes to the maturation of spermatozoa is unknown. In some marsupials, such as the North American opossum, the sperm form pairs in the epididymis. Transit time through the epididymis is about 3 to 10 days in most animals, and about 7 days for humans.

Ductus Deferens

KEY WORDS: mucosa, pseudostratified columnar, stereocilia, lamina propria, muscularis, adventitia, ampulla

The ductus deferens unites the ductus epididymidis and the prostatic urethra. It is characterized by a thick wall consisting of a mucosa, a muscularis, and an adventitia. The **mucosa** is thrown into longitudinal folds that project into the lumen and consists of **pseudostratified columnar** epithelium resting on a thin basal lamina. The epithelium bears **stereocilia** on the luminal surface. The surrounding **lamina propria** is dense and contains numerous elastic fibers. The **muscularis** is the dominant feature of the ductus deferens and consists of three layers of smooth muscle arranged longitudinally in the inner and outer layers and circularly in the middle layer (see atlas figure 17-16). The muscularis is surrounded by the loose connective tissue of the **adventitia,** which blends with neighboring structures and anchors the ductus deferens in place. Powerful contractions of the muscular wall propel sperm from the distal ductus epididymidis and rapidly transport them through the ductus deferens during ejaculation.

Near its termination, the ductus deferens dilates to form the **ampulla.** The lumen expands and the mucosa is folded, creating a labyrinth of pocketlike recesses (see atlas figure 17-17). The

lining epithelium is pseudostratified columnar. The muscular coat of the ampulla is thinner and the layers are less distinct than in other parts of the ductus deferens. Each smooth muscle cell in the muscularis of the ductus deferens receives direct sympathetic innervation. This accounts for the rapid, forceful contractions of the ductus during ejaculation.

Ejaculatory Duct

KEY WORDS: pseudostratified or simple columnar epithelium

A short, narrow region of the ductus deferens extends beyond the ampulla and joins the duct of the seminal vesicle. This combined duct forms the ejaculatory duct, which empties into the prostatic urethra. It is about 1 cm long and is lined by a **pseudostratified or simple columnar epithelium** (see atlas figure 17-21). The mucosa forms outpockets that are similar to, but not as well developed as, those in the ampulla. The remainder of the wall of the ejaculatory duct consists only of fibrous connective tissue (see atlas figure 17-20).

Prostatic Urethra

KEY WORDS: transitional epithelium, colliculus seminalis, prostatic utricle

The ejaculatory duct penetrates the prostate gland and opens into the prostatic part of the urethra. The prostatic urethra is lined by a thin **transitional epithelium** and bears a dome-shaped elevation, the **colliculus seminalis,** on its posterior wall. A small blind diverticulum called the **prostatic utricle** lies on the summit of the colliculus and represents a remnant of the müllerian duct in the male. The two ejaculatory ducts, one draining each testis, empty into the prostatic urethra on either side of the utricle. Numerous glands from the surrounding prostate also empty into this part of the urethra.

Accessory Sex Glands

Male accessory sex glands include the seminal vesicles, prostate, and bulbourethral glands. The secretion from each of these glands is added to the testicular fluid and forms a substantial part of the semen.

Seminal Vesicles

KEY WORDS: **folds, honeycombed appearance, pseudostratified columnar epithelium**

The seminal vesicles are elongated, saclike structures that lie posterior to the prostate gland. Each joins with the distal end of the ductus deferens to form the ejaculatory duct. The mucosa of the seminal vesicles is thrown into numerous complex primary **folds** that give rise to secondary and tertiary folds (see atlas figure 17-18). These project into the lumen to subdivide it into many small, irregular compartments that give the lumen a **honeycombed appearance.** All the compartments communicate with the central lumen, although in sections the impression is one of individual chambers.

The mucosal folds are lined mainly by **pseudostratified columnar epithelium** consisting of rounded basal cells interposed between cuboidal or columnar cells (see atlas figure 17-19). Regions of simple columnar epithelium may be present also. The mucosal cells contain numerous granules, some lipid droplets, and lipochrome pigment, which first appears at sexual maturity and increases with age. The ultrastructural features indicate a cell that is active in protein synthesis. The cytoplasm contains abundant granular endoplasmic reticulum, a prominent supranuclear Golgi complex, and conspicuous, dense secretory granules in the apical cytoplasm.

The epithelium rests on a thin lamina propria of loose connective tissue with many elastic fibers. A muscular coat is present and consists of an inner layer of circularly arranged smooth muscle cells and an outer layer in which the muscle fibers have a longitudinal orientation. Both layers of muscle are thinner than those in the ductus deferens (see atlas figure 17-18). External to the muscle coat is a layer of loose connective tissue rich in elastic fibers.

Secretions from the seminal vesicles form a substantial part of the total ejaculate. It is a yellowish, viscid secretion that contains much fructose and prostaglandins. It provides a source of energy for sperm. In sections the secretions appear as deeply stained, coagulated masses, often with a netlike structure. The seminal vesicles depend on testosterone, and removal of the hormone, as by castration, results in their involution and loss of secretory function.

Prostate

KEY WORDS: **composite gland, compound tubuloalveolar, capsule, septa, prostatic concretion**

The prostate is the largest of the accessory sex glands in the male and surrounds the urethra at its origin from the bladder. It is a **composite gland,** made up of 30 to 50 small, **compound tubuloalveolar** glands from which 20 or more ducts drain independently into the prostatic urethra. These small glands appear to form strata around the urethra and consist of the periurethral mucosal glands, submucosal glands, and the main or principal prostatic glands, which lie peripherally and make up the bulk of the prostate (see atlas figures 17-22 and 17-23). The prostate is contained within a vascular, fibroelastic **capsule** that contains many smooth muscle fibers in its inner layers. Broad **septa** extend into the prostate from the capsule and become continuous with the dense fibroelastic tissue that separates the individual glandular elements.

The secretory units of the glands are irregular and vary greatly in size and shape. The glandular epithelium differs from gland to gland and even within a single alveolus. It usually is simple or pseudostratified columnar but may be low cuboidal or squamous in some of the larger saccular cavities. The epithelium is limited by an indistinct basal lamina and rests on a layer of connective tissue that contains dense networks of elastic fibers and numerous capillaries. The cells contain abundant granular endoplasmic reticulum and many apical secretory granules. The lumina of secretory units may contain spherical bodies, the **prostatic concretions,** that are thought to result from condensation of secretory material (see atlas figure 12-23). The concretions appear to increase with age and may become calcified. The connective tissue surrounding the individual glandular units contains much smooth muscle (a fibromuscular stroma), which aids in the discharge of prostatic fluid at ejaculation.

The prostatic secretion is a thin, milky fluid of pH 6.5 that is rich in zinc, citric acid, phosphatase, and proteolytic enzymes, one of which, fibrinolysin, is important in the liquefaction of semen. In several species of rodents, some of the prostatic glands are specialized to provide a secretion that coagulates seminal fluid to form a vaginal plug that prevents loss of semen from the female reproductive tract. These modified glandular units have been called coagulating glands. Like seminal vesicles, the development and functional maintenance of the prostate depends on testosterone and its metabolites.

Bulbourethral Glands

KEY WORDS: compound tubuloalveolar, simple cuboidal to simple columnar

The bulbourethral glands are a pair of pea-sized structures located in the urogenital diaphragm, close to the bulb of the urethra. They are **compound tubuloalveolar glands** whose long ducts drain into the proximal part of the penile urethra. Each gland is limited by a connective tissue capsule from which septa, containing elastic fibers and smooth and skeletal muscle cells, extend into the glands, dividing them into lobules.

The ducts and secretory portions are irregular in shape and size, and at their terminations, the secretory parts may form cystlike enlargements. The glandular epithelium varies from **simple cuboidal to simple columnar** depending on the functional state, but in distended alveoli the epithelium may be flattened. Active cells show a lightly stained cytoplasm filled with mucinogen granules that confine the nucleus to the base of the cell. Excretory ducts are lined by simple columnar epithelium that becomes pseudostratified near the urethra. In smaller ducts, the epithelium appears to be secretory. The surrounding connective tissue contains an incomplete layer of circularly arranged smooth muscle.

Bulbourethral glands produce a clear, viscid fluid that is rich in amino sugars and contains sialoprotein. It is secreted in response to erotic stimulation and serves as a lubricant for the penile urethra.

Semen

The final product formed by the exocrine secretions of the testes and accessory glands is a whitish fluid called seminal fluid or semen. The average ejaculate in human males consists of about 3 ml of semen which, in addition to about 300 million sperm, contains degenerating cells exfoliated by the ductal system, occasional wandering cells from connective tissues, pigment granules, and prostatic concretions. Hyaline bodies of unknown origin, lipid granules, fat, and protein also are present.

External Genitalia

In the male, the two structures that make up the external genitalia are the scrotum and penis.

Scrotum

KEY WORDS: skin, tunica dartos, spermatic cord, pampiniform plexus

The scrotum is a pendulous, cutaneous pouch situated at the base of the penis and below the symphysis pubis. It is divided into two compartments, each of which houses a testis, an epididymis, and the lower part of the spermatic cord. The scrotum consists only of skin and a closely associated tunica dartos.

The scrotal **skin** is thin, pigmented, and commonly thrown into folds. It contains many sweat glands, sebaceous glands that produce an odorous secretion, and some coarse hairs, the follicles of which are visible through the skin. The **tunica dartos** underlies the skin and forms the septum that divides the scrotum into its two compartments. It is firmly attached to the skin and consists largely of smooth muscle and collagenous connective tissue. The appearance of the scrotum varies with the state of contraction of the smooth muscle. Under influence of cold, exercise, or sexual stimulation, the muscle contracts and the scrotum becomes short and wrinkled.

The **spermatic cord** consists of several thin layers of connective tissue that are acquired from the anterior abdominal wall as the testes descend from the abdominal cavity into the scrotal sac during development. It contains the ductus deferens, nerve fibers, lymphatic channels, testicular artery, and **pampiniform plexus** of testicular veins. As the testicular artery nears the testis, it becomes highly convoluted and is surrounded by the venous plexus. The proximity of the surrounding, cooler venous blood causes the arterial blood to lose heat and provides a thermoregulatory mechanism for precooling incoming arterial blood. In this way the temperature of the testes is maintained a few degrees below body temperature, a condition necessary for production of sperm. The temperature can be elevated by drawing the testes closer to the abdominal wall by contraction of the layer of striated muscle (cremaster muscle) that invests the spermatic cord.

The testes in some animals (e.g., elephant) descend into the scrotum only during the breeding season, after which the testes return to the abdominal cavity and are inactive. In humans, failure of the testes to descend (cryptorchidism) results in sterility.

Penis

KEY WORDS: **erectile tissue, corpora cavernosa penis, pectiniform septum, tunica albuginea, cavernous spaces, corpus cavernosum urethrae (corpus spongiosum), glans penis, prepuce**

The penile urethra serves as a common channel for conducting urine and seminal fluid to the exterior. It is contained within a cylinder of **erectile tissue,** the corpus cavernosum urethrae (corpus spongiosum) that lies ventral to a pair of similar erectile bodies called the corpora cavernosa penis. Together, the three structures make up the bulk of the penis, the copulatory organ of the male.

The **corpora cavernosa penis** begin as separate bodies along the rami of the pubis on either side and join at the pubic angle to form the shaft of the penis. They are united by a common, connective tissue septum called the **pectiniform septum,** and each corpus is surrounded by a thick fibrous sheath, the **tunica albuginea.** Trabeculae of collagenous and elastic fibers with numerous smooth muscle cells extend into the corpora from the tunica albuginea and divide the central regions of the corpora cavernosa into numerous **cavernous spaces,** those near the center being the larger. These spaces are endothelial-lined vascular spaces and are continuous with the arteries that supply them and with draining veins. The cavernous tissue of each corpus cavernosum penis communicates with the other through numerous slitlike openings in the pectiniform septum.

The ventrally placed **corpus cavernosum urethrae (corpus spongiosum)** ends in an enlargement, the **glans penis,** which forms a cap over the ends of the corpora cavernosa penis. Structurally, corpus spongiosum is similar to the corpora cavernosa penis, but the tunica albuginea is thinner and contains more elastic fibers and smooth muscle, and the trabeculae are thinner and contain more elastic tissue (see atlas figure 17-24).

The three corpora are bound together by subcutaneous connective tissue that contains numerous smooth muscle cells but is devoid of fat. The shaft of the penis is covered by a thin, mobile skin that shows a slight increase in pigmentation. The skin of the distal shaft, unlike that of the root, lacks hair but does contain scattered sweat glands. The hairless skin of the glans penis is fused to the underlying connective tissue and is nonmobile. Unusual sebaceous glands not associated with hair follicles occur in this region. The glans penis is covered by a fold of skin called the **prepuce** or foreskin, the inner surface of which is moist and resembles a mucous membrane. Numerous free nerve endings are present in the epithelium of the glans penis, prepuce, and subepithelial connective tissue of the urethra and skin. Meissner's corpuscles are associated with the epidermis of the genitals and Vater-Pacini corpuscles are present in the deeper layers of the dermis.

A section through the penis is shown in Fig. 17-5.

Arterial Supply

KEY WORDS: helicine arteries, intimal ridge

The principal arterial supply to the penis is from two arteries that lie dorsal to the corpora cavernosa penis and deep arteries that run within the erectile tissue of these structures. Branches from the dorsal arteries penetrate the tunica albuginea and enter the cavernous tissue, where the arteries branch and either form capillary plexuses or course distally in the cavernous tissue. These **helicine arteries** are highly convoluted in the flaccid penis and take a spiral course through the trabeculae of the cavernous tissue. The intima of most of these arteries, even before they enter the cavernous tissue, have long, ridgelike thickenings that project into and partially occlude the lumina. These **intimal ridges** are most frequent where vessels branch. They consist of loose connective tissue that contains many smooth muscle cells. Blood from the large central lacunae drains peripherally toward the smaller vascular spaces and finally into a plexus of veins at the periphery. The veins run along the interior of the tunica albuginea, pierce the limiting tunica, and drain into the deep dorsal vein of the penis.

The arterial blood supply to the corpus spongiosum is similar to that of the corpora cavernosa

Fig. 17-5. Section through the penis.

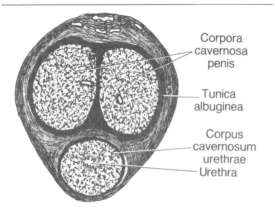

Corpora cavernosa penis

Tunica albuginea

Corpus cavernosum urethrae

Urethra

penis, except for the venous drainage. Beginning at the lacunae, the veins of the corpus spongiosum have large openings and immediately penetrate the tunica albuginea to drain to the exterior.

The structure and arrangement of the blood vessels in the cavernous tissues provide the mechanism for erection. During erotic stimulation, the smooth muscle of the arterial and trabecular walls relaxes and blood pressure overcomes the elastic resistance of the arteries. The helicine arteries dilate and straighten, and the vascular spaces of the cavernous tissues quickly fill with blood. The lacunae, especially near the center of the cavernous bodies, become engorged with blood, thus compressing the small peripheral spaces and veins against the tunica albuginea, retarding the egress of blood; the erectile tissues of corpora cavernosa penis become enlarged and rigid. Corpus spongiosum does not become as rigid as the corpora cavernosa penis because there is less compression of the venous drainage and the tunica albuginea is thinner and more yielding. The lesser rigidity of corpus spongiosum allows the urethra to remain patent, which is essential for the passage of semen during ejaculation.

After cessation of sexual activity, the smooth muscle in the arteries and cavernous tissue regains its tone. The intimal ridges once again partially occlude the lumina of the arteries, thus reducing the volume of incoming blood. Excess blood in the vascular spaces of the erectile tissue is forced out by contraction of smooth muscle cells in the trabeculae and by recoil of surrounding elastic tissue. Gradually, the normal route of blood flow through the penis is restored and the penis returns to the flaccid condition.

Development of the Male Reproductive System

The indifferent gonad arises in the urogenital ridge, a thickened area of mesoderm that contains primordia for the kidneys and gonads. Proliferation of peritoneal epithelium (mesothelium) on the ventromedial aspect of the ridge gives rise to the genital ridge, a longitudinal thickening several cells deep that runs parallel to the mesonephric ridge. The indifferent gonad consists of a superficial epithelium and an internal gonadal blastema made up of ill-defined cords of cells derived from the superficial epithelium.

Testes

In the male, the gonad rounds up, increases in size, and acquires a network of branched (testis) cords and a tunica albuginea, which identify it as a testis. With the appearance of tunica albuginea, the germinal epithelium reverts to a typical peritoneal mesothelium and no longer plays a part in testicular development. Primordial germ cells migrate from the yolk sac during the fifth week of gestation in the human and give rise to gonocytes; with cells from the gonadal blastema, they form testis cords (see atlas figures 17-27 and 17-28). By the third month in humans, fetal spermatogonia are present. The testis cords extend radially toward the mesorchium (gonadal mesentery) and a dense region that will become the rete testis. The two become continuous and the testis cords elongate and differentiate into seminiferous tubules. Where they join the rete testis, the tubules remain straight and form the tubuli recti. The seminiferous tubules contain only spermatogonia and Sertoli cells (see atlas figure 17-29). The number of Sertoli cells remains constant from birth, but spermatogonia increase markedly between about 10 years of age and puberty. The full sequence of spermatogenic cells from spermatogonia to spermatids does not appear until puberty.

The mesenchymal tissue in which the testis cords develop forms the septula testes, connective tissue of the mediastinum testis, and tunica albuginea. Cells in the mesenchymal stroma differentiate into interstitial cells. These are large and abundant from the fourth to sixth months of development in humans but then regress only to increase again in number and size at puberty.

Specific development of exocrine ducts does not occur in the male. As the mesonephric kidney degenerates and is resorbed, its ducts are incorporated into the reproductive system and transformed into genital ducts. In some amphibians, the mesonephric dust persists, the upper region being associated with the testis and the lower part with the kidney. In these species, the mesonephric duct conducts sperm and urine to the cloaca. In higher animals, this arrangement begins, but as the mesonephros is resorbed, the cranial mesonephric tubules are modified and unite with tubules of the rete testis. These efferent ductules are continuous with mesonephric ducts whose proximal region becomes highly convoluted to form the ductus epididymidis. In the opossum, efferent ductules evaginate from the proximal part of the mesonephric duct and unite with the rete testis in a manner reminiscent of the ureteric bud and its subdivisions during differentiation of the metanephros.

Distally, the mesonephric duct remains straight, forming the ejaculatory duct and ductus deferens, which, near its distal end, dilates to form the ampulla. Just beyond the ampulla, the epithelium of the ductus evaginates to provide the primordia for the seminal vesicles. Muscle coats are derived from surrounding mesenchyme. In humans the seminal vesicles attain the adult pattern by the seventh fetal month and slowly grow until puberty, after which the adult proportions are reached.

The prostate develops from multiple outgrowths of the urethral epithelium, above and below the entrance of the ejaculatory duct. Some 60 glands develop in humans, organized into five groups that will become the lobes of the prostate. The mesenchyme into which the prostatic glands grow provides the fibromuscular stroma. The glands remain small until puberty when, under the influence of testosterone, development is completed.

The bulbourethral glands also arise as buds of ectodermal epithelium, but in the region of the urogenital sinus that forms the membranous urethra. The outgrowths evaginate through the investing mesenchyme to lie in the urogenital diaphragm. Mucous cells appear at about four months in humans. The bulbourethral glands, also influenced by testosterone, grow throughout puberty. The urethal glands develop from outgrowths of the epithelium that lines the urethra.

External Genitalia

Early in development, the cloacal membrane becomes surrounded by mesenchyme and forms two folds that unite anteriorly to form the cloacal swelling. From the anterior part of the swelling, the genital (urethal) folds develop, while the posterior part forms the anal folds. The cloacal swelling increases in size, giving rise to a genital tubercle, at which time the genital swellings become visible just lateral to the genital fold. In the male, the swellings are called scrotal swellings, which move caudally, fuse, and form the scrotum (see atlas figures 17-30 and 17-32).

The genital tubercle elongates to form a phallus, pulling the genital fold forward as it does. The folds form the lateral walls of the urogenital groove, which extends along the caudal surface of the phallus. The genital folds close over, fuse, and form the penile urethra, the tip of which lacks an orifice. Ectodermal cells at the tip grow inward as a solid cord that later canalizes to establish continuity with the remainder of the urethra. Corpora cavernosa penis and urethrae develop from paired and single columns of mesenchyme, respectively. The single column forms around the penile urethra within the shaft and also gives rise to the glans (see atlas figures 17-30 and 17-31). The external genitalia develop slowly after birth, then grow rapidly during puberty.

Functional Summary

The primary function of the male reproductive system is to provide haploid germ cells for procreation, and one of the consequences of meiotic division is to reduce the number of chromosomes to half that present in somatic cells. This ensures that on union of gametes, the normal diploid number of chromosomes will be maintained. A second consequence of meiosis that is of great importance is provision of genetic variation as the result of the exchange of genetic material between homologous chromosomes and from the random distribution of homologous chromosomes between daughter nuclei. The unequal division of cytoplasm among ova provides one cell with sufficient material to nourish the zygote until other forms of nourishment can be established.

Production of sperm occurs in the germinal epithelium of the seminiferous tubules and represents a holocrine (exocrine) secretion of the testes. Spermatogenesis and spermiogenesis depend on high concentrations of testosterone, the endocrine secretion of the testes produced by interstitial cells.

Germinal epithelium essentially contains two major classes of cells: a mobile population of germ or spermatogenic cells and a stable population of supporting (Sertoli) cells. Seminiferous epithelium is unique in that it is divided into basal and adluminal compartments, each differing in their cellular content and environments. The basal compartment contains stem cells (spermatogonia) and newly formed primary spermatocytes that are exposed to an environment similar to that of blood plasma. The primary spermatocytes soon migrate into the adluminal compartment, where, along with secondary spermatocytes, spermatids, and spermatozoa, they are exposed to an environment rich in ions that contains amino acids not found in the basal compartment and has a high concentration of testosterone. The two different environments are established and maintained by Sertoli cells, and the tight junctions between them constitute — at least in part — a blood-testis barrier. Any substances that enter or leave the adluminal compartment must pass through the cytoplasm of the Sertoli cells.

Under the influence of gonadotropic hormone (FSH), Sertoli cells release androgen-binding protein that complexes with testosterone to maintain a high concentration of hormone in the adluminal compartment. The blood-testis barrier also prevents escape of developing germ cells out of the adluminal compartment and into general body tissues. If this escape occurred, the haploid germ cells might be interpreted as foreign elements, resulting in immunologic responses directed against developing germ cells in the germinal epithelium and thus causing sterility.

Development of germ cells occurs in the adluminal compartment, in the embrace of the complex cytoplasmic processes of Sertoli cells. As spermatogenic cells develop and differentiate, the Sertoli cell is thought to move them actively along its lateral surfaces toward the lumen, where they are released from the apical surface of the Sertoli cell. Gap junctions permit communication between Sertoli cells and allow for coordinated release of spermatozoa from a given segment of a seminiferous tubule. Testosterone is present in the adluminal compartment of the seminiferous tubules and in the proximal duct system as far as the lower regions of the ductus epididymidis. Thus, there exists the unusual circumstance of an endocrine secretion of the testis (testosterone) not only entering the bloodstream but also passing through the lumen of the proximal duct system to have effect on the ductus epididymidis. Systemic concentrations of testosterone are essential for development and functional maintenance of the rest of the excretory duct system and for the male secondary sex characteristics. In some instances, testosterone serves primarily as a prohormone and its metabolites are the active factors. Dihydrotestosterone, for example, is the active agent for the prostate and epididymis.

Much testicular fluid is produced by the germinal epithelium and serves as a vehicle for the transport of spermatozoa out of the seminiferous tubules and into the excretory duct system. Spermatozoa released into the seminiferous tubules are nonmotile and are moved into the tubuli recti by the flow of testicular fluid and the shallow peristaltic movements of the seminiferous tubules. The ciliated epithelium and the increased smooth muscle in the walls of the ductuli efferentes contribute to the movement of spermatozoa into the proximal epididymis. Most of the testicular fluid is absorbed in the ductuli efferentes and proximal ductus epididymidis.

Sperm entering the epididymis show weak, random movement, and for the most part they are incapable of fertilization; spermatozoa from the distal epididymis show strong, unidirectional motility and are capable of fertilization. Sperm are slowly propelled through the long ductus epididymidis by peristaltic contractions of its muscular walls. During their passage through the epididymis, spermatozoa of some species show continued differentiation of the acrosome and sperm head, as well as progressive increase in the fertilizing capacity. Sperm require the environment provided by the epididymis to become physiologically mature and viable. Although the maturation process is androgen-dependent, how the various segments of the epididymis control and regulate the physiological maturation of spermatozoa is unknown. The distal ductus epididymidis stores sperm. Because of its thick muscular wall, it can contract forcibly and, in coordination with the wall of the ductus deferens, empty stored sperm into the prostatic urethra.

During ejaculation, the primary accessory sex glands contribute successively to the seminal fluid. The bulbourethral and intraepithelial urethral glands secrete fluids that lubricate the urethra during sexual arousal and erection of the penis. At the onset of ejaculation, muscular tissue of the prostatic stroma contracts, discharging the secretory product into the prostatic urethra. The abundant, thin secretion is slightly acidic and contains acid phosphatase. Sperm and their suspending fluids are expelled from the distal ductus epididymidis and ductus deferens. The last component added to the ejaculate is the viscous secretion of the seminal vesicles. This secretion is rich in fructose, an important energy source for the active, motile spermatozoa. Seminal vesicles also secrete prostaglandins in high concentration, but the role of these agents in the female tract is unknown. The final phase of physiologic maturation of spermatozoa is capacitation and occurs in the female reproductive tract, substantially increasing the number of spermatozoa that are capable of fertilization.

Testosterone is vital for the male reproductive system to develop properly and to maintain normal structure and function. It is synthesized and released by interstitial (Leydig) cells of the testis. Secretion is controlled by circulating levels of testosterone that are monitored by neurons within the hypothalamic region of the brain that, through releasing factors, influence the secretion of ISCH (LH) by cells of the anterior pituitary. It is through this feedback system that normal testosterone levels are maintained. Sertoli cells, which are under the influence of FSH, produce androgen-binding protein that functions to concentrate testosterone within the seminiferous tubules and the genital duct system. Secretion of FSH by cells of the anterior pituitary also is controlled by releasing factors from neurons with the hypothalamus. Inhibin released by Sertoli cells suppresses FSH secretion and, through this negative feedback loop, functions to control the rate of spermatogenesis.

Clinical Correlations

Infections of the male genital tract are often transmitted sexually. Inflammatory lesions of the urethra can ascend to the prostate, enter the vas deferens and epididymis, and extend to the testis. Gonococcal infection may spread to the bladder and even into the ureters. Scarring and obstruction of the posterior urethra may occur with dilatation and hypertrophy of the bladder. The most common blood-borne infection of the testis is mumps, which causes a diffuse inflammation and can lead to fibrosis and atrophy of the seminiferous tubules.

If the testes do not descend from the abdomen during development, spermatogenesis is defective, even if germ cells are present. The seminiferous tubules are atrophic and contain only Sertoli cells and the occasional spermatogonium. Probably as a result of inadequate stimulation by testosterone in utero, the male external genitalia may be imperfectly developed. Minor conditions such as bifid scrotum or hypospadias (urethral opening on the underside of the penis) also may be associated with temporary inadequacy of testosterone.

Testicular tumors are rather uncommon and usually occur early in adult life. Primary testicular tumors may arise from the epithelium of the seminiferous tubule (germinal tumors) or originate in the Leydig cells or less specific cells of the testicular stroma (nongerminal tumors). Seminomas are the most common type and consist of an admixture of lymphocytes and uniform round cells with clear cytoplasm and prominent nuclei and nucleoli. Electron micrographs show evidence of spermatocytic differentiation. Teratomas occur at all ages and are derived from totipotent cells (spermatogonia) so their form and malignant potentials are varied. Adult teratoma contain tissues representing each embryonic layer of tissue; such tumors may contain neural tissue, thyroid, skin, cartilage, and so forth. Interstitial (Leydig) cell tumors and Sertoli cell tumors form the bulk of the nongerminal tumors of the testis. Leydig cell tumors are associated with endocrinologic dysfunctions, and androgenic, estrogenic, and corticosteroidogenic effects have been reported.

Benign enlargement of the prostate is a common aspect of aging. The central and periurethral glands are most frequently involved; the more posterior lobe may be unaffected. The gland shows nodules of hyperplasia involving the stroma and glandular tissue. The acinar units are dilated and since they are lined by columnar epithelium, squamous metaplasia may occur; proliferation of the fibromuscular stroma may be a prominent feature. As a result of the enlargement of the periurethral glands, compression of the prostatic urethra may occur with disruption of the sphincter mechanism and retention of urine in the bladder. The residual urine predisposes the bladder to infection, and back pressure in the ureters and calyces can dilate these structures and eventually impair renal function.

Atlas and Table of Key Features

Key Features of the Male Reproductive Tract

	Epithelial Lining	Support	Muscle
Seminiferous tubule	Germinal epithelium containing spermatogenic cells (spermatogonia, primary and secondary spermatocytes, spermatids) and Sertoli cells	Peritubular connective tissue; collagen fibers and myoid cells	
Tubuli recti	Simple columnar	Loose connective tissue	
Rete testis	Simple cuboidal. Short microvilli, single cilium on each cell	Dense, vascular connective tissue	
Ductuli efferentes	Tall, ciliated columnar and short ciliated or nonciliated cuboidal. Lining has irregular contour	Loose connective tissue between tubules	Thin, circular smooth muscle
Ductus epididymidis	Pseudostratified columnar: tall principal cells with stereocilia; short basal cells	Thin lamina propria	Primarily circular smooth muscle, three layers appear distally
Ductus deferens	Pseudostratified columnar, thrown into longitudinal folds; stereocilia	Dense lamina propria; collagen and elastic fibers; adventitia of loose connective tissue	Three layers: inner longitudinal, middle circular, outer longitudinal smooth muscle
Ampulla of ductus deferens	Pseudostratified columnar with stereocilia; complex folds form extensive pocketlike recesses	Lamina propria and adventitia less well defined	Thinner, less distinct layers of smooth muscles

Key Features of the Male Reproductive Tract (continued)

	Epithelial Lining	Support	Muscle
Ejaculatory duct	Pseudostratified or simple columnar; forms pockets but less prominent than in ampulla	Dense collagenous connective tissue with many elastic fibers	
Seminal vesicles	Honeycombed appearance; pseudostratified columnar with regions of simple columnar	Thin lamina propria with many elastic fibers; external layer of loose connective tissue rich in elastic fibers	Inner circular, outer longitudinal smooth muscle
Prostate	Variable; usually simple columnar or pseudostratified columnar. Low cuboidal or squamous may occur	Vascular connective tissue with dense network of elastic fibers	Smooth muscle fibers in connective tissue surround individual glandular units
Bulbourethral glands	Variable; simple cuboidal to simple columnar; flattened in distended alveoli; ducts lined by simple columnar, pseudostratified near urethra	Fibroelastic connective tissue around each glandular structure	Smooth and skeletal muscle fibers in interstitial tissue between glandular elements
Corpora cavernosa penis	Endothelium of vascular spaces	Fibroelastic connective tissue	Smooth muscle cells in trabeculae between cavernous spaces
Corpora cavernosa urethrae	Cavernous spaces lined by endothelium, penile urethrae lined by pseudostratified columnar, nonkeratinized stratified squamous	Fibroelastic connective tissue rich in elastic fibers	Smooth muscle cells more abundant

Testis

Interstitial cells

Germinal epithelium

Peritubular tissue

Seminiferous tubule

Fig. 17-6. Seminiferous tubules from a human testis. (LM, ×100.)

Sertoli cell nucleus

Primary spermatocytes

Peritubular tissue

Primary spermatocytes

Spermatogonium

Spermatids

Sertoli cell

Fig. 17-7. The cell types comprising the germinal epithelium of seminiferous tubules. (LM, ×250.)

Fig. 17-8. A fractured seminiferous tubule illustrating the three-dimensional nature of cell types shown in 17-7. (SEM, ×500.)

Fig. 17-9. Cell types that make up the germinal epithelium. (LM, ×250.)

Spermatogonium

Primary spermatocytes

Capillary

Spermatogonia

Sertoli cell

Lumen

Spermatids

Spermatids

Spermatogonium

Fig. 17-10. Cell types that make up the germinal epithelium. (LM, ×250.)

Spermatids

Spermatids

Tails of spermatids

Spermatids

Spermatids

Fig. 17-11. Tails of late spermatids in the germinal epithelium project into the lumen of a seminiferous tubule. (SEM, ×2,000.)

Fig. 17-12. Interstitial (Leydig) cells that exhibit crystals of Reinke from human testis. (LM, ×400.)

Excretory Ducts

Fig. 17-13. A region of human rete testis. Note the adjacent seminiferous tubules. (LM, ×40.)

Smooth
muscle

Lumen

Epithelium

Fig. 17-14. A tubule from human ductuli efferentes. (LM, ×250.)

Basal
cells

Spermatozoa

Principal
cells

Smooth
muscle

Clumps of
stereocilia

Arteriole

Connective
tissue

Pseudostratified
columnar
epithelium

Fig. 17-15. A portion of ductus epididymidis showing both basal
and principal cells of the lining epithelium. Stereocilia of the
principal cells project into the lumen. (LM, ×250.)

Pseudostratified columnar epithelium

Lumen

Lamina propria

Outer longitudinal smooth muscle

Middle circular smooth muscle

Inner longitudinal smooth muscle

Fig. 17-16. Three distinct layers forming the muscular wall of the human ductus deferens. (LM, ×150.)

Muscularis

Mucosal folds

Lumen

Fig. 17-17. The ampulla of human ductus deferens. Note the elaborate mucosal folds projecting into the lumen. Compare the mucosa of this region with that shown in 17-16. (LM, ×100.)

Accessory Sex Glands

Smooth muscle coat

Mucosal folds

Lumen

Lamina propria

Smooth muscle coat

Fig. 17-18. Elaborate mucosal folds and well-defined smooth muscle wall characterize the human seminal vesicle (compare with 17-17). (LM, ×40.)

Capillary

Pseudostratified columnar epithelium

Lamina propria

Lumen

Fig. 17-19. The pseudostratified columnar epithelium lining the seminal vesicle. (LM, ×250.)

Lumen

Spermatozoa

Prostate gland

Ejaculatory duct

Fig. 17-20. A region of human prostate containing the ejaculatory ducts. (LM, ×250.)

Capillaries

Fibrous connective tissue

Pseudostratified columnar epithelium

Capillary

Arteriole

Fig. 17-21. Pseudostratified columnar epithelium lining a human ejaculatory duct. (LM, ×250.)

Lumen of
prostatic
alveolus

Simple
columnar
epithelium

Fig. 17-22. Submucosal glands of the human prostate. (LM,
×250.)

Epithelium

Prostatic
concretion

Smooth
muscle
cells

Fig. 17-23. Principal glands of the human prostate. Note the
smooth muscle cells in the surrounding fibromuscular stroma.
(LM, ×250.)

Penis

Smooth muscle

Blood sinuses

Fig. 17-24. Erectile tissue from the corpus spongiosum of a human penis. (LM, ×30.)

Spermatozoa

Head

Articular fossa

Connecting piece

Middle piece

Principal piece

Fig. 17-25. Subcomponents of an opossum spermatozoon. (SEM, ×5,000.)

Fig. 17-26. Subcomponents of a human spermatozoon. (SEM, ×10,000.)

Development

Fig. 17-27. A developing testis adjacent to a degenerating mesonephros. Note that the mesonephric duct remains well established, whereas the müllerian duct is being resorbed. (LM, ×100.)

Testis cord

Tunica
albuginea

Fig. 17-28. Cords within a developing testis. (LM, ×450.)

Seminiferous
tubules

Spermatogonium

Sertoli cells

Fig. 17-29. A prepubertal human testis illustrates established
seminiferous tubules comprised primarily of Sertoli cells. Occasional spermatogonia also are observed. (LM, ×15.)

Fig. 17-30. Developing external genitalia from a 40-day male human embryo. (LM, ×15.)

Fig. 17-31. The penile urethra within the developing penis of a 40-day human embryo. (LM, ×200.)

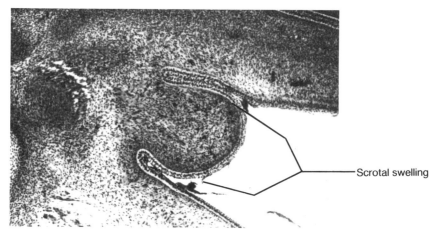

Fig. 17-32. A scrotal swelling from a 40-day human embryo. (LM, ×200.)

—————— *Review Questions and Answers* ——————

Questions

88. Briefly discuss the role of the Sertoli cells.
89. What is the effect of testosterone on the male reproductive system?
90. What is meant by the terms *spermatogenesis* and *spermiogenesis*?
91. Relate the ultrastructural features of the interstitial cells (of Leydig) to their function.
92. What role does the pampiniform plexus play in the physiology of the testis?

Answers

88. The Sertoli cell is a tall columnar cell that spans the entire depth of the germinal epithelium. Tight junctions occur between adjacent Sertoli cells near their bases and subdivide the germinal epithelium into basal and adluminal compartments. The basal compartment extends from the basal lamina of the germinal epithelium to the tight junctions, while the adluminal compartment lies between the tight junctions and the lumen of the seminiferous tubule. The basal compartment contains spermatogonia and newly formed primary spermatocytes, exposed to an environment similar to that of blood plasma. Cells of the adluminal compartment (primary and secondary spermatocytes, spermatids, and spermatozoa) differentiate in an environment that is rich in ions, contains amino acids not found in the basal compartment, and has a relatively high concentration of testosterone. Sertoli cells are responsible for establishing and maintaining these two different environments, and the tight junctions contribute to the blood-testis barrier between the two compartments. Substances that enter or leave the adluminal compartment must first pass through the cytoplasm of the Sertoli cells.

    Sertoli cells synthesize androgen-binding protein, which complexes with testosterone to maintain a high concentration of the hormone in the adluminal compartment. High levels of testosterone are necessary for the differentiation and development of germ cells. The Sertoli cells and blood-testis barrier also may prevent the escape of spermatogenic cells from the adluminal compartment and into the general body tissues, thus preventing an immunologic response against the forming germ cells.

    In addition to providing nutritional and mechanical support for the developing germ cells, Sertoli cells also control the movement of germ cells through the epithelium and play an important role in their release into the lumen of the seminiferous tubules. Sertoli cells phagocytose degenerating germ cells and the residual cytoplasm that normally is shed during the release of germ cells. Inhibin released by Sertoli cells suppresses FSH secretion and through this negative feedback loop, controls the rate of spermatogenesis.

89. Testosterone, the male hormone produced by the interstitial cells of the testes, is essential for the proliferation and differentiation of germ cells, for the structural development of the excretory ducts and accessory sex glands, and for the maintenance of these structures in a functional state. In addition, testosterone influences other tissues of the body and is responsible for the development and maintenance of the male secondary sex characteristics: growth of the beard, low pitch of the voice, muscular build, and male pattern of pubic hair. Production of testosterone is under the control of a gonadotropic hormone called interstitial cell–stimulating hormone, secreted by cells in the anterior pituitary.

90. The term *spermatogenesis* encompasses the entire sequence of events in the transformation of the diploid spermatogonia at the base of the germinal epithelium into the haploid spermatozoa that are released into the lumen of the seminiferous tubule. In humans this process takes about 64 days. Spermiogenesis, on the other hand, refers to the elaborate sequence of events by which the spermatids differentiate into slender, motile spermatozoa.

91. The interstitial cells (of Leydig) commonly are found in groups or nests and constitute the endocrine portion of the testis, producing the male hormone testosterone. They usually contain a single large, spherical nucleus, although binucleate cells are not uncommon. The cytoplasm is characterized by an abundance of smooth endoplasmic reticulum and well-developed Golgi complexes. Mitochondria are numerous, and in several species their cristae are of the tubular rather than the lamellar form. These are features characteristic of a cell type that is actively engaged in steroid synthesis. Testosterone is a steroid hormone. All enzymes (except one) needed for the conversion of acetate to testosterone are associated with membranes of the smooth endoplasmic reticulum. Enzymes for one step — cleavage of the side chain of cholesterol — are found in the mitochondria. Thus, in this particular cell type, acetate is synthesized to cholesterol on the membranes of the smooth endoplasmic reticulum. Cholesterol then enters surrounding mitochondria, where its side chain is removed enzymatically and the resulting pregnenolone molecule then diffuses out of the mitochondria. The synthesis of pregnenolone to testosterone is completed on the membranes of the smooth endoplasmic reticulum.

92. Each testicular vein forms an extensive plexus, the pampiniform plexus, which surrounds the testicular artery as it nears the testis. The close proximity of the surrounding cooler venous blood causes the arterial blood to lose heat and provides a thermoregulatory mechanism for the precooling of the incoming arterial blood. In this way the temperature of the testis in the scrotal sac is maintained a few degrees below the body temperature, a condition necessary for the production of germ cells.

18 Female Reproductive System

The female reproductive system consists of internal organs — the ovaries, oviducts, uterus, and vagina — and external structures (external genitalia), which include the labia majora, labia minora, and clitoris. Although not genital organs, the mammary glands are important accessory organs of the female reproductive tract. For the first 10 or 11 years of life, the reproductive organs remain immature and growth parallels that of the body generally. During the 2 to 3 years prior to the first menstrual period, the generative organs increase in size, the breasts enlarge, and pubic and axillary hair appears. Following the first menses and thereafter throughout the reproductive period, the ovaries, oviducts, uterus, vagina, and mammary glands undergo cyclic changes in function and structure associated with the menstrual cycle and pregnancy. During menopause, the cycles become irregular and eventually cease; in the postmenopausal period the reproductive organs atrophy.

Ovaries

The ovaries are paired oval bodies that lie on each side of the uterus, suspended from the broad ligament by a mesentery, the mesovarium. The ovaries are homologous with the testes and are compound organs with exocrine and endocrine functions. The exocrine secretion consists of whole cells — the ova — and thus the ovary can be classed as a holocrine or cytogenic gland. In cyclic fashion it secretes female sex hormones directly into the bloodstream and therefore is an endocrine gland.

Structure

KEY WORDS: surface epithelium, cortex, ovarian follicle, tunica albuginea, medulla

Each ovary is covered by a mesothelium that is continuous with that of the mesovarium. As this membrane extends over the surface of the ovary, the squamous cells become cuboidal and form the **surface epithelium** of the ovary. Sections of the ovary show an outer cortex and an inner medulla, but the boundary between the two regions is indistinct. The stroma of the **cortex** consists of a compact feltwork of fine collagenous fibers and numerous fibroblasts. Elastic fibers are associated mainly with blood vessels and otherwise are rare in the cortex. Scattered throughout the cortical tissue are the **ovarian follicles,** whose size varies with their stage of development. Immediately below the surface epithelium, the connective tissue of the cortex is less cellular and more compact, forming a dense layer called the **tunica albuginea** (see atlas figure 18-4).

The stroma of the **medulla** consists of a loose connective tissue that is less cellular than that of the cortex and contains many elastic fibers and smooth muscle cells. Numerous large, tortuous vessels, lymphatics, and nerves also are present in the medulla.

Ovarian Follicles

KEY WORDS: cortex, ovum, epithelial cell

The follicles are located in the **cortex** of the ovary, deep to tunica albuginea, and consist of an immature **ovum** surrounded by one or more layers of **epithelial cells.** At birth, the human ovary contains 300,000 to 400,000 ova embedded in the cortical stroma, but only a few reach maturity and are ovulated. During the menstrual cycle, several follicles begin to grow and develop, but only one attains full maturity; the rest degenerate. The size of the follicle and the thickness of the epithelial envelope vary with the stage of development. During their growth, the follicles undergo a sequence of changes in which primordial, primary, secondary, and mature follicles can be distinguished.

Primordial Follicles

KEY WORDS: unilaminar, follicular cell, primary oocyte, diplotene

In the mature ovary, follicles are present in all stages of development. Most, especially in young females, are primordial or **unilaminar** follicles, which are found in the peripheral cortex, just beneath tunica albuginea (see atlas figures 18-4 and 18-5). These follicles consist of an immature ovum surrounded by a single layer of flattened **follicular cells** that rest on a basement membrane. At this stage, the ovum is a **primary oocyte,** suspended in the **diplotene** stage of the meiotic prophase. The primary oocyte is a large cell with a prominent vesicular nucleus and nucleolus. The Golgi apparatus is well developed, and spherical mitochondria tend to concentrate in the region of the centrosome. As the primordial folicle develops into a primary follicle, changes occur in the ovum, follicular cells, and adjacent connective tissue of the cortex.

Primary Follicles

KEY WORDS: zona pellucida, granulosa cell, stratum granulosum, theca folliculi, theca interna, theca externa

During growth of a primary follicle, the oocyte increases in size and the Golgi complex, originally a single organelle next to the nucleus, becomes a multiple structure scattered throughout the cytoplasm. Free ribosomes increase in number, mitochondria become dispersed, and granular endoplasmic reticulum, although not prominent, becomes more extensive. A few lipid droplets and lipochrome pigments appear in the cytoplasm, and yolk granules accumulate; these, however, are smaller and less numerous than in nonprimate species. As the oocyte grows, a clear refractile proteoglycan membrane, the **zona pellucida,** develops between the oocyte and adjacent follicular cells (see atlas figures 18-5, 18-6, and 18-10). The origin of this membrane generally is attributed to the follicular cells, but the oocyte also might contribute to its formation. Microvilli extend from the oocyte into the zona pellucida.

As the ovum grows, the flattened follicular cells of the primordial follicles become cuboidal or columnar in shape and proliferate to form several layers. These cells now are **granulosa cells,** and the layers of stratified epithelium that they form is called **stratum granulosum** (see atlas figures 18-5 and 18-6). Mitochondria, free ribosomes, and endoplasmic reticulum increase and the Golgi element becomes prominent. Irregular, slender cytoplasmic processes extend from the granulosa cells and penetrate the zona pellucida to make contact with processes from the oocyte. There is no cytoplasmic continuity between the oocyte and cells of the stratum granulosum, but the processes of the granulosa cells sometimes penetrate into the cytoplasm of the oocyte.

While these changes occur in the oocyte and follicular cells, the adjacent stroma becomes organized into a sheath, the **theca folliculi,** which surrounds the growing primary follicle. The theca folliculi is separated from the stratum granulosum by a distinct basement membrane. The cells differentiate into an inner secretory layer, the **theca interna,** and an outer fibrous layer, the **theca externa,** but the boundary between the layers is somewhat indistinct. The theca externa merges imperceptibly into the surrounding stroma (see atlas figure 18-6). Many small blood vessels penetrate the theca externa to provide a rich vascular network to the theca interna. The stratum granulosum remains avascular until after ovulation.

Secondary Follicles

KEY WORDS: liquor folliculi, follicular antrum, antral follicle, cumulus oophorus, corona radiata

As the follicular cells continue to proliferate, the growing follicle assumes an ovoid shape and gradually sinks deeper into the cortex. When the stratum granulosum has become 8 to 12 layers thick, fluid-filled spaces appear between the granulosa cells. The fluid, the **liquor folliculi,** increases in amount and the spaces fuse to form a single cavity called the **follicular antrum** (see atlas figure 18-7). The follicle is now a secondary or **antral follicle** and the oocyte has reached its full size and undergoes no further growth. The follicle, however, continues to increase in size, due in part to continued accumulation of liquor folliculi. The ovum is eccentrically placed in the follicle, surrounded by a mass of granulosa cells that project into the fluid-filled antrum, forming the **cumulus oophorus** (see atlas figure 18-7). The cells of the cumulus are continuous with those lining the antral cavity. Granulosa cells that surround the oocyte form the **corona radiata** and are anchored to the zona pellucida by cytoplasmic processes.

Mature Follicles and Ovulation

KEY WORDS: endocrine gland, aromatase enzyme complex, secondary oocyte, ovulation, stigma (macula pellucida)

In the human female, a follicle requires 10 to 14 days to reach the stage of maturity. At maximum size, the follicle occupies the thickness of the cortex and bulges from the surface of the ovary. Fluid spaces appear between granulosa cells of the cumulus oophorus, and the connection between the ovum and stratum granulosum is weakened. The theca folliculi has attained its greatest development, and the theca interna assumes the cytologic characteristics of a steroid-secreting

endocrine gland. Androstenedione and testosterone are important androgens secreted by the theca interna that serve as substrates for estrogen biosynthesis by the granulosa cells. An **aromatase enzyme complex** within the granulosa cells converts the substrates to estradiol, a form of estrogen. Just before ovulation, the oocyte completes the first meiotic division and gives off the first polar body. Thus, at ovulation a **secondary oocyte** is liberated.

Rupture of the mature follicle and liberation of the ovum constitute **ovulation,** which normally occurs at the middle of the menstrual cycle. Immediately before ovulation, further expansion of the follicle occurs due to increased secretion of liquor folliculi. Where the follicle bulges from the ovary, its wall becomes thinner and a small, avascular, translucent area appears. This is the **stigma** or **macula pellucida.** The tunica albuginea thins out and the surface epithelium of the ovary becomes discontinuous in this area. A collagenase produced by granulosa cells adjacent to the tunica albuginea appears to be responsible for the breakdown of collagen fibers at the site of the stigma. The stigma protrudes as a small blister and ruptures, and the ovum, with its adherent corona radiata, is extruded along with follicular fluid.

Corpus Luteum

KEY WORDS: estrogen, progesterone, granulosa lutein cell, theca lutein cell, luteinization, corpus albicans, relaxin

Following ovulation, the follicle is transformed into a temporary endocrine gland, the corpus luteum, which elaborates both **estrogens** and **progesterone.** The walls of the follicle collapse and stratum granulosum is thrown into folds. Bleeding from capillaries in the theca interna may result in a blood clot in the center of the corpus luteum. Granulosa cells increase greatly in size, take on a polyhedral shape, and transform into pale-staining **granulosa lutein cells.** Lipid accumulates in the cytoplasm of the cells, smooth endoplasmic reticulum becomes abundant, and mitochondria show tubular cristae. Cells of the theca interna also enlarge and become epithelioid in character to form **theca lutein cells** (see atlas figures 18-8 and 18-9). The lutein cells derived from the theca interna are somewhat smaller than granulosa lutein cells. The process of formation of granulosa and theca lutein cells is called **luteinization.**

With the depolymerization of the basement membrane between the theca interna and the granulosa cells, capillaries from the theca interna invade the lutein tissue to form a complex vascular network throughout the corpus luteum. Connective tissue from the theca interna also penetrates the mass of lutein cells and forms a delicate network about them. The fully formed corpus luteum secretes estrogens and progesterone; secretion of progesterone increases rapidly during luteinization, and high levels are maintained until the corpus luteum involutes.

If the ovum is not fertilized, the corpus luteum persists for about 14 days, then undergoes involution. The cells decrease in size, accumulate much lipid, and degenerate. Hyaline material accumulates between the lutein cells, the connective tissue cells become pyknotic, and the corpus luteum gradually is replaced by an irregular white scar, the **corpus albicans** (see atlas figure 18-10). Over the following months, the corpus albicans itself disappears. If fertilization occurs, the corpus luteum enlarges further and persists for about the first 6 months of pregnancy, then gradually declines. The corpora lutein cells of pregnancy secrete a polypeptide known as **relaxin.** Relaxin is thought to suppress uterine contractile activity during pregnancy and late in pregnancy enhances softening of the cervix and relaxation of the pelvic ligaments, resulting in a slight separation of the pubic symphysis prior to birth. Following delivery, involution of the corpus luteum is accelerated, resulting in the formation of a corpus albicans.

Atresia of Follicles

KEY WORDS: atresia, glassy membrane

During the early part of each menstrual cycle, several primordial follicles begin to grow, but usually only one attains full development and is ovulated. The remainder undergo a degenerative process called **atresia,** which may occur at any stage in the development of a follicle. In atresia of a primary follicle, the ovum shrinks, degenerates, and undergoes cytolysis; the follicular cells show similar degenerative changes. The follicle is resorbed, and the small space that is left is rapidly filled by connective tissue from the stroma. Similar degenerative changes occur in larger follicles, but the zona pellucida may persist for a time after dissolution of the oocyte and follicular cells. Macrophages invade the atretic follicle and engulf the degenerating material, including fragments of the zona pellucida.

Cells of the theca interna persist longer than those of the stratum granulosum but also show degenerative changes. The theca cells increase in size, lipid droplets appear in the cytoplasm, and the cells assume an epithelioid character, similar to that of lutein cells. The cells assume a cordlike arrangement, the cords being separated by connective tissue fibers and capillaries. The basal lamina between granulosa cells and the theca interna frequently becomes thicker and forms a hyalized, corrugated layer, the **glassy membrane.** This structure is characteristic of growing follicles that have undergone atresia and aids in distinguishing a large atretic follicle from a corpus luteum (see atlas figure 18-11). Other differences include degenerative changes in the granulosa cells and the presence of fragments of zona pellucida at the center of a follicle without an associated oocyte. Ultimately, the degenerated remains of the follicle are removed and a scar resembling a small corpus albicans is left. This, too, eventually disappears into the stroma of the ovary.

In some mammals, especially rodents, clusters of epithelioid cells are scattered in the stroma of the cortex. These interstitial cells contain small lipid droplets and bear a marked resemblance to luteal cells. It is thought that these interstitial cells arise from the theca interna of follicles that are undergoing atresia. In the human, interstitial cells are most abundant during the first year of life, the period during which atretic follicles are most numerous. In the adult they are present only in widely scattered, small groups. Their exact role in ovarian physiology is unknown; in humans they elaborate androgens.

Other large epithelioid cells, the hilus cells, are found associated with vascular spaces and unmyelinated nerves in the hilus of the ovary. The cells appear similar to the interstitial cells of the testis and contain lipid, lipochrome pigments, and cholesterol esters. Hilus cells are most commonly found during pregnancy and at menopause, but their function is unknown. Tumors arising from these cells have a masculinizing effect.

The Ovarian Cycle

KEY WORDS: follicle-stimulating hormone, luteinizing hormone, inhibin

Maturation of ovarian follicles, their endocrine functions, and the phenomenon of ovulation are regulated by follicle-stimulating hormone (FSH) and luteinizing hormone (LH). These are gonadotropic hormones elaborated by the anterior pituitary. **Follicle-stimulating hormone** is responsible for maturation of follicles and stimulates the aromatase enzyme complex within granulosa cells to produce estrogens. Initial development of follicles is self-regulated and does not require FSH, but the hormone is essential for their maturation. Together with FSH, **luteinizing hormone** induces ripening of the mature follicle and ovulation. Alone, LH converts the mature follicle to a corpus luteum and induces it to secrete estrogen and progesterone. The cyclic nature of follicle formation and ovulation is the result of reciprocal interaction between pituitary gonadotropins and ovarian hormones.

As production of estrogens by the granulosa cells increases, release of FSH from the pituitary is inhibited and the level of FSH falls below that needed for maturation of new follicles. However, the rising level of estrogen stimulates release of LH from the pituitary, resulting in ovulation, formation of a corpus luteum, and secretion of progesterone and estrogen by this body. Increasing levels of progesterone now inhibit release of LH

from the pituitary, and as the level of LH declines, the corpus luteum no longer is maintained. With decline of the corpus luteum, estrogen levels diminish, the pituitary no longer is inhibited from secreting FSH, and a new cycle of follicle formation is initiated. The ovarian steroid hormones have only minor effects on the pituitary directly; their primary action is mediated through neurons in the hypothalamus. Both FSH and ovarian androgens stimulate granulosa cells to synthesize and release a glycoprotein called **inhibin.** Inhibin preferentially suppresses the synthesis and secretion of FSH by cells in the anterior pituitary.

Oviducts

The oviducts (uterine tubes) are a pair of muscular tubes that extend from the ovary to the uterus along the upper margin of the broad ligament. One end of the tube is closely related to the ovary and, at this end, is open to the peritoneal cavity. The other end communicates with the lumen of the uterus. The oviduct delivers the ovum, released at ovulation, to the uterine cavity and provides an environment for fertilization and initial segmentation of the fertilized ovum.

Structure

KEY WORDS: infundibulum, fimbria, ampulla, isthmus, intramural (interstitial) part

The oviduct is divided into several segments. The ovarian end, the **infundibulum,** is funnel-shaped, and its margin is drawn out in numerous tapering processes called **fimbria** (see atlas figure 18-12). The infundibulum opens into the tortuous, thin-walled **ampulla** of the tube, which makes up slightly more than half the length of the oviduct. The ampulla is continuous with the **isthmus,** a narrower, cordlike portion that makes up about the medial one-third. The **intramural (interstitial) part** is the continuation of the tube where it passes through the uterine wall. As in other hollow viscera, the wall of the oviduct consists of several layers: an external serosa, an intermediate muscularis, and an internal mucosa.

Mucosa

KEY WORDS: plica, columnar epithelial cell, lamina propria, ciliated cell, nonciliated cell, cyclic change

The mucosa of the oviduct presents a series of longitudinal folds called **plicae.** In the ampulla the plicae have secondary and even tertiary folds to create a complex labyrinth of epithelial-lined spaces. In the isthmus, the plicae are shorter with little branching, while in the intramural part the plicae form only low ridges. Throughout the tube, the plicae consist of a single layer of **columnar epithelial cells** resting on an incomplete basement membrane, and a **lamina propria** of richly cellular connective tissue that contains a network of reticular fibers and fibroblasts. The epithelium decreases in height from ampulla to uterus and contains ciliated and nonciliated cells (see atlas figures 18-13 through 18-15). The **ciliated cells** are most numerous on the surface of the fimbria and progressively decrease in number through the ampulla, isthmus, and intramural portions. The **nonciliated cells** appear to be secretory and may help establish an environment that is suitable for the survival and fertilization of the ovum and for maintenance of the zygote. A third cell type, an undifferentiated cell with a darkly staining nucleus, may represent a precursor of the secretory cells or an exhausted secretory cell.

The epithelium shows **cyclic changes** associated with ovarian cycles. During the follicular phase, ciliated cells increase in height, reaching their maximum at about the time of ovulation, and there is evidence of increased preparations in the secretory cells. In the luteal phase, ciliated cells decrease in height and lose their cilia, and there is augmented secretory activity by the secretory cells. Loss of cilia is greatest in the fimbria and least in the isthmus. The cilia are responsive to steroid hormones: Estrogen appears to be responsible for the appearance and maintenance of cilia, and progesterone increases the rate at which they beat. Other ciliated cells of the body show no such hormone responsiveness.

Muscular Coat and Serosa

KEY WORDS: no submucosa, inner circular muscle, outer longitudinal muscle

The mucous membrane rests directly on the muscle coat and there is **no submucosa.** The muscle coat consists of two layers of smooth muscle, but the layers are not sharply defined. The **inner layer is circular** or closely spiralled; the **outer layer of longitudinal muscle** is the thinner (see atlas figure 18-14). The muscularis increases in thickness toward the uterus due to the increased depth of the inner layer. Externally, the oviduct is covered by a serosa that represents the peritoneal covering of the organ.

Uterus

The human uterus is a single, hollow, pear-shaped organ with a thick muscular wall, it lies in the pelvic cavity between the bladder and rectum. The nonpregnant uterus varies in size depending on the individual but generally is about 7 cm in length, 3 to 5 cm at its widest (upper) part, and 2.5 to 3.0 cm thick. It is slightly flattened dorsoventrally, and the cavity corresponds to the overall shape of the organ. The uterus receives the fertilized ovum and nourishes the embryo and fetus throughout its development until birth.

Structure

KEY WORDS: body, cervix, cervical canal, endometrium, myometrium, perimetrium

Several regions of the uterus can be distinguished. The bulk of the organ consists of the **body,** which comprises the upper expanded portion. The dome-shaped part of the body between the junctions with the oviduct constitutes the fundus. Below, the uterus narrows and becomes more cylindrical in shape: This region forms the **cervix,** part of which protrudes into the vagina. The **cervical canal** passes through the cervix from the uterine cavity and communicates with the vagina at the external os.

The wall of the uterus is made up of several

layers that have special names: The internal lining or mucosa is called the **endometrium**; the middle muscular layer forms the **myometrium**; and the external layer is referred to as the **perimetrium.** The perimetrium is the serosal or peritoneal layer that covers the body of the uterus and supravaginal part of the cervix posteriorly, and the body of the uterus anteriorly.

Myometrium

KEY WORDS: smooth muscle, internal layer, middle layer, stratum vasculare, outer layer

The bulk of the uterine wall consists of the myometrium, which forms a thick coat about 15 to 20 mm in depth. The myometrium consists of bundles of **smooth muscle** fibers separated by thin strands of connective tissue that contain fibroblasts, collagenous and reticular fibers, mast cells, and macrophages. The muscle forms several layers that are not sharply defined because of the intermingling of fibers from one layer to another. Generally, however, internal, middle, and outer layers can be distinguished. The **internal layer** is thin and consists of longitudinal and circular fibers. The **middle layer** is the thickest and shows no regularity in the arrangement of the muscle fibers, which run longitudinally, obliquely, circularly, and transversely. This layer also contains many large blood vessels and has been called the **stratum vasculare.** The **outer layer** of muscle consists mainly of longitudinal fibers, some of which extend into the broad ligament, oviducts, and ovarian ligaments. Elastic fibers are prominent in the outer layer but are not present in the inner layer of the myometrium except around blood vessels.

In the nonpregnant uterus, the smooth muscle cells are 30 to 50 μm long, but during pregnancy they hypertrophy to reach lengths of 500 to 600 μm or greater. New smooth muscles are produced in the pregnant uterus from undifferentiated cells and possibly from division of mature cells also. The connective tissue of the myometrium also increases in amount during pregnancy. In spite of a total increase in muscle mass, the layers are thinned during pregnancy as the uterus becomes distended. After delivery, the muscle cells rapidly decrease in size, but the uterus does not regain its original, nonpregnant dimensions.

The myometrium normally undergoes intermittent contractions that, however, are not intense enough to be perceived. The intensity may increase during menstruation to result in cramps. The contractions are diminished during pregnancy, possibly in response to the hormone relaxin. At parturition, strong contractions of the uterine musculature occur, causing the fetus to be expelled. Uterine contractions increase after administration of oxytocin, a hormone produced by the neurohypophysis, and in response to prostaglandins. A rise in the level of prostaglandins occurs just prior to delivery.

Endometrium

KEY WORDS: endometrial stroma, simple columnar epithelium, uterine gland, stratum basale, stratum functionale, radial artery, straight artery, spiral artery, lacuna

The endometrium is a complex mucous membrane that, in the human female, undergoes cyclic changes in structure and function in response to the ovarian cycle. The cyclic activity begins at puberty and continues until menopause. In the body of the uterus, the endometrium consists of a thick lamina propria **(endometrial stroma)** and a covering epithelium (see atlas figures 18-16 and 18-18). The stroma resembles mesenchymal tissue and consists of loosely arranged stellate cells with large, round or ovoid nuclei, supported by a network of fine connective tissue in which lymphocytes, granular leukocytes, and macrophages are scattered. There is no submucosa, and the stroma lies directly on the myometrium, to which it is firmly attached.

The stroma is covered by a **simple columnar epithelium** that contains ciliated cells and nonciliated secretory cells. The epithelium dips into the stroma to form numerous **uterine glands** that extend deeply into the stroma, occasionally penetrating into the myometrium (see atlas figures 18-16 and 18-17). Most are simple tubular glands, but some may branch near the muscle. There are fewer ciliated cells in the glands than in the covering epithelium. A basement membrane underlies the glandular and surface epithelia.

The endometrium can be divided into a stratum basale (basal layer) and a stratum functionale (functional layer), which differ in their structure, function, and blood supply. The **stratum basale** is the narrower, more cellular, and more fibrous layer and lies directly on the myometrium (see atlas figure 18-17). Occasionally, small pockets of stratum basale may extend into the myometrium, between muscle cells. This layer undergoes few changes during the menstrual cycle and is not shed at menstruation but serves as the source from which the functional layer is restored.

The **stratum functionale** extends to the lumen of the uterus and is the part of the endometrium in which cycle changes occur and which is shed during menstruation (see atlas figure 18-16). The stratum functionale sometimes is divided into the compacta, a narrow superficial zone, and the spongiosa, a broader zone that forms the bulk of the functionalis.

The blood supply of the endometrium (Fig. 18-1) is unique and plays an important role in the events of menstruation. Branches of the uterine artery penetrate the myometrium to its middle layer, where they furnish arcuate arteries that run circumferentially in the myometrium. One set of branches from these arteries supplies the superficial layers of the myometrium, while other branches, the **radial arteries,** pass inward to supply the endometrium. At the junction of myometrium and endometrium, the radial branches provide a dual circulation to the endometrium. **Straight arteries** supply the stratum basale while stratum functionale is supplied by highly coiled **spiral arteries** (see atlas figure 18-17). As the latter pass through the functional layer, they provide terminal arterioles, which unite with a complex network of capillaries and thin-walled, dilated vascular structures, the **lacunae.** The venous system forms an irregular network of venules and veins with irregular sinusoidal enlarge-

ments, then drains into a plexus at the junction of myometrium and endometrium. During menstrual cycles, the spiral arteries constrict periodically, subjecting the functional layer to intermittent periods of anoxia. The distal portions of the arterial supply in the functionalis undergo degeneration and regeneration with each menstrual cycle, whereas the straight arteries of the basal layer show no such changes.

Cyclic Changes in the Endometrium

KEY WORDS: proliferative phase, maturation of follicle, secretory phase, corpus luteum, ischemic (premenstrual) phase, menstrual phase

During a normal menstrual cycle, the endometrium undergoes a continuous sequence of changes in which four phases can be described. The phases correlate with the functional activities of the ovaries and constitute the proliferative, secretory, ischemic (premenstrual), and menstrual phases.

The **proliferative phase** begins at the end of the menstrual flow and extends to about the middle of the cycle. This stage is characterized by rapid regeneration and repair of the endometrium. Epithelial cells in the remnants of the glands in the stratum basale proliferate and migrate over the raw surface of the mucosa; stromal cells also proliferate. In the early part of this period, the endometrium is of limited thickness, and its glands are sparse and fairly straight and have small lumina. The epithelium of the glands and surface is simple cuboidal to low columnar, and mitoses are present in the glandular lining. As the proliferative phase advances, the endometrial glands increase in number and length and become more tortuous and more closely spaced, and the lumina widen. Toward the end of the proliferative phase, glycogen accumulates in the basal region of the glandular epithelium. The surface and glandular epithelia now are tall columnar with fewer ciliated and more secretory cells. The secretory cells have large numbers of small mitochondria, but the endoplasmic reticulum and Golgi complex are poorly developed. Microvilli are present on the free borders of the cells.

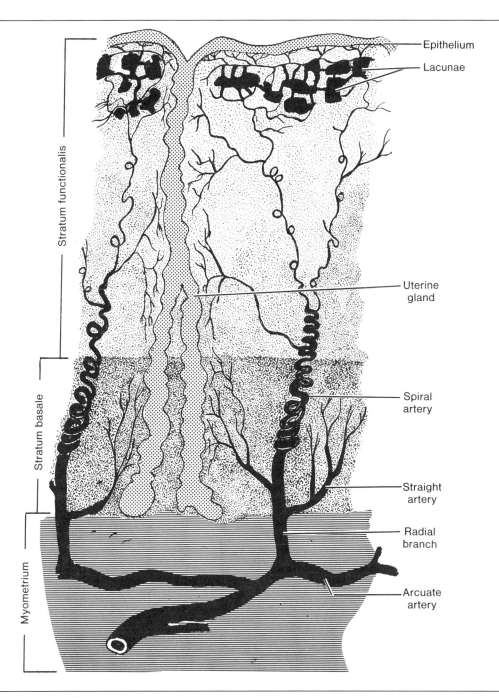

Fig 18-1. Arrangement of blood vessels in the endometrium.

The nuclei are round or oval and contain finely granular chromatin with one or more nucleoli. The spiral arteries lengthen but are lightly coiled and do not extend into the superficial third of the endometrium.

The proliferative phase corresponds to the **maturation of the ovarian follicle** up to the time of ovulation. Estrogen, secreted by the developing follicle, stimulates growth of the endometrium; some growth may continue for a day or two after ovulation.

During the **secretory phase,** the endometrium continues to increase in thickness as a result of hypertrophy of stromal and glandular cells, stromal edema, and increased vascularity. The glands lengthen and become irregularly coiled and convoluted and show wide, irregular lumina. The epithelial cells become larger and their free surfaces show many long microvilli. Mitochondria are large, there is a rich endoplasmic reticulum, and the Golgi apparatus is prominent. Nuclei are enlarged and contain a distinct nucleolus. Glycogen and mucoid materials rapidly increase, first in the bases of the glandular cells, then in the apical portions of the cells, and then into the lumina of the glands. Elongation and coiling of the spiral arteries continue, and the vessels extend into the superficial part of the endometrium.

The secretory phase is associated with development of a **corpus luteum** and is maintained as long as the corpus luteum remains functional. Progesterone secreted by the corpus luteum is responsible for the secretory changes in the endometrium.

The **ischemic (premenstrual) phase** is characterized by intermittent constriction of the spiral arteries, resulting in vascular stasis and reduced blood flow to the functional layer. The outer zone of the endometrium is subjected to anoxia for hours at a time, resulting in breakdown of the stratum functionale. The stroma becomes increasingly edematous and infiltrated by leukocytes.

In the **menstrual phase,** the functional layer become necrotic and is shed. The spiral arteries also become necrotic and blood is lost from the arteries and veins. Small lakes of blood form and coalesce, and overlying patches of mucosa are detached, leaving a denuded stromal surface. Sloughing of the endometrium continues until the entire functional layer has been discarded. Blood oozes from veins torn during the shedding of the endometrial tissue. The menstrual discharge consists of arterial and venous blood, autolyzed and degenerated epithelial cells, and glandular secretions. The straight arteries of stratum basale do not constrict during menstruation, thus preserving the basal layer to provide for restoration of the endometrium during the following new proliferative stage.

The onset of the menstrual cycle coincides with the beginning involution of a corpus luteum. The hormonal relationships of the ovary and uterine mucosa are shown in Figure 18-2.

Cervix

KEY WORDS: dense connective tissue, endocervix, nonkeratinized stratified squamous epithelium, secretory change

The wall of the cervix differs considerably from that of the body of the uterus. Little smooth muscle is present, and the cervical wall consists mainly of **dense connective tissue** and elastic fibers. In the part that protrudes into the vaginal canal, smooth muscle is lacking. The cervical canal is lined by a mucosa, the **endocervix,** which forms complex, branching folds. The epithelial lining consists of tall, mucus-secreting columnar cells along with a few ciliated columnar cells. Numerous large, branched glands are present that are lined by mucus-secreting columnar cells similar to those of the lining epithelium. The cervical canal usually is filled with mucus. Occasionally the glands become occluded and filled with secretion, forming nabothian cysts.

The portion of the cervix that protrudes into the vaginal canal, the exocervix, is covered by a **nonkeratinized stratified squamous epithelium** whose cells contain much glycogen. The transition from the columnar epithelium of the cervical canal is fairly abrupt and usually occurs just inside the external os. The cervical mucosa does

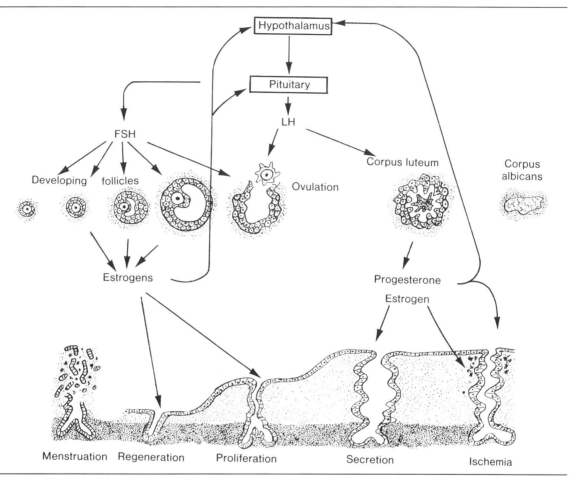

Fig. 18-2. Hormonal relationships of the ovary and uterine mucosa. (FSH = follicle-stimulating hormone; LH = luteinizing hormone.)

not take part in the cyclic changes of the body of the uterus and is not shed. The glandular elements do show **changes in secretory activity,** however. At midcycle there is a copious secretion of a thin alkaline fluid, probably the result of increased stimulation by estrogen. After ovulation and establishment of a corpus luteum, the amount of secretion decreases and the mucus becomes thicker and more viscous.

Vagina

The vagina is the lowermost portion of the female reproductive tract and is a muscular tube that joins the uterus to the exterior of the body. It represents the copulatory organ of the female. Ordinarily the lumen is collapsed and the anterior and posterior walls make contact.

Structure

KEY WORDS: mucosa, rugae, nonkeratinized stratified squamous epithelium, lamina propria, muscularis, adventitia

The vaginal wall consists of a mucosa, a muscularis, and an adventitia. The **mucosa** is thrown into folds **(rugae)** and consists of a thick surface layer of **nonkeratinized stratified squamous epithelium** overlying a lamina propria (see atlas figures 18-19 through 18-21). The epithelial cells contain abundant glycogen, especially at midcycle. The **lamina propria** consists of a fairly dense connective tissue that becomes more loosely arranged near the muscle coat. Immediately below the epithelial lining, elastic fibers form a dense network. Diffuse and nodular lymphatic tissues are found occasionally, and many lymphocytes, along with granular leukocytes, invade the epithelium. The vagina has no glands and the epithelium is kept moist by secretions from the cervix.

The **muscularis** consists of bundles of smooth muscle fibers that are arranged circularly in the inner layer and longitudinally in the outer part. The longitudinal fibers become continuous with similarly oriented fibers in the myometrium.

The **adventitia** is a thin outer layer of dense connective tissue and elastic fibers. It merges imperceptibly into the surrounding loose connective tissue around other organs.

Cytology of the Cervical Canal

KEY WORDS: basal cell, parabasal cell, intermediate squamous cell, superficial squamous cell

The stratified squamous epithelium that lines the vagina and covers the exocervix is arranged in layers similar to those of the epidermis. Deepest is the basal layer (stratum germinativum), followed by an intermediate (spinous) layer and a superficial layer (stratum corneum) from which cells are shed. Desquamated cervical cells can be recovered from vaginal secretions, or cells can be obtained more directly by gentle abrasion of the exocervix. The cells can be studied in smear preparations and examination of Papanicolaou's ("Pap") smears has become a standard procedure for early detection of cervical cancer.

In the normal adult female, four types of cells usually are recognized cytologically, loosely corresponding to the layers of the cervicovaginal epithelium. These include basal (lower basal) cells, parabasal (outer basal) cells, intermediate (precornified) squamous cells, and superficial (cornified) squamous cells. Germinal cells from the basal layer are exceedingly rare in smears from normal adults, and the basal and parabasal cells recognized cytologically are derived from different levels of the intermediate layer. They do represent less mature cells, and their presence indicates that immature cells are at higher than normal levels in the epithelium. These cells are associated with marked deficiency of estrogens and are common before puberty and during menopause.

Basal cells arise from the lower levels of the transitional zone and are rounded or oval cells, about 4 to 5 times the size of a granular leukocyte. The central nucleus is deeply stained, but a pattern of fine chromatin granules and dense patches can be made out. In some cells a Barr body is distinctly visible. The moderate amount of basophilic cytoplasm stains deeply and evenly. **Parabasal cells** arise higher up in the transitional zone and also are round or oval cells, but they are larger than basal cells with a more abundant cytoplasm that is less basophilic and often shows a somewhat "blotchy" pattern. The central nucleus remains about the same size but may be more dense than that of a basal cell. **Intermediate squamous cells** vary in size, but all appear as thin, polygonal plates with abundant transparent cytoplasm. The nucleus is smaller, vesicular, and centrally placed. The cytoplasm stains somewhat variably and may be lightly basophilic or show some degree of eosinophilia. **Superficial squamous cells** represent dead surface cells. They are large, with voluminous eosinophilic cytoplasm that is thin and transparent with sharply defined borders. Because of the thinness, the cytoplasm often is curled, wrinkled, and folded. The nucleus is very small — about one-half to one-third of that of an intermediate squamous cell — and is densely stained and pyknotic. The superficial and intermediate squamous cells are the largest cells seen in a routine preparation and range from 40 to 50 μm in diameter. Occasionally, anucleate squamous cells may be found. They have a somewhat shrivelled appearance, and the site of the nucleus is suggested by a pale central zone. They represent cells that are more completely keratinized.

Cells that originate from the endocervix also may be present and often occur in small sheets or strips; their appearance depends on the orientation. From end on, the cells appear as groups or nests of small polyhedral or round cells with sharp cell boundaries and relatively large central nuclei. In profile, the cells show their columnar shape with the nuclei close to one pole. Strips of these cells give a "picket fence" appearance.

External Genitalia

The external genitalia of the female consist of the labia, clitoris, and vestibular glands.

Labia

KEY WORDS: **labia majora, homologue of the scrotum, labia minora**

The **labia majora** consist of folds of skin covering an abundance of adipose tissue. In the adult the outer surface is covered by coarse hair with many sweat and sebaceous glands. The inner surface is smooth and hairless and also contains sweat and sebaceous glands. The labia majora are the **homologue of the scrotum** in the male. The **labia minora** consist of a core of highly vascular, loose connective tissue covered by stratified squamous epithelium that is deeply indented by connective tissue papillae. The deeper layers of epithelium are pigmented. Both surfaces of the labia minora are devoid of hair, but large sebaceous glands are present.

Clitoris

KEY WORDS: **erectile, corresponds to dorsal penis, corpora cavernosa, glans clitoridis, no corpus spongiosum**

The clitoris is an **erectile** body that **corresponds to the dorsal penis.** It consists of two **corpora cavernosa** enclosed in a layer of fibrous connective tissue and separated by an incomplete septum. The free end of the clitoris terminates in a small, rounded tubercle, the **glans clitoridis,** which consists of spongy erectile tissue. The clitoris is covered by a thin layer of stratified squamous epithelium with high papillae associated with many specialized nerve endings. The clitoris has **no corpus spongiosum** and therefore does not contain the urethra.

Vestibular Glands

KEY WORDS: **stratified squamous epithelium, mucous cell, major vestibular gland, tubuloalveolar gland**

The vestibule is the cleft between the labia minora and in it are the vaginal and urethral openings. It is lined by **stratified squamous epithelium** and contains numerous small vestibular glands concentrated about the openings of the vagina and urethra. The glands contain **mucous cells** and resemble the urethral glands of the male. A pair of larger glands, the greater or **major vestibular glands,** are present in the lateral walls of the vestibule. They are **tubuloalveolar glands** that secrete a mucoid lubricating fluid. The major glands correspond to the bulbourethral glands of the male.

Pregnancy

Pregnancy involves implantation of a blastocyst into a prepared uterine endometrium and subsequent formation of a placenta to nourish and maintain the developing embryo. Prior to implantation, fertilization of the ovum and cleavage of the resulting zygote occur in the oviduct.

Fertilization

KEY WORDS: **female pronucleus, male pronucleus**

Before an ovum can be fertilized, it must undergo maturational changes, chief of which is reduction of the chromosome complement to the haploid number. The oocyte passes through the early stages of the first meiotic division during fetal life, and it is only just before ovulation that the division is completed and the first polar body is given off. The resulting secondary oocyte immediately enters the second meiotic division, which, however, proceeds only to metaphase and is not completed until fertilization occurs.

At the time of ovulation, the oviduct shows active movements that bring the ampulla and fimbria close to the ovary. Cilia on the surface of the fimbria sweep the ovum into the ampulla of the oviduct where fertilization, if it is to occur, takes place. The human ovum probably remains fertilizable for about 1 day, after which it degenerates if fertilization does not occur.

Of the millions of sperm deposited in the female tract, only one penetrates the ovum. There is no evidence for chemotactic attraction, and random movement brings sperm and ovum together. The successful sperm pierces the corona radiata and zona pellucida, possibly by lysis of the membrane by enzymes in the sperm acrosome, and the entire spermatozoon is engulfed by the cytoplasm of the ovum. Electron micrographs suggest that the plasma membranes of the sperm and ovum fuse, that of the spermatozoon being left at the surface of the ovum. Penetration is followed by release of electron-dense, cortical granules that underlie the plasmalemma of the ovum and by immediate changes in the permeability of the zona pellucida, which thereafter excludes entry by competing sperm.

The ovum now completes the second maturation division and extrudes the second polar body. The remaining chromosomes (23) reconstitute and form the **female pronucleus.** The nucleus (head) of the spermatozoon swells and forms the **male pronucleus,** and the body and tail are re-sorbed. The two pronuclei move to the center of the cell and two centrioles, supplied by the anterior centriole of the spermatozoon, appear. The chromatin of each pronucleus resolves into a set of chromosomes that align themselves on a spindle to undergo a normal mitotic division of the first cleavage. Each cell resulting from this division receives a full diploid set of chromosomes.

Cleavage

KEY WORDS: **blastomere, morula, blastocele, blastocyst, inner cell mass, trophoblast**

The zygote undergoes a series of rapid divisions called cleavage that result in a large number of cells, the **blastomeres.** The cells are bounded by the zona pellucida, and a mulberry-like body, the **morula,** is formed (see atlas figures 18-22 through 18-24). Cleavage is a fractionating process: No new cytoplasm is formed, and at each division the cells become smaller until a normal, predetermined, cytoplasmic/nuclear ratio is reached. Thus, the total size of the morula is not increased. Cleavage occurs as the morula slowly is moved along the oviduct by the waves of peristaltic contractions in the muscle coat. When the morula reaches the uterine cavity, it is at the 12- to 16-cell stage. At about this time, fluid penetrates zona pellucida and diffuses between the cells of the morula. The fluid increases in amount, the intercellular spaces become confluent, and a single cavity, the **blastocele,** is formed. The morula has now become a **blastocyst** that forms a hollow sphere containing, at one pole, a mass of cells called the **inner cell mass** that will form the embryo proper (see atlas figures 18-25 through 18-27). The capsule-like wall of the blastocyst consists of a single layer of cells, the **trophoblast.** After reaching a critical mass, the blastocyst breaks through the surrounding zona pellucida and remains free in the uterine cavity for about a day, then attaches to the endometrium, which is in the secretory phase.

Implantation

KEY WORDS: secretory phase, syncytial trophoblast, cytotrophoblast, lacunae

At the time of implantation, the endometrium is in the **secretory phase** and, having been under the influence of progesterone from the corpus luteum for several days, has reached its greatest thickness and development. Implantation is initiated by close approximation of the trophoblast to the microvilli and surface projections of the uterine epithelial cells. At the points of contact, the trophoblast shows patches of coated vesicles and numerous lysosomes. The microvilli shorten and disappear and the trophoblast extends fingerlike processes between the uterine epithelial cells, and the two layers become closely locked by numerous tight junctions that develop between them. The epithelial cells degenerate and are engulfed by the trophoblast, the cellular debris appearing in phagosomes within the trophoblast cytoplasm. Where it is fixed to the endothelium, the trophoblast proliferates to form a cellular mass between the blastocyst and maternal tissues. No cell boundaries can be made out in this cell mass, which is called the **syncytial trophoblast** (see atlas figures 18-28 and 18-29). The syncytium continues to erode the endometrium at the point of contact, creating a ragged cavity into which the blastocyst sinks, gradually becoming more deeply embedded until it entirely lies within the endometrial stroma. The surface defect in the endometrium is closed temporarily by a fibrin plug. Later, proliferation of surrounding cells restores the surface continuity of the endometrial lining.

As the blastocyst sinks into the endometrium, the syncytial trophoblast rapidly increases in thickness at the original site of attachment and progressively extends to cover the remainder of the blastocyst. When completely embedded, the entire wall of the blastocyst consists of a thick outer syncytial trophoblast and an inner **cytotrophoblast,** which is composed of a single layer of cells with well-defined boundaries (see atlas figure 18-28). The cytotrophoblast shows active mitosis and contributes cells to the syncytial trophoblast,

where they fuse with and become part of that layer. The syncytial trophoblast continues to erode the uterine tissues, opening up the walls of maternal blood vessels. Spaces appear in the syncytial trophoblast and these **lacunae** expand, become confluent, and form a labyrinth of spaces. Many of the spaces contain blood extravasated from eroded maternal blood vessels; this blood supplies nourishment for the embryo and represents the first step in the development of uteroplacental circulation.

Placenta

KEY WORDS: primary villus, chorion, secondary villus, chorionic plate, chorion frondosum, chorion laeve, tertiary placental villus, decidua, chorionic gonadotropin

As the lacunae enlarge, intervening strands of trophoblast form the **primary villi** that cover the entire periphery of the blastocyst. Each villus consists of a core of cytotrophoblast covered by a layer of syncytial trophoblast. Trophoblastic cells at the tips of the villi apply themselves to the endometrium and form a lining for the cavity in which the blastocyst lies. When the embryonic germ layers have been established, mesoderm grows out from the embryo as the **chorion** and forms a lining for the trophoblast that surrounds the blastocyst. Mesoderm extends into the primary villi to form a core of connective tissue and convert the villi to **secondary villi.** The deeply embedded portion of the chorion constitutes the **chorionic plate** from which numerous villi project to form the **chorion frondosum.** Villi on that part of the chorion facing the uterine cavity grow more slowly and are less numerous; ultimately these villi disappear, leaving a smooth surface that forms the **chorion laeve.** Blood vessels develop in the mesenchymal cores of the secondary villi and soon make connection with the fetal circulation. With vascularization, the secondary villi become the definitive or **tertiary placental villi** (see atlas figure 18-29).

At parturition, all but the deepest layers of the endometrium are shed; thus, the superficial part of the endometrium is called the **decidua.** A feature of the stroma is the alteration of its cells to form enlarged, decidual cells that contain much glycogen. According to the relationship with the implantation site, three areas of the decidua are recognized. The *decidua capsularis* is the part that lies over the surface of the blastocyst, while the *decidua basalis* underlies the implantation site and forms the maternal component of the placenta. The endometrium lining the remainder of the pregnant uterus is the *decidua parietalis*. As the embryo grows, the decidua capsularis becomes increasingly attenuated. Eventually, the decidua capsularis makes contact with decidua parietalis on the opposite surface of the uterus and the uterine cavity is obliterated.

The mature placenta consists of maternal and fetal components. The maternal part is decidua basalis; the fetal portion consists of the chorionic plate and the villi arising from it. Maternal blood circulates through the intervillous spaces and bathes the villi, of which there are two types. Some pass from the chorionic plate to decidua basalis as anchoring villi from which secondary and tertiary branches float in the intervillous spaces as the floating villi. Both types of villi consist of a core of loose connective tissue in which lie fetal capillaries. Covering each villus is an inner layer of cytotrophoblast cells, which have large nuclei and lightly basophilic cytoplasm containing considerable glycogen. External to the cytotrophoblast is a layer of syncytial trophoblast of variable thickness. The cells of the cytotrophoblast decrease in number in the latter half of pregnancy, and only a very few are present at term. The syncytial trophoblast also thins out to form a narrow layer.

The structure of the placenta is shown diagrammatically in Figure 18-3.

The placenta transfers oxygen and nutrients from the maternal to the fetal circulation and waste products from the fetal to the maternal circulation. Although maternal and fetal circulations are closely apposed, they remain separated by the syncytial trophoblast (and early in pregnancy by the cytotrophoblast also), a basement membrane, the connective tissue of the villi, and the wall of the fetal blood vessels. Transport of material between fetal and maternal blood ap-

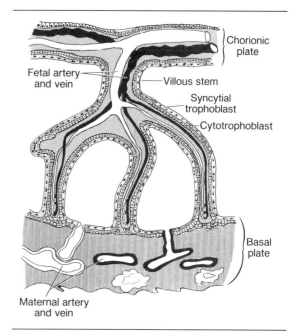

Fig. 18-3. Diagram of the structure of the placenta.

pears to be regulated by the syncytial trophoblast. Being without cell boundaries and intercellular spaces, any materials passing into or out of the fetal blood must pass through the cytoplasm of the syncytium. The cytotrophoblast appears to serve as the source of cells for the syncytial trophoblast. The placenta also is a multipotential endocrine organ, supplying estrogens, progesterone, and **chorionic gonadotropin.** The latter is produced by the syncytial trophoblast and possibly by the cytotrophoblast; it stimulates secretion of estrogen and progesterone by the corpus luteum during early pregnancy.

Development of the Female Reproductive Tract

Early development of the female reproductive tract is related closely to that of the urinary system and of the male reproductive tract. All arise in the mesoderm of the urogenital ridges within epithelial thickenings on each side of the midline. Initially, the ovaries and testes are indistinguishable and form a primitive, indifferent gonad that does not acquire male or female morphology until the seventh week of development.

Ovary

The first indication of gonads appears at four weeks, when a pair of longitudinal ridges, the genital (gonadal) ridges, appear. These are divided into lateral and medial parts, and only the medial portion gives rise to the ovary. No germ cells are present in the gonadal ridges until the sixth week of development. The epithelium of the gonadal ridge proliferates, and in places, clumps of cells become thickened to form a number of cellular gonadal cords that penetrate the underlying mesenchyme. The cords at the periphery form a primary ovarian cortex, while centrally, proliferation of mesenchyme establishes a primary medulla (see atlas figures 18-34 through 18-36). The gonadal cords break up into irregular clusters separated by strands of mesenchyme, an extension of which cuts off the cell clusters from the surface epithelium and eventually forms the tunica albuginea. A second proliferation of the surface epithelium gives rise to new cellular cords that invade the primary cortex, dissociate into isolated clusters, and form the definitive cortex. The cell clusters surround one or more primitive germ cells (primary oocytes) that enter prophase of the first meiotic division. The primary medulla is replaced by a fibroelastic stroma to establish a permanent medulla.

Primordial germ cells, which give rise to the definitive oogonia, are segregated early in development. They appear first in the yolk sac, then migrate to the dorsal mesentery and then to the genital ridges. It is uncertain whether the primordial cells arise from a group of special blastomeres during cleavage or as clones of a single blastomere. Their early association with endoderm has suggested this as the tissue of origin.

Oviducts, Uterus, and Vagina

By six weeks' gestation in the human, male and female embryos have paired mesonephric and paramesonephric ducts. In the female embryo,

paramesonephric ducts become predominant, giving rise to oviducts, uterus, and possibly vagina. Unlike the male, the mesonephric ducts are not part of the female system. Mesonephric ducts regress, except for a few remnants.

Paramesonephric ducts begin to form at about 35 or 36 days. Each duct begins as an invagination on the lateral side of the mesonephric ridge. The ingrowing mesothelium forms a short groove that sinks beneath the surface and seals off to form a tube. The anterior end develops first and opens into the coelomic cavity as a funnel-shaped structure that gives rise to the fimbriated and ampullary parts of the oviduct. Caudally, the paramesonephric tubes from each side lengthen and descend, then turn medially to meet each other and form a single structure, the utero-vaginal canal. At first the two lumina are separate, but the intervening walls degenerate and a single cavity is formed. The descending part forms the body and cervix of the uterus. Mesenchyme surrounding the utero-vaginal canal supplies the endometrial stroma and myometrium.

The vagina arises from an epithelial proliferation, the sinovaginal bulb, on the posterior wall of the uterogenital sinus. It is not certain whether this epithelium is true sinus epithelium or epithelium of the mesonephric duct that descended into this region. The proliferating epithelium extends cranially as a solid bar that forms the vaginal plate. Beginning at the caudal end, cells in the center of the plate degenerate and a vaginal lumen is formed. In humans, canalization is complete by the fifth month. The fetal vaginal epithelium is under the influence of maternal hormones and in late fetal life becomes markedly hypertrophied. It regresses after birth and assumes its inactive childhood form.

External Genitalia

The external genitalia also pass through an indifferent stage before they develop their definitive sexual characteristics. The caudal end of the primitive hindgut is closed by a cloacal membrane around which the urogenital folds develop. The folds unite at their cranial ends to form the genital tubercle, which, in the female, elongates only slightly to give rise to the clitoris. A pair of genital swellings develops along each side of the genital folds; in the female these remain separate and form the labia majora. Similarly, the urogenital folds do not fuse in the female, and these give rise to the labia minora.

Functional Summary

The ovary is a cytogenic gland releasing ova and also acts as a cyclic endocrine gland. During its growth in the follicles, the oocyte is nourished by blood vessels of the ovary via the theca interna. When a corpus luteum is formed after ovulation, estrogens and progesterone are produced and are responsible for development of the uterine mucosa prepared for reception of the blastocyst. The periodic nature of hormone production by the ovary establishes the menstrual cycle during which, in the absence of pregnancy, the uterine mucosa is shed. If pregnancy occurs, the corpus luteum persists and its hormonal activity maintains the endometrium in a prepared state.

Female reproductive function is regulated primarily by positive and negative feedback loops on neurons in the hypothalamic region of the brain and on cells of the anterior pituitary. The hypothalamic neurons release a single factor (gonadotropin-releasing factor) that regulates the release of both FSH and LH from cells of the anterior pituitary. Follicle-stimulating hormone influences the growth of late primary and secondary follicles and promotes the formation of estrogens. Luteinizing hormone stimulates ovulation and promotes corpus luteum formation. Estrogen suppresses FSH secretion by acting on both cells of the anterior pituitary and neurons within the hypothalamus. Inhibin secreted by follicular granulosa cells suppresses secretion of FSH directly by acting on cells of the anterior pituitary. Progesterone inhibits LH release; therefore the corpus luteum lacks the stimulus essential for its maintenance and soon degenerates.

The oviduct is the site of fertilization of an ovum and also transports the zygote to the uterus as the result of muscular and ciliary actions. Conditions within the oviduct sustain the zygote as it undergoes cleavage during passage through the tube. Nutrition for the zygote is provided by material stored in the cytoplasm of the ovum.

On entering the uterine cavity, the blastocyst lies in secretions produced by the endometrium. The secretion is rich in glycogen, polysaccharides, and lipids, providing an excellent "culture medium" for the dividing cells of the blastocyst. The uterine endometrium, to which the blastocyst attaches, provides for the sustenance of the embryo throughout its development. A rich food supply for the implanting blastocyst comes from the secretions of the uterine glands and from products of the uterine stroma as the blastocyst burrows into the endometrium. These products are absorbed by the syncytial trophoblast and diffuse to the developing embryo. As the trophoblast continues to erode into the endometrium, blood-filled spaces form and the blastocyst is bathed by pools of maternal blood that supply the embryo with nourishment. When a placenta has been established, the nutritional, respiratory, and excretory needs of the embryo are met by this fetal-maternal membrane. The placenta also has protective functions, preventing passage of particulate matter to the embryo. It also has endocrine functions, elaborating gonadotropins, estrogens, and progesterone. Gonadotropins are produced very early and maintain the corpus luteum during early pregnancy.

The basal layer of the myometrium is not shed at parturition or at menstruation and provides for the restoration of the uterine mucosa after these events have occurred. The myometrium, by its muscular contractions, expels the fetus at birth.

Changes in the secretory activities of cervical glands during the menstrual cycle may have some significance in fertility. During most of the cycle, the glands produce a thick, viscous mucus that appears to inhibit passage of sperm. The thin, less viscid mucus elaborated at midcycle appears to favor the migration of sperm.

Clinical Correlations

The ovary is especially subject to formation of cysts derived from ovarian follicles. Follicular cysts arise from mature follicles and appear as multiple, small cysts filled with a clear watery fluid. The cysts are lined by one or more layers of cuboidal or columnar epithelium, the remnants of the stratum granulosum of a mature follicle. Corpus luteum cysts usually are single and are formed by hemorrhage or exudation into corpora lutea. The fibrous wall may lack a distinct lining, or granulosa lutein cells may form a thick yellowish layer, especially at one area. The cells are large and rounded and contain much lipid and yellow pigment. Theca lutein cysts usually are small and multiple, causing enlarged cystic ovaries. They arise from granulosa cells of atretic follicles that have come under the influence of gonadotropin.

Benign cystic tumors include mucinous and serous (papillary) cystadenomas. The mucinous type is the more frequent and forms a rounded, usually single mass filled with thick, viscous fluid. The cyst is lined by a single layer of tall, nonciliated columnar cells that show a clear cytoplasm. The lining is thrown into folds and may form papillary ingrowths. The serous type often appears single, but small secondary cysts frequently occur within the capsule. The cyst is lined by low columnar epithelium, and papillary growth is characteristic, often to such an extent that the cyst cavity is nearly filled. True carcinoma develops more frequently in serous than mucous cysts. The origin of the cystic tumors is uncertain, but they may arise from surface epithelium that has invaginated into the ovarian stroma during adult life.

Endometriosis is the presence of functioning endometrial tissue in sites other than the uterine mucosa. Ectopic endometrium may occur in the vagina, ovaries, uterosacral ligament, peritoneum, and, less commonly, the appendix, ileum, or rectum. The extrauterine tissue appears as small cysts that contain thick, black, tarry material derived from cyclic episodes of bleeding. The cysts are lined by endometrium. After menopause, the cysts usually atrophy.

The most common uterine tumor is the leiomyoma, a benign tumor of the myometrium. Interlacing bundles of smooth muscle cells run in every direction, producing a whorled pattern. Fibrous tissue may become plentiful and make up a large part of the tumor, hence the alternate name *fibroid.* Rarely does a leiomyoma become malignant, but the tumors are space-occupying lesions, can become quite large, and may physically interfere with pregnancy and the normal functioning of the uterus.

Cervical erosion is a term given to reddened areas around the external uterine os, extending onto the exocervix. It may represent actual replacement of the normal squamous epithelium or an unusual junctional site of exocervix and cervical canal. The exposed columnar epithelium is more prone to injury and infection than is stratified squamous epithelium.

Most of the invasive carcinomas of the cervix arise in the area of the squamocolumnar junction and appear as irregular ulcerations and indurations of one lip of the cervix, followed by the appearance of an irregular, infected growth with a nodular surface. The tumor may appear well-differentiated, with sheets and cords of cells often variably keratinized — an aberrant form of differentiation since normal cervical epithelium does not keratinize. Adenocarcinomas arise from the columnar epithelium of the endocervical canal and glands.

Hydatidiform mole is a benign tumor of the placenta. The terminal chorionic villi enlarge and form discrete, grapelike masses that consist of edematous, mucoid connective tissue. As the chorionic epithelium proliferates, the cytotrophoblast becomes several layers thick and the syncytiotrophoblast also becomes prominent. There usually is no trace of a fetus, and the mole consists entirely of altered villi. Although the fetus dies early, abortion does not occur. Trophoblastic epithelium may become malignant, giving rise to the rare choriocarcinoma, a very invasive tumor that erodes into and may penetrate the uterine wall, spreading early and widely. Hydatidiform mole and choriocarcinoma secrete large amounts of chorionic gonadotropin and commonly are associated with theca-lutein cysts in the ovary.

Cytodiagnosis

The presence of granular leukocytes in vaginal smears usually indicates an infection, but granulocytes also are present in large numbers during the late proliferative and menstrual phases of the normal menstrual cycle. Thus, the significance of leukocytes in vagino-cervical smears often depends on the physiologic status. Lymphocytes generally indicate a chronic inflammation and are numerous in chronic cervicitis.

Cancer of the cervix can be detected by examination of vagino-cervical smears. The abnormal cells in invasive cancer appear smaller than normal squames and show much wider variation in size and shape. Elongated, irregular, or tailed forms may be seen. The most reliable changes are referable to the nuclei and include increase in the nuclear/cytoplasmic ratio, enhanced staining, thickening of the nuclear envelope, change in chromatin pattern characterized by irregular distribution of heterochromatin, and irregularities in shape. Prominent nucleoli are associated with malignant change but not all malignant cells reveal nucleoli.

There is no one, single cytologic feature that will invariably identify tumor cells. All of the cytologic changes seen in cancer can be found at one time or another in other, noncancerous conditions and even in normal individuals. However, a neoplastic process is indicated by the multiplicity of the changes occurring in a large number of cells, and cytodiagnosis can be a valuable and precise screening method.

Mammary Glands

Mammary glands are present in both sexes but in males remain rudimentary throughout life. In the female, the size, shape, and structure vary with age and functional status. Prior to puberty, the female breasts are undeveloped but enlarge rapidly at puberty due mainly to accumulation of adipose tissue. They reach their greatest development at late pregnancy and lactation. In the adult female, the mammary glands are variably hemispherical and conical in shape, each surmounted by a cylindrical projection, the nipple. Surrounding the nipple is a slightly raised, circular area of pigment, the areola.

The mammary gland is a compound tubuloalveolar gland and is considered to be of cutaneous origin, representing a modified apocrine sweat gland.

Structure of the Resting Gland

KEY WORDS: duct, simple cuboidal epithelium, lactiferous sinus, stratified cuboidal epithelium, stratified squamous epithelium, alveolus, myoepithelial cell

Each mammary gland consists of 15 to 20 individual pyramid-shaped lobes that radiate from a nipple. The lobes are separated by septa of dense connective tissue. Each lobe represents an individual gland and contains glandular tissue drained by its own ductal components, embedded in the intralobular connective tissue. The proportions of glandular and nonglandular tissue vary with functional status.

In the resting gland, the principal glandular elements are the **ducts,** which are grouped together to form lobules (see atlas figure 18-30). The smallest branches of the ductal system are lined by **simple cuboidal epithelium,** but the lining increases in height as the ducts unite and pass toward the nipple. Just beneath the areola, the ducts expand to form the **lactiferous sinuses,** which are lined by a two-layered **stratified cuboidal epithelium.** As the duct ascends through the nipple, it becomes lined by **stratified squamous epithelium.**

Secretory units consist of clusters of **alveoli** surrounding a small duct. The alveolar wall consists of simple cuboidal epithelium resting on a basement membrane. Between the epithelial cells and the basement membrane are highly branched **myoepithelial cells** whose long, slender processes embrace the alveolus in a basketlike network. Alveoli are not prominent in the resting gland, and there is some question as to whether they are present at all. When present, they usually occur as small, budlike extensions of the terminal ducts.

The intralobular connective tissue around the ductules and alveoli is loosely arranged and cellular, whereas that surrounding the larger ducts and lobes (interlobular connective tissue) is variably dense and contains much adipose tissue.

Nipple and Areola

KEY WORDS: **keratinizing stratified squamous epithelium, lactiferous duct, smooth muscle, areolar gland**

The nipple is covered by **keratinizing stratified squamous epithelium** continuous with that of the skin overlying the breast. The dermis projects deeply into the epithelium, forming unusually tall dermal papillae. The skin of the nipple is pigmented and contains many sebaceous glands but is devoid of hair and sweat glands. The nipple is traversed by many **lactiferous ducts,** each of which drains a lobe and empties onto the tip of the nipple. The outer parts of the ducts also are lined by keratinizing stratified squamous epithelium. The dense collagenous connective tissue of the nipple contains bundles of elastic fibers, and much **smooth muscle** is present. The smooth muscle fibers are arranged circularly and radially

and on contraction, produce erection of the nipple.

The areola is the pigmented area of skin that encircles the base of the nipple. During pregnancy, the areola becomes larger and more deeply pigmented. It contains sweat, sebaceous, and **areolar glands.** The latter appear to be intermediate in structure between apocrine sweat glands and true mammary glands.

Pregnancy and Lactation

KEY WORDS: **proliferation of glandular tissue, colostrum, apocrine secretion**

During pregnancy, mammary glands undergo extensive development in preparation for their role in lactation. During the first half of pregnancy, the terminal portions of the ductal system grow rapidly, branch, and develop terminal buds that expand to become alveoli (see atlas figure 18-31). **Proliferation of glandular tissue** takes place at the expense of the fat and stromal connective tissue, which decrease in amount. The connective tissue becomes infiltrated with lymphocytes, plasma cells, and granular leukocytes. During late pregnancy, proliferation of glandular tissue subsides, but the alveoli expand and there is some formation of secretory materials. The first secretion, **colostrum,** is thin and watery. It is poor in lipid but contains a considerable amount of antibodies that may give some degree of passive immunity to the newborn.

True milk secretion begins a few days after parturition, but not all the breast tissue is functioning at the same time. In some areas, alveoli are distended with milk, the epithelial lining is flattened, and the lumen is distended; in other areas, the alveoli are resting and are lined by tall columnar epithelial cells (see atlas figures 18-32 and 18-33). Secreting cells have abundant granular endoplasmic reticulum, moderate numbers of relatively large mitochondria, and supranuclear Golgi complexes. Milk proteins are elaborated by the granular endoplasmic reticulum and in association with the Golgi body form membrane-bound vesicles. These are carried to the apex of the cell, where the contents are released by exocytosis. Lipid arises as cytoplasmic droplets that coalesce to form large spherical globules. The droplets and globules, apparently with portions of the plasmalemma and apical cytoplasm, are cast off into the lumen. This method of release is a form of **apocrine secretion,** but only minute amounts of cytoplasm are lost. Passage of milk from alveoli into and along the ducts is due to contraction of the myoepithelial cells.

With weaning, lactation soon ceases and the glandular tissue returns to its resting state. However, regression is never complete and not all of the alveoli completely disappear.

Hormonal Control

KEY WORDS: estrogen, progesterone, somatotropin, prolactin, adrenal corticoid, neurohormonal reflex, oxytocin

Before puberty, growth of the mammary gland parallels general body growth, but as the ovaries become functional, the mammary tissue comes under the influence of estrogen and progesterone. While some structural changes can be observed, the cyclic response of the breast is minor. During pregnancy, the glands are continuously stimulated by **estrogen** and **progesterone** from the corupus luteum and placenta. Generally, growth of the ductal system depends on estrogen, but for alveolar development, both progesterone and estrogen are required. To attain the full development in pregnancy, other hormones — **somatotropin, prolactin,** and **adrenal corticoids** — appear to be necessary.

At the end of pregnancy, the levels of circulating estrogen and progesterone fall abruptly, and increased output of prolactin by the hypophysis results in the secretion of milk. Maintenance of lactation requires continuous secretion of prolactin, which results from a **neurohormonal reflex** established by suckling. Periodic suckling also causes release of **oxytocin** from the neurohypophysis, which stimulates contraction of myoepithelial cells, resulting in release of milk from alveoli into and along the ducts.

Development of Mammary Glands

Mammary glands represent modified apocrine sweat glands and are derived from ectodermal outgrowths. Primordia of mammary glands arise as two ventral bands of ectoderm, the mammary ridges, that extend from axilla to the inguinal region. In the human female, a single pair of glands develops in the pectoral region, and the remainder of the mammary ridges usually disappear. As the gland develops, 15 to 20 solid buds of ectoderm invade the underlying mesenchyme. Each bud will form the branching lactiferous ducts of one mammary lobule. The ducts are lined by columnar epithelial cells, and myoepithelial cells can be distinguished early. Alveoli do not develop until puberty and even then are small and scarce. Further expansion of the ductal system occurs during pregnancy and some alveoli form, but they reach their greatest development during lactation. The surrounding mesenchyme forms the supporting connective tissue and at puberty becomes infiltrated with fat cells.

Functional Summary

The mammary glands provide nourishment for the newborn, which is delivered in an immature and dependent state. The first secretion, colostrum, has a high content of antibodies and may give passive immunity to the suckling young. Passage of milk from the alveoli to and along ducts is accomplished by contraction of myoepithelial cells under the influence of the hormone oxytocin.

Clinical Correlations

Infections of the breast are called mastitis and may be acute or chronic. Most occur via the ducts and through abrasions of the nipple and often are associated with lactation.

Mammary duct ectasia is marked by progressive dilatation of ducts, beginning in the lactiferous sinus and extending to the lactiferous duct. The walls of the dilated duct are thickened and surrounded by infiltrating lymphocytes and plasma cells. Chronic low-grade infection of the distended ducts may lead to accumulation of macrophages and giant cells. Increase in interlobular connective tissue (fibrosis) may occur and cause retraction of the nipple.

In fibrocystic disease, the breast contains numerous firm nodules but overall is not enlarged, and clusters of small cysts may be present. The connective tissue is dense but often is not increased in amount. The cysts are due to local distentions of ducts and alveoli, and some may contain papilla-like spurs of epithelium. The lining cells usually are cuboidal or flattened, but several layers of cells may form and fill the cyst. Some cysts are lined by large cuboidal cells with eosinophilic cytoplasm and resemble the cells of apocrine sweat glands.

Several types of carcinomas have been described but all are manifestations of one disease process. Scirrhous carcinoma is the most common form of breast cancer, forming a hard nodular tumor that consists of groups and thin columns of spheroidal cells separated by dense collagenous stroma. The tumor becomes adherent to the skin, causing shrinking of the breast, distortion or retraction of the nipple, and puckering of the skin. Encephaloid (medullary) carcinoma forms a soft "brainlike" tumor of relatively rapid growth. Masses of spherical tumor cells, many showing aberrant mitoses, are separated by scanty stroma.

Key Features of Structures Contained Within the Ovary

	Ovum	Cells of Wall	Other
Primordial follicle	Dominates follicle; nucleus large, central, and vesicular; prominent nucleolus	Unilaminar layer of flattened follicular cells	
Primary follicle	Large with central vesicular nucleus; zona pellucida may be visible	Two or more layers of granulosa cells; cuboidal in shape	Surrounding stroma organized into theca interna and externa
Secondary follicle	Ovum with large vesicular nucleus; zona pellucida prominent	Stratum granulosum 8 to 12 layers thick; large spaces between cells; formation of antrum	Well defined theca interna and externa
Mature follicle	Ovum eccentric in large follicle located near surface of ovary	Cells organized into cumulus oophorus and corona radiata; very large antrum	Well defined theca interna and externa; cells of theca interna plump
Atretic follicle	May or may not be present — shows signs of degeneration	Show degenerative changes; macrophages usually present; connective tissue infiltration	Cells of theca interna show degenerative changes; appearance of glassy membrane
Corpus luteum	Absent	Prominent granulosa lutein cells; smaller theca lutein cells	
Corpus albicans	Absent	Thin, dark staining nuclei of fibroblasts	Large bundles of thin collagen fibers; hyaline material

Atlas and Table of Key Features

Key Features of the Female Reproductive Tract

	Epithelial Lining	Support	Muscle
Oviduct	Simple columnar; ciliated and nonciliated cells	Lamina propria, cellular, thin collagen, and reticular fibers	Well-defined inner circular smooth muscle; outer layer of scattered longitudinal fibers
Uterus	Simple columnar with groups of ciliated cells; extends into lamina propria to form tubular glands	Lamina propria = endometrial stroma, similar to mesenchyme; richly cellular, fine reticular fibers, few collagen fibers. *Note:* The oviduct and uterus are the only hollow organs with this type of lamina propria	Myometrium; thick coat of smooth muscle in 3 intermingling layers
Cervix	1. Tall columnar; some ciliated, some mucus-secreting cells 2. Vaginal part covered by nonkeratinized stratified squamous	Dense collagenous and elastic connective tissue	Smooth muscle much reduced in amount, lacking in vaginal part
Vagina	Stratified squamous nonkeratinized epithelium	Lamina propria of dense collagenous connective tissue. Dense elastic network below epithelial layer	Inner circular smooth muscle, outer longitudinal smooth muscle

Ovary

Primordial follicle

Follicular cell

Nucleus of primary oocyte

Surface mesothelium of ovary

Tunica albuginea

Fig. 18-4. A region of ovarian cortex illustrating the surface mesothelium and the tunica albuginea. (LM, ×250.)

Primordial follicle

Granulosa cells

Primary follicle

Oocyte

Zona pellucida

Ovarian stroma

Fig. 18-5. Follicles within the ovarian cortex. (LM, ×250.)

Theca externa

Mitotic figure

Granulosa cells

Nucleus of oocyte

Zona pellucida

Fig. 18-6. Components of a primary ovarian follicle. (LM, ×250.)

Theca interna

Granulosa cells

Cumulus oophorous

Zona pellucida

Corpus albicans

Corona radiata

Theca externa

Antrum of follicle

Fig. 18-7. Components of a secondary ovarian follicle. (LM, ×100.)

Granulosa lutein cells

External surface of ovary

Theca lutein cells

Corpus luteum

Theca lutein cells

Loose connective tissue

Fig. 18-8. A human corpus luteum. (LM, ×25.)

Granulosa lutein cells

Theca lutein cells

Lumen of venule

Fig. 18-9. Granulosa lutein and theca lutein cells of a human corpus luteum. (LM, ×100.)

Primordial
follicles

Corpus
albicans

Primary
follicle

Corpus
albicans

Fig. 18-10. A region of ovarian cortex showing follicles as well as two corpus albicans. (LM, ×100.)

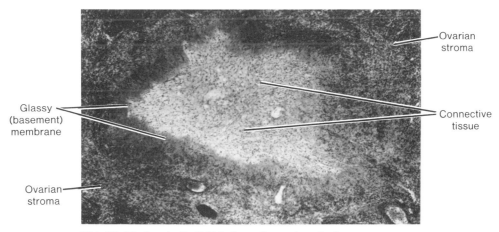

Ovarian
stroma

Glassy
(basement)
membrane

Connective
tissue

Ovarian
stroma

Fig. 18-11. An atretic follicle from the cortex of a human ovary. (LM, ×40.)

Oviduct

Lumen

Fimbria

Fig. 18-12. The infundibulum of a human oviduct. (LM, ×40.)

Ciliated cells

Nonciliated cells

Fig. 18-13. Apices of ciliated cells lining the mucosal surface of the oviduct. (SEM, ×2,000.)

Inner circular layer

Outer longitudinal layer

Muscularis

Fig. 18-14. The ampulla of the oviduct. Note the smooth muscle layers forming the muscularis. (LM, ×100.)

Lamina propria

Lamina propria

Ciliated epithelial cells

Fig. 18-15. The ciliated simple columnar epithelium lining the ampullary region of the oviduct. Note the ciliated epithelial cells and compare to those shown in 18-13. (LM, ×250.)

Uterus

Lumen of uterus

Simple columnar epithelium

Uterine gland

Stroma

Fig. 18-16. A section of human endometrium showing the lining epithelium, a uterine gland, and numerous stromal cells. (LM, ×100.)

Endometrial stroma

Uterine glands

Spiral arteries

Bundles of smooth muscle

Fig. 18-17. The stratum basale of human endometrium. Note the spiral arteries. (LM, ×100.)

Fig. 18-18. Stromal cells of the endometrium from a pregnant woman. (LM, ×250.)

Vagina

Fig. 18-19. The mucosal surface of the vagina showing numerous rugae. (SEM, ×50.)

Fig. 18-20. Surface cells lining the mucosa of the vagina. (SEM, ×1,000.)

Fig. 18-21. The mucosal lining of the vagina. Note the surface cells and compare to 18-20. (LM, ×250.)

Development
Zygote

Fig. 18-22. A pig zygote at the two-cell stage. Note the heads of spermatozoa embedded in the surrounding zona pellucida. (LM, ×300.)

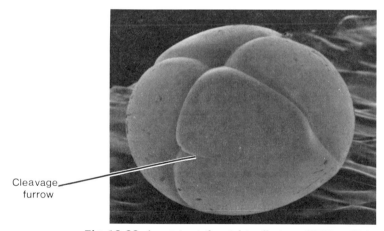

Cleavage furrow

Fig. 18-23. A zygote at the eight-cell stage. (SEM, ×50.)

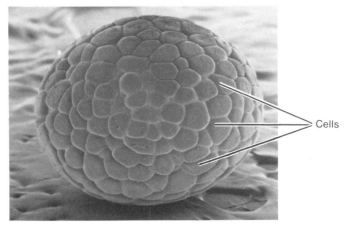

Fig. 18-24. A zygote formed by many cells. (SEM, ×50.)

Embryos

Fig. 18-25. A nine-day opossum embryo. (LM, ×100.)

Pharyngeal arches

Developing eye

External nares

Heart

Forelimb (limb bud stage)

Fig. 18-26. The head region of a 9-mm pig embryo. (SEM, ×20.)

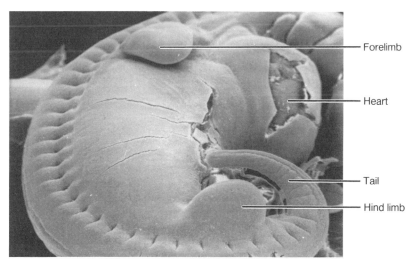

Forelimb

Heart

Tail

Hind limb

Fig. 18-27. The caudal region of a 9-mm pig embryo. Note the position of the heart and the limb buds. (SEM, ×20.)

Placenta

Syncytial trophoblast

Cytotrophoblast

Nucleated erythrocytes

Fig. 18-28. Human placenta at the third week of gestation showing syncytial trophoblast and cytotrophoblast layers. (LM, ×250.)

Syncytial trophoblast

Fetal erythrocytes in capillary

Placental villus

Maternal erythrocytes

Fig. 18-29. Human placenta at the sixth month of gestation. Note that only the syncytial trophoblast remains covering placental villi. (LM, ×250.)

Mammary Gland

Lobule —

Duct —

Connective
tissue —

Fig. 18-30. A lobule from an inactive human mammary gland.
(LM, ×100.)

Interlobular
duct —

— Developing
alveoli

Fig. 18-31. A lobule from a mammary gland in a pregnant
woman (compare with 18-30). (LM, ×40.)

Interlobular duct

Alveoli

Fig. 18-32. A portion of a lobule from a lactating human mammary gland. Note the abundant alveoli. Compare with 18-30 and 18-31. (LM, ×100.)

Alveoli

Fig. 18-33. Increased magnification of alveoli from a lactating human mammary gland. (LM, ×250.)

Ovary

Fig. 18-34. Developing ovary and adjacent resorbing mesonephros. Note the development of the müllerian duct. (LM,
×200.)

Fig. 18-35. Gonadal cords in the primary cortex of the developing
ovary. (LM, ×250.)

Fig. 18-36. Surface epithelium and gonadal cords from a developing ovary. (LM, ×400.)

Review Questions and Answers

Questions

93. What is the appearance of the ovarian follicle at the time of ovulation? Describe the ovum immediately after ovulation.
94. Describe the endometrium during the proliferative and secretory phases and relate the events to the ovarian cycle.
95. What parts of the placenta are derived from fetal components and what parts from maternal components?
96. Outline the nutritional supply to a newly developing organism from fertilization to birth.
97. What changes occur in the mammary gland as the result of pregnancy? How is lactation maintained?

Answers

93. At the time of ovulation, the ovum is contained within a mature or graafian follicle, which occupies the thickness of the cortex and bulges from the surface of the ovary. The ovum becomes loosened from its attachment to the cumulus oophorus as fluid-filled spaces appear between the granulosa cells of the cumulus. The cells of the theca interna have assumed the characteristics of an endocrine gland and secret androgens, which are converted to estrogens by aromatase enzymes of the granulosa cells. At the point where the follicle bulges from the ovary, its wall thins and the stigma, a small avascular, translucent area, appears and protrudes as a small blister.

    With rupture of the stigma, ovulation occurs. The ovum has completed the first meiotic division and so a secondary oocyte is released, complete with its corona radiata and zona pellucida.
94. During the proliferative stage, the epithelial cells of the glandular remnants in the stratum basale proliferate rapidly and migrate to cover the denuded mucosal surface. The stromal cells also proliferate and the endometrium increases in thickness. These events are stimulated by estrogens elaborated by the developing follicles. In the secretory phase, the glandular elements elongate, become tortuous and coiled, and begin to secrete. Stromal edema and an increase in the vascularity of the endometrium also occur. The secretory phase is associated with the production of large amounts of progesterone by the corpus luteum.
95. The fetal components of the mature placenta consist of the chorionic plate (established from mesoderm of the embryo) and its villi. The maternal component consists of the decidua basalis, the superficial part of the endometrium that lies beneath the implantation site.
96. In the oviduct, the nutrition for the dividing zygote is derived from the cytoplasm of the ovum. Within the uterine cavity and prior to implantation, the blastocyst lies within the secretions of the endometrium, which are rich in glycogen, polysaccharides, and lipids. As the blastocyst implants in the endometrium it encounters a rich food supply in the glandular secretions and products of the breakdown of the uterine stroma. Later in the process of implantation, the blastocyst becomes surrounded by blood-filled spaces in the endometrium that supply the nutritional needs. When the placenta has been fully established, the nutritional needs of the embryo are met by diffusion of materials between the closely related maternal and fetal circulations.
97. During the first half of pregnancy the terminal portions of the ducts branch and de-

velop terminal buds that will become the secretory alveoli. In later pregnancy the glandular portions increase in size and some slight secretion occurs. Growth of the ducts depends on stimulation by estrogens; development of the alveoli requires proges- terone, estrogen, and other hormones. Lac- tation is maintained by a neurohormonal reflex established by suckling; prolactin and oxytocin are released by the pituitary, resulting in milk secretion and release.

19 Endocrine Glands

Endocrine glands lack ducts, and their secretory products (hormones) generally pass into the blood or lymphatic circulation. However, hormones also may be secreted directly into the intercellular space (paracrine secretion) to elicit a local effect on adjacent cells. In some instances cells may secrete a chemical messenger that acts on its own receptors and is self-regulatory (autocrine secretion). Hormones that are secreted into the vascular system eventually enter the tissue fluids and, depending on the specificity of the hormone, can alter the activities of just one organ or influence several. The organs that respond to a specific hormone are the target organs of that hormone. Hormones may be biogenic amines, steroids, polypeptides, proteins, or glycoproteins, depending on their gland of origin.

In some glands, such as the liver, the epithelial cells have exocrine and endocrine functions. Hepatocytes fulfill the definition of endocrine cells since they release glucose, proteins, and other substances directly into the hepatic sinusoids, but the same hepatocytes also secrete bile into adjacent canaliculi (the beginnings of the liver duct system) and thus are exocrine cells also. The pancreas, kidney, testis, and ovary are mixtures of endocrine and exocrine components in which separate or isolated groups of cells secrete directly into the vasculature and form the endocrine portion. The rest of the gland makes up the exocrine portion that usually is drained by ducts. The placenta is a unique, temporary endocrine gland that persists only for about nine months in the pregnant human female. The brain and heart also have aspects of endocrine organs.

What are termed *classic endocrine glands* consist of discrete masses of cells with a relatively simple organization into clumps, cords, or plates supported by a delicate vascular connective tissue. Endocrine glands have a rich vascular supply, and the secreting cells have direct access to capillaries. The classic endocrine system consists, in part, of pineal, parathyroid, thyroid, adrenal, and pituitary glands.

A vast system of unicellular endocrine cells (glands) also exists, and collectively these cells form a diffuse endocrine system. It is represented by scattered unicellular glands that often lie at some distance from one another, separated by cells of a different type. These cells are present through much of the gastrointestinal tract, in the ducts of the major digestive glands, and in the conducting airways of the lungs. When the cells of this system are considered collectively, they form a mass larger than many of the individual organs of the classic endocrine system.

Pineal Gland

The human pineal gland is a somewhat flattened body 5 to 8 mm long and 3 to 5 mm wide. It is attached to the brain (roof of the diencephalon) by a short stalk that contains some nerve fibers and their supportive elements.

671

Structure

KEY WORDS: pinealocyte, glial cell, corpora arenacea (brain sand), melatonin, serotonin

The pineal is covered by a thin connective tissue capsule that is continuous with the surrounding meningeal (pial) tissue. Richly vascularized and innervated septa extend into the parenchyma of the gland and subdivide it into poorly defined lobules (see atlas figure 19-13). Two types of cells, pinealocytes and glial cells, are present and form clumps and cords.

Pinealocytes have relatively large lobulated nuclei. Long cytoplasmic processes often radiate from the cell body to form club-shaped endings near adjacent perivascular spaces or pinealocytes. Small, membrane-bound vesicles, some with electron-dense cores, are present in the swollen ends of the processes. Synaptic ribbons may be present also. Nearer the cell body, the cytoplasm contains abundant, fairly large mitochondria, numerous free ribosomes, profiles of smooth endoplasmic reticulum, lipid droplets, lipochrome pigment, lysosomes, and large numbers of microtubules and intermediate filaments. Numerous gap junctions link groups of pinealocytes electrically and metabolically. Although light and dark forms have been described, it is unknown whether each forms a distinct cell type or whether they represent differences in the activity of a single cell type.

Glial cells form an interwoven network within and around the parenchymal cords and clumps of the pineal gland. They are fewer in number than pinealocytes, and their nuclei are smaller and stain more deeply. Glial cells show long cytoplasmic processes and often are regarded as a form of astrocyte. The cytoplasm contains many fine filaments, 5 to 6 nm in diameter, which may form large bundles.

Corpora arenacea (brain sand) are concretions found in the pineal gland of humans and some animals such as ungulates. These irregularly shaped structures occur in the capsule and substance of the gland. They consist mainly of calcium carbonates and phosphates within an organic matrix. In humans they increase with age, but their significance is unknown.

The mammalian pineal gland has an extensive blood supply and is provided with many postganglionic sympathetic nerve fibers from neurons in the superior cervical ganglia.

The pineal gland produces **melatonin,** an indolamine, which in some amphibians causes blanching of melanophores. In mammals such as the rat, pinealocytes synthesize **serotonin,** a precursor of melatonin that varies cyclically (circadian and seasonal) in amount and changes in relation to the amount of light. Serotonin levels fall and melatonin levels rise during darkness. These circadian rhythms are controlled by the release of norepinephrine from the sympathetic fibers that enter the pineal from the superior cervical ganglia, which in turn is controlled by the light perceived by the retina. In some rodents and birds the pineal, through secretion of melatonin, plays an active role in the reproductive cycles, which are influenced by the length of daylight (photoperiod). The pineal in these species acts as a neuroendocrine organ, influencing the gonads in response to light. The function of melatonin in humans, however, is unknown. Pineal-specific peptides such as arginine vasotocin are thought to influence or mediate hypophyseal function, but their exact role is uncertain.

Parathyroid Glands

The parathyroid glands are small, brownish, oval bodies 4 to 8 mm long and 2 to 5 mm wide. There usually are four in humans, but as many as six or more may lie within the capsule of the thyroid gland or may be embedded in the substance of the middle third of the thyroid. In about 8 percent of the human population, additional parathyroid tissue is present in the thymus, the association being due to the common developmental origin of these structures from the third pharyngeal pouch. Parathyroid glands are present in all mammals and most vertebrates except for fishes and gill-bearing amphibians.

Structure

KEY WORDS: chief (principal) cell, oxyphil cell, parathyroid hormone

Each parathyroid gland is surrounded by a thin connective tissue capsule and is subdivided by delicate trabeculae that extend from the capsule. Blood vessels, lymphatics, and nerves course through the trabeculae to enter the substance of the parathyroid. In older persons fat cells often are abundant and may form about 50 percent of the gland. The parenchyma consists of closely packed groups or cords of epithelial cells supported by a delicate framework of reticular fibers that contains nerve fibers and a rich capillary network.

The parenchyma contains two types of cells. **Chief (principal) cells** are the more numerous and measure 8 to 10 μm in diameter. They have round, centrally placed, vesicular nuclei, and the cytoplasm contains the usual organelles as well as large accumulations of glycogen and lipid droplets. In addition to small, dense, membrane-bound granules, lipofuscin granules often are present also.

Oxyphil cells form only a small part of the cell population and may occur singly or in groups (see atlas figure 19-19). This type of cell has been reported only in humans, macaque monkeys, and cattle. It is not present in significant numbers until puberty, then increases with age. Oxyphil cells are larger than chief cells, and their cytoplasm stains intensely with eosin and is packed with large, elongated mitochondria that show numerous cristae. Between the mitochondria are small accumulations of glycogen and occasional profiles of granular endoplasmic reticulum. The small nuclei stain deeply and often appear pyknotic.

Numerous cells that are intermediate in appearance between chief and oxyphil cells also have been described. Chief cells may be the primary parenchymal element of the parathyroid gland, and other cell types (such as the oxyphil and intermediate cells) may represent a modification or a stage of development of the chief cell.

The parathyroid secretes **parathyroid hormone** (PTH), a polypeptide hormone that regulates the calcium level of the blood. Nearly half the blood calcium is bound; the remainder is present as free ions. It is the concentration of calcium ion that governs the secretion of parathyroid hormone. If the concentration drops below normal, the hormone is secreted and acts directly on osteoclasts and osteocytes to mobilize calcium ion from bone and on the renal tubules to promote absorption of calcium ion and inhibit absorption of phosphate ion from the glomerular filtrate. Parathyroid hormone also promotes synthesis and release of 1,25-vitamin D_3 by the proximal convuluted tubules of the kidney. This form of vitamin D_3 increases calcium absorption in the small intestine. Increase in the concentration of calcium ion in the blood results in a decrease in the amount of PTH released. Blood levels of calcium are kept from exceeding the optimum by a second calcium-regulating hormone, calcitonin, produced by the parafollicular cells of the thyroid gland.

Parathyroid hormone is essential for life. Complete removal of the parathyroid glands results in a precipitous drop in blood calcium followed by tetany and death.

Thyroid Gland

The thyroid gland normally weighs between 25 and 40 g in humans and is located in the anterior of the neck, below the cricoid cartilage. It consists of two lateral lobes and an isthmus that forms a narrow bridge across the trachea between the two lobes.

Structure

KEY WORDS: follicle, colloid, principal (follicular) cell, colloid resorption droplet, thyroglobulin, triiodothyronine, tetraiodothyronine (thyroxin), binding protein, parafollicular cell (light cell, C cell), calcitonin (thyrocalcitonin)

The parenchyma of the thyroid gland is enclosed in a connective tissue capsule and organized into spherical structures, the **follicles,** which vary considerably in diameter and contain a gelatinous material called **colloid** (see atlas figures 19-14 and 19-15). The walls of the follicles consist of a simple epithelium that rests on a thin basal lamina, about 50 nm thick. Each follicle is supported by a delicate reticular network that contains a vast capillary plexus, numerous nerve fibers, and blindly ending lymphatic vessels.

The follicular epithelium consists mainly of **principal (follicular) cells,** which usually are squamous to cuboidal in shape; depending on the functional status of the thyroid, the cells may become columnar. The nuclei are spherical, contain one or more nucleoli, and have a central position. The lateral cell membranes are united at the apex by junctional complexes, and the luminal surfaces bear short microvilli. The basal plasmalemma is smooth, with no infoldings. Mitochondria are evenly distributed throughout the cytoplasm and vary in number according to the activity of the cell. Active cells take on a cuboidal shape and show many profiles of granular endoplasmic reticulum. Inactive cells are squamous and granular endoplasmic reticulum is sparse. Golgi complexes usually have a supranuclear location in active cells, and the apical cytoplasm contains numerous small vesicles, lysosomes, and multivesicular bodies. **Colloid resorption droplets** also are found in the apical cytoplasm (see atlas figures 19-15 and 19-16).

The thyroid is a unique endocrine gland in that the secretory product, colloid, is stored extracellulary in the lumen of the follicle. Colloid consists of mucoproteins, proteolytic enzymes, and a glycoprotein called **thyroglobulin,** the primary storage form of thyroid hormone. Synthesis of thyroglobulin occurs in the principal cells along the same basic intracellular pathway as glycoprotein in cells elsewhere in the body. Amino acids are synthesized into polypeptides in the granular endoplasmic reticulum and then carried in transport vesicles to the Golgi complex, where the carbohydrate moiety is conjugated to the protein. From the Golgi complex, the glycoprotein (noniodinated thyroglobulin) is transported to the apical surface in small vesicles, from which it is discharged by exocytosis into the follicular lumen and stored as part of the colloid.

While thyroglobulin is being synthesized, thyroperoxidase is assembled in the granular endoplasmic reticulum, then passes through the Golgi complex and is released by small vesicles at the apical surface of the cells. Follicular cells have a unique ability to take up iodine from the blood and concentrate it. The iodine subsequently is oxidized to iodide by intracellular peroxidase and used in the iodination of tyrosine groups in thyroglobulin. Formation of monoiodotyrosine and diiodotyrosine is thought to occur in the follicle, immediately adjacent to the microvillus border of the follicular cells. When one molecule of monoiodotyrosine is linked to one of diiodotyrosine, a molecule of **triiodothyronine** is formed. Coupling of two molecules of diiodotyrosine results in the formation of **tetraiodothyronine (thyroxin).** The thyronines make up a small part of the thyroglobulin complex but represent the only constituents with hormonal activity. Thyroglobulin and the thyronines are stored in the lumen of the follicle until needed.

When thyroid hormone is required, droplets of colloid are sequestered from the follicular lumen by endocytosis and enter the apical cytoplasm of the follicular cells. Lysosomes coalesce with the vacuoles and hydrolyse the contained thyroglobulin, liberating mono-, di-, tri-, and tetraiodothyronine into the cytoplasmic matrix. The mono- and diiodotyrosines are deiodinated and the iodine is reused by the cell. Thyroxin and triiodothyronine molecules are the thyroid hormone and are released at the base of the cell into blood and lymphatic capillaries. Thyroxin is transported in the blood plasma complexed to a binding protein. Triiodothyronine, which hormonally is the more potent of the two but is not as abundant, is not as firmly bound to the protein.

Synthesis of thyroid hormone is shown in Figure 19-1.

Binding protein is important in regulating the amount of free hormone that circulates in the blood plasma. Thyroxin and triiodothyronine are released from the binding protein only in response to metabolic needs, thus preventing rapid fluctuations in the levels of these hormones. As they are released and elicit their effects, the hor-

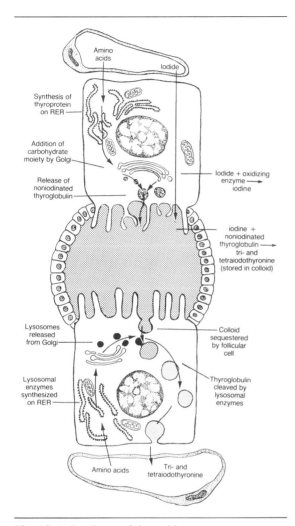

Amino
acids
Iodide

Synthesis of
thyroprotein
on RER

Addition of
carbohydrate
moiety by Golgi

Release of
noniodinated
thyroglobulin

Iodide + oxidizing
enzyme ──→
iodine

iodine +
noniodinated
thyroglobulin ──→
tri- and
tetraiodothyronine
(stored in colloid)

Lysosomes
released
from Golgi

Colloid
sequestered
by follicular
cell

Lysosomal
enzymes
synthesized
on RER

Thyroglobulin
cleaved by
lysosomal
enzymes

Amino acids   Tri- and
tetraiodothyronine

Fig. 19-1. Synthesis of thyroid hormone.

mones are replaced by other thyroxin and triio-dothyronine molecules from the thyroid. The activity of the thyroid is regulated by a thyroid-stimulating hormone (TSH) secreted by the anterior lobe of the pituitary.

Thyroid hormone has general effects on the metabolic rate of most tissues and among its functions are influencing carbohydrate metabolism, the rate of intestinal absorption, heart rate, body growth, and mental activities.

The mammalian thyroid also contains a smaller number of cells variously called **parafollicular, light,** or **C cells,** which are present in the follicular epithelium and in the delicate connective tissue between follicles (see atlas figure 19-17). The C cells in the follicular epithelium appear to be sandwiched between follicular cells and lie immediately adjacent to the basal lamina; parafollicular cells never directly border on the lumen of the follicle. Between follicles, the cells may occur singly or in small groups. In electron micrographs, the parafollicular cells show numerous moderately dense, membrane-bound secretory granules that measure 10 to 50 nm in diameter. The cytoplasm also contains occasional profiles of granular endoplasmic reticulum, scattered mitochondria, and poorly developed Golgi complexes (see atlas figure 19-18).

Parafollicular cells secrete **calcitonin (thyrocalcitonin),** another polypeptide hormone that regulates blood calcium levels. Calcitonin lowers blood calcium by acting on osteocytes and osteoclasts to suppress resorption of calcium from bone and its release into the blood. Thus, calcitonin has an effect opposite that of PTH, serves to control the action of PTH, and helps regulate the upper levels of calcium concentration in the blood.

In fishes, amphibians, and birds, C cells form a separate epithelial mass called the ultimobranchial body, and calcitonin is secreted from this body, not the thyroid.

Adrenal Gland

The adrenal glands in humans are a pair of flattened, triangular structures with a combined weight of 1 to 2 g. One adrenal is situated at the upper pole of each kidney. The mammalian adrenal is a complex organ consisting of a cortex and medulla, each differing in function, structure, and embryonic origin. The distinct relationship of outer cortex and inner medulla is found only in mammals. In lower vertebrates such as sharks and teleost fishes, the cortex and medulla occur as separate entities; in amphibians the cortex and medulla may lie next to one another or (depending on the species) may show some intermingling of the two tissues. Islets of medullary tissue generally are scattered throughout the cortex in the adrenals of reptiles and birds.

Adrenal Cortex

KEY WORDS: zona glomerulosa, zona fasciculata, zona reticularis, mineralocorticoid, glucocorticoid

The adrenal gland is surrounded by a thick capsule of dense irregular connective tissue that contains scattered elastic fibers. In some species a few smooth muscle cells may be present also. The capsule contains a rich plexus of blood vessels — mainly small arteries — and numerous nerve fibers. Some blood vessels and nerves enter the substance of the gland in the trabeculae that extend inward from the capsule, then leave the trabeculae to enter the cortex.

The parenchyma of the adrenal cortex consists of continuous cords of secretory cells that extend from the capsule to the medulla, separated by blood sinusoids. The cortex is subdivided into three layers according to the arrangement of the cells within the cords. These layers consist of an outer zona glomerulosa, a middle zona fasciculata, and an inner zona reticularis (see atlas figure 19-20). The cytologic changes from one zone to the next are gradual.

Zona glomerulosa forms a narrow band just beneath the capsule. The columnar cells are arranged into ovoid groups or arcades and have centrally placed, spherical nuclei (see atlas figure 19-21). In electron micrographs, the cells show a well-developed smooth endoplasmic reticulum and numerous mitochondria that are evenly distributed throughout the cytoplasm. Occasional lipid droplets and scattered profiles of granular endoplasmic reticulum also are present.

Zona fasciculata forms the widest zone of the cortex and consists of long cords that usually are one or two cells thick (see atlas figure 19-21). The cords run parallel to one another, separated by sinusoids that are lined by an attenuated endothelium. The cells of zona fasciculata are larger than those of the other two zones and have a polyhedral shape, and their spherical nuclei are centrally placed; binucleate cells are common.

The cytoplasm contains numerous rounded mitochondria with tubular cristae, abundant smooth endoplasmic reticulum, and well-developed granular endoplasmic reticulum. Many lipid droplets also are present and contain neutral fat, fatty acids, and fatty acyl esters of cholesterol; these represent stored precursors for the synthesis of the steroid hormones secreted by the zona fasciculata. Short microvilli often are present on the plasmalemma adjacent to sinusoids.

Zona reticularis forms the innermost zone and is made up of a network of irregular, anastomosing cords that also are separated by sinusoids (see atlas figure 19-22). In general, the cells of this zone resemble those of zona fasciculata except that they are smaller, the cytoplasm contains fewer fat droplets, the nuclei stain more deeply, and lipofuscin granules are prominent. Light and dark forms of the cells have been described but their significance is not known.

The adrenal cortex synthesizes and secretes various steroid hormones, which generally can be placed in two broad categories: mineralocorticoids that control water and electrolyte balance and glucocorticoids that affect carbohydrate metabolism. Both are derived from cholesterol. Enzymes for the synthesis of the hormones are located mainly in the smooth endoplasmic reticulum and mitochondria of the adrenal cortical cells. The pathway involves transfer of precursor molecules and intermediate products back and forth between the two organelles. Adjacent lipid droplets provide the substrates needed for the biosynthetic processes.

The **mineralocorticoids** (aldosterone and deoxycorticosterone) are secreted mostly by zona glomerulosa. Aldosterone acts on the distal tubules of the kidney to increase the rate of sodium absorption from the glomerular filtrate and, at the same time, to increase potassium excretion. It also lowers the concentration of sodium in the secretions of sweat and salivary glands and intestinal mucosa. Aldosterone secretion is controlled primarily by the renin-angiotensin system, which is sensitive to changes in blood pressure and to the concentration of sodium and potassium in the blood plasma. The exact mechanism is unknown, but it has been suggested that the juxtaglomerular apparatus of the kidney receives signals created by decreased arterial renal blood pressure (which reduces the degree of stretch on the juxtaglomerular cells) or by a decrease in the amount of sodium detected by the macula densa. In response to the signal, juxtaglomerular cells release renin, which, together with a converting enzyme, ultimately transforms angiotensinogen to angiotensin II. The latter stimulates the zona glomerulosa to secrete aldosterone. Angiotensin II also is a vasoconstrictor and directly increases blood pressure; aldosterone increases blood pressure by increasing the sodium ion concentration. Both agents influence juxtaglomerular cells and the release of renin. Adrenocorticotropic hormone from the pituitary may have a minor role in the activity of the zona glomerulosa.

Glucocorticoids (cortisol, cortisone, and corticosterone) are secreted by zona fasciculata and zona reticularis. The hormones act mainly on the metabolism of fats, proteins, and carbohydrates, resulting in an increase in blood glucose and amino acid levels and in the movement of lipid into and out of fat cells. Cortisol also suppresses the inflammatory response and some allergic reactions. A weak androgen called dehydroepiandrosterone also is secreted by cells of the zona fasciculata and zona reticularis, although cells of the reticularis are said to be the more active in androgen secretion.

Secretion by zona fasciculata and zona reticularis is controlled by adrenocorticotropic hormone (ACTH), a polypeptide hormone secreted by the anterior pituitary. Adrenocorticotropic hormone stimulates the synthesis and release of steroids, increases blood flow through the cortex, and promotes growth of the two inner zones of the adrenal cortex. The adrenal cortex is essential for life.

Adrenal Medulla

KEY WORDS: chromaffin cell, catecholamine, epinephrine, norepinephrine

The adrenal medulla is composed of large round or polyhedral cells arranged in clumps or short cords (see atlas figures 19-20 and 19-23). These are the **chromaffin cells,** so named because they show numerous brown granules when treated with chromium salts (the chromaffin reaction). The parenchyma is supported by a framework of reticular fibers, and this stroma contains numerous capillaries, veins, and nerve fibers. Sympathetic ganglion cells are present also and may occur singly or in small groups. Chromaffin cells secrete **catecholamines.** By special histochemical means, two types of chromaffin cells have been identified, one containing **epinephrine** and the other **norepinephrine.**

Ultrastructually, chromaffin cells are characterized by numerous electron-dense granules, 100 to 300 nm in diameter, that are limited by a membrane. The granules from cells that secrete norepinephrine have intensely electron-dense cores, whereas cells that elaborate epinephrine have homogeneous, less dense secretory granules. Both cell types show profiles of granular endoplasmic reticulum, scattered mitochondria, and well-developed Golgi complexes that lie close to the nucleus.

Although not essential for life, hormones of the adrenal medulla help the organism meet stressful situations. Epinephrine increases cardiac output, elevates blood glucose, and increases the basal metabolic rate. Norepinephrine acts primarily to elevate and maintain blood pressure by causing vasoconstriction in the peripheral segments of the arterial system. Secretion of both hormones is controlled by the sympathetic nervous system.

Blood Supply

The rich plexus of small arteries in the capsule of the adrenal provides cortical arteries that enter the parenchyma of the adrenal to empty into the vast network of cortical sinusoids that surrounds the cords of epithelial cells. The attenuated endothelium of the sinusoids has numerous fenestrations and is supported only by a thin basal lamina and a delicate network of reticular fibers. The sinusoids pass through all three layers of the cortex and near the corticomedullary junction begin to merge to form large collecting veins. These drain the medulla and finally empty into a single, large suprarenal vein that drains the entire gland. The cortex has no separate venous drainage. Some arteries enter the cortex in the trabeculae and provide a direct arterial supply to the medulla. Hence, the medulla receives blood from cortical sinusoids and medullary arteries. The capillaries that surround the medullary cords also are lined by a thin, fenestrated endothelium.

In addition to their systemic effects, adrenocorticosteroids (especially glucocorticoids) may affect the adrenal medulla, and the steroid-rich blood from the cortex may influence the secretion of epinephrine or norepinephrine by the chromaffin cells. Some experimental evidence indicates that glucocorticoids induce an enzyme that converts norepinephrine to epinephrine. In lower forms such as the shark, the cortex and medulla exist as separate entities with no interconnecting blood supply, and norepinephrine is the primary catecholamine secreted by the chromaffin tissue. In mammals, where the adrenal is a composite gland, epinephrine is the major catecholamine secreted.

Paraganglia

KEY WORDS: chief cell, norepinephrine, supporting cell

Clusters of chromaffin cells enclosed in thick capsules of dense irregular connective tissue normally occur outside the adrenal medulla associated with the sympathetic nervous system. These form the paraganglia, which are highly vascularized structures that contain two types of cells: chief and supporting cells. **Chief cells** contain numerous membrane-bound, electron-dense granules that are similar to those of chromaffin cells of the adrenal medulla. They are believed to secrete **norepinephrine.** The chief cells are surrounded, in part or completely, by elongated **supporting cells** that lack secretory granules. Some paraganglia, such as aortic chromaffin bodies, are paired and quite large. Paraganglia can be important clinically if they secrete abnormally high amounts of catecholamine.

Hypophysis

The hypophysis or pituitary is a complex endocrine gland located at the base of the brain, lying in the sella turcica, a small depression in the sphenoid bone. It is attached to the hypothalamic region of the brain by a narrow stalk and has vascular and neural connections with the brain. The gland weighs about 0.5 g in the adult but is slightly heavier in females and in multiparous women may exceed 1 g in weight. Despite its small size, the pituitary gland produces several hormones that directly affect other endocrine glands and tissues.

Organization

KEY WORDS: adenohypophysis, neurohypophysis, pars distalis (anterior lobe), pars intermedia, pars tuberalis, pars nervosa, infundibular stalk, median eminence

The hypophysis consists of two major parts, an epithelial component called the **adenohypophysis** and a nervous component that forms the **neurohypophysis** (see atlas figure 19-3). The adenohypophysis is further subdivided into the **pars distalis (anterior lobe)** that lies anterior to the residual lumen of Rathke's pouch; **pars intermedia,** which forms a thin partition behind the residual lumen; and **pars tuberalis,** which is an extension of pars distalis surrounding the neural stalk (Fig. 19-2).

The neurohypophysis also contains three portions. The major part is **pars nervosa,** which lies just posterior to pars intermedia and is continuous with the **infundibular stalk** and the **median eminence** (see atlas figures 19-3 and 19-11). Pars intermedia of the adenohypophysis and the pars nervosa of the neurohypophysis often are regarded collectively as forming a posterior lobe. The hypophysis is surrounded by a thick connective tissue capsule.

Vascular Supply

KEY WORDS: superior, middle, and inferior hypophyseal arteries; common capillary bed

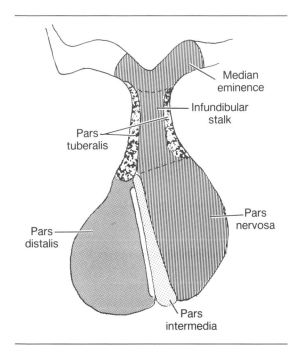

Fig. 19-2. Subdivisions of the hypophysis and their relationships.

The pituitary is supplied by three pairs of arteries: the **superior, middle,** and **inferior hypophyseal arteries,** all of which supply directly to the neurohypophysis. The middle hypophyseal artery previously was believed to traverse the parenchyma of the adenohypophysis, but other evidence has shown that it too passes directly to the neurohypophysis. Thus the adenohypophysis has no direct arterial blood supply but is linked to the neurohypophysis by a **common capillary bed** that extends throughout all three regions of the hypophysis and connects with the capillary bed of the hypothalamus. Large-bore, thin-walled veins (portal veins) also have been described and may play a role in forming a link between the capillary plexus associated with the median eminence and infundibular stalk and that of the pars distalis.

Venous drainage occurs through confluent pituitary veins that carry blood from the adenohypophysis, pars intermedia, and neurohypophysis through a common trunk to the venous systemic circulation. Only a few lateral hypophyseal veins extend directly from the adenohypophysis to the cavernous sinus. The only direct drainage of the neurohypophysis is by the neurohypophyseal limbs of the confluent veins located at the lower end of the neurohypophysis. Pars intermedia is relatively avascular and few capillaries traverse it. The most prominent vessels of pars intermedia are confluent pituitary veins.

Pars Distalis (Anterior Lobe)

KEY WORDS: chromophilic cell, acidophilic cell, somatotrope, somatotropin (growth hormone), mammotrope, prolactin, basophilic cell, corticotropes, adrenocorticotropic hormone, thyrotrope, thyrotropin (thyroid-stimulating hormone), gonadotrope, follicle-stimulating hormone, luteinizing hormone, interstitial cell-stimulating hormone, chromophobe

Pars distalis makes up about 75 percent of the hypophysis and primarily consists of epithelial cells arranged in clumps or irregular cords (see atlas figure 19-4). The parenchyma and surrounding sinusoids are supported by a delicate network of reticular fibers. The parenchymal elements mostly consist of chromophobic and chromphilic cells, distinguished by whether or not they take up stain. **Chromophilic cells** are further subdivided into acidophilic and basophilic cells according to the staining properties of their secretory granules. All three cell types — chromophobes, acidophils, and basophils — are present in pars distalis.

Acidophilic cells are large round or ovoid cells, 14 to 19 μm in diameter, with well-developed juxtanuclear Golgi bodies. The secretory granules stain with eosin in standard preparations. Two types of acidophils are present in most mammals: somatotropes and mammotropes. The cytoplasm of **somatotropes** contains a well-developed granular endoplasmic reticulum and numerous spherical, electron-dense secretory granules that measure 350 to 400 nm in diameter. Somatotropes produce **somatotropin (growth hormone),**

a peptide hormone that is important in controlling body growth and acts primarily on epiphyseal cartilage (see atlas figure 19-6). The second type of acidophil, the **mammotrope,** tends to be more scattered within the cellular cords. Active cells contain granular endoplasmic reticulum, Golgi complexes, and scattered lysosomes. The cytoplasm also contains irregular granules that measure 550 to 615 nm in diameter. Mammotropes secrete **prolactin,** which promotes mammary gland development and lactation. The concentration of prolactin rises progressively during pregnancy but is kept from showing its lactogenic effect by the high concentration of progesterone and estrogen. The titer of these hormones decreases after birth, and the lactogenic properties of prolactin are expressed. In rodents prolactin helps to maintain the corpora lutea, hence its alternative name, luteotropic hormone.

Basophilic cells of pars distalis consist of three types of cells: corticotropes, thyrotropes, and gonadotropes. **Corticotropes** generally are round or ovoid and larger than most acidophilic cells (see atlas figure 19-7). They are most numerous in the central anterior portion of pars distalis. In humans the cells contain numerous secretory granules, 350 to 400 nm in diameter, that are similar in appearance to the granules of somatotropes. The cytoplasm often contains lipid droplets and small filaments ranging from 6 to 8 nm in diameter. Corticotropes synthesize a glycoprotein prohormone, protropin, that is then cleaved to form ACTH, beta-lipotropic hormone (LPH), melanocyte-stimulating hormone (alpha-MSH), and beta-endorphin. The different hormones produced by acidophils and basophils in the adenohypophysis also are produced as prohormones, but how these are cleaved to form the active hormone is not understood. **Adrenocorticotropic hormone** stimulates the zona fasciculata and zona reticularis of the adrenal to produce glucocorticoids.

The **thyrotrope** type of basophil often is angular in shape and may form small groups deep in the parenchymal cords, at some distance from the sinusoids (see atlas figure 19-8). At 130 to 150 nm in diameter, their secretory granules are the smallest of any granules in the parenchymal cells of the hypophysis. Thyrotropes secrete a glycoprotein, **thyrotropin (thyroid-stimulating hormone),** which stimulates the thyroid to produce and release thyroid hormone.

Gonadotropes are the third type of basophil cells in the pars distalis (see atlas figures 19-9 and 19-10). They are generally smaller than corticotropic basophils, often show only a scattering of granules, and usually are round in shape. They often lie immediately adjacent to sinusoids. The cytoplasm shows profiles of granular endoplasmic reticulum, prominent Golgi complexes, and scattered lysosomes. The few spherical secretory granules are about 150 nm in diameter. This type of basophil secretes two glycoprotein hormones. **Follicle-stimulating hormone** (FSH) stimulates growth of ovarian follicles in the female and, in the male, stimulates synthesis of androgen-binding protein by Sertoli cells in the seminiferous epithelium, thereby activating and promoting spermatogenesis. **Luteinizing hormone** (LH) is essential for ovulation, for stimulating secretion of estrogen by ovarian follicles, and for promoting luteinization of follicles following development induced by FSH. The male equivalent of luteinizing hormone, **interstitial cell-stimulating hormone** (ICSH), is secreted by this type of basophil also. It stimulates production of testosterone by the interstitial cells of the testis. Testosterone is essential for sperm maturation and for development and maintenance of secondary sex organs and characteristics.

The remaining general cell type, the **chromophobes,** usually are small and are confined to the interior of the parenchymal cords. Lacking granules, they fail to color with routine stains, hence their name. Their existence as a separate type has been debated, and they may represent a reservoir of cells from which chromophilic cells originate. This accords with the hypothesis that cells of the pars distalis cycle, first accumulating secretory granules, then releasing them.

Occasionally, cystlike follicles, lined by nonsecretory (follicular) cells and filled with a colloid type of material, may be seen in the pars distalis. Microvilli and occasional tufts of cilia extend from the apices of the cells into the follicular lumen. The follicular cells are unusual in that they also have long basal processes that extend between adjacent secretory cells. Similar cells (stellate cells) that are not organized into follicles extend long branching processes between secretory cells. Both forms may represent glial cells. Their function is unknown.

Pars Tuberalis

Pars tuberalis has been identified in all vertebrates studied and forms a sleeve, up to 60 μm thick, around the infundibular stalk. It is thickest anteriorly and may be incomplete posteriorly. Pars tuberalis is characterized by longitudinally arranged cords of parenchymal cells, separated by sinusoids. The parenchyma of pars tuberalis is continuous with that of pars distalis and consists of acidophils, basophils, and undifferentiated cells. The latter usually are columnar, and their cytoplasm shows numerous small granules and large amounts of glycogen. Nests of squamous cells may be present. Pars tuberalis has no known distinct hormonal function.

Pars Intermedia

KEY WORDS: chromophobe, basophil, melanocyte-stimulating hormone

Pars intermedia is absent in some vertebrates (whale, porpoise, manatee, and some birds) and is rudimentary in humans, in whom it forms only about 2 percent of the hypophysis. It consists of **chromophobe** and **basophil cells,** the latter often encroaching into pars nervosa. Colloid-filled cysts lined by chromophobic or basophilic cells also may be present, and remnants of Rathke's cleft may persist as fluid-filled cysts lined by ciliated columnar epithelium (see atlas figures 19-3 and 19-5). Pars intermedia in some species is responsible for the secretion of **melanocyte-stimulating hormone** (MSH), a polypeptide hormone. In amphibians the hormone causes dispersion of melanin granules in the melanophores of the skin, resulting in increased pigmentation. Its role in mammals is unknown, but it may be involved in

melanocyte production. In some species, MSH occurs in alpha and beta forms, but only the precursor molecule for MSH occurs in humans. Both forms of MSH contain amino acid sequences that are identical to portions of the ACTH molecule, and the occurrence of these structurally similar regions is believed to account for the melanocyte-stimulating effect of ACTH.

Control of the Adenohypophysis

KEY WORDS: hypothalamus, releasing hormone, inhibitory hormone, somatostatin

Secretions from target endocrine glands that are under control of the adenohypophysis influence cells in the adenohypophysis through regulatory neurons in the median eminence of the **hypothalamus.** These neurons produce **releasing hormones,** small peptides that enter the capillaries surrounding the infundibular stalk and then are transported to the capillaries of pars distalis, where they stimulate specific cells to release hormones. Releasing factors are known for somatotropin, thyrotropin, corticotropin, and gonadotropin, and their amino acid sequences have been determined. **Inhibitory hormones** such as **somatostatin** (a peptide of 14 amino acids) also are secreted by hypothalamic neurons. Somatostatin inhibits secretion of growth and thyrotropic hormones. Inhibitory hormones affecting the remaining cell types are said to be produced by hypothalamic neurons, but their biochemical structure and nature are unknown.

Neurohypophysis

KEY WORDS: hypothalamo-hypophyseal tract, Herring bodies, pituicytes, neurophysin, oxytocin, antidiuretic hormone

Macroscopically, the neurohypophysis consists of the median eminence, infundibular stalk, and infundibular process (pars nervosa). The greater part of the neurohypophysis consists of unmyelinated nerve fibers of the **hypothalamo-hypophyseal tract,** which originates mainly from neurons in the supraoptic and paraventricular nuclei. The tract receives additional nerve fibers from other hypothalamic regions. The fibers end blindly in the pars nervosa, close to a rich capillary plexus. The axons comprising the hypothalamo-hypophyseal tract commonly contain spherical masses of secretory material that vary considerably in size (see atlas figure 19-12). These are the **Herring bodies,** which consist of large accumulations of dense secretory granules that vary from 120 to 200 μm in diameter. Hormones are thought to be synthesized in the perikarya of neurons in the supraoptic and paraventricular nuclei. They are then passed down the axons to be stored in the nerve terminals that form the pars nervosa. When released, the hormones cross a thin, fenestrated endothelium to enter the capillaries in the pars nervosa, thence into hypophyseal veins to finally enter the systemic circulation.

Scattered among the nerve fibers are cells called **pituicytes,** which vary in size and shape and may contain pigment granules. Pituicytes are considered to be the equivalent of neuroglial cells of the central nervous system, but whether they have only a supportive function or actively participate in the secretory processes of adjacent nerve terminals is not known.

Two cyclic polypeptide hormones, oxytocin and antidiuretic hormone (vasopressin), are stored and released from the pars nervosa. During axonal transport, each hormone is bound to a carrier protein called **neurophysin,** and it is the neurophysin-hormone complex that forms the major part of the Herring bodies. **Oxytocin** is released in lactating mammals by means of a neuronal reflex that is initiated during suckling and transmitted to the hypothalamus through the cerebral cortex. Oxytocin causes contraction of myoepithelial cells around the alveoli of the mammary gland and helps to express milk into the ductal system. Large exogenous doses of oxytocin enhance the contraction of uterine muscles during parturition, but it is not certain that this is a normal, physiologic function. **Antidiuretic hormone** (ADH) acts primarily on the collecting tubules of the kidney to increase their permeability to water, thus promoting its resorption from the glomerular filtrate. The perikarya of neurons in

the supraoptic and paraventricular nuclei are thought to act as osmoreceptors and to secrete in response to an increase in the osmolarity of the body fluids. Pharmacologic doses of ADH cause contraction of vascular smooth muscle and elevate blood pressure. This hormone is sometimes called vasopressin.

Development of Endocrine Glands

Classic endocrine glands develop from invaginations of epithelium (ectoderm, endoderm, and mesoderm) into underlying mesenchyme. Connection with the epithelium of origin is lost.

The pineal gland arises from the roof of the developing brain by fusion of a solid anterior growth near the habenular commissure with a hollow, saccular evagination from the roof of the diencephalon. Cell proliferation first begins and is more extensive in the anterior region, where the differentiating pineal neuroepithelial cells form a network of anastomosing cords and follicles within the mesenchyme. Together with contributions from the neural crest, the mesenchyme forms the connective tissue capsule, trabeculae, and stroma of the gland. Neuroepithelial cells differentiate into pinealocytes and neuroglial cells. As the gland matures, the lobules become more distinct and are composed mainly of pinealocytes.

The parathyroids develop in the ectodermal epithelium of the third and fourth branchial pouches. Dorsolateral thickenings of each pouch form solid masses of cells, each of which represents a primordium of a parathyroid gland. As they invaginate, each cell mass forms a vesicle that loses its connection to the epithelium of the pharyngeal floor. The paired primordia from the third pouches migrate with the thymic rudiment to the caudal border of the thyroid to become the inferior parathyroids. The pair associated with the fourth pouches remains at the cranial border of the thyroid and forms the superior pair.

The cells of the primordia mainly differentiate

into chief cells, which form anastomosing cords and sheets. Growth of the gland occurs as the cords of cells expand by addition of new cells derived by mitosis. The thin capsule and vascular stroma of each parathyroid originate from the surrounding mesenchyme. Initially, the stroma is relatively inconspicuous and free of fat, which accumulates with age. In humans oxyphils appear at about six years of age but are not present in appreciable numbers until after puberty and continue to increase with age.

Generally, thyroid development can be divided into three main stages: formation and separation of the thyroid anlagen, early differentiation (prefollicular stage), and follicle formation.

The thyroid is derived from ventral outpockets of the endodermal epithelium over the floor of the pharynx. These outgrowths form the median thyroid, which fuses with smaller caudal-lateral outpockets (the lateral thyroid) of the pharynx. The latter contribute to the ultimobranchial bodies of the thyroid. The median thyroid enlarges and forms an epithelial-lined vesicle that separates from the pharyngeal floor. As the vesicle migrates caudally, it expands laterally to form two lobes that fuse with tissues of the developing ultimobranchial bodies. The lumen of the thyroid vesicle is lost, epithelial cells in the wall of the vesicle proliferate, and numerous anastomosing cords expand into the surrounding mesenchyme (see atlas figures 19-24 and 19-25A). A minute lumen lies in the center of each cord. These features characterize the prefollicular stage. As a result of the secretory activities of the epithelial cells, the lumen expands and segmentation of the epithelial cords results in formation of follicles. Secondary follicles arise by budding and/or further subdivision and growth of the primary follicles (see atlas figure 19-25B). The capsule and stroma develop from the surrounding mesenchyme.

The origin of parafollicular (C) cells is obscure. They may be derived from neural crest or endoderm associated with the ultimobranchial bodies.

The adrenal cortex is a derivative of mesoderm, and the medulla arises from neural ectoderm. A provisional fetal cortex arises first from the mesothelial cells over the dorsal mesentery. The cells proliferate and invade adjacent vascular mesenchyme, which subsequently forms the capsule and stroma of the gland. Differentiation of the epithelial cells gives rise to a thick zone of large, acidophilic cells that form the provisional cortex (see atlas figures 19-27 through 19-29). This soon is enveloped by an outer, compact layer of smaller, densely staining cells that will form the permanent cortex. The provisional cortex continues to grow and at birth makes up almost 80 percent of the cortex. Immediately after birth, it begins to involute and disappears within the first few weeks of postnatal life. As the provisional cortex regresses, the cells of the definitive cortex differentiate and advance centrally. At birth, the zona glomerulosa is present and the zona fasciculata is in its initial stage of development. Zona fasciculata and zona reticularis become well defined and assume adult form during the first few months of postnatal life.

The medulla arises during the seventh week in humans by migration of cells from developing ganglia in the region of the celiac plexus. The cells invade the medial side of the cortical primordium, which subsequently envelops them (see atlas figure 19-27). As a result, the presumptive chromaffin cells take a central position in the adrenal late in fetal life. Ultimately, the chromaffin cells become arranged into cords and plates separated by sinusoids.

The neurohypophysis develops as an outgrowth of the floor of the diencephalon while the adenohypophysis arises from an ectodermal epithelial invagination of the developing oral cavity (Rathke's pouch). The vesicle loses its connection with the epithelium and comes to abut the rostral surface of the infundibulum. It differentiates into the three primary epithelial subdivisions of the adenohypophysis. The rostral wall thickens to become pars distalis, the caudal wall thins to form pars intermedia, and bilateral outgrowths of the dorsolateral wall wrap around the infundibular stem to become pars tuberalis (see atlas figure 19-26).

As these events occur, the lumen of Rathke's

pouch is obliterated or may form a residual lumen that appears as cysts in the adult. Thickenings of the rostral wall occur at a time when the parenchyma of the developing pars distalis differentiates into cords or plates of cells that are separated by sinusoids. The latter arise from surrounding mesenchyme that is incorporated into the parenchyma as the two major subdivisions blend into one. The capsule and septae arise from the surrounding mesenchyme. By the tenth week in humans, the major cell types have differentiated.

Functional Summary

The parenchymal cells of the endocrine glands synthesize hormones that may regulate specific tissues or have more general, systemic effects. Endocrine glands control and coordinate many of the physiologic activities of the body and often act in concert with the nervous system. Neurons often perform endocrine functions by secreting peptides directly into the bloodstream. Antidiuretic hormone and oxytocin are synthesized by neurons in the supraoptic and paraventricular nuclei of the hypothalamus, travel down their respective axons, and are released into the vasculature of the pars nervosa. From here they enter the hypophyseal veins and make their way into the general circulation. Antidiuretic hormone promotes absorption of water from the glomerular filtrate, thus conserving body water and concentrating the urine. The stimulus for secretion of ADH is an increase in the osmolality of the blood plasma. The cell bodies of neurons in the paraventricular and supraoptic nuclei are thought to act as osmoreceptors and to secrete ADH in response to this stimulus, as well as to stimuli from other pressure-sensitive regions of the vascular system. Oxytocin, which is released in response to the suckling reflex, stimulates contraction of myoepithelial cells and helps to express milk from the secretory units into the ductal system of the mammary gland.

Other hypothalamic neurons act on mediator cells, the gonadotropes of the adenohypophysis, and through them control follicular growth, ovulation, and hormone production in the female and spermatogenesis and hormone production in the male. Several hypothalamic neurons, acting through releasing hormones, influence somatotropes and thyrotropes of the pars distalis to control the levels of growth hormone and thyroid hormone, which control body growth and metabolism, respectively.

Adrenocorticotropic hormone elaborated by corticotropes of the pars distalis stimulates the zona fasciculata and zona reticularis of the adrenal cortex to secrete and release glucocorticoids. Like other epithelial cells in the pars distalis, corticotropes are controlled by inhibitory and releasing hormones secreted by hypothalamic neurons.

Unlike most of the classic endocrine glands, the chromaffin cells of the adrenal medulla are under the direct control of the sympathetic nervous system. When stimulated to secrete, the chromaffin cells release two active catecholamines — epinephrine and norepinephrine — which, although not essential for life, are important in meeting stressful "fight or flight" situations by increasing cardiac output, metabolic rate, and blood pressure.

Other classic endocrine glands are not under direct nervous stimulation or control by neural hormones. The activity of the parathyroid gland, for example, is influenced primarily by the concentration of calcium ion in the circulating blood. If the concentration falls below a specific level, PTH is secreted and acts on the following: osteocytes and osteoclasts to promote release of calcium ion from bone; kidney tubules to increase calcium absorption from the glomerular filtrate; and proximal convoluted tubules to release 1,25-vitamin D_3, which increases calcium absorption in the small intestine. Blood calcium is kept from rising above optimum levels by the hormone calcitonin, which is released by the parafollicular cells of the thyroid gland. Calcitonin counters the action of PTH by suppressing the resorptive activities of osteoclasts and osteocytes. Thus, regulation of the concentration of calcium ion in the blood is controlled by two endocrine glands that act in opposition to one another.

Parathyroid hormone is the major hormone regulating the excretion of phosphate and retention of calcium ion by the kidney, but it also controls the synthesis of 1,25-dihydroxy-vitamin D_3 by cells in the proximal tubules of the kidney. 1,25-dihydroxyvitamin D_3 is the hormonal form of vitamin D_3, which is now considered to be a prohormone. Like vitamin D_3, 1,25-dihydroxyvitamin D_3 is lipid soluble and its mechanism of action is similar to that of steroid hormones. In the proximal small intestine, it induces an increase in mucosal weight and the length of villi and microvilli and accelerates the rate of mucosal turnover. It also is involved in regulating calcium stores in the skeleton. Receptors for the hormone occur in a variety of tissues, including differentiating cells of the immune system.

The hypothalamus is the major neuroendocrine regulatory region of the brain and is restricted by the blood-brain barrier, whereas the neurohypophysis is not. This may explain why oxytocin, ADH, and the releasing and inhibitory hormones released by neurons in the hypothalamic region must travel considerable distances along axons before being released into capillaries in the region of the median eminence, infundibular stalk, and infundibular process finally to enter the hypophyseal or systemic circulations.

Clinical Correlations

Endocrine organs normally balance themselves and each other, regulating their activities through a number of effective feedback mechanisms. Generally, endocrine diseases result from too much or too little of one or more of the hormones. Elevated secretion may result from hyperactivity without clear morphologic change in the gland or from non-neoplastic hyperplasia of a specific organ or group of cells within an organ. Abnormally high levels of a specific hormone may indicate a neoplasm of an endocrine gland. Inadequate or lack of secretion of a hormone can result from congenital aplasia, hypoplasia, or atrophy of the endocrine organ. Because of the reciprocal interplay of the endocrine glands, insufficient stimulus from one organ may result in inadequate production and secretion by another.

Excessive production of hormones by the adenohypophysis usually is the result of tumor (adenomas) but can occur without tumor involvement. Tumors can arise in any of the three cell types in the pituitary (chromophobes, basophils, or eosinophils). Tumors involving somatotropes (one type of acidophil) can cause gigantism in children and acromegaly in adults due to excess production of growth hormone. Chromophobe adenomas also have been implicated in these conditions, but in either case somatotropin can be demonstrated in the tumor cells. Basophil adenomas usually remain small and are a rarer type of pituitary tumor. They may cause or be involved in Cushing's disease, which is associated with hyperactivity of the adrenal cortex.

Hyposecretion of all hormones associated with the adenohypophysis (panhypopituitarism) usually results from destruction of the adenohypophysis by tumors, trauma, infection, or ischemic necrosis. Destruction must be widespread before noticeable hormonal deficiencies occur, because of the resiliency of the adenohypophysis. Decreased production of growth hormone in childhood results in dwarfism; decreased production or absence of other tropic hormones has effects on the tropic organs and secondary effects from the lack of secretion by the target organ.

Secretory tumors of the neurohypophysis generally do not arise. Destruction of the neurohypophysis from any cause results in deficient secretion of ADH, which in turn results in uncontrolled water diuresis characteristic of diabetes insipidus.

Goiter is an abnormal enlargement of the thyroid. It may be diffuse or nodular and may be associated with normal, deficient, or excessive hormone production. The goiter may be composed of large distended follicles filled with colloid and lined by a low cuboidal or flattened, inactive type of epithelium. These are called colloid goiters and have been preceded by stages of hyperplasia. In some cases, simple goiter is composed of small inactive follicles without excess colloid formation. These types of nontoxic goiter can arise from any interference with synthesis of thyroxin, including dietary deficiency of iodine.

Hyperthyroidism results from hyperplastic overactivity of the thyroid with excess hormone released into the circulation. The epithelial cells of the follicles are tall columnar; nuclei are closely packed and basally located in the cells. Mitotic figures are not uncommon, and fingers of hyperplastic epithelium project into the lumen. Colloid is decreased in amount, pale-staining, and vacuolated. Increased hormonal activity is associated with increased metabolic rate, nervous excitability, and changes in muscular and mental activity.

Deficiency of parathyroid hormone is characterized by low calcium and high phosphorus levels in the blood and may result from neck injury, idiopathic disease (autoimmune disorders), and congenital deficiency. The low levels of calcium are associated with tetany, muscular spasms and tremors brought on by minor stimuli that may become widespread convulsions. Hyperplasia of the parathyroid glands may occur, in which the normal architecture may not be markedly altered. Occasionally, the hyperplastic glands consist of small chief cells. Adenomas are the most frequent tumor of the parathyroid and may consist of chief and oxyphil cells: Pure oxyphil-cell adenomas may occur. Hyperparathyroidism is associated with elevated levels of serum calcium and low phosphorus. The bones lose calcium, renal calculi are frequent, and the bone marrow may progressively be replaced by fibrous tissue.

Adrenal cortical hyperfunction is important because of the associated functional disorders. Excess cortisol production from zona fasciculata results in Cushing's syndrome and may arise from basophil tumors of the hypophysis, adrenocortical tumors, or hyperplasia. Hyperplasia or functional adenomas involving the zona glomerulosa result in hypertension and depletion of potassium (Conn's syndrome). Elevated secretion of ketosteroids, commonly involving androgens, occurs in some adrenal tumors and reflects involvement of zona fasciculata and reticularis. The elevated levels of sex steroids result in precocious puberty in males and virilism in females.

Atlas and Table of Key Features

Key Features of Classic Endocrine Glands

	Arrangement of Cells	Cell Types	Other Features
Neurohypophysis	Vary in size; arranged around unmyelinated nerve fibers	Pituicytes	Herring bodies
Adenohypophysis	Irregular cords and plates	Basophils, acidophils, chromophobes	Numerous capillaries between cords
Parathyroids	Irregular cords and plates	Chief cells (majority), oxyphils; occur singly or in nests	Abundant fat in interlobular connective tissue
Thyroid	Follicles	Follicular cells, parafollicular cells; single (adjacent to follicles) or in small interfollicular nests	Colloid in follicular lumen
Adrenal cortex			
Zona glomerulosa	Ovoid groups or arcades	Columnar cells, occasional lipid droplets	Near capsule
Zona fasciculata	Long cords	Polyhedral cells, numerous lipid droplets	Cords of cells separated by sinusoids
Zona reticularis	Irregular, anastomosing cords	Polyhedral cells, few lipid droplets	Cords of cells separated by sinusoids
Adrenal medulla	Irregular clumps or short cords	Large, pale-staining chromaffin cells	Ganglion cells, "sympathetic neurons"; sinusoids
Pineal	Poorly defined lobules, clumps, and cords	Pinealocytes, glial cells	Corpora arenacea

Hypophysis

Fig. 19-3. A sagittal section of human hypophysis. (LM, ×20.)

Fig. 19-4. Epithelial cells of human pars distalis. (LM, ×250.)

Pars nervosa

Colloid-filled cysts of pars intermedia

Pars distalis

Fig. 19-5. Cysts of human pars intermedia. (LM, ×100.)

GH-containing cells

Fig. 19-6. Growth hormone (GH)-containing cells in pars distalis as shown by immunohistochemistry. (LM, ×400.)

ACTH-containing
cells

Fig. 19-7. ACTH-containing cells in pars distalis as shown by immunohistochemistry. (LM, ×400.)

TSH-containing
cells

Fig. 19-8. TSH-containing cells in pars distalis as shown by immunohistochemistry. (LM, ×400.)

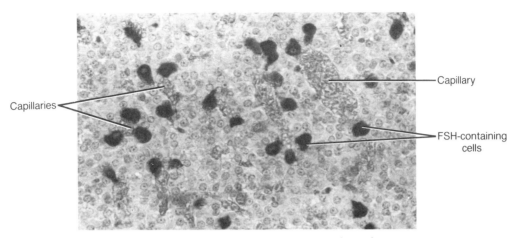

Fig. 19-9. FSH-containing cells in pars distalis as shown by immunohistochemistry. (LM, ×400.)

Fig. 19-10. LH-containing cells in pars distalis as shown by immunohistochemistry. (LM, ×400.)

Median Eminence

Fig. 19-11. Neurophysin-containing nerve fibers in the median eminence as shown by immunohistochemistry. (LM, ×100.)

Infundibular Stem

Fig. 19-12. Herring body in the infundibular stem of a human hypophysis. (LM, ×250.)

Pineal

Septa

Capsule

Corpora arenacea

Pineal lobule

Fig. 19-13. A region of human pineal showing corpora arenacea and lobules. (LM, ×400.)

Thyroid

Thyroid follicle

Follicular cells

Colloid

Fig. 19-14. Human thyroid. Note the colloid in each follicle. (LM, ×100.)

Nuclei of
follicular
cells

Colloidal
droplets

Colloid in
lumen of
follicle

Fig. 19-15. Follicular cells of a human thyroid follicle, some of
which contain colloidal resorption droplets. (LM, ×400.)

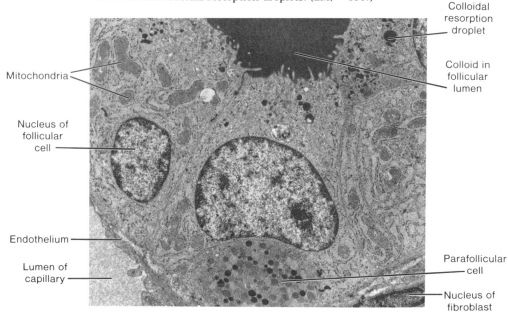

Mitochondria

Nucleus of
follicular
cell

Endothelium

Lumen of
capillary

Colloidal
resorption
droplet

Colloid in
follicular
lumen

Parafollicular
cell

Nucleus of
fibroblast

Fig. 19-16. Follicular cells and a portion of a parafollicular cell in
a thyroid follicle. (LM, ×3,500.)

Colloid

Parafollicular
cells

Lumen of
thyroid
follicle

Fig. 19-17. Parafollicular cells in a thyroid gland. (LM, ×250.)

Nucleus of
follicular
cell

Secretory
granules

Golgi
complex

Nucleus

Fig. 19-18. Secretory granules within the parafollicular cell of a
thyroid. (TEM, ×4,000.)

Parathyroid

Capillary

Chief cells

Fat cells

Nest of oxyphil cells

Capillaries

Fig. 19-19. Human parathyroid exhibiting both chief and oxyphil cells. (LM, ×100.)

Adrenal

Zona glomerulosa

Arterioles

Capsule

Zona fasciculata

Medullary vein

Medulla

Zona reticularis

Fig. 19-20. Human adrenal showing the three zones of the cortex as well as the medulla. (LM, ×40.)

Capsule

Cells of zona fasciculata

Sinusoid

Zona glomerulosa

Zona fasciculata

Fig. 19-21. A region of adrenal cortex showing the capsule, zona glomerulosa, and zona fasciculata. (LM, ×250.)

Cell of zona fasciculata

Adrenal medullary cells

Zona reticularis

Fig. 19-22. Zona reticularis of the adrenal. (LM, ×250.)

Erythrocytes in medullary sinusoid

Sinusoid

Nucleus of endothelial cell

Chromaffin cells

Fig. 19-23. Chromaffin cells and sinusoids of adrenal medulla. (LM, ×325.)

Development

Capillary

Prefollicular cord

Fig. 19-24. Thyroid early in development consists only of growing parafollicular cords. (LM, ×250.)

Anastomosing epithelial cords

Budding secondary follicle

Primary follicle

Secondary follicle

A   B

Fig. 19-25. A. Epithelial cords of a developing thyroid. (LM ×200.) B. Forming follicles of a developing thyroid. (LM, ×400.)

Brain

Infundibular stalk

3rd ventricle

Developing pars distalis

Developing pars tuberalis

Hyaline cartilage

Fig. 19-26. Hypophysis early in development. Note the relationship between the infundibular stalk, pars distalis, and pars tuberalis. (LM, ×100.)

Fig. 19-27. Adrenal in a 40-day human embryo. Note the position of the developing medulla. (LM, ×15.)

Fig. 19-28. Fetal adrenal cortex from a 40-day human embryo. Note the position of the capsule. (LM, ×250.)

Fig. 19-29. Cords of cells separated by sinusoids in deep adrenal cortex of a 40-day human embryo. (LM, ×250.)

Review Questions and Answers

Questions

98. Briefly discuss the relationship that exists (1) between the hypophysis and the adrenal and (2) between the adrenal and the kidney.

99. In what way is the thyroid unique among endocrine glands?

100. Describe the functional relationship between the thyroid and parathyroid glands with regard to blood calcium levels.

101. What is a common capillary bed? How is it important?

102. How is secretion by the pars distalis controlled?

Answers

98. (1) Secretory neurons in the hypothalamic region of the brain synthesize and secrete a small peptide known as corticotropin-releasing hormone. This hormone is synthesized in the perikaryon, transported down the axon, and released in the region of the infundibular stem. Here it passes into a rich capillary plexus stemming from the superior hypophyseal arteries and enters the portal veins of the hypophyseal portal system, which conduct it to the sinusoids of the pars distalis. The corticotropin-releasing hormones pass through the thin, fenestrated endothelium of the sinusoids and enter the intercellular fluids of the pars distalis, where they elicit the secretion of adrenocorticotropic hormone (ACTH) from the corticotropes, a specific population of basophils. Adrenocorticotropic hormone passes from the hypophysis by way of the hypophyseal veins to enter the general systemic circulation. Ultimately, it reaches the zona fasciculata and zona reticularis of the adrenal cortex and stimulates these specific zones to synthesize and release glucocorticoids. (2) The zona glomerulosa of the adrenal cortex is functionally related to the juxtaglomerular apparatus of the kidney. It is thought that either the juxtaglomerular cells sense changes in renal arterial pressure and/or that cells of the macula densa sense differences in sodium ion concentration in the glomerular filtrate. Whatever the case, the juxtaglomerular cells release an enzyme called renin that, acting through the renin-angiotensin system, stimulates the zona glomerulosa to release mineral corticoids, principally aldosterone. Aldosterone has its primary activity on the distal convoluted tubules of the kidney, where it promotes sodium absorption and potassium excretion. Aldosterone also promotes sodium retention by the salivary glands, sweat glands, and intestinal mucosa.

99. The thyroid is unique among endocrine glands in its ability to store secretory products extracellulary in the lumen of a follicle. Individual follicular cells synthesize thyroglobulin, which is then transported to and temporarily stored in the lumen of the follicle in a complex of materials called colloid. When stimulated to secrete their endocrine product (thyroid hormone), the follicular cells sequester colloid from the lumen of the follicle by pinocytosis. The resulting colloid droplets, which contain iodinated thyroglobulin, fuse with lysosomes whose hydrolytic enzymes act on the thryoglobulin to release triiodothyronine and tetraiodothyronine (thyroxine) into the cytoplasm. Other iodinated compounds released during this process are broken down intracellularly, and the iodine is reutilized by the follicular cells. Thyroxine and triiodothyronine are released at the base of the cell and enter

surrounding capillaries and lymphatics. The thyroid also has a unique ability to concentrate iodine.

100. The parathyroid glands secrete parathyroid hormone in direct response to lowered calcium ion levels in the circulating blood plasma. Parathyroid hormone stimulates osteocytes and osteoclasts to resorb calcium from the bone matrix and also acts on the tubules of the kidney to promote calcium ion absorption from the glomerular filtrate. At the same time it decreases the retention of phosphate, which is lost in the urine. It is through these mechanisms that parathyroid hormone functions to elevate the level of blood calcium.

Parafollicular cells (C cells) of the thyroid gland, on the other hand, secrete a peptide hormone called calcitonin that inhibits bone resorption by osteocytes and osteoclasts, thereby preventing blood calcium levels from rising above optimal levels. Calcitonin counters the action of parathyroid hormone and keeps the circulating levels of blood calcium within normal limits.

101. A common capillary bed forms a vital link between the hypothalamic neurons of the brain and the epithelial cells of the pars distalis. It consists of two capillary plexuses, one in the area of the median eminence and infundibular stalk and one in the pars distalis. These are united to some extent by a series of thin-walled, large-bore veins called the portal veins. Neurohormones released from axons in the region of the infundibular stalk enter the surrounding capillary plexus, and via this vascular network enter the sinusoids that surround the epithelial cells of the pars distalis. In this way neurohormones (releasing and inhibiting hormones) released in the region of the infundibular stem have a direct vascular pathway to target cells in the pars distalis.

102. The cells of the pars distalis are controlled by releasing and inhibitory hormones that are secreted from the axons of the hypothalamic neurons. It is thought that there are chemically distinct releasing and inhibitory hormones for most hormones secreted by the pars distalis.

Appendix: Key Features in the Recognition of Structures with Similar Morphology

Appendix Table 1. Key Features in Identifying Cartilage, Bone, and Tendon

	Arrangement of Cells and Lacunae	Other Features
Hyaline cartilage	Glasslike matrix; lacunae randomly distributed, slitlike in appearance near perichondrium	Isogenous groups; territorial matrix
Elastic cartilage	Matrix more fibrous in appearance; elastic fibers (need to be stained selectively)	Large isogenous groups
Decalcified bone	Lacunae show organization within lamellae of osteons; haversian canals	Tide marks; bone marrow; caniculi
Ground bone	Haversian systems; interstitial and circumferential lamellae	Canaliculi between lacunae
Fibrocartilage	Dense fibrous connective tissue a dominant feature with a small amount of ground substance; lacunae few in number and scattered between fibers	Round chondrocytes
Tendon	Fibroblast nuclei are densely stained and elongate; lie in parallel rows between fibers of collagen	Lacunae absent

Appendix Table 2. Key Features in the Recognition of Connective Tissue, Muscle, and Nerve

	Characteristics of Nuclei	Shape and Orientation of Cells and Fibers	Additional Features
Loose areolar connective tissue	Fibroblast nuclei stain either intensely or lightly, appear scattered within extracellular material	Fibroblasts and extracellular fibers are randomly oriented. Extracellular fibers stain intensely.	Scattered fat cells, adipose tissue
Peripheral nerve	Numerous Schwann cell nuclei, stain lightly, may be stippled in appearance	Schwann cells (nuclei) parallel to nerve axons	Undulating or wavy appearance of discrete bundles; limited by perineurium; nodes of Ranvier and axons may be visible
Smooth muscle	Single, oval-shaped, light-staining	Small, spindle-shaped cells; single central nucleus; well-stained cytoplasm	Cells organized into sheets or layers; scant intervening connective tissue
Dense regular connective tissue	Dense-staining; elongate fibroblast nuclei organized in rows	Large, dense-staining fibers arranged parallel; fibers and fibroblasts orderly arranged in same direction	
Skeletal muscle	Numerous light-staining peripheral nuclei within each cell	Cells arranged in same direction per fascicle; striations of cell visible in longitudinal section	Connective tissue visible around individual cells, organizes several cells into fascicles
Cardiac muscle	Usually a single, large, light-staining central nucleus; occasional cell (fiber) shows 2–3 nuclei	Large branching cells oriented in same direction as others in a specific layer; cross striations as for skeletal muscle	Intercalated discs

Appendix Table 3. Key Features in Identifying Major Glandular Structures

	Secretory Units	Ductal System	Other Features
Parotid	All acini (alveoli) and tubules are serous	Prominent intercalated ducts; intralobular duct system prominent	Numerous fat cells in humans
Pancreas	Acini and tubules are serous; cells pyramidal	Centroacinar cells, prominent intralobular ducts	Islets of Langerhans
Lacrimal gland	All acini and tubules are serous; cells low columnar	Inconspicuous	Occasional fat cells; gland small in size
Submandibular gland	Most acini and tubules are serous; some mucous tubules capped with serous demilunes	Very prominent intralobular duct system, especially striated ducts; numerous profiles in each lobule	Occasional fat cells
Sublingual gland	Mucous and serous acini and tubules equal in abundance; mucous tubules capped by serous demilunes	Duct system not prominent	Occasional fat cells
Thyroid	Large follicles filled with gelatinous colloid	Absent	Nests of parafollicular cells between follicles
Lactating mammary gland	Large, expanded alveoli contain thin secretion	Ducts visible in interlobular connective tissue	Lobulated
Nonlactating mammary gland	Alveoli poorly developed	Intralobular and interlobular ducts visible	Lobulated, loose connective tissue and fat abundant
Parathyroid gland	Irregular cords of serous cells; individual or clumps of oxyphil cells	Absent	Abundant fat cells in gland and surrounding connective tissue
Adenohypophysis	Irregular cords or clumps of epithelial cells; basophils, acidophils, chromophobes	Absent	Abundant capillaries in surrounding connective tissue
Adrenal	Cortex: cells arranged into epithelial cords separated by sinusoids; three zones Medulla: large, light-staining cells	Absent	Cortex: dark-staining Medulla: light-staining
Ovary	Ovarian follicles in cortex	Absent	Surface covering mesothelium; cortex; medulla of connective tissue and blood vessels

Appendix Table 3. Key Features in Identifying Major Glandular Structures (continued)

	Secretory Units	Ductal System	Other Features
Kidney	Parenchyma consists of tubules forming the nephrons; large scattered, renal corpuscles	Large, light-staining collecting ducts in medulla and medullary rays	Cortex: dark-staining tubules Medulla: light-staining tubules running in parallel
Testis	Seminiferous tubules, spermatogenic cells	Rete testis, efferent ductules	Tunica albuginea, septae, interstitial cells

Appendix Table 4. Key Features of Major Tubular Structures

Organ	Epithelial Lining	Muscle Coats	Special Features
Esophagus	Nonkeratinized stratified squamous	Prominent muscularis mucosae; muscularis externa of inner circular and outer longitudinal layers; skeletal (upper ¼), mixed smooth and skeletal (middle ¼), smooth (lower ½)	Glands present in submucosa; may occur in lamina propria at distal and proximal ends
Small intestine	Simple columnar, striated border; goblet cells	Muscularis mucosae and externa, inner circular, outer longitudinal smooth muscle	Villi; intestinal glands; glands in submucosa of duodenum; Peyer's patches in ileum
Colon	Simple columnar, striated border; more goblet cells	Outer longitudinal layer of muscularis externa thinner except for taeniae coli	No villi, smooth luminal surface, intestinal glands
Appendix	Simple columnar, goblet cells	Muscularis mucosae obscured by lymphocytic infiltration	No villi; much nodular and diffuse lymphatic tissue, small size
Trachea and main bronchi	Ciliated pseudostratified columnar; goblet cells	Thin muscularis mucosae	Cartilage rings
Aorta	Simple squamous (endothelium)	Tunica media dominant layer; smooth muscle and elastic laminae	Lumen usually circular in outline; vasa vasorum
Muscular artery	Endothelium	Prominent muscular tunica media	Internal and external elastic laminae
Vena cava and large veins	Endothelium	Tunica adventitia is main layer; collagen, elastic, and smooth muscle fibers	Lumen often irregular
Vagina	Nonkeratinized stratified squamous	No muscularis mucosae; external coat of inner circular and outer longitudinal smooth muscle	Prominent venous plexus in lamina propria; no glands
Oviduct	Simple ciliated columnar	External muscle: inner circular, outer longitudinal smooth muscle; cellular lamina propria	Ampulla: mucosa elaborately branched, lumen complex Isthmus: mucosa less branched, lumen a single space

Appendix Table 4. Key Features of Major Tubular Structures (continued)

Organ	Epithelial Lining	Muscle Coats	Special Features
Ureter	Transitional epithelium	Proximal ⅔, inner longitudinal, outer circular smooth muscle	
		Distal ⅓, inner longitudinal, middle circular, outer longitudinal	Stellate lumen
Vas deferens	Pseudostratified columnar	Inner longitudinal, middle circular, outer longitudinal smooth muscle	Small, irregular lumen bounded by a thick muscle coat

Appendix Table 5. Key Features in Identifying Major Abrupt Junctions

	Changes in Epithelium	Other Features
Olfactory: respiratory junction of nasal cavity	Olfactory *to* ciliated pseudostratified columnar with goblet cells	Thick lamina propria containing nerves, serous glands, and venous sinuses *to* a thin, vascular lamina propria
Oropharynx: nasopharynx junction at edge of soft palate	Nonkeratinized stratified squamous *to* ciliated pseudostratified columnar with goblet cells	Central core of skeletal muscle, mucous/seromucous glands in connective tissue underlying epithelium
Integument: oral mucosal junction at vermillion border of lip	Typical thin skin with hair follicles, sebaceous glands, and sweat glands *to* a thick, nonkeratinized stratified squamous	Typical dermis of thin skin *to* a thick submucosa with tall connective tissue papillae extending into the oral epithelium; labial salivary glands; skeletal muscle core between the skin and oral mucosa
Esophageal: gastric junction	Thick, nonkeratinized stratified squamous *to* simple columnar	Branched tubular glands of esophagus *to* gastric pits and simple branched tubular cardiac glands of stomach
Gastrointestinal junction	Simple columnar *to* simple columnar with striated (microvillus) border and goblet cells	Gastric pits, pyloric glands *to* villi, intestinal glands, Brunner's glands in submucosa
Rectoanal junction	Simple columnar with striated border and goblet cells *to* nonkeratinized stratified squamous epithelium	Intestinal glands and muscularis mucosae of rectum *lost* at rectoanal junction
Vaginal-cervical junction	Nonkeratinized stratified squamous *to* tall, light-staining simple columnar	Coarse, vascular lamina propria devoid of glands, muscularis of smooth muscle *to* dense connective tissue wall containing cervical glands, nabothian cysts

Board-Style Final Exam

———————— *Multiple Choice Questions* ————————

Chapter 1. The Cell

Pick the one correct answer.

1. Organelles most notable for producing and degrading hydrogen peroxide are
   A. lysosomes.
   B. mitochondria.
   C. Golgi bodies.
   D. peroxisomes.
   E. genomes.

2. Dense granules of RNA typically occur, among other places, within the
   A. pars granulosa of cytoplasmic nucleoli.
   B. pars granulosa of membrane-bound nucleoli.
   C. pars fibrosa of nuclear nucleoli.
   D. pars granulosa of nuclear nucleoli.
   E. nucleolus-associated chromatin.

3. Euchromatin of a cell is
   A. active in controlling the cell's metabolic processes.
   B. concentrated within the cell's karyosomes.
   C. metabolically active during mitosis.
   D. more heavily stained by nuclear stains than is heterochromatin.
   E. typically complexed chemically with histones.

4. The nucleus is
   A. always found one per cell.
   B. an essential organelle present in all cells.
   C. enclosed within a nucleolar membrane.
   D. enclosed within inner, intermediate, and outer unit membranes.
   E. completely covered externally by the fibrous lamina.

5. Which set of items below includes only those that are either cytoplasmic inclusions or that are found within some kind of cytoplasmic inclusion?
   A. lipofuscin, glycogen, karyosome, lipid droplets
   B. melanin, lipid droplets, endoplasmic reticulum, glycogen
   C. hemosiderin, secretory granules, glycogen, lipofuscin
   D. endoplasmic reticulum, melanin, lipid droplets, Golgi bodies
   E. secretory granules, lipofuscin, melanosome, autosome

6. Which one of the characteristics below is *not* true for messenger RNA (mRNA) in typical living human cells?
   A. contains a message encoded in successive sets of three nucleotides called codons
   B. functionally the same as transfer RNA
   C. attaches to ribosomes in the cytoplasm
   D. formed within the nucleus
   E. formation occurs on a template of DNA

7. Fluid-phase micropinocytosis is a cellular process that
   A. employs pseudopodia.
   B. is directly visible with the aid of a light microscope.
   C. occurs with the formation of small fluid-filled vesicles.
   D. is narrowly selective or specific in the materials it takes in.
   E. characterizes cell breakdown.
8. Granular endoplasmic reticulum is most abundant in cell types that are involved in
   A. transport of calcium ions.
   B. producing steroid hormones.
   C. lipid metabolism.
   D. detoxification of foreign compounds.
   E. protein synthesis.

Chapter 2. Epithelium

Pick the one correct answer.

1. Which of the following statements is true of the basal lamina of mammalian epithelia?
   A. It is the same as an epithelium's basement membrane.
   B. It is a product of the underlying connective tissue.
   C. It normally constitutes a barrier to the diffusion of nutrients and electrolytes to basal epithelial cells.
   D. It is composed of laminin, a proteoglycan rich in heparan sulfate and collagen.
   E. It has a lamina densa directly adjacent to the basal surface of overlying epithelial cells.
2. Which one of the epithelial subtypes listed below typically is also simple squamous?
   A. mesothelium
   B. distended transitional
   C. germinal
   D. keratinized
   E. pseudostratified
3. In epithelia, a junctional complex

A. is the same as a desmosome.
B. consists of two adjacent sets of internal laminae.
C. generally consists of three regions: zonula occludens, zonula adherens, and macula adherens.
D. usually contains a hemidesmosome.
E. is composed of the peripheral cytoskeletons of two or more adjacent cells.
4. Microvilli of epithelial cells
   A. are restricted in occurrence to the lining of the digestive system.
   B. are generally visible with light microscopy.
   C. develop into cilia.
   D. increase the absorptive capacity of the cells.
   E. are motile appendages, chiefly of the basal plasma membrane.
5. Myoepithelial cells
   A. are simple squamous epithelial cells that have contractile ability.
   B. consist of actin-containing contractile cells associated with some gland cells.
   C. represent striated muscle cells that lie adjacent to certain epithelial cells.
   D. generally lie outside the basement membrane of the adjacent epithelial cells.
   E. are incompletely differentiated mesenchymal cells.

Chapter 3. General Connective Tissue

Pick the one correct answer.

1. Name the material *not* formed by connective tissue.
   A. adipose tissue
   B. scar tissue
   C. stroma of a gland
   D. parenchyma of a gland
   E. elastic fibers
2. Mature general connective tissue consists *chiefly* of
   A. intercellular material that contains only ground substance.

B. matrix that contains fibers and ground substance.

C. connective tissue cells.

D. tissue fluid (under normal conditions).

E. mesenchyme.

3. In loose connective tissue, collagen fibers
   A. provide the greatest tensile strength.
   B. are composed of unit fibrils showing repeating transverse bands at 340-nm intervals.
   C. are composed of macromolecules of tropocollagen consisting of three globular proteins.
   D. contain alpha units that have uniform amino acid compositions and sequences in different parts of the body.
   E. can be synthesized only by fibroblasts.

4. Which *one* of the following is true of reticular fibers?
   A. concentration into bundles
   B. secreted by reticulocytes in the red bone marrow
   C. a major fibrous component of scar tissue
   D. well seen with light microscopy after routine histology/pathology staining procedures (e.g., hematoxylin-eosin, Masson's, etc.)
   E. with electron microscopy they are seen to have the same banding pattern as collagen fibers

5. Which *one* of the following is true of elastic fibers?
   A. are more variable in diameter than collagen fibers
   B. their microfibrils are composed of cross-banded lengths of elastin
   C. their elastin contains glycine and hydroxylysine
   D. their elastin contains glycine and proline
   E. their microfibrillar protein differs from elastin itself in containing desmosine and isodesmosine

6. Ground substance of general connective tissue

A. typically has a large content of free water, the intercellular fluid.

B. contains glycoproteins, glycosaminoglycans, and proteoglycans.

C. does not contain collagen or tropocollagen.

D. owes its changeability in viscosity and permeability to its content of glycoproteins.

E. retards the spread of microorganisms, chiefly because of its contained network of long-chain carbohydrates.

Chapter 4. Special Connective Tissue: Cartilage, Bone, and Joints

Each question has one to five correct answers among the choices A through E.

1. Which of the following are characteristic of hyaline cartilage?
   A. matrix that contains ground substance and collagen fibers
   B. capable of interstitial growth
   C. incapable of appositional growth
   D. chondrocytes within lacunae
   E. where exposed to synovial fluid it usually is covered by a perichondrium

2. Elastic cartilages of the human body include those within the
   A. external ear (pinna).
   B. epiglottis.
   C. intervertebral discs.
   D. symphysis pubis.
   E. growing ends of long bones.

3. The periosteum of a diaphysis
   A. can proliferate bone, increasing shaft length.
   B. can proliferate bone, increasing shaft diameter.
   C. can proliferate bone in an epiphyseal ossification center.
   D. can proliferate bone on the outer surface of the bone marrow cavity.
   E. enables strong tendon attachments during bone growth and repair.

4. Osteocytes in compact bone
   A. lie in lacunae.
   B. arc interconnected by canaliculi housing their cytoplasmic processes.
   C. have nexus junctions with their neighbors.
   D. show cytoplasmic constituents suggesting active protein synthesis.
   E. are metabolically inert.

5. Adult bone is
   A. rigid and, in its composition and microarchitecture, is fixed for life.
   B. preceded developmentally by a cartilage precursor or model, as in the flat bones of the skull.
   C. without internal blood vessel channels.
   D. cancellous within the centers of the epiphyses of long bones.
   E. subject to resorption by osteoclasts.

6. Specific "structural units" of compact bone are the
   A. interstitial lamellae.
   B. circumferential lamellae.
   C. osteons.
   D. haversian systems.
   E. Volkmann's canals.

7. Major chemical constituents of bone matrix include:
   A. calcium phosphate.
   B. calcium carbonate.
   C. type I collagen.
   D. type III collagen.
   E. minerals in the form of hydroxyapatite crystals.

8. Joints or articulations that involve skeletal elements that have little if any movement in relation to each other include:
   A. fibrous joints.
   B. sutures.
   C. synostoses.
   D. gomphoreses.
   E. diarthroses.

9. Synovial fluid within synovial joints is
   A. in direct contact with articular cartilage.
   B. elaborated by the synovial membrane.
   C. an important route for nutrients to the deeper chondrocytes of the neighboring articular cartilage(s).
   D. an ultrafiltrate of blood plasma, plus added mucin.
   E. very viscous, due especially to its content of highly polymerized hyaluronic acid.

Chapter 5. Special Connective Tissue: Blood

Each question has one to five correct answers among the choices A through E.

1. Polychromatophilic erythrocytes
   A. are also called reticulocytes.
   B. have typically lost their nucleus.
   C. have patches of bluish cytoplasm (after usual staining procedures) due to some remaining ribonucleoprotein material.
   D. have areas of acidophilic, hemoglobin-rich cytoplasm.
   E. in peripheral blood can provide an indication of the rate of erythrocyte proliferation.

2. Blood platelets of mammals
   A. are small but are the *most* numerous of the formed elements of blood.
   B. are released by megakaryocytes as cytoplasmic fragments.
   C. have a granulomere with alpha particles containing a wide variety of platelet-specific and platelet-nonspecific proteins.
   D. have a marginal bundle formed by a system of microtubules.
   E. are in many ways the functional equivalents of the thrombocytes of some other classes of vertebrates.

3. As a group, granular leukocytes in humans
   A. have a nonlobate nucleus.
   B. have a multilobate nucleus in some cell subtypes.
   C. have nuclear lobation that usually increases in distinctness and number with cellular development and aging.

D. include blood monocytes having cyto-plasmic granules.

E. are normally formed in the adult by re-ticular cells in the spleen.

4. Human neutrophil granulocytes normally
   A. comprise 5 to 15 percent of the circu-lating leukocytes.
   B. comprise 20 to 45 percent of the cir-culating leukocytes.
   C. comprise 55 to 70 percent of the cir-culating leukocytes.
   D. contain a myeloperoxidase that com-plexes with peroxide to produce acti-vated oxygen, having bactericidal activity.
   E. have specific granules (type B granules) that contain lysozyme, an enzyme com-plex that can act against components of bacterial cell walls.

5. Human eosinophil granulocytes normally
   A. comprise 10 to 13 percent of the cir-culating leukocytes.
   B. comprise 20 to 35 percent of the cir-culating leukocytes.
   C. have a decrease in numbers in relation to the alarm reaction and adrenocortical endocrine secretion.
   D. have large cytoplasmic granules con-taining a high content of myeloperoxi-dase.
   E. have large cytoplasmic granules con-taining a major basic protein that is re-sponsible for their eosinophilia.

Chapter 6. Special Connective Tissue: Hemopoietic Tissue

Each question has one to five correct answers among the choices A through E.

1. Bone marrow in adult humans is a major organ for proliferation of cells maturing into
   A. lymphocytes.
   B. monocytes.

C. plasma cells.
D. red blood cells.
E. granular leukocytes.

2. Adult human red bone marrow
   A. contains a network of reticular fibers.
   B. contains primarily regions of well-vas-cularized adipose tissue.
   C. is anatomically continuous with endos-teum.
   D. lies within the Howship's lacunae.
   E. contains both fixed tissue cells and free cells of blood.

3. Primitive stem cells of adult human red bone marrow
   A. include pluripotent stem cells.
   B. include cells that when transfused can give rise to splenic colony-forming units
   C. include restricted stem cells, destined to proliferate only one specific cell line.
   D. can be increased numerically by the ap-propriate administration of particular antimitotic drugs.
   E. include some that resemble lymphoid cells.

4. In human proerythroblasts
   A. hemoglobin synthesis has not begun.
   B. nuclear chromatin masses are large and dense appearing.
   C. mitotic divisions no longer occur.
   D. some cytoplasmic regions are eosino-philic.
   E. the cytoplasm is basophilic and rela-tively small in volume.

5. The loss of a nucleus from precursor cells of the erythrocytes
   A. gives rise to the normoblasts.
   B. may involve an active expulsion me-diated by contractile protein.
   C. is preceded by nuclear pyknosis.
   D. is preceded by nuclear vesiculation.
   E. can be followed by loss of the expelled nuclei through the activity of phago-cytes.

6. *The* fundamental stimulus for production of erythrocytes is
   A. erythropoietin.
   B. the kidney.

C. the spleen.

D. hypoxia.

E. hyperoxygenation.

7. *Myelocyte* is a cell category and maturational stage

A. normally found in circulating blood.

B. that precedes metamyelocyte in the sequence of stages leading to mature granular leukocytes.

C. at which the differentiation of specific cytoplasmic granules can first be seen.

D. at which mitotic activity normally still occurs.

E. that contributes to erythropoiesis.

8. Lymphocytes from pluripotent stem cells in bone marrow emigrate and then they and/ or certain of their daughter cells can be found in

A. blood.

B. spleen.

C. lymph nodes.

D. Peyer's patches.

E. tonsils.

9. Cells commonly within or adjacent to lymphatic (lymph) nodules include

A. reticular cells.

B. small lymphocytes.

C. macrophages.

D. plasma cells.

E. lymphoblasts.

10. Germinal centers of lymphatic nodules

A. start in development during the third trimester of fetal life.

B. are inhibited during later development by antigenic stimuli.

C. are inhibited in their development in experimental laboratory mammals that are raised and maintained in a germ-free environment.

D. are centers of lymphocyte production.

E. are essential for antibody production.

Chapter 7. Muscle

Each question has one to five correct answers among the choices A through E.

1. A skeletal muscle fiber is

A. a multinucleated cell.

B. in direct contact with the endomysium.

C. the smallest independent structural unit of the muscle.

D. *not* changed in size by degree of use or disuse.

E. composed of contractile units called sarcomeres.

2. Tissues and tissue components closely associated within a fascicle of skeletal muscle include

A. reticular fibers.

B. collagen fibers.

C. capillaries.

D. motor end plates.

E. sarcolemmas.

3. Myofibrils of skeletal muscle fibers

A. do not run the length of the fiber.

B. are too small for resolution by the light microscope.

C. have a cross-banding pattern identical to that of the whole fiber.

D. individually (each one) lie *within* a membrane-encircled sarcotubule.

E. have A-I band junctions at which a pair of dilated sarcotubules, the terminal cisternae, pass around the sarcoplasmic reticulum.

4. The triad of skeletal muscle is composed of

A. three sarcomeres.

B. two sarcosomes and one T-tubule.

C. two terminal cisternae and one T-tubule.

D. two T-tubules and one terminal cisterna.

E. a set of three closely adjacent T-tubules.

5. In smooth muscle cells

A. only very thin myofibrils have been found.

B. there is no distinct sarcomere organized.

C. strong contractions cannot be maintained for long without muscle fatigue.

D. a structurally organized tubule system of the sarcoplasmic reticulum is generally present.

E. cell boundaries inhibit the free intercellular passage of electrical impulses.

Chapter 8. Nervous Tissue

Each question has one to five correct answers among the choices A through E.

1. The physiologic activities of a neuron depend in part on the _____ within the perikaryon.
   A. chromatin
   B. melanosomes
   C. lipofuscin granules
   D. neurotubules
   E. Nissl substance

2. Neuronal cytoplasmic processes called dendrites
   A. do *not* contain Nissl substance.
   B. do not contain microtubules.
   C. often have spines or gemmules on their surface.
   D. have synapses that may sometimes number hundreds of thousands per cell.
   E. do not contain neurofilaments.

3. Axons near their parent neuron cell body generally differ from dendrites in
   A. being more numerous.
   B. conducting impulses away from the perikaryon.
   C. having more ribonucleoprotein bodies.
   D. being more slender and smoother.
   E. being more nearly constant in diameter.

4. Cytoplasmic transport within axoplasm typically can be
   A. antigrade and fast, transferring membranous organelles to the telodendria.
   B. antigrade and slow, transferring small nutrient molecules and calcium to the axon terminals.
   C. retrograde, transferring some proteins and small molecules to the telodendria.
   D. aided by neurotubules.
   E. retrograde, facilitating invasion of the central nervous system by some toxins and viruses.

5. Within the central nervous system, gray matter differs from white in containing per unit volume
   A. more neuronal cell bodies.
   B. fewer small blood vessels.
   C. more axons covered with thick myelin sheaths.
   D. more axons covered with thin myelin sheaths.
   E. fewer interneuronal synaptic contacts.

6. The neuroglia of the human central nervous system
   A. are less abundant than the neurons.
   B. account for less than one-fourth of brain weight.
   C. include Schwann cells.
   D. include cells that form myelin sheaths.
   E. include the microglia.

7. The ependymal cells of the adult human central nervous system
   A. typically form a simple cuboidal to columnar epithelium.
   B. line the spinal cord's central canal and the brain's ventricles.
   C. have long, thin cytoplasmic processes (extensions) basally.
   D. line the subarachnoid space.
   E. where they adjoin the tela choroidea, contribute to choroid plexuses.

8. Gray matter of the human spinal cord
   A. has two dorsal and two ventral horns.
   B. contains perikarya of multipolar sensory neurons, particularly in the ventral horns.
   C. contains dorsal horn motor neurons of very large size.
   D. includes the intermediolateral horns containing preganglionic sympathetic fibers.
   E. is subdivided into anterior, lateral, and posterior funiculi.

9. Tracts in the adult human central nervous system
   A. collectively predominate in the contents of the gray matter.
   B. are composed chiefly of dendrites.

C. contain neuroglia.

D. contain many myelin sheaths.

E. contain many perikarya of motor neurons.

10. Following transection of a peripheral nerve

A. degenerative changes occur only in the peripheral axonal processes.

B. the axon and its myelin sheath show wallerian degeneration distal to the transection.

C. within a few hours mitochondria and neurofilaments become vesicular and begin to break up.

D. Schwann's cells degenerate along with the adjacent myelin layers.

E. myelin degenerates distally into droplets of simpler lipids that are phagocytized there by microglia.

Chapter 9. The Eye

Each question has one to five correct answers among the choices A through E.

1. The layers of the eye's cornea include

A. Bowman's membrane, which lies between the inner surface of the substantia propria and the corneal epithelium.

B. the stratefied squamous corneal epithelium.

C. the pseudostratified columnar corneal epithelium.

D. the substantia propria or stroma, containing keratocytes.

E. Descemet's membrane, lying between the outer surface of the substantia propria and the corneal epithelium.

2. The middle and vascular coat of the eyeball

A. is called the uvea.

B. includes the choroid.

C. includes the ciliary body.

D. includes the sclera.

E. includes the iris.

3. The ciliary epithelium

A. covers the inner surface of the ciliary body.

B. elaborates vitreous humor that flows into the anterior chamber of the eye.

C. elaborates aqueous humor, which is similar to blood plasma in its relative percentage concentrations of proteins and electrolytes.

D. lines the ciliary processes from which zonule fibers extend, holding the lens in place.

E. produces zonule fibers, mainly by its nonpigmented cell portion.

4. The neural retina

A. is chiefly anchored within the eyeball by a cellular interdigitation with the pigment epithelium.

B. posteriorly has an exactly central region containing the macula lutea.

C. posteriorly has a small depression called the fovea centralis, where photoreceptor cells are most tightly clustered and most precisely organized.

D. about 3 mm lateral to the macula lutea has a "blind spot."

E. contains an optic disc about 3 mm medially (nasal side) from the macula lutea.

5. The photoreceptor cells of the human retina

A. are represented by rod cells and cone cells.

B. include rod cells whose outer segments each have hundreds of flattened membranous sacs or discs containing rhodopsin.

C. include rod cells that after exposure to light have rhodopsin that changes from cis to trans and breaks down.

D. include rod cells that with exposure to light undergo a hyperpolarization of the plasmalemma.

E. include cone cells that, as a group, respond to light of relatively low intensity through effects on a single kind of visual pigment.

Chapter 10. The Ear

Each question has one to five correct answers among the choices A through E.

1. The tympanic cavity of the middle ear
   A. contains ossicles that convey vibrations from the tympanic membrane to the inner ear via the round window.
   B. contains ossicles that consist of fibro-cartilages suspended by connective tissue ligaments.
   C. is normally filled with a serous fluid that circulates through middle and inner ear chambers.
   D. lacks muscles affecting movement of the ossicles.
   E. is connected to the nasopharynx via the eustachian tube.

2. The membranous labyrinth of the inner ear
   A. contains perilymph.
   B. contains endolymph that, like extracellular fluid, has contents of sodium and potassium ions that are low and high, respectively.
   C. contains endolymph produced by the stria vascularis of the cochlear duct.
   D. has a portion known as the vestibular labyrinth, important in containing the cochlea and its sensory apparatus for hearing.
   E. is tightly bound to the petrous part of the temporal bone.

3. In the inner ear, the sensory neuroepithelial region of a semicircular canal
   A. is a crista ampullaris.
   B. is a macula of the utricle.
   C. contains type I and type II sensory hair cells.
   D. contains a gelatinous cupula supporting crystalline otoliths.
   E. contains a gelatinous cupula in which the microvilli of the hair cells are embedded.

4. The modiolus of the adult human cochlea
   A. contains afferent multipolar neurons of the spiral ganglion.
   B. is composed of spongy bone.
   C. has a spiral lamina extending from it into the cochlear duct.
   D. has a spiral ligament extending from it to the basilar membrane.

   E. has a spiral lamina extending from it to the stria vascularis.

5. Cells of the organ of Corti
   A. transform vibrations of the basilar membrane into nerve impulses.
   B. are isolated from the vibrations transmitted along small blood vessels.
   C. lie on the vestibular membrane.
   D. lie within the scala vestibuli.
   E. include the inner and outer phalangeal cells that support hair cells.

Chapter 11. Cardiovascular and Lymph Vascular Systems

Each question has one to five correct answers among the choices A through E.

1. Muscle tissues of the heart wall
   A. are composed entirely of cardiac muscle.
   B. include large amounts of smooth muscle in the atrial endocardium.
   C. include part of the conduction system of the heart.
   D. are mainly concentrated in the myocardium.
   E. include the pectinate muscles spiralling in the walls of the ventricles.

2. Tissue structures of the epicardium include
   A. mesothelium.
   B. fat.
   C. fibro-elastic connective tissue.
   D. visceral pericardium.
   E. parietal pericardium.

3. The so-called "skeleton of the heart" in adult humans
   A. is composed of a mixture of hyaline, elastic, and fibrous cartilages.
   B. is formed in part by the annuli fibrosi, composed of Purkinje fibers.
   C. includes the septum membranaceum.
   D. is composed chiefly of dense irregular connective tissue.
   E. is structurally supported by the atrioventricular bundle (of His).

4. Within a normal adult human heart, impulses for cardiac muscle contraction
    A. are transmitted directly from one cardiac muscle fiber to another.
    B. typically pass in this sequence: sinoatrial node to atrial cardiac muscle to atrioventricular node to atrioventricular bundle.
    C. typically pass in this sequence: Purkinje cells to A-V node to atrial cardiac muscle fibers to sinoatrial node to atrioventricular bundle.
    D. depend on innervations from the autonomic nervous system.
    E. involve a "pacemaker" in the epicardium next to the right atrium.
5. The innermost tissue layer of blood vessels is
    A. the lamina propria.
    B. the tunica intima.
    C. the tunica adventitia.
    D. continuous with the endocardium of the heart.
    E. lined with endothelium.

Chapter 12. Lymphatic Organs

Each question has one to five correct answers among the choices A through E.

1. Human tonsils that
    A. are single and medial in position are the palatine and lingual.
    B. have the deepest crypts are the pharyngeal and lingual.
    C. filter lymph have the most extensively branching crypts.
    D. are functionally active proliferate lymphocytes.
    E. are functionally active have afferent lymph vessels.
2. Mammalian lymphatic organs with distinctive tissue capsules include
    A. nodules with independent fibroelastic capsules.
    B. the spleen, having a capsule containing

much smooth muscle, depending on the animal group.
    C. the thymus, located in the dorsal mesogastrium.
    D. Peyer's patches within the intestinal lamina propria.
    E. the appendix.
3. Human lymph nodes have
    A. their afferent lymphatic vessels collected at the hilus.
    B. their efferent lymphatic vessels collected within the cortical rays.
    C. a cortex containing trabeculae, lymphatic nodules, and diffuse lymphatic tissue.
    D. a medulla containing medullary cords with numerous plasma cells, macrophages, and lymphocytes.
    E. B-lymphocytes that are concentrated typically in the nodular regions.
4. The human spleen serves
    A. to filter the lymph that passes through it from afferent to efferent lymph vessels.
    B. to filter blood that passes through it.
    C. to release lymphocytes, especially those produced in the red pulp.
    D. to release lymphocytes, especially those produced in the white pulp.
    E. to remove from the blood aged and defective erythrocytes whose remains are phagocytized.
5. The human thymus
    A. after puberty typically shows gradual involution, accompanied by replacement of lymphoid tissue by connective and adipose tissues.
    B. contains thymic corpuscles consisting of concentric layers of epithelial reticular cells.
    C. contains widespread macrophages that can be seen to have engulfed degenerating cells.
    D. attains its greatest relative size by the time of birth.
    E. contains reticular cells only in its medulla.

6. Lymphocytes of the human thymus
   A. appear to be functionally inert until after they are released and then pass through the spleen.
   B. include a great many that are produced there as T cells and that are themselves and their daughter cells elsewhere involved in cell-mediated immune responses.
   C. after release have a relatively short life span.
   D. after release circulate and recirculate through the other lymphatic organs via lymph and blood flows.
   E. are active in mitosis and give rise to daughter cells that will emigrate and engender immunologic responses to certain bacteria, viruses, and fungi.
7. Lymphocytes of the T cell series
   A. do not typically nor directly elaborate conventional antibodies.
   B. can cooperate with B cells to produce antibodies against foreign erythrocytes.
   C. can be readily distinguished from those of the B cell series when studied with routine staining procedures and light microscopy.
   D. participate in the mechanism of rejection of tissue grafts of significantly different genetic source(s).
   E. give rise to immunologic "memory cells" at widespread systemic sites.
8. Endocrine (hormonal) activity of the thymus is
   A. suggested by the characteristic secretory granules of the T cells.
   B. known best in terms of peptide factors or fractions isolated and tested from thymic extracts.
   C. known best in terms of steroidal factors or fractions extracted and tested from thymic tissue.
   D. believed to include some regulatory and stimulatory actions on the thymus itself.
   E. known in part in relation to thymosin and its restoration of T cell deficiencies in thymectomized mice.

Chapter 13. Skin

Each question has one to five correct answers among the choices A through E.

1. Normal cells within the human epidermis include
   A. stratified squamous epithelial cells.
   B. keratinocytes.
   C. Langerhans' cells.
   D. endothelial cells.
   E. melanocytes.
2. Human epidermis proliferates epithelial cells in the
   A. stratum basale.
   B. stratum lucidum.
   C. stratum corneum.
   D. stratum granulosum.
   E. stratum germinativum.
3. Melanocytes in human skin
   A. can be found in the dermis.
   B. originate from cells derived from the neural crest cells of early development.
   C. contain melanosomes.
   D. when absent, constitute the usual basis for complete albinism.
   E. when unable to synthesize melanin, constitute the usual basis for complete albinism.
4. "Appendages" of human skin include
   A. lanugo.
   B. sebaceous glands.
   C. apocrine glands.
   D. nails.
   E. eccrine sweat glands.

Chapter 14. Respiratory System

Each question has one to five correct answers among the choices A through E.

1. Pseudostratified columnar epithelium in the human nasal cavity
   A. contains, in part, goblet cells that have a serous secretion.
   B. contains, in part, goblet cells that have mucous secretion.

C. contains, in part, ciliated cells.
D. lines the vestibule.
E. includes the olfactory epithelium.

2. Olfactory cells of the olfactory epithelium in humans
   A. are bipolar neurons.
   B. are unipolar sensory cells.
   C. can regenerate.
   D. apically have modified nonmotile cilia, the olfactory hairs.
   E. basally have thin dendritic processes that combine to form the fila olfactoria.

3. Intrapulmonary bronchi
   A. are supported by C-shaped cartilages in their walls.
   B. are not supported by cartilages in their walls.
   C. are lined with simple columnar epithelium through which the ducts of compound mucous glands pass.
   D. are lined with pseudostratified ciliated columnar epithelium with goblet cells.
   E. have a layer of spiralling smooth muscle external to the submucosa.

4. Terminal bronchioles
   A. are lined with ciliated cuboidal cells mixed with goblet cells.
   B. are lined with a mixture of ciliated and nonciliated cells.
   C. do not contain any visible mucus-secreting cells or glands.
   D. support some respiratory alveoli from their walls.
   E. distally connect directly with alveolar ducts.

5. Interalveolar septa of the human lung
   A. normally contain a rich capillary network.
   B. contain a supporting framework of elastic and collagenous fibers.
   C. lack perforations or pores.
   D. contain, as the thinnest blood-air barrier of the lung, in sequence: capillary endothelial cell, fused basal laminae of the latter and next epithelium, attenuated epithelium of the alveolar lining cell, and a thin film of fluid.
   E. contain, as the thinnest blood-air barrier of the lung, in sequence: basal lamina of capillary endothelial cell, interstitial tissue, basal lamina of alveolar lining cell, attenuated epithelial cell of the alveolar wall, and a thin film of fluid.

Chapter 15. Digestive System

Each question has one to five correct answers among the choices A through E.

1. In which two layers below are ganglion cells of the autonomic nervous system most common?
   A. epithelium of the mucosal lining
   B. lamina propria
   C. submucosa
   D. between muscle layers of the muscularis externa
   E. adventitia

2. Unicellular glands of the alimentary tract's lining epithelium and a segment in which they are common:
   A. goblet cells, middle part of the esophagus
   B. neutral mucus-secreting cells, fundic stomach
   C. goblet cells, colon
   D. Paneth cells, fundic stomach
   E. goblet cells, ileum

3. Submucosal glands of the alimentary tract and a tract segment in which they are common in humans:
   A. gastric glands, fundic stomach
   B. Brunner's glands, duodenum
   C. Brunner's glands, ileum
   D. intestinal glands, colon
   E. goblet cell glands, appendix

4. The mucosa of the fundic stomach contains:
   A. Peyer's patches.
   B. parietal cells.
   C. mucous neck cells.

D. chief cells.

E. gastric pits.

5. Villi of the alimentary tract occur in the:

A. large intestine.

B. appendix.

C. stomach.

D. jejunum.

E. ileum.

6. The liver's blood vascular system includes:

A. branches of the portal vein from the kidney.

B. branches of the portal vein from the gastrointestinal tract.

C. hepatic sinusoids that receive blood from branches both of the portal vein and the hepatic artery.

D. hepatic sinusoids that transmit blood to the branches of the hepatic vein.

E. hepatic sinusoids that transmit blood to the central veins.

7. Hepatocytes

A. occur in plates within liver lobules.

B. commonly include some that are polyploid, as can be recognized from variation in nuclear size.

C. have microvilli bordering bile canaliculi.

D. have microvilli bordering bile ducts.

E. produce and secret bile.

8. The exocrine pancreas is

A. a compound tubuloacinar gland containing holocrine secretory cells.

B. composed of secretory cells of several types and duct cells that transmit their secretions to the duodenum.

C. dominated by zymogenic secretory cells with abundant granular endoplasmic reticulum.

D. active in secreting amylase, which breaks down starch and glycogen to disaccharides.

E. active in secreting several kinds of proteolytic enzymes.

9. In the development and growth of human teeth, formative cells and a product from each:

A. mesenchyme cells, odontoblasts

B. ameloblasts, dentin

C. odontoblasts, dentinal fibers

D. mesenchyme cells, cementoblasts

E. ameloblasts, enamel

10. Which are the correctly paired cell products and their cellular sources in the endocrine pancreas?

A. secretin, S cells

B. cholecystokinin, I cells

C. glucagon, alpha cells

D. insulin, delta cells

E. pancreatic polypeptide, beta cells

Chapter 16. Urinary System

Each question has one to five correct answers among the choices A through E.

1. In the following pairs select those that show a direct proximal to distal sequence.

A. urethra, urinary bladder

B. renal sinus, minor calyx

C. glomerular capsule, proximal convoluted tubule

D. loop of Henle, medullary collecting duct

E. papillary ducts, minor calyces

2. Contents of the juxtaglomerular apparatus include the

A. macula densa.

B. vascular pole of the glomerular capsule.

C. efferent arteriole of the glomerulus.

D. renin-producing cells.

E. angiotensinogen-producing cells.

3. A simple cuboidal epithelium typically lines the lumen of

A. a minor calyx.

B. the thin part of Henle's loop.

C. the proximal convoluted tubule.

D. the urethra.

E. the arched collecting duct.

4. Factors and one of their direct and cellular targets that contribute to the production of a hypertonic urine:

A. antidiuretic hormone, some collecting ducts

B. renin, glomerular capsule cells
C. increased cellular permeability, thin part of Henle's loop
D. vascular countercurrent exchange system, medullary vasa recta
E. Vascular countercurrent exchange system, cortical vasa recta

5. Surface specializations and the epithelial cells in which they occur in the urinary system include:
   A. microplicae and large numbers of apical cytoplasmic vesicles, principal (light) cells of some collecting ducts.
   B. apically a central cilium surrounded by short microvilli, intercalated cells of some collecting ducts.
   C. apically a brush border consisting of closely packed cilia, cells of the proximal convoluted tubules.
   D. apically a brush border consisting of closely packed microvilli, cells of the proximal convoluted tubules.
   E. pores (fenestrations), glomerular capillaries.

Chapter 17. Meiosis and Male Reproductive Organs

Each question has one to five correct answers among the choices A through E.

1. Meiosis
   A. is characterized by two cell divisions, but only one includes replication of DNA.
   B. in its first cell division produces haploid cells.
   C. in its second cell division produces sister chromatids.
   D. in its first prophase is similar to that of mitosis.
   E. in its first prophase has tetrads formed, each representing homologous chromosomes.

2. Each testis
   A. functions in part as a holocrine gland.
   B. functions in part as an endocrine gland.

C. is covered anteriorly and laterally with mesothelium.
D. has a thick fibrous capsule that is part of the visceral layer of the tunica vaginalis.
E. contains about 250 elongate compartments called lobuli testis.

3. Interstitial tissue of the testis contains
   A. fibroblasts.
   B. macrophages.
   C. testosterone synthesizing and secreting the Leydig cells.
   D. mast cells.
   E. mesenchyme cells.

4. Synthesis of testosterone in certain testicular cells depends on
   A. enzymes of the smooth endoplasmic reticulum.
   B. mitochondrial enzymes.
   C. cytoplasmic crystals of Reinke.
   D. a gonadotropic hormone, ICSH, from the pars distalis of the anterior pituitary gland.
   E. sufficient growth of the beard.

5. In the seminiferous tubules there are
   A. contractile myoid cells.
   B. Sertoli cells that proliferate precursors of spermatozoa.
   C. spermatogonia that have a supportive function primarily.
   D. cells secreting testicular fluid.
   E. cells releasing androgen-binding protein.

6. The blood-testis barrier separates
   A. the adluminal compartment from the spermatogonia.
   B. the adluminal compartment from the basal compartment.
   C. the adluminal compartment from haploid cells differentiating into sperm cells.
   D. the basal compartment of the seminiferous tubules from blood vessels of the interstitial tissue.
   E. the basal compartment of the seminiferous tubules from small vascular channels within the peritubular membrane.

7. Lining epithelium of the tubuli recti is
   A. stratified columnar.
   B. simple squamous.
   C. in direct contact with that of the efferent ductules.
   D. in direct contact with that of the rete testis.
   E. a pavement of undifferentiated primary spermatocytes.

8. The ductus deferens is
   A. lined with stratified columnar epithelium.
   B. lined with pseudostratified columnar epithelium.
   C. functionally active in muscular propulsion of sperm during ejaculation.
   D. connected directly to the prostatic urethra by its ampulla, which has a thicker muscularis.
   E. swollen proximally, forming the colliculus seminalis.

9. Among the human male's accessory sex glands,
   A. the seminal vesicles' secretory cells are active in protein synthesis.
   B. the seminal vesicles are significant in storing the semen prior to ejaculation.
   C. the seminal vesicles' secretion provides a source of energy for sperm.
   D. the prostate contains 30 to 50 compound tubuloalveolar glands, whose numerous main ducts drain independently into the membranous urethra.
   E. the prostate gland's lumina commonly contain concretions, especially around the time of puberty.

10. Mesenchymal tissue in which the testis cords develop later forms the
    A. septuli testis.
    B. tunica albuginea.
    C. connective tissue of the mediastinum.
    D. interstitial tissue.
    E. cells of Leydig.

Chapter 18. Female Reproductive System

Each question has one to five correct answers among the choices A through E.

1. Human ovarian follicles typically lie
   A. within capsules, each one of which is formed and surrounded by the tunica albuginea.
   B. within the medullary stroma.
   C. within the cortical stroma.
   D. within a mesothelial epithelium that surrounds each follicle individually.
   E. in grapelike clusters called uveal tracts.

2. Of the types or stages of human ovarial follicles,
   A. primordial follicles reach their maximum number at a woman's age of 20 to 30 years.
   B. primordial follicles reach their maximum number around the time of birth.
   C. primordial follicles have a primary oocyte surrounded by a two- to three-celled layer of cuboidal follicle cells.
   D. primary follicles contain a primary oocyte surrounded by simple squamous epithelium of granulosa cells.
   E. secondary follicles have reached maximum follicle size.

3. Ovulation in the human female
   A. in its timing centers around the middle of the menstrual cycle.
   B. most commonly involves the release from the follicle of a primary oocyte.
   C. most commonly involves follicular release of a secondary oocyte.
   D. is immediately preceded by a marked increase in liquor folliculi.
   E. involves a follicular rupture facilitated by collagenase produced by certain of the granulosa cells.

4. Ovarian follicular atresia occurs
   A. chiefly at menopause.
   B. chiefly with the formation of corpora lutea.
   C. as the fate of a minority of the follicles

growing during each menstrual cycle.

D. generally only in early stages of follicular development.

E. with a relatively thick glassy membrane forming from the basal lamina of the granulosa cell epithelium.

5. The distal to proximal sequence of named segments of the oviduct is:

A. fimbria, ampulla, isthmus, infundibulum.

B. infundibulum, ampulla, isthmus, pars interstitialis.

C. isthmus, ampulla, infundibulum, uterine tube.

D. fimbria, infundibulum, isthmus, ampulla, pars interstitialis.

E. ampulla, infundibulum, isthmus, pars interstitialis.

6. In comparison with the body of the uterus, the adult cervix has

A. a wall composed chiefly of dense connective tissue.

B. a junctional zone between smooth and skeletal muscle layers in its muscularis.

C. a copious secretion of thin alkaline fluid, especially during menses.

D. a nonkeratinized stratified squamous epithelium throughout its length.

E. a cyclic shedding of only the proximal part and superficial layer of its mucosa.

7. The vaginal wall of mature women typically has

A. a keratinized stratified squamous epithelium.

B. a mucosa containing plicae circulares.

C. short branched tubular mucous glands in its lamina propria.

D. a serosal outer covering over about one-half its length anteriorly.

E. a muscularis of smooth muscle formed by inner circular and outer longitudinal layers.

8. Tissue components of the human clitoris include

A. a corpus spongiosum of erectile tissue.

B. a glans clitoridis containing spongy erectile tissue.

C. a single corpus cavernosum containing dense irregular connective tissue.

D. a covering of pseudostratified columnar epithelium.

E. an abundance of high connective tissue papillae containing sensory nerve endings.

9. Fertilization in the human female

A. takes place in the isthmus of the oviduct.

B. takes place in the ampulla of the uterine tube.

C. involves a single spermatozoon penetrating the ovum.

D. involves the oocyte just prior to the second maturation division.

E. is rapidly followed by reduction in permeability of the penetrated ovum's zona pellucida, which thereafter blocks entry by contending sperm.

10. A human blastocyst

A. forms from a morula 5 to 10 days after fertilization.

B. has an inner cell mass that will form the embryo proper.

C. has a capsule-like wall, the trophoblast, consisting of a layer one cell thick.

D. after being freed in the uterine cavity, will implant in the endometrium during the proliferative phase of the endometrial cycle.

E. during implantation extends fingerlike processes of its trophoblast between uterine epithelial cells; numerous tight junctions then form, locking them together.

Chapter 19. Endocrine Glands

Each question has one to five correct answers among the choices A through E.

1. Human parathyroid glands

A. contain chief cells that constitute the most numerous of its endocrine cells.

B. have oxyphil endocrine cells, notable after puberty, and then increasing with further aging.

C. secrete parathyroid hormone, whose action on calcium metabolism is nearly opposite to that of calcitonin.

D. secrete parathyroid hormone, which raises blood levels of calcium.

E. secrete parathyroid hormone, which promotes synthesis and release of 1,25-vitamin D_3 by the kidney.

2. Thyroid follicles

A. most commonly have a simple cuboidal to simple squamous epithelium formed of principal (follicular) cells.

B. generally have follicular cells that are lower (squamous) in height when they are most active in synthesis and transport of thyroid hormone.

C. surround a lumen containing colloid, representing primarily stored lipid materials.

D. store halogen salts in their colloidal droplets.

E. contain parafollicular cells that lie outside the principal cells and that secrete iodine salts.

3. Endocrine cells of the adrenal

A. cortex are developmentally derived from neural crest cells.

B. medulla secrete hormones that are catecholamines.

C. cortex secrete hormones that are steroids.

D. cortex are arranged in irregular parenchymal cords, between which chromaffin cells are common.

E. medulla can regenerate after trauma or surgical removal.

4. The pituitary adenohypophysis

A. embryologically develops from the infundibulum of the diencephalon.

B. contains chromophilic and chromophobic endocrine cells.

C. contains somatotropes and mammotropes, both of which have cytoplasmic secretory granules that are acidophilic.

D. includes the pars intermedia and the pars tuberalis.

E. contains some basophilic endocrine cells; two of these that have basophilic cytoplasmic secretory granules are thyrotropes and gonadotropes.

5. The hypothalamo-hypophyseal tract

A. contains axons from the neurosecretory neuroendocrine cells of the supraoptic and paraventricular nuclei of the hypothalamus.

B. transports oxytocin and antidiuretic hormone to the neurohypophysis, where they are stored and released.

C. contains neuroglia.

D. contains abundant neuronal perikarya.

E. descends the pituitary stalk.

Answer Key

Chapter 1. The Cell

1. D
2. D
3. A
4. B
5. C
6. B
7. C
8. E

Chapter 2. Epithelium

1. D
2. A
3. C
4. D
5. B

Chapter 3. General Connective Tissue

1. D
2. B
3. A
4. E
5. D
6. B

Chapter 4. Special Connective Tissue: Cartilage, Bone, and Joints

1. A, B, D, E
2. A, B
3. B, E
4. A, B, C
5. D, E
6. C, D
7. A, B, C, E
8. A, B, C, D
9. A, B, C, D, E

Chapter 5. Special Connective Tissue: Blood

1. A, B, C, D, E
2. B, C, D, E
3. B, C
4. C, D, E
5. C, D, E

Chapter 6. Special Connective Tissue: Hemopoietic Tissue

1. A, B, C, D, E
2. A, C, E
3. A, B, C, D, E
4. D, E
5. B, C, E
6. D
7. B, C, D
8. A, B, C, D, E

9. A, B, C, D, E
10. C, D

Chapter 7. Muscle

1. A, B, C, E
2. A, B, C, D, E
3. C
4. C
5. B

Chapter 8. Nervous Tissue

1. A, D, E
2. C, D
3. B, D, E
4. A, D, E
5. A
6. D, E
7. A, B, C, E
8. A, D
9. C, D
10. B, C

Chapter 9. The Eye

1. B, D
2. A, B, C, E
3. A, D, E
4. B, C, E
5. A, B, C, D

Chapter 10. The Ear

1. E
2. C
3. A, C, E
4. B
5. A, B, E

Chapter 11. Cardiovascular and Lymph Vascular Systems

1. C, D
2. A, B, C, D
3. C, D

4. A, B, E
5. B, D, E

Chapter 12. Lymphatic Organs

1. D
2. B
3. C, D, E
4. B, D, E
5. A, B, C, D
6. A, B, D, E
7. A, B, D, E
8. B, D, E

Chapter 13. Skin

1. A, B, C, E
2. A, E
3. A, B, C, E
4. A, B, C, D, E

Chapter 14. Respiratory System

1. B, C, E
2. A, C, D
3. D
4. B, C
5. A, D

Chapter 15. Digestive System

1. C, D
2. B, C, E
3. B
4. B, C, D, E
5. D, E
6. B, C, D, E
7. A, B, C, E
8. C, D, E
9. A, C, D, E
10. C

Chapter 16. Urinary System

1. C, E
2. A, D
3. C, E
4. A, D
5. D, E

Chapter 17. Meiosis and Male Reproductive Organs

1. A, C, E
2. A, B, C, E
3. A, B, C, D, E
4. A, B, D
5. A, D, E
6. A, B
7. D
8. B, C
9. A, C
10. A, B, C, D, E

Chapter 18. Female Reproductive System

1. C
2. B
3. A, C, D, E
4. E
5. B
6. A
7. E
8. A, B, E
9. B, C, D, E
10. B, C, E

Chapter 19. Endocrine Glands

1. A, B, C, D, E
2. A
3. B, C
4. B, C, D, E
5. A, B, C, E

INDEX

Page numbers in *italics* refer to illustrations.